BSAVA Manual of Raptors, Pigeons and Passerine Birds

T0203390

Editors:

John Chitty

BVetMed CertZooMed CBiol MIBiol MRCVS
Strathmore Veterinary Clinic, Andover, Hants SP10 2PH

and

Michael Lierz

Dr.med.vet DZooMed(avian) MRCVS
Institute for Poultry Diseases,
Freie Universität Berlin, Berlin, Germany

Published by:

British Small Animal Veterinary Association
Woodrow House, 1 Telford Way, Waterwells
Business Park, Quedgeley, Gloucester GL2 2AB

A Company Limited by Guarantee in England.
Registered Company No. 2837793.
Registered as a Charity.

Copyright © 2021 BSAVA
First published 2008
Reprinted 2019, 2021 twice

All rights reserved. No part of this publication may be reproduced, stored in a retrieval system, or transmitted, in form or by any means, electronic, mechanical, photocopying, recording or otherwise without prior written permission of the copyright holder.

Figures 14.7, 14.16 and 14.17 were drawn by S.J. Elmhurst BA Hons (www.livingart.org.uk) and are printed with her permission.

A catalogue record for this book is available from the British Library.

ISBN 978 1 905319 04 6

The publishers and contributors cannot take responsibility for information provided on dosages and methods of application of drugs mentioned in this publication. Details of this kind must be verified by individual users from the appropriate literature.

Printed in the UK by Severn, Gloucester GL2 5EU – a carbon neutral printer
Printed on ECF paper made from sustainable forests

17091PUBS21

Contributors

Tom Bailey BSc BVSc CertZooMed MSc(Wild Animal Health) PhD DipECAMS MRCVS
Falcon and Wildlife Veterinarian, Dubai Falcon Hospital, PO Box 23919, Dubai,
United Arab Emirates

René Becker DVM
Aspastrasse 41, D-59394, Nordkirchen, Germany

J.R. Best BVSc MRCVS
Quantock View Farmhouse, Steart, Somerset TA5 2PX

John Chitty BVetMed CertZooMed CBiol MIBiol MRCVS
Strathmore Veterinary Clinic, London Road, Andover, Hants SP10 2PH

John E. Cooper DTVM FRCPath FIBiol DipECVP FRCVS
School of Veterinary Medicine, The University of the West Indies (UWI), St Augustine,
Trinidad & Tobago

Bob Doneley BVSc FACVSc(avian medicine)
West Toowoomba Veterinary Surgery, 194 West Street, Toowoomba, Queensland 4350, Australia

Gerry M. Dorrestein DVM Veterinary Pathologist Honorary Member ECAMS
Dutch Research Institute for Avian and Exotic Animals (NOIVBD), Wintelresedijk 51,
NL-5507 PP Veldhoven, The Netherlands

Kevin Eatwell BVSc(Hons) DZooMed(reptilian) MRCVS
Birch Heath Veterinary Clinic, Birch Heath Road, Tarporley, Cheshire CW6 9UU

Neil A. Forbes BVetMed CBiol MIBiol RFP DipECAMS FRCVS
Great Western Referrals, Unit 10 Berkshire House, County Park Estate, Shrivenham Rd, Swindon,
Wiltshire, SN1 2NR

Jean-Michel Hatt Dr.med.vet MSc DipECAMS
Division of Zoo Animals and Exotic Pets, Vetsuisse Faculty, University of Zurich,
Winterthurstrasse 260, 8057 Zurich, Switzerland

J. Jill Heatley DVM MS DipABVP(avian)
Clinical Associate Professor, Zoological Medicine, College of Veterinary Medicine,
Texas A&M University, College Station, TX 77843-4474, USA

Ruth Maria Hirschberg Dr.med.vet
Institute of Veterinary Anatomy, Department of Veterinary Medicine, Freie Universität Berlin,
Koserstrasse 20, D-14195 Berlin, Germany

Michael P. Jones DVM DipABVP(avian)
Associate Professor, Avian and Zoological Medicine, The University of Tennessee,
College of Veterinary Medicine, Department of Small Animal Clinical Sciences, 2407 River Drive,
Room C247, Knoxville, TN 37996, USA

Richard G. Jones BVSc MSc MRCVS
Birch Heath Veterinary Clinic, Birch Heath Road, Tarporley, Cheshire CW6 9UU

Alistair M. Lawrie BVMS MRCVS
The Lawrie Veterinary Group, 25 Griffiths Street, Falkirk, Central Scotland, FK1 5QY

Michael Lierz Dr.med.vet DZooMed(avian) MRCVS
Institute for Poultry Diseases, Freie Universität Berlin, Königstrasse 63, 14163 Berlin, Germany

Christopher Lloyd BVSc MSc (Wild Animal Health) CertZooMed MRCVS
Nad Al Shiba Veterinary Hospital, Dubai, United Arab Emirates

Jemima Parry-Jones MBE
The International Centre for Birds of Prey, Eardisland, Herefordshire HR6 9AS

Michael Pees Dr.med.vet DipECAMS
University of Leipzig, Clinic for Birds and Reptiles, An den Tierkliniken 17, 04103 Leipzig, Germany

Tom Pennycott BVM&S CertPMP MRCVS
Veterinary Centre Manager, SAC Veterinary Services, Auchincruive, Ayr KA6 5AE

Romain Pizzi BVSc MSc DZooMed FRES MACVSc(Surg) MRCVS
Special Lecturer in Zoo and Wildlife Medicine, University of Nottingham School of Veterinary Medicine and Science, Sutton Bonington Campus, Leicestershire LE12 5RD

Aidan Raftery MVB CertZooMed CBiol MIBiol MRCVS
Avian and Exotic Animal Clinic, 221 Upper Chorlton Road, Manchester M16 0DE

Ron Rees Davies BVSc CertZooMed ESVetS MRCVS
Essex Gardens, Hornchurch, Essex RM11 3EH

Peter W. Scott MSc BVSc FRCVS
Vetark Professional, PO Box 60, Winchester SO23 9XN

Michael Stanford BVSc FRCVS
Birch Heath Veterinary Clinic, Birch Heath Road, Tarporley, Cheshire CW6 9UU

Brian Stockdale BVM&S MRCVS
Meadow Lane Veterinary Centre, 9 Meadow Lane, Loughborough, Leicestershire LE11 1JU

David L. Williams MA VetMB PhD CertVOphthal FRCVS
Fellow and Director of Studies, Veterinary Medicine and Pathology, St John's College, Cambridge CB2 1TP
Associate Lecturer in Veterinary Ophthalmology, Department of Veterinary Medicine, Madingley Road, Cambridge CB3 0ES

Foreword

The first BSAVA *Manual of Raptors, Pigeons and Waterfowl* was published in 1996. And as the first Foreword noted, at some stage in their life most veterinary surgeons will be asked to treat these birds. The truth of that statement remains the same; however, time moves on and this new version of the Manual has been produced. The whole book is a great improvement.

Only four of the original authors remain, and both the editors are new. The senior editor (showing how times change) is John Chitty, who is well known as an avian veterinarian and previous editor of the most recent (and excellent) *BSAVA Manual of Psittacine Birds*; he deserves a medal for his efforts! Michael Lierz will not be immediately recognized by most UK practioners but is a very experienced avian vet, as well as a falconer and falcon breeder. He is also a teacher in the University of Berlin and, in addition to his other roles, runs an avian clinic within the university. His editorship is a notable achievement for a man who does not have English as his first language. Between them they have mapped out a comprehensive set of chapters, each authored by an authority on their subject. They have managed an excellent balance between experience and new information and ideas.

The substitution of Passerine Birds for Waterfowl is an excellent one. Many more general practitioners will be asked to see canaries and zebra finches than ducks and geese, and a wealth of concise information about this huge group of birds is very welcome.

As is the norm for more exotic BSAVA Manuals, the book is aimed at all levels of knowledge. For the less experienced vets there are chapters that cover basic knowledge, such as anatomy and physiology, husbandry and handling. However, experienced avian vets will benefit from the information provided by the many experts writing about their favourite subjects, for example the ophthalmology and imaging chapters.

This manual has also benefitted greatly from the superior layout now adopted for BSAVA Manuals, which includes the use of modern technology to produce a wealth of coloured images beyond the means and scope of the previous manual.

I am sure that the *BSAVA Manual of Raptors, Pigeons and Passerine Birds* will find a place on most veterinary practice's bookshelves, where it will be of immense help for years to come.

Nigel Harcourt-Brown BVSc DipECAMS FRCVS
May 2008

Preface

The first incarnation of this book, the *BSAVA Manual of Raptors, Pigeons and Waterfowl,* was published twelve years ago. While this new edition looks to update the previous one in terms of raptors and pigeons, it features passerine birds for the first time.

This volume, therefore, attempts to summarise a huge diversity of different birds. Fortunately, not all the three thousand plus species of raptor, pigeon and passerine are kept in captivity, but the range is complex enough! Therefore, the book focuses on the more commonly kept species and the problems seen in daily veterinary practice. Contributing authors have considerable practical experience in their subject and we trust that this has resulted in a practical and easy-to-use manual. More detailed information and references are also quoted for those looking to study to greater depth.

The manual is divided into several distinct parts. The first four chapters describe the natural history and captive husbandry of these groups of birds. They present a summary of the keeping of these species in various countries, as well as the purposes for which they are kept.

The next section covers general clinical techniques. All three groups of birds are covered in these chapters, as there is a significant overlap. Starting with transport and handling, the section also includes clinical examination, basic techniques and diagnostic procedures – clinical pathology and imaging – as well as anaesthesia and surgery. The surgery chapters include basic requirements and descriptions of common techniques.

The third section is devoted to raptors. Given the wealth of knowledge now available on these species, and the fact that they are usually high value birds (both financially and emotionally) belonging to often well-informed falconers, this section is detailed and covers raptor diseases by system rather than presenting sign. Raptor reproduction is covered in depth as captive breeding is a rapidly expanding area.

The next two sections cover pigeons and passerines, respectively. These birds are normally kept as flocks rather than as individuals so the emphasis here is more on flock medicine than diagnosis and therapy of the individual bird. There has also, traditionally, been less veterinary involvement with these species than with raptors. Therefore these chapters are more arranged as per clinical approach to a particular presentation or problem. The final chapter covers legal and ethical aspects of all the species.

The editors could not have produced this book without a lot of help. We are very grateful for the hard work of all the authors – they have been very punctual, and have tolerated a lot of editorial interference and changes of approach! Gerry Dorrestein has given great assistance in editing the passerine chapters. We would also like to thank Marion Jowett and her team at BSAVA for all their encouragement and technical assistance. We would like to thank Nigel Harcourt-Brown for writing the Foreword and for all his help and advice – not only in editing this book, but throughout the editors' careers.

In particular we would both like to thank our wives and families for tolerating absentee husbands/ fathers, and for their support and encouragement.

John Chitty and Michael Lierz
May 2008

Introduction

John E. Cooper

Terminology

An understanding of terminology is important. The word 'raptor' is an ancient one. It is Latin for a bird with a hooked beak and sharp claws and is perpetuated in (for example) the French *rapace* and Italian *rapaci*. In theory, the term could embrace a range of different species, but in practice it is normally used for birds of prey of the Orders Falconiformes (hawks, falcons, eagles, vultures) (Figure 1.1) and Strigiformes (owls) (Figure 1.2). Sibley and Ahlquist (1990) suggested an alternative classification for raptors, based on DNA studies, but such an approach to taxonomical detail would not significantly alter the situation. There remains some disagreement as to the contemporary use of the term raptor, as it is taken from an Order (abandoned in the Victorian era) used as a classification of owls, hawks, falcons and vultures; however, it is a word that continues to be used regularly, as evidenced by the title of this Manual. Other terminology reflects the nature and appearance of these birds: for instance, the word 'falcon' comes from the Latin *falx* (a sickle), probably on account of the curved appearance of the talons.

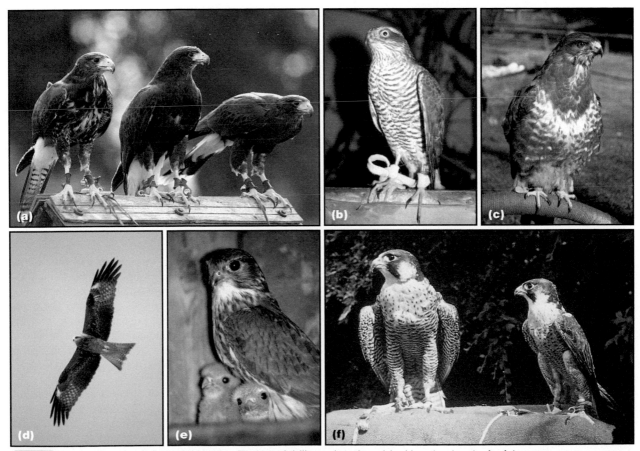

1.1 Falconiformes. **(a)** Harris' Hawks. Their sociability makes them ideal hunting hawks for falconers. **(b)** Sparrowhawk. **(c)** Eurasian Buzzard. **(d)** Black Kite, the most common raptor in the world. **(e)** Merlin with chicks. **(f)** Peregrine Falcon: the female is larger than the male. (b–e, © Michael Lierz; f, © John Chitty, reproduced from *BSAVA Manual of Exotic Pets, 4th edition*) (continues)

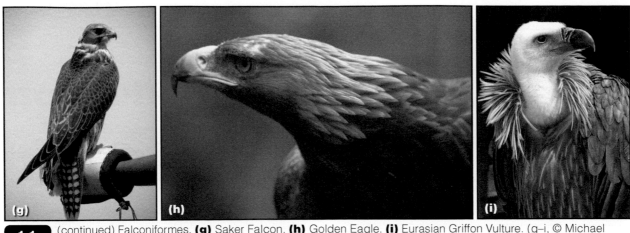

1.1 (continued) Falconiformes. **(g)** Saker Falcon. **(h)** Golden Eagle. **(i)** Eurasian Griffon Vulture. (g–i, © Michael Lierz)

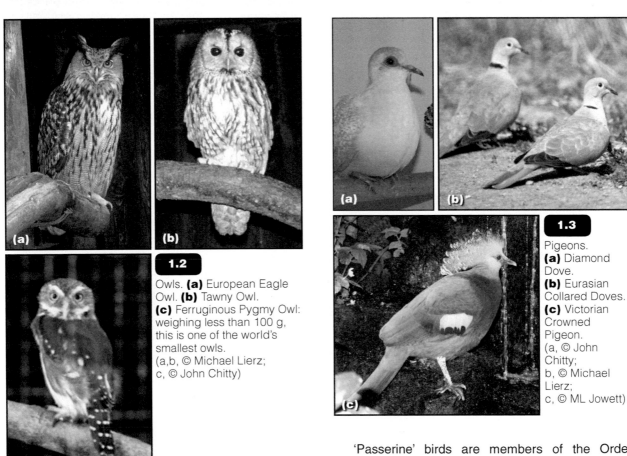

1.2 Owls. **(a)** European Eagle Owl. **(b)** Tawny Owl. **(c)** Ferruginous Pygmy Owl: weighing less than 100 g, this is one of the world's smallest owls. (a,b, © Michael Lierz; c, © John Chitty)

1.3 Pigeons. **(a)** Diamond Dove. **(b)** Eurasian Collared Doves. **(c)** Victorian Crowned Pigeon. (a, © John Chitty; b, © Michael Lierz; c, © ML Jowett)

The word 'pigeon' is taken to include 'dove' (Figure 1.3). The distinction between the two is perpetuated in many English names, often implying a smaller species or an ornamental variety, but is artificial. These birds all belong to the Order Columbiformes. Domesticated pigeons have been described as our 'oldest feathered friends' (Powers, 2005) and have served the human race in a variety of ways. Pigeons and doves are considered to comprise nearly 50% of all birds kept in captivity (Hooimeijer and Dorrestein, 1997).

'Passerine' birds are members of the Order Passeriformes, the largest group of birds (nearly 6000 of the 9000 known extant species) (Figure 1.4). The word comes from the Latin *passer*, meaning 'sparrow', and is a reminder of the fact that these are the perching or song birds, many of them either familiar in gardens or popular in captivity. Numerous passerine species have been kept in captivity, some for decades or centuries.

Another aspect of terminology is also important. Because they have a long association with humans, the three groups of birds covered by this Manual have attracted their own descriptive words and phraseology – part of the 'culture' of bird-keeping, an understanding of which can be important when a veterinary surgeon is dealing with these species and needs to communicate with their owners. Examples

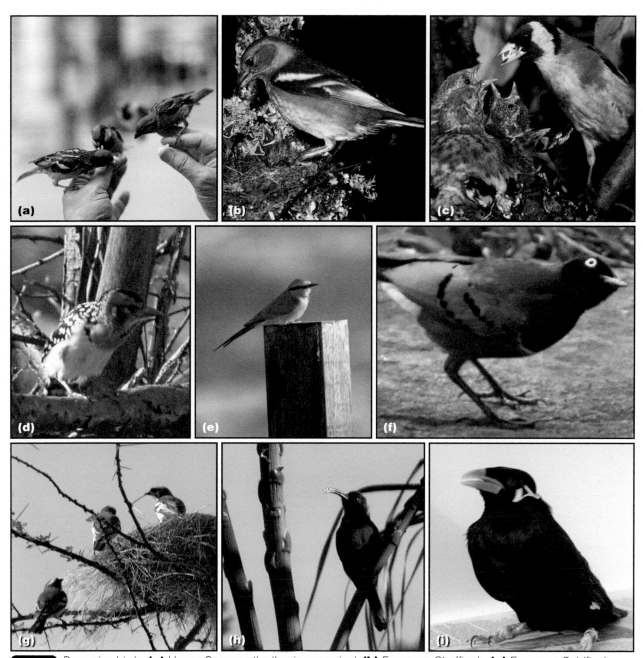

1.4 Passerine birds. **(a)** House Sparrow, the 'basic passerine'. **(b)** European Chaffinch. **(c)** European Goldfinch. **(d)** Bearded Barbet. **(e)** European Bee-eater. **(f)** Superb Starling. **(g)** Weavers, often kept because of the beauty and complexity of their nests rather than for the bird's appearance. **(h)** Sunbird, a nectivorous species. **(i)** Greater Hill Mynah. (a,b,c, courtesy of Brian Stockdale; d,f,g,h,i, © John Chitty; e, © Michael Lierz)

concerning pigeons and doves and birds of prey, respectively, are given by Hooimeijer and Dorrestein (1997) and Cooper (2002) and in Chapters 2 and 3. Terms relating to passerine birds are given in Chapter 4 and in most avicultural texts. It is not possible in one Manual to cover this aspect in detail; reference should be made to more specialized publications.

Biology and natural history

As with other 'exotic' species, an understanding of the biology and natural history of a bird is important in investigation, in diagnosis and in treatment. For that reason, the best avian practitioners are usually those veterinary surgeons who are keen birdwatchers, or who keep birds in captivity themselves.

The main biological characteristics of raptors, pigeons and passerines are given in Figure 1.5.

The behaviour of different species cannot be discussed in any detail: there is much variation. Whether a bird is generally solitary or social in the wild influences how it should be kept in captivity or housed when undergoing veterinary attention. Other aspects of behaviour are relevant to feeding practices, to captive breeding and to rehabilitation of sick and injured birds (for the latter, see *BSAVA Manual of Wildlife Casualties*).

Feature	Raptors		Columbiformes	Passeriformes
	Falconiformes	Strigiformes		
Lifestyle	Generally diurnal. Spend much of time on land, perching, or in flight	Mainly nocturnal. Spend much of time on land, perching, or in almost noiseless flight	Diurnal. Spend much of time on land, perching, or in flight	Generally diurnal
Diet	Carnivorous – whole animals, including vertebrates, invertebrates and (some species) carrion. Generally fed only once a day in captivity	Carnivorous, including mammals, birds, fish and invertebrates; rarely carrion. Generally fed only once a day in captivity	Herbivorous – seeds, leaves, fruit. Young birds fed on crop 'milk'. Usually fed *ad libitum* in captivity or offered food several times a day	Some species predominantly carnivorous (including insectivorous), some herbivorous, some omnivorous. Diet sometimes reflected in popular terminology. In UK, those that eat fruit, nectar and insects are called 'softbills'; those with heavier bills (beaks) that eat seeds are 'hardbills'. Small birds have high basal metabolic rate and need food several times a day
Moult	Usually annual, after breeding season. In sequence, gradual. Large raptors such as vultures may take 2–3 years to complete moult	Usually annual, after breeding season. In sequence, gradual	Usually annual, after breeding season. Moult patterns variable	Usually annual, after breeding season, but variations. Some tropical species may moult more than once in a year
Reproduction	Sexual dimorphism sometimes pronounced in markings and colour (e.g. Common and American Kestrels), often slight (e.g. *Buteo* spp.). Size differences often especially pronounced: male Peregrine termed tiercel because one-third smaller than female. Young altricial	Sexual dimorphism generally slight but exceptions (e.g. Snowy Owl) and size often distinct (e.g. Eagle Owl). Young altricial	Close sexual monomorphism but depends on species (e.g. differences in colour in *Columbina* spp. and in appearance of cere in *Columba* spp.); pigeon fanciers can usually readily sex birds used for racing. Young altricial	Sexual dimorphism often marked. Young altricial. Some species used as foster parents
Anatomy	Hooked beak (bill) and claws (talons) for holding and eating whole animals	Hooked beak and claws for holding and eating whole animals	Relatively slender beak for holding vegetable matter; short claws	Much variability in beak shape, depending upon feeding habits
	Crop present	Crop absent	Crop present	Crop variable: not present in some tropical softbills
	Generally no grit in small gizzard (thin-walled)	Generally no grit in small gizzard (thin-walled)	Grit in large gizzard (thick-walled)	Grit in large gizzard (thick-walled) in hardbills; little or no grit in softbills
	Caeca small	Caeca large	Caeca small or absent	Caeca vary
	Preen gland pointed with feather(s)	Preen gland rounded, no feather(s)	Preen gland varies, usually no feathers	Preen gland varies
	Anisodactyl – perch with three digits forward, one back (Osprey semi-zygodactyl)	Owls perch with two digits forward and two back but are semi-zygodactyl – can be two toes cranial and two caudal or three cranial and one caudal (digit IV rotates)	Anisodactyl – perch with three digits forward, one back	Anisodactyl, palmate – perch with three digits forward, one back
Habitat in wild and use of special senses	Land birds (but some species have adopted lifestyle involving catching fish or seabirds). Usually excellent eyesight. New World vultures can detect food by smell. Limited vocalization	Land birds, a few adapted to aquatic environments. Acute hearing, good eyesight. Generally poor sense of smell. Vocalization varied, depending upon species; some have different calls (hoots, sharp cries) for hunting and for courtship	Land or coastal birds. Good eyesight and hearing. Traditionally not thought to have well developed sense of smell, but recent research on racing pigeons suggests may use olfactory cues to navigate. Limited vocalization but distinctive quality. Magnetic sense for orientation	Predominantly land birds, some adapted to coastal and aquatic habitats. Good eyesight and hearing. Probably poor sense of smell. Very well developed vocalization, especially in songbirds (musical notes)
Behaviour	Essentially solitary, except during breeding season. A few species social (gregarious), e.g. Harris' Hawk, Eleonora's Falcon	Solitary or in loose pairs except during breeding season	Generally social, in flocks	Vary; many are social, in flocks

1.5 Biology and natural history of the four Orders. The information given in this table is broad and general in its scope. In each group there are exceptions, especially within the Passeriformes, which is a large Order and within which many anatomical and behavioural adaptations are seen.

Attention to the behavioural needs of captive birds can do much to enhance their health and welfare. Many of the stressors that birds encounter in captivity can be minimized if the veterinary surgeon understands how birds live and the ways in which they respond to stimuli. Examples of stressors that can be very deleterious include:

- Close exposure to humans. Birds have their own, different, 'fright, fight and flight' distances and allowance should be made for this by providing accommodation of a suitable size, partly covered (so that the bird can retreat from view) and elevated so that the bird is in a high vantage point, as most would be in the wild
- Unfamiliar or threatening sounds such as doors slamming, dogs barking, cats climbing aviaries, or people wearing bright clothing, speaking loudly or gesticulating wildly
- Contact with members of the same species where this may present a threat. A male canary that is kept close to others of the same sex may serve as a challenge. A large female raptor may kill (and devour) a male if they are housed together in unsatisfactory accommodation, especially on a poor diet
- Incorrect environmental conditions. Birds can be affected by a change in photoperiod; for example, they may refuse to feed. Incorrect temperatures can prove fatal to small passerine birds, which have a high basal metabolic rate (BMR) and are therefore particularly susceptible to hypothermia.

Longevity of a species is an important consideration in veterinary practice, where decisions have to be made about the ethics of treating a particular condition or prolonging the life of an apparently geriatric bird.

As a general rule, larger birds live for longer than do small ones. Thus a large raptor, such as an eagle or vulture, may survive for decades; a medium-sized pigeon is likely to have a lifespan of less than a decade; while a very small passerine bird may die after just a few years (Cooper, 2003). Life expectancy in captivity usually exceeds that in the wild.

It will be seen that, although they have much in common as members of the Class Aves, the three groups also show significant differences that are of relevance to their care, examination and treatment.

One feature that the three groups do share is that some members of each have long been associated with humans. Certain pigeons and passerine birds have been truly 'domesticated', in the sense that their breeding and maintenance have been continuously controlled by humans (Wood-Gush, 1985). Raptors have only relatively recently been regularly bred in captivity, but, with selection for specific traits and changes in appearance and behaviour, a number are clearly on their way to domestication. Insofar as pet (companion) species, including passerine birds, are concerned, the human–avian bond is increasingly being recognized and discussed. An understanding of what this entails can help the practitioner to deal with both birds and their owners (Harris, 1997).

Although this Manual covers the three groups, it must not be forgotten that only a relatively small number of species from each Order are regularly kept in captivity. Those genera that are in the latter category and therefore likely to come to the attention of the practising veterinary surgeon, including species specifically referred to elsewhere in this Manual, are listed in Figure 1.6. The nomenclature and taxonomy are taken mainly from *The Howard and Moore Complete Checklist of the Birds of the World* (Dickinson, 2003).

Order	Species	Origins	Adult weight (g)	Comments
Falconiformes	Common Kestrel	Eurasia	(M) 250–320 (F) 300–350	Widespread species. Breeds readily in captivity
	Peregrine Falcon	Worldwide	(M) 500–800 (F) 900–1000	Used on its own, or as hybrid, for falconry
	Saker Falcon	Palaearctic regions, eastern Europe to central/eastern Asia	(M) 730–950 (F) 970–1300	Used on its own, or as hybrid, for falconry
	Gyrfalcon	Holarctic regions Old and New World	(M) 800–1320 (F) 1130–2100	Used on its own, or as hybrid, for falconry
	Harris' Hawk	Southern USA, Central and South America	(M) 550–880 (F) 825–1200	Most commonly used hunting hawk, due to unique social structure
	Eurasian Buzzard	Europe and large parts of Asia; some races migrate to southern Africa	(M) 430–1000 (F) 500–1400	Not very effective hunting bird but often used as training bird for beginners
	Red-tailed Hawk	North America	(M) 900–1100 (F) 1000–1400	Excellent hunting hawk
	Northern Goshawk	Holarctic regions, Old and New World	(M) 530–750 (F) 800–1200	Excellent hunting hawk, but use limited to experienced handlers due to *Accipiter* temperament
	Golden Eagle	Nearctic and Palaearctic regions, extending to northern Africa and southern China	(M) 2800–4600 (F) 3800–6700	Much prized hunting eagle across its entire range

1.6 Some more detailed information about raptors, pigeons and passerine birds that are often kept in captivity. (continues)

Order	Species	Origins	Adult weight (g)	Comments
Strigiformes	Tawny Owl	Eurasia	400	Widespread species; breeds readily in captivity
	Barn Owl	Ubiquitous (different subspp.)	350	Breeds readily in captivity
	Eurasian Eagle Owl	Eurasia	(M) 1620–3000 (F) 2280–4200	Large impressive species, often kept and bred in captivity
Columbiformes	Domestic Pigeon	Europe	250–500	Derived from Rock Dove. Much variation in appearance relating to whether used for racing or show (ornamental)
	Eurasian Collared Dove	Europe and Asia	150–220	One of the 'turtle doves' (of which there are 8 spp.). Popular in captivity on account of apparent gentle nature and characteristic soft calls
	Victoria Crowned Pigeon	Northern New Guinea	Up to 2500	Largest living pigeon. Found in many zoological collections
	Diamond Dove	Australia	40–50	One of smallest doves. Commonly kept in avicultural collections, especially alongside finches
Passeriformes	Canary	Canary Islands, Madeira and Azores	10–40	Many different varieties, e.g. Border, Norwich, Fife. Selected for song, colour and shape
	Zebra Finch	Australia	10–20	Breeds readily in captivity. Many colour forms
	Gouldian Finch	Northern Australia	16–20	Popular with aviculturists. One of the 'Australian finches'
	European Greenfinch	Europe	15–25	One of a number of finches that can be crossed with canaries to produce 'mules'
	Java Sparrow	South-east Asia	20–35	Popular aviary species. Several colour forms. Breeds readily
	Orange-cheeked Waxbill	Africa	10–20	Popular species; inexpensive and hardy
	Greater Hill Mynah	Asia	180–250	Typical 'softbill', feeds on fruit and insects. Popular pet, good mimic

1.6 (continued) Some more detailed information about raptors, pigeons and passerine birds that are often kept in captivity.

Acknowledgements

I am grateful to my Trinidadian colleague, Dr Gabriel Brown, for helpful comments and discussions on many occasions.

References and further reading

Cooper JE (1984) A veterinary approach to pigeons. *Journal of Small Animal Practice* **25**, 505–516
Cooper JE (2002) *Birds of Prey: Health & Disease*. Blackwell, Oxford
Cooper JE (2003) *Captive Birds in Health and Disease*. World Pheasant Association UK/Hancock Publishers, Surrey, B.C., Canada
Del Hoyo J, Elliot A and Sargison J (in preparation) *Handbook of the Birds of the World*. Lynx Edicions, Barcelona (Vols 1–11 published, 12–16 in preparation)
Dickinson EC (ed.) (2003) *The Howard and Moore Complete Checklist of the Birds of the World, 3rd edn*. Christopher Helm, London
Dorrestein GM (2000) Passerines and exotic softbills. In: *Avian Medicine*, ed. TN Tully *et al.* pp. 144–179. Butterworth-Heinemann, Oxford
Ferguson-Lees J and Christie DA (2001) *Raptors of the World*. Christopher Helm, London
Gotch AF (1981) *Birds – Their Latin Names Explained*. Blandford, Poole
Harris JM (1997) The human–avian bond. In: *Avian Medicine and Surgery*, ed. RB Altman *et al.*, pp. 995–998. WB Saunders, Philadelphia
Hooimeijer J and Dorrestein GM (1997) Pigeons and doves. In: *Avian Medicine and Surgery*, ed. RB Altman *et al.*, pp. 886–905. WB Saunders, Philadelphia
Lockwood WB (1984) *The Oxford Book of British Bird Names*. Oxford University Press, Oxford
Mullineaux E, Best D and Cooper JE (eds) (2003) *Manual of Wildlife Casualties*. BSAVA Publications, Gloucester
Powers LV (2005) Veterinary care of Columbiformes. *Proceedings of the Association of Avian Veterinarians*, p. 171
Sibley CE and Ahlquist JE (1990) *Phylogeny and Classification of Birds: a Study in Molecular Evolution*. Yale University Press, New Haven, CT

2

Raptor husbandry and falconry techniques

Jemima Parry-Jones

Introduction

Raptors have been kept in captivity for many centuries. While the original purpose was for falconry, to obtain meat for the pot, they are now kept for a more diverse range of reasons (Figure 2.1). This has great relevance to the clinician, as husbandry has a considerable impact on disease.

Methods of keeping vary according to purpose. They are also frequently dictated by tradition and this may vary from country to country. Falconers use many terms that may not always be familiar to veterinary surgeons (Figure 2.2).

Group	Reasons
Falconers and raptor keepers	Hunting; demonstration flying and education; airfield and rubbish dump clearance; pest control; conservation and commercial breeding of endangered species
Zoos	Education (e.g. flying demonstrations); conservation and captive breeding of endangered species
Private breeders	Commercial breeding; conservation breeding
'Pet' keepers (mainly owls)	Limited flying; personal pleasure; 'line' breeding (e.g. for colour variants)

2.1 Reasons for keeping birds of prey.

Accipiter	Hawk of a group with short broad wings and relatively long legs, adapted for fast flight in wooded country. Includes *Accipiter* spp. and related genera within the family Accipitridae, e.g. Northern Goshawk, Eurasian Sparrowhawk, Cooper's Hawk
Austringer	Flyer of short-wings
Aylmeri	Most popular type of jess: bracelet joined by riveted brass ring
Bate, bating off	Excitable or panicked flight attempt by tethered bird on fist or on block/perch
Bell	Quality audible bell to assist in locating bird in flight or sitting still; can be place on leg (above jesses and ring) or on tail
Bewit	Thin leather strap used to attach bell to bird's leg
Block perch	Perch used for falcons
Bow perch	Perch used for hawks, buzzards and eagles
Buteo	Bird of prey of a group with broad wings used for soaring. Includes *Buteo* spp. and related genera within the family Accipitridae, e.g. buzzards, Red-tailed Hawk, Harris' Hawk
Cadge	Portable perch for more than one bird (usually a padded wooden frame)
Cast (*noun*)	Two or more birds flown together
Cast (*verb*)	1. To regurgitate a pellet 2. To grab and hold bird for examination (see Figure 6.8)
Casting	Indigestible part of diet
Cast off	To release bird from the fist
Cope (*verb*)	To trim beak or talons
Crab (*verb*)	Term relating to one bird of prey footing (striking with feet) another
Creance	Light line used to fly a bird during training
Crop, put over	Food to pass over from crop towards proventriculus

2.2 Some useful falconry terms. (continues) ▶

Deck feathers	Central two tail feathers
Diurnal	Daytime hunting
Eyass	Bird taken from nest in first year
Foot (*verb*)	To strike with the feet
Furniture	Collective term for jesses, bell, telemetry, etc.
Hack (*verb*)	To allow eyasses to fly free for a few weeks before starting training
Hard-penned, hard down	State of plumage once a young bird has become fully feathered and the blood supply in the quill has dried up; or when bird has completed the annual moult
Gauntlet	Traditional glove used on falconer's left hand (unless left-handed)
Hood	Close-fitting leather cap used to blindfold and calm ('hoodwink') bird
Imp	Replacement of damaged feather by gluing new tip on to old broken feather
Imprinted	Usually meaning birds raised by hand believing humans are their parents (but a range of imprinting exists)
Jack	Male Merlin
Jerkin	Male Gyrfalcon
Jesses	Leather thongs around bird's ankles for restraint
Keen, to be	State in which a bird's weight has been slightly reduced so that it responds well and is eager to fly or hunt
Lure	Imitation bird on a line, used during training
Make in	To approach a hawk that is on a lure or kill in order to pick it up
Man (*verb*)	To tame a bird so that it will accept handling and training
Mantle (*verb*)	To spread wings over food
Mews	Building within which trained tethered birds are kept at night or during bad weather, or outside but under shelter
Musket	Male Sparrowhawk
Mutes	Droppings
Passage	Applied to a bird taken from the wild
Rangle	Indigestible material (e.g. stones) sometimes ingested accidentally; formerly given deliberately to clean out the crop
Rouse	Vigorous shaking of feathers, usually just before flight
Stoop	Attack method used by falcons – a steep fast dive
Swivel	Rotating metal joint between jesses and leash
Telemetry	Radio tracking equipment, often used when flying birds in case of loss of bird
Tiercel	Male Peregrine
Wait on	Falcons circling over falconer waiting for game to be flushed
Weathering	Area where birds may be placed outside on perch during day to sun themselves
Yarrack	Keen, i.e. hungry and ready for work

2.2   (continued) Some useful falconry terms.

Tethered birds

In many countries the typical husbandry technique for a 'flying' bird (i.e. one used for hunting, pest control, or for demonstration purposes) is tethering to a block (falcons) (Figure 2.3) or bow perch (hawks) during the flying season, which is usually winter for hunting and summer for public demonstration.

Blocks and bow perches are often covered in cork or artificial turf in the belief that these materials will reduce the occurrence of bumblefoot (see Chapter 16). It is important to keep perches and equipment clean and well maintained to avoid injury to the bird's feet. The perch is generally placed outside during the day (if dry) and in a covered bay at night or during wet days (Figure 2.4). Ideally a bird should have access

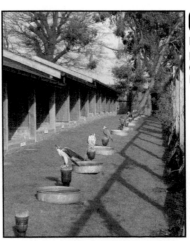

2.3

Falcons on block perches. Note the essential water bowls.

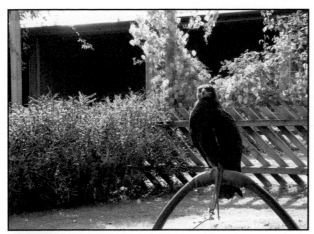

2.4 Classic husbandry of Steppe Eagle tethered on bow perch in the day. Bays for tethering at night or in poor weather are in the background.

to sunshine and rain, yet be sheltered from sudden weather extremes. In countries where wild predators are around, it is important to remember that tethered birds must be kept behind netting.

The bird is tethered by a leash connected to equipment (known as 'furniture' – see later) attached to the legs. There is variety in the traditions and methods used to accomplish this, but the basic principle is to fit leather material to the legs to which a leash can be attached via a swivelling metal joint.

The length of leash can vary according to species of bird and its temperament; for example, a nervous flighty bird on a long leash is very likely to injure itself as it may attempt to fly, generating a good velocity by the time it reaches the end of the leash. Fracture of the tibiotarsus is very common in young Harris' Hawks for this reason, but this can be prevented by using a short leash when initially training the bird.

Birds will be flown on most days. Ideally they are flown every day when tethered. Zoo legislation in the UK requires that all tethered birds should be flown at least five days out of seven. In Germany tethered birds must be flown every other day; other countries have their own regulations.

Tethering allows for excellent observation and good control of the bird, especially considering that the well managed falconry bird will be picked up several times a day so that the perch can be moved. It will also be handled regularly when it is weighed, examined and checked for body condition, and when it is put away safely at night.

During the close season tethered birds should be moved into an aviary and allowed to moult prior to being caught up and tethered when being re-manned (tamed) for the following season. However, there are many variations on this, even within the UK.

- Many birds are now being housed all year round in aviaries and are flown from the aviary ('free-lofting'). This is particularly true for owls and vultures, many of which find tethering stressful. It is also the method of choice for keeping of birds in zoological parks, where tethering is positively discouraged, though not banned in the relevant

legislation. It should be noted that it can be potentially dangerous to handlers to free-loft some eagles when in hunting condition.
- Some birds may be tethered to longer lines allowing as much room for manoeuvre as in a small aviary while maintaining the degree of control permitted by tethering. This method can be very useful for eagles (Figure 2.5) and *Buteo* species. The line used is very specialized; it is not simply a very long leash.
- Some birds are tethered and flown year-round (e.g. for pest control, or for year-round flying demonstrations) without a break for moulting. It needs to be kept in mind that energy and food content requirements are different in the moulting period: if the condition of the bird is not watched closely while flying and moulting, this technique might carry the risk of poor moulting and feather condition in the long term.

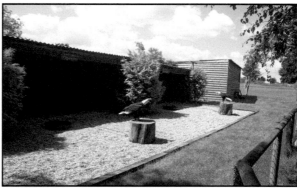

2.5 Bald Eagles on line tethers: there is a bow perch under cover and large block in the open. Although the leash is short, it is attached by a moving ring to a fixed long rod, allowing greater movement for the birds without the dangers (to the handler/falconer) of flying from the aviary. (© John Chitty)

Aviaries

Aviaries may be used for flying birds (as above) as well as for breeding birds and for those displayed in zoological collections. While there are some differences in design criteria (for example, an aviary in a zoo must allow greater visibility of the bird than a typical private breeder's aviary) there are many similarities. Design needs will vary according to species (for example, accipiters tend to require a much more secluded aviary) and geographical location (e.g. prevailing winds, ambient temperature) and the interaction between the two (such as keeping a tropical species in a temperate climate, or vice versa).

The standards for an aviary should not be skimped. Poor planning and poor-quality materials will result in health problems.

Size

Some countries have legislated or recommended minima; others have no limit on minimum size, saying only that aviaries should be as large as possible. In the UK the minimum requirement is that the bird is able to stretch its wings fully in all directions.

While large aviaries may be appropriate when displaying birds to the public in zoos (for reasons of perception, as well as allowing some increase in privacy for the birds), this is not the case for all situations. For example, when flying non-tethered birds, larger aviaries may make management more difficult. Additionally, birds may reach higher speeds in larger aviaries when frightened, thus increasing the occurrence and severity of injuries when hitting the wall or roof (though round aviaries can be huge, as birds tend not to hit the walls). In summary, it is fair to say that aviaries should be as large as practicable for good management of the birds.

Design

This will vary according to species and need. For example, accipiters are nervous species and are better in more secluded aviaries with solid sides and limited viewing panels for them to see out (Figure 2.6). More confident birds (e.g. Harris' Hawk) may be perfectly content in more open aviaries. Nonetheless, a balance should always be struck between privacy and lack of disturbance, especially for breeding birds (see Chapter 21), and good viewing and access by the keeper.

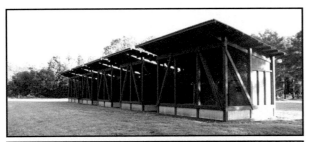
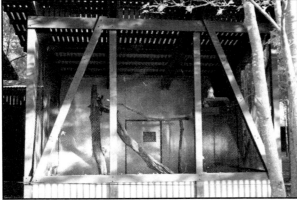

2.6 Covered aviaries.

Materials

Walls

Walls may be solid (timber, fence panels, metal), netted, meshed/wired, or a combination of these materials, according to the species being kept and their purpose. For example, keeping flighty birds in wired enclosures is a recipe for disaster as they will fly into the wire, causing feather, foot and facial injuries. Netting or, preferably, solid wooden walls (Figure 2.7) would be more sensible.

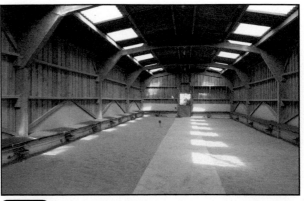

2.7 Indoor weatherings.

Where wire is used, the gauge (thickness of the strands) should be the widest available, to avoid foot injuries; plastic-coated mesh is definitely recommended. Mesh size should be such that birds with large feet cannot become entangled. The spacing diameter depends not only on species size but also on the size of wild birds that may attempt to get in, and it should be small enough to prevent the entry of rodents. All aviaries should be rodent-proofed, which may require the lower parts of the walls to be brick.

Roof

Ideally, for security and shelter, a good part of the roof should be covered (wood, felt, Onduline or Eternit plastic roofing) but part may be open (wire or netting) to allow access to sunshine and rain as the bird wishes (Figure 2.8). In some cases double layers of mesh, wire or netting may be used for roofs and walls in order to reduce entry by other animals and conflict between captive and wild raptors (especially grasping injuries). However, in the event of an outbreak of avian influenza in the area the roof should be able to be covered to stop cross-contamination from wild birds' droppings.

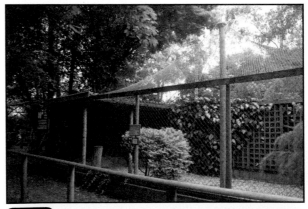

2.8 Part-netted, part-covered aviary. (© John Chitty)

Base

Many choose a concrete base for ease of cleaning and rodent-proofing. Concrete should always be covered with a substrate. It can be difficult to make natural flooring rodent-proof; wire or netting walls should be buried, or brick bases built.

Perches

Perching should be selected on the basis of the species being kept (falcons prefer ledges but most other species prefer branch-type structures). Falconers will debate the choice of material heatedly, but the most important aspects are that the perches should be well maintained and cleaned, or replaced at regular intervals, and that they are the correct width and design for the species being housed. If in doubt, a variety of perches should be provided *at each height in the aviary*. Many birds will select the highest perch and so may be forced to use a perch that is not so good for their feet. Low perching is not recommended during winter (whether birds are kept in an aviary or tethered) as the risk of wing-tip oedema and necrosis syndrome is increased (see Chapter 24).

The traditional perching for disabled birds is either very low, so that they can hop up on to it, or laddering, so that they can climb up. Laddering perches are often steep, narrow and put up in a corner, which is a recipe for broken feathers. Large branches should be used and set at the shallowest angle possible. Because the branch is wide the birds learn to run up it, keeping their bodies horizontal and wings out; therefore it should be sited in the middle of the enclosure, so that wings do not hit the walls, with subsequent damage to the feathers, and the tail can be held away as they run up.

Substrate

There are many opinions and choices regarding substrates. Some of these are summarized in Figure 2.9.

Substrate	Advantages	Disadvantages
Concrete	Easy to clean	Not good for feet. Unattractive
Bare earth	Cheap	Varies with wetness: muddy when wet, concrete-like when dry. Hard to replace. Risk of endoparasitism, as will harbour invertebrates and parasite eggs
Sand	Absorbent. Looks 'clean and attractive'. Cheap. Easy to replace. Low risk of aspergillosis and endoparasitism	Need to maintain good equipment: sand trapped under jesses will cause severe problems. Gut impaction of birds fed on floor. May cause foot problems if bird spends a lot of time on floor
Gravel	Easy to clean and replace. Low risk of aspergillosis and endoparasitism	May cause feather or foot damage if bird spends time on floor. Some birds will ingest gravel as 'rangle', causing gut impaction; size of gravel pieces must be large enough to avoid this
Grass	Attractive. Good for feet. Low risk of aspergillosis	Hard to clean. High risk of endoparasitism. Grass is soon killed off
Shavings, mulch, bark chip	Attractive. Low risk of endoparasitism. Cheap and easy to replace	High risk of aspergillosis. Poor drainage. Risk of ingestion and gut impaction

2.9 Substrates used for raptors.

Siting

Aviaries should be sited such that the bird is sheltered from prevailing winds and, thus, from the worst of the weather conditions. External factors such as disturbance (e.g. people, noise, potential predators – especially cats) should also be taken into account, as well as local building regulations and possible annoyance to neighbours.

Nest boxes

Owls generally prefer nest boxes, as do smaller diurnal species such as kestrels. Most larger diurnal species are best with a high ledge in a sheltered 'private' part of the aviary (see Chapter 21). All nest boxes and ledges should be in a dry position with a soft substrate as a base to protect the eggs. Nesting materials can be provided but care must be taken, as rotting organic materials provide a high risk for aspergillosis in young raptors.

Security

Theft is not rare and so good security should be employed. As a minimum, all doors should be padlocked. This is also to ensure against escape, to prevent which double doors are essential (these should always open inwards).

Heating

It is unlikely that any aviary can be adequate year-round for all species. In temperate climates, for example, small tropical raptors will probably need to be brought inside during winter. Indoor heated rooms attached to aviaries may be used instead. Few external heating methods are satisfactory, but the heated perches produced in the United States for parrots work well, as do the heated wall plates used by the Peregrine Fund.

Feeding in aviaries

Methods and equipment used in aviaries for feeding are compared in Figure 2.10.

Method	Advantages	Disadvantages
Place food on perches	None	Disturbs birds. Food falls to ground
Drop food down tube on to platform	Lack of disturbance for breeding birds	Food falls on platform and can become contaminated
Use feed drawers	Excellent way to feed – keeps food out of sight and off ground, and easy to deal with leftovers	None
Use plastic dishes inside aviaries	Keeps food clean and off ground	Entrance to aviaries required, leading to disturbance with nervous birds

2.10 How to feed in aviaries.

Baths

All birds need to be able to bathe and drink on a daily basis. They may not use the bath that frequently, but they must have access to clean water all the time. Baths should be large enough for the bird to get in and extend its wings.

Baths need to be cleaned at least once a week in the winter months and twice in the summer, depending on the birds.

With tethered birds, baths should be removed at noon in winter to ensure that the bird has time to dry off before night, thus reducing the risk of wing-tip oedema and necrosis syndrome.

Falconry equipment

Typical falconry equipment (Figure 2.11) includes the following:

- Weighing machine
- Glove
- Bag
- Catch-up net
- Jesses
- Swivel
- Leash
- Correct perch for species kept
- Hood if necessary
- Creance (training line)
- Lures
- Travel box.

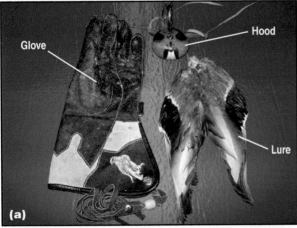

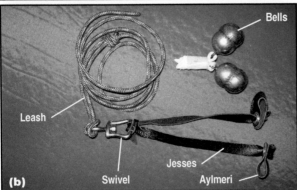

2.11 Falconry equipment. This varies between countries according to the falconry tradition. For example, the lure shown here is not typical of that used in the UK. (© Michael Lierz)

Training

Falconry is the art of training a bird to hunt. Many purist falconers do not consider that keeping a bird and not hunting with it can be described as falconry. However, the training procedure is much the same, whatever the end result.

To train a bird (other than an imprint, i.e. a bird that has become imprinted on humans from being reared by hand), its weight is reduced to get the bird keen enough to want to feed on the fist and overcome its natural fear of humans. All raptors should be weighed daily during training and flying, but they should also be felt physically, around the breast muscles, to check for condition.

1. The first step is to tether the bird, so that the trainer does not have to chase it round an aviary each day. Once tethered the work of training begins.
2. To reduce stress levels in early training (and thus reduce the risk of stress-related diseases), no attempt should be made to try to persuade it to feed on the fist immediately. The trainer should initially wait until the bird is feeding while tethered and then try to pick it up.
3. Once a bird is feeding readily on the fist, the training consists of encouraging it to jump or fly to the fist for food. This is done daily and the weight and feeding of the bird are manipulated according to the readiness of the bird to respond.
4. Once the bird is coming from a distance of more than a leash length, a creance or training line is used to control the bird before it is ready to go loose.

The training diverges at this point:

- *Buteo* spp., owls and accipiters are kept flying to the fist, with the distance increasing daily
- Falcons are introduced to a lure (a piece of meat dressed with wings) on a line that is swung to simulate a flying bird (Figure 2.12)

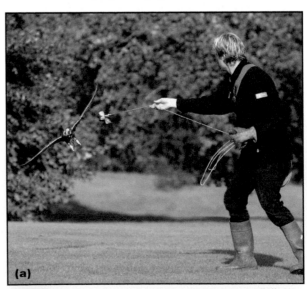

2.12 Falcons exercised and trained to lures. Different types of lure are used in different countries: **(a)** rope lure. (continues) ▶

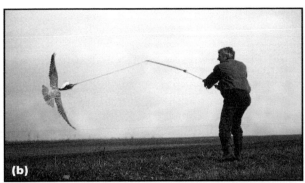

2.12 (continued) Falcons exercised and trained to lures. Different types of lure are used in different countries: **(b)** pole lure. (b, courtesy of W Bednarek)

- Eagles are best not flown to the fist, but to a perch or the ground. Calling a young eagle to the fist for food can lead to aggression later on.

Time spent in the early stages of training manning (holding the bird on the fist), walking with the bird and introducing it to all that it might meet in the future (e.g. dogs, children, umbrellas, wheelchairs, lawnmowers) will make for a more settled bird in the long term. Sitting inside in artificial light does not help much; once taken outside, birds are inclined to be just as wild as previously.

If a bird is being kept for hunting, the time to introduce it to quarry is once it is fully trained and flying free. It is necessary to have permission to hunt over the land, to fly a bird at quarry species within that species' legal hunting season and to keep in mind the laws of the land.

Telemetry
All birds should be flown with telemetry (radio tracking equipment). There are now mounting methods and weights of telemetry to fit almost any bird.

3

Pigeon husbandry and racing management

René Becker

Pigeon husbandry

History of pigeon domestication

All domesticated European pigeons descend from the wild Rock Pigeon (*Columba livia*) of Asia and the Mediterranean. Around 7000 to 8000 years ago pigeons began to affiliate with humans, whose buildings resembled the birds' natural habitat in respect of nesting and roosting places. Domestication and selection for certain characteristics marked the beginning of pigeon husbandry. The earliest accounts of domesticated pigeons come from what are now Iran, Syria, Israel and Egypt.

Much later, around 100BC to AD100, the domesticated pigeon spread across modern Greece and Italy and further into Europe. By then pigeon breeding was already being practised on a large scale in, for example, Italy.

The pigeon was highly symbolic and was used in sacrifices; it was also used as a message carrier and for the production of meat and guano as well as for pleasure. Regional preferences generated wide variety in the domesticated pigeon.

Modern husbandry

Pigeon husbandry differs according to the purpose for which the birds are kept. There are four main areas of interest:

- Since the beginning of pigeon breeding there have been varieties in colour, physique and build, which have been deliberately developed in **exhibition** breeds
- **Pigeon racing** arose in Belgium, which is therefore known as the original home of the sport. Racing pigeons, bred in a variety of colours and physiques, were developed in the mid 19th century, with international exhibitions and the creation of race standards for competitions
- Of lesser importance than for racing and as carriers are pigeons bred for **performance-flying** feats such as tumbling (turning over in the air), staying in the air for as long as possible (endurance) or flying at high altitudes
- The breeding of pigeons for **meat** production is more widespread in the United States, where it is practised on an agricultural scale, whereas in Europe it is now less important and most of the meat pigeons are consumed by those who rear them.

In addition, ever since their domestication pigeons have been used as message carriers, especially by the military.

Carrier and racing pigeon lofts

The quality of the environment within the pigeon loft is an important factor in the health and condition of the birds throughout the year. Humidity, temperature and ventilation all influence their physical state. Healthy-looking birds with sleek plumage and a good general constitution reflect good accommodation. Poor body condition and vulnerability to infection are consequences of lofts with an insufficient air supply, high exposure to dust, high humidity and inadequate protection from fluctuating weather conditions (see Chapter 30). This is particularly important in the case of birds maintained permanently in aviaries, such as those kept only for breeding.

Dovecotes on poles have been known from ancient times (Figure 3.1) but do not play any part in contemporary pigeon husbandry. They are only used for smaller flocks on farms and in gardens. Instead, birds are kept in lofts of different sizes and designs. Often these are still in attics, garages or stables, much as they were when the sport first developed, but the most up-to-date lofts are free-standing (Figure 3.2). Their construction allows for optimum ventilation, while good insulation avoids fluctuations in temperature, providing an optimal and consistent climate within the loft.

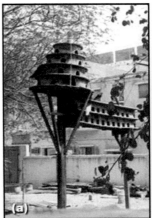 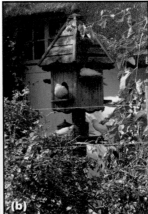

3.1 Traditional dovecotes. **(a)** From the Arabic region. **(b)** An English dovecote, from which fancy doves are allowed to fly freely. (b, © John Chitty)

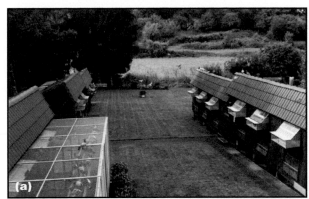

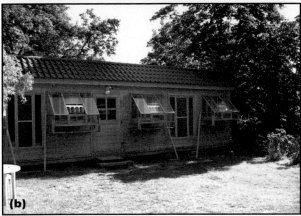

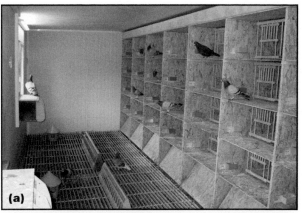

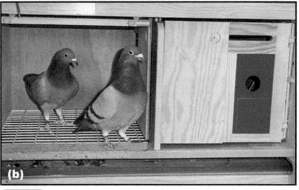

3.2 Modern free-standing systems. **(a)** A set-up with several lofts, some with attached aviaries. **(b)** The loft exits can be seen at the front. (b, courtesy of E and R Schmölz)

3.3 Interiors of modern lofts for racing pigeons. **(a)** This arrangement has timber grating on the floor. Pigeons can be prevented from leaving the cells. **(b)** A breeding pair in their cell, which has a grating floor above a conveyor belt for removing excrement.

The modern loft is efficient. It consists of several compartments, in each of which different groups (e.g. 'old' birds, 'young' birds, breeding pairs) are housed. The interior is fitted with perches or boards with an individual space for each bird (Figure 3.3a). The compartments for breeding stock and those for male pigeons that are sent out racing have nest cells or nest boxes built into the back wall in which the female pigeon and her partner can be confined for breeding (Figure 3.3b). The cell mimics the breeding caves of wild Rock Doves and forms the male pigeon's territory. Each cell has an adjustable partition so that it can be used for pairs or for single birds.

At the front of the loft are openings for each compartment through which the birds enter and leave. These 'traps' can be adjusted so that birds can enter a compartment but not leave. Registration antennae, triggered by an electronic-chip ring on the bird's leg, are installed to record the return of each individual after a race.

Breeding pigeons

Pigeon breeding is relatively problem-free. Pairs form quickly once males and females are brought together. Egg laying commences after about 10 days of display behaviour (during which the male will constantly seek to urge the hen into his nest box). In the space of two days, each female lays two eggs in a prepared nesting bowl within the nest box (Figure 3.4a). These are incubated in shifts by both partners for 17 days until hatching (Figure 3.4b).

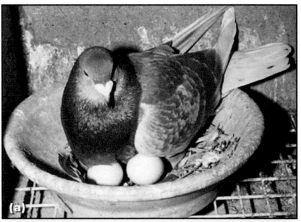

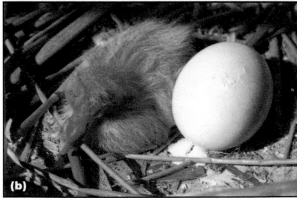

3.4 **(a)** Breeding pigeon with a clutch of two eggs. **(b)** Newly hatched pigeon chick; hatching of the second egg is imminent.

Selective breeding

Exhibition and racing pigeons are bred selectively, with each pairing carefully chosen for particular breeding targets. For exhibition pigeons there are breed standards to be met. With racing pigeons, two important criteria are competitive flying strength and a good homing instinct, but many racing pigeons are also exhibited during the winter months and so colour, wing shape and plumage quality are important. In both cases, lineage is a major criterion. Some breeders of racing pigeons keep a special stock of breeding birds, used solely for the production of a new generation; these are often the most valuable birds in the loft.

To achieve selective breeding, males and females are kept separately after the end of the previous breeding period. Pairing usually takes place in the winter or early spring and at this time each pair of chosen partners is confined to a cell. Bonding is established after a day or two and then the birds can again move freely. The cell is now used for breeding. Usually there will be several successive broods.

Management of young

After approximately 5–8 days each young pigeon (or 'squeaker' colloquially) receives a metal leg ring stamped with an individual number supplied by the breeder's federation, so that the bird can be identified clearly throughout its life. Further growth inhibits the removal of the ring after a few days. The ring identifies the individual bird and contains a country code, the number of the local pigeon association, the year of hatching and the individual number of the bird. All rings are produced centrally, which allows the bird to be traced back to its breeder. Each ring comes with a passport, which is given to the new owner if a bird is sold. Some fanciers also stamp their contact details on a primary feather.

For show pigeons the ring contains only the country code, year of hatching and the individual bird number. Passports are not issued for each ring.

After approximately 25 days in the nest, during which they are fed with 'crop milk' by both parents (see Chapter 27), the young pigeons are removed to a separate compartment for young birds. By now they can eat independently and they begin to fly. After a few more days they leave the loft for the first time and explore their environment. This loft becomes their homing loft, to which they will find the way back even over large distances throughout their lives.

For racing pigeons the first 'Young Bird' races take place in late summer (late July in the UK), when the young birds, by then 3–6 months of age, are sent on their first race, having been gradually trained in the meanwhile to fly back to their own loft after a series of 'tosses'. In the autumn the current year's offspring of exhibition pigeons are sent to their first shows.

Management of racing pigeons

Breeders

Breeders are either the offspring of successful parents or have themselves achieved success, and they are often purchased for high amounts by the fanciers. The birds are placed in a special breeding compartment, with attached aviary. They do not usually have access to free flight, since their sole purpose is to breed.

Racers

Racers enter Young Bird races at the age of approximately 3–6 months, as described above. In the following year they settle into the Old Bird compartment and remain there for several years. The males are placed in compartments with cells, as described above; each bird has its own cell, which it quickly recognizes and defends as own territory. Racing females are accommodated in a simply furnished compartment with box-perches or shelves.

Many fanciers also let their racers raise offspring. This happens in the spring before the beginning of the racing season. Alternatively, to avoid placing a strain on them for the coming season, the birds are allowed to breed for only a few days and the eggs are then removed.

Each year the older pigeons progress from Young Bird races to Old Bird races.

The racing season

The timing of the racing season depends on the region. In Central Europe, for example, it opens with Old Bird races in April (usually the last Saturday in April in the UK). The season continues until perhaps late September.

At first the length of the races may be about 100 km; thereafter the distances are gradually increased with each race, reaching perhaps 700 km by mid July (which is also about the time of the first Young Bird races). In many countries the majority of breeders specialize in races of only 100–200 km, but there are long-haul specialists who send their pigeons on flights of up to 1200 km. The latter require specially bred lines that have the physical constitution and predisposition to master these distances.

The older birds are often prepared by being separated according to sex during the week of the race and trained daily in separate groups of males and females by taking part in regular but time-limited free flights. Just before the birds are placed into travel baskets prior to a flight, partners can meet for a short time (which will encourage them to return to the home loft). Then they are separated and taken to the flight. Prior to the flight the electronic chip-ring on the pigeon's leg (Figure 3.5) is registered and the documentation is completed.

The pigeons are placed in boxes or baskets of approximately 20–30 birds. These are taken to the release point in large purpose-built pigeon transporters. In a single release there are usually several thousand competing pigeons. When they return home their arrival time is recorded (either electronically or by 'clocking in'). The data from different breeders are collected and evaluated by computer and, after several flights have been accomplished, championships and best performances of individual pigeons are determined.

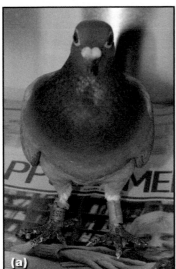

3.5

(a) Rubber racing leg-bands on a pigeon. **(b)** An electronic racing ring. The pigeon is registered when placed in the racing cabin and again automatically when entering the loft after the race. (a, courtesy of Alistair Lawrie; b, courtesy of E and R Schmölz)

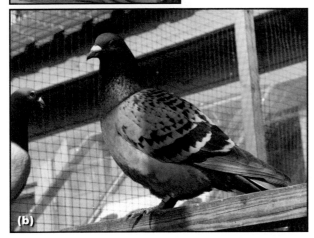

On returning to the home loft a pigeon may see its partner again and remain with it for some time. Usually only one partner is sent on the journey, generally the male. This is known as the jealousy incentive or widower system, since the travelling males do not usually see their partners during the week (Figure 3.6a). The method is not employed for young pigeons (Figure 3.6b) and the sexes are not separated, since the mating impulse is not yet present in most of the young birds.

Delayed moult

In many countries it is common to retard the moult of young pigeons, which often otherwise would begin at start of the Young Bird racing season. Delaying the moult means that the young bird is more competitive with a more complete plumage. For this purpose the photoperiod is shortened artificially by deferring 'springtime' to the middle of June and reducing the day length to 10 hours of brightness by simply darkening the loft.

Care of the racing team

As well as the basic requirements for successful pigeon sport, which are primarily an efficient loft and good-quality high-performance birds, the general care of the birds is of crucial importance. This includes appropriate nutrition, high standards of loft hygiene and sound health precautions to keep the birds in top racing condition.

Nutrition: Feeding should be adapted to specific requirements according to the season (see Chapter 27). There are relevant feed mixtures for each phase of the pigeon year, i.e. for young birds during rearing, for the racing season, for the moult period and for the resting phase in the winter. There is also a multiplicity of different supplementary feeds to tackle nutritional deficits. These are marketed as a package and contain adequate nutritional elements for the appropriate phase. The manufacturers also supply appropriate feeding plans and recommendations.

Hygiene: Loft hygiene is a substantial factor in maintaining the birds' health, particularly in the racing season. In general the loft should be cleaned daily where the floor and the cells are lined with timber. In modern systems the floor often comprises gratings, which permit the excrement to fall through, so that cleaning beneath the grating becomes necessary only every few months. Sometimes there are conveyor belts to remove the excrement (Figure 3.7).

General disinfection of the loft is common in spring. In addition, disinfection measures are essential after the treatment of parasitic and bacterial infections, in order to break the infection chain. Choice of the correct disinfectant is important.

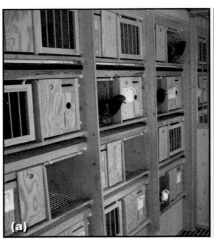

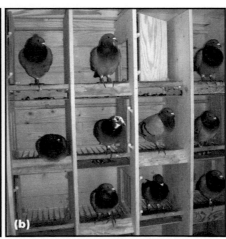

3.6 **(a)** The widower system, with females waiting in their nest cells (which can be divided) offering an added incentive for racing males to come home. **(b)** In contrast, the widower system is not used for young racing pigeons; they have no nest cells, just simple box-perches. (Courtesy of E and R Schmölz)

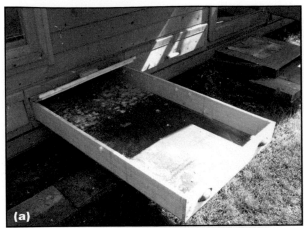

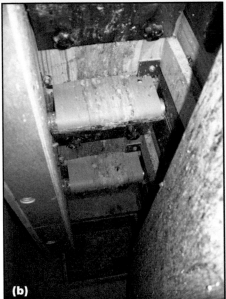

3.7 Removal of droppings is an essential part of loft hygiene. **(a)** The bottom-drawer system enables easy regular removal. **(b)** Modern systems use automated conveyor belts. (Courtesy of E and R Schmölz)

As an alternative to wet disinfectant, a gas burner is used in many lofts to 'flame' the floor and is preferable during the racing season. This method is used, for example, after treatment of coccidia. It must be used with care, however.

Health: Pigeon breeders pay particular attention to the health of their birds in the racing season. Hence in early spring many will consult a veterinary surgeon, who should determine the health status of the pigeons and prescribe appropriate treatments to be carried out before the racing begins (see Chapters 28 to 32). Due to the stress of weekly flights and the high risk of cross-infection from pigeons from other lofts in the transport van, specific treatments are required both before and after the flights in order to ensure the birds' wellbeing. Sometimes these treatments are carried out under veterinary direction but many breeders have their own methods. Most have acquired a good basic knowledge of potential health problems during the racing season and will treat their own flock before consulting a veterinary surgeon.

Veterinary examination prior to racing should proceed as follows.

1. First the bird is handled (see Chapter 6) for a general physical examination.
2. Plumage quality, body weight and condition and any ectoparasite burden are evaluated (see Chapter 7).
3. Crop swabs and faecal samples are taken.
4. The condition of the throat is checked (see Chapter 31). The crop swab gives information about the possible existence of *Trichomonas* infection and allows an assessment of the crop mucosa. For young pigeons in particular, the faecal sample is examined to detect the presence of *Spironucleus* spp.
5. A bacteriological throat smear is taken and is assessed for any pathogens that might require treatment. It also provides an overview of the resistance situation within the flock and might hint that the owner has been using excessive antibiotic treatment.
6. A bacteriological and parasitological faecal examination completes the analysis.

On the basis of the results the veterinary surgeon draws up an appropriate treatment plan. During the racing season this comprises regular treatment of *Trichomonas* infection, because these organisms often pave the way for further illnesses, particularly bacterial throat infections. Depending on the bacteriological result, antibiotic treatment may be carried out before the start of the season. These treatments are repeated frequently by many breeders during a short period after a race, in order to regain good condition in their animals; hence in many cases there is inappropriate treatment. Parasitic pathogens found in the faeces should be treated according to results of the analysis.

The veterinary surgeon's recommendations after clinical examination before the racing season should include regular examination of the birds during the season, ideally every few weeks.

Tracing lost birds

Lost racing pigeons may be traced through the relevant national pigeon racing association. In the UK this is the Royal Pigeon Racing Association at The Reddings, Cheltenham GL51 6RN (www.rpra.org) (tel. 01452 713529); there are also regional Homing Unions in Scotland, Wales, Ireland, the North of England and the North West. In Germany the equivalent national association's website is www.brieftaube.de

4

Passerine bird husbandry and show management

Brian Stockdale

Introduction

Passerine birds range in size from a few grams to over 1.5 kg (see Chapter 1). They inhabit a wide range of habitats and have a variety of diets. Their life histories and reproductive behaviour are often unique. They include some of the most colourful and melodic songsters within the bird world.

For ease of description, passerine birds are divided into two main types: *hardbills* and *softbills*. This division reflects the nature of their diets, the former being basically hard-coated seeds and the latter soft fruit and insects (see Chapter 33); it has no bearing on the physical strength of their anatomical bill.

The passerine species most likely to be seen in general practice are finches of the Fringillidae family (Canary, Greenfinch and Bullfinch) and of the Estrildidae family of Asia, Africa and Australia (Zebra Finch, Java Sparrow, Gouldian Finch and Bengalese Finch) (Figure 4.1).

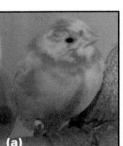

4.1 **(a,b)** Different colour variants of domesticated Canaries. The true 'wild' form is rarely seen. **(c)** Zebra Finches are found in many different colour varieties; the natural form is seen here on the left. (© John Chitty)

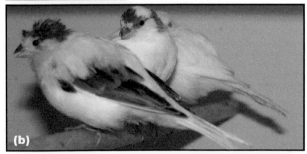

(b)

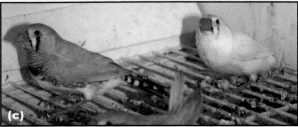

(c)

Sexing passerine birds

Whilst not possessing any external genitalia, male passerine birds can sometimes be identified by the presence of a 'cloacal promontory'. The caudal end of the ductus deferens enlarges during the breeding season into a mass called the seminal glomerulus, which pushes the cloacal wall into a small projection. Females do not develop this projection. Some species show differences in direction of the cloaca, with females pointing backwards and males pointing downwards.

Many passerines are sexually dimorphic and can be easily sexed visually. Many others have more subtle characteristics that may only be apparent once maturity is reached or during the breeding season, and experience is required to differentiate accurately between the sexes. Species that appear to be sexually monomorphic include the Canary; however, male Canaries tend to have a rich melodic song when in breeding condition whereas female vocalization tends to be small chirps and whistles. Many softbill species are also monomorphic (Figure 4.2) and DNA sexing is practical in some of these species.

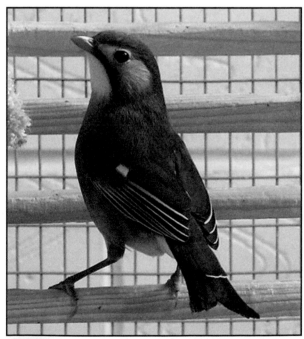

4.2 Pekin Robin. The cock's song is a means of distinguishing between the sexes. Import bans have led to a marked increase in economic value for the Pekin Robin. (Courtesy of Kevin Eatwell)

Careful observation of 'pairs' of monomorphic birds will often give a good indication as to the sex of the individual, especially if it is a male. The majority of male birds, both hardbills and softbills, perform courtship displays. Females will often perform copulation-soliciting displays when in sight and sound of male birds.

Breeding and management of hardbills

Canaries typify the group of hardbill finches and can be divided into three main types: those bred for their song (e.g. Roller Canary); those bred for their colour (see Figure 4.1); and 'type' Canaries (e.g. Border, Gloster, Fife, Yorkshire and Norwich) bred to conform to a prescribed size, shape and posture. Breeders of Canaries and other finches that are commonly exhibited are often referred to as belonging to 'the fancy'.

Canaries can be bred communally in outdoor or indoor aviaries (Figure 4.3a), but for serious fanciers controlled breeding in box-type cages is necessary. Many fanciers now have sophisticated purpose-built bird rooms (Figure 4.3b).

Photoperiod

The breeding cycle of northern temperate birds, including the Canary and European finches, is induced by an increase in photoperiod. To bring their birds into breeding condition earlier, most breeders in Europe house their birds indoors and artificially extend the daily photoperiod incrementally from December onwards, lengthening the light period by about 15–30 minutes each week until the required photoperiod of 14–15 hours a day is achieved. The use of natural daylight bulbs also helps to increase reproductive activity.

Most fanciers attempt to get their hens to lay their first round of eggs in late March or early April, which is about 4–6 weeks earlier than they might naturally. This ensures that, before the show season starts in September, the young from the current year's breeding are of a good size and maturity and the adult birds have completed their moult.

Housing

Canaries are usually bred in wooden box-type cages with wire fronts. Whilst as much space as is practical should be allowed, a pair will happily breed in a cage 50 × 40 × 40 cm (Figure 4.3c). For easier management, access to food, water and grit is usually provided from the outside of the cage.

Cage-floor substrate is a matter of choice. Many breeders use shavings or sawdust in a deep-litter system, cleaning out periodically between clutches. This reduces disturbance to the incubating or rearing hen. Another method is to use sheets of newspaper, removing a layer as it becomes soiled by means of a sliding drawer in the bottom of the cage. On the Continent (though rarely in the UK), silver sand and crushed shells are used to cover the bottom of the cages. Some breeders use white or river sand from construction sites or children's play areas, but this practice must be discouraged because of the risk of toxoplasmosis from cat faeces.

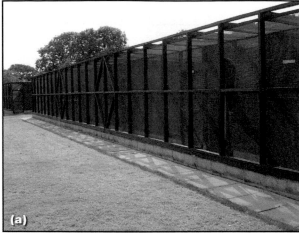

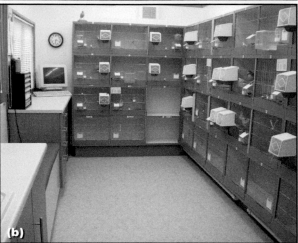

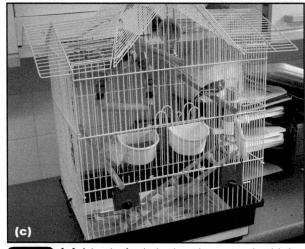

4.3 **(a)** A bank of aviaries housing passerine birds undergoing rehabilitation for release into the wild. **(b)** A modern bird room. The floor and all the surfaces and cages are made from easily disinfected material. Electricity and water are provided. Heating is from tubular heaters situated under the cages and lighting is both natural and artificial by means of 'natural light' fluorescent tubes (on a time switch for photoperiod control). Additional ventilation is provided by a wall-mounted extraction fan. In this bird room the nest-pans are situated on the outside of the cages for ease of management. A computer helps with data management, breeding records, feeding etc. **(c)** This typical pet finch cage held two Zebra Finches. Such cages are often small, with inappropriate toys and vast quantities of seed.
(a, courtesy of Kevin Eatwell; b, courtesy of Alan Harper; c, © John Chitty)

Nesting

Canaries construct open cup-shaped nests. Nest bowls made from plastic or clay (materials easily cleaned and disinfected between rounds of chicks) or wooden trays form the base for the nest. A circular piece of felt secured in the bottom of the nest bowl provides anchorage for nesting material. The felt is usually treated with an appropriate acaricide to prevent red mite infestations.

Many breeders initiate the nest, hollowing out nesting material and providing additional material for the hen to refine the structure herself. Suitable materials include: teased-out pieces of sisal, string or hessian; strips of paper; cotton wool; or coconut fibre (hay is now generally not used as nesting material, because of the risk of contamination with fungal spores and *Toxoplasma* oocysts). Care must be taken when using animal hair or synthetic fibres, as these can wrap themselves around the chicks' legs and cause the loss of toes.

In most designs, nest bowls are within the breeding cage. Sometimes they are outside, in a small box attached to the cage front (see Figure 4.3b). This allows for easier access to the nest and causes less disturbance when checking eggs and ringing young birds.

Breeding systems

Sexual maturity in the Canary is usually reached around 10 months of age.

A pair of birds can be kept together for the breeding period, or a quality cock bird may be mated with a number of hens. If both birds are in full breeding condition, mating usually takes place within a few minutes of his introduction.

Breeding as a trio, with the cock bird housed between two hens and allowed to 'run' with each hen for a period during the day, allows for easy management. The sections of these triple-breeder cages are divided by a removable slide.

Allowing a cock to mate with more than one hen maximizes the genetic potential of the best cock birds and also reduces the number of birds a fancier needs to keep. Top studs usually try to breed from all their hens in a season but use only a limited number of cock birds, keeping some as backups. Whilst not common, pair incompatibility does occur and the birds bicker constantly or, occasionally, there is actual trauma.

Egg laying, incubation and rearing

Canaries usually lay from three to five eggs in a clutch. The eggs are pale blue, heavily mottled in green and black. The last egg laid in a clutch is often a paler colour, giving an indication that laying has finished.

In the Canary only the hen incubates the eggs. Incubation starts with the laying of the first egg and hatching would be asynchronous if allowed to occur naturally. Canaries are not good at bringing up broods of asynchronistically hatched chicks. Male parents, in particular, tend to feed the most energetic feeders and the smaller chicks get pushed to one side and often squashed, especially in larger clutches.

Synchronized hatching helps to ameliorate this problem. To achieve this, breeders usually remove the eggs the morning after they are laid and replace them with plastic dummy eggs until the clutch is complete. The removed eggs are kept in a cool place (optimally 8–11°C) and then replaced in the nest on the day when the fourth egg is laid; hatching will then be more or less synchronous. This procedure is also used when cage-breeding European finches.

At around 7–8 days of incubation most fanciers test each clutch for fertility by 'candling', i.e. shining a bright light through the egg to assess embryo development. Blood vessels radiating across the inner shell membrane can be detected in fertile eggs but not in infertile ones, which appear clear. A clear round of eggs is usually removed and the hen will recycle, laying another clutch. Some fanciers allow the hen to 'sit' for the natural incubation period, believing that it better 'tunes' the natural hormonal balance for recycling.

Incubation lasts 12–14 days. Being altricial, passerine chicks are blind and naked at hatching but grow quickly. Canary chicks reach around 50% of their adult weight by 8 days and fledge at around 15 days. They are fed by both parents for a further 2 weeks or so, during which period the hen will usually lay a second clutch.

A third or even a fourth clutch could be laid in a season, but breeders usually take only two rounds of young. Stopping the hens from breeding by removing the nest (and denying access to the cock) hastens the onset of the moult and prepares the birds for the show season. In continental Europe only birds that are hatched in the same year as the show are able to enter competitions.

Reproductive problems

Reproductive problems are common in Canaries bred indoors, with an overall fertility rate of 55–60% over the season. Losses include clear (i.e. infertile) eggs, early embryonic death and 'dead-in-shell' (where the chick develops to the point of hatching and then dies).

A high percentage of eggs laid in the first round may be infertile. Hen Canaries generally come into breeding condition before males and often lay a round of eggs without mating. Clear eggs also represent 25–50% of problems in other rounds. Whilst management and nutrition do play a role in infertility, the author is of the opinion that genetic selection for other traits, particularly size, has had an adverse effect on natural fertility levels.

There are many possible reasons for dead-in-shell embryos (see Chapter 33).

Rings and ringing

For the purposes of identification, most passerine birds are ringed (Figure 4.4). In the UK this is a legal requirement and captive-bred birds that are to be sold or exhibited must be fitted with a closed ring. This ring must be of the correct size as laid down by governmental authorities and has a unique code number and year of issue on it (see Chapter 37). As closed rings can only be fitted when the chick is a few days old, they are deemed testimony that the bird

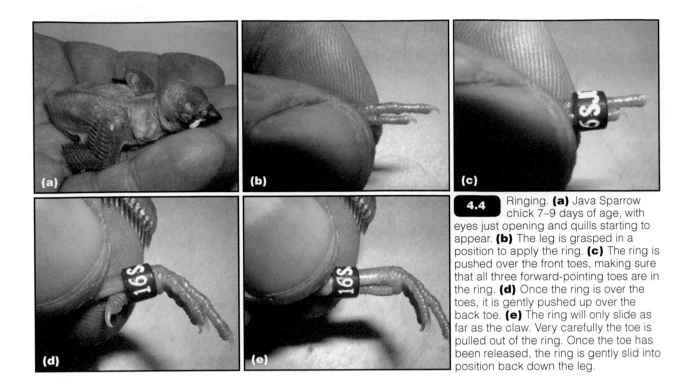

<table>
</table>

(a)	(b)
(c)	
(d)	(e)

4.4 Ringing. **(a)** Java Sparrow chick 7–9 days of age, with eyes just opening and quills starting to appear. **(b)** The leg is grasped in a position to apply the ring. **(c)** The ring is pushed over the front toes, making sure that all three forward-pointing toes are in the ring. **(d)** Once the ring is over the toes, it is gently pushed up over the back toe. **(e)** The ring will only slide as far as the claw. Very carefully the toe is pulled out of the ring. Once the toe has been released, the ring is gently slid into position back down the leg.

was captive bred and not wild caught. Ringing must be done while the chick is still small enough to allow easy passage of the ring over the tarsus. Canary chicks are usually ringed around days 6–8.

One disadvantage of fitting closed rings is intrusion into the nest, potentially causing a bird to desert her brood. Breeders try to wait until the chicks are defecating over the edge of the nest, as at this stage the parents are much less likely to remove the ring – with the chick attached – whilst cleaning the nest.

With foreign finches and Canaries there is no stipulated need to fit closed (as opposed to split) rings, though many breeders do fit them. Birds without closed rings cannot be shown in many countries and this should always be checked with the show standard rules in the relevant country. Canary rings are colour coded depending on the year.

Appropriately sized coloured or numbered split identity rings can be applied at any age. These are either plastic or light alloy and are expanded to fit around the bird's tarsometatarsal bone and then allowed to reform in the case of the plastic rings or crimped into shape with a small pair of pliers for the alloy ones.

Breeding rules

Certain 'rules' govern the breeding of 'type' Canaries. Canaries have two forms of feathering: a loose feathering termed '*buff*' and a tight feathering termed '*yellow*', irrespective of the actual colour of the bird. The feather form arises due to the physical structure of the barbules. When breeding Canaries the aim should be to pair 'buff' to 'yellow' to ensure a normal feather structure. Pairing 'yellow' to 'yellow' produces a tight contoured bird lacking a rounded shape. Paring 'buff' to 'buff' ('double buffing') produces an open-feathered fluffy bird which, again, will have poor shape definition and feather quality; double

buffing is also reported to predispose to the formation of feather cysts.

A similar 'feather rule', but for different reasons, applies to the breeding of Gloster Canaries. Glosters come as two types: *consorts*, which have a normal head appearance; and *coronas*, which have a crest of heavy feathering on their heads. The corona gene is dominant and is lethal when homozygous; therefore all phenotypic coronas are heterozygous. Pairing a corona with a consort will result in 50% corona and 50% consort. Pairing two corona phenotypes gives 25% consort, 50% corona and 25% dead chicks. To prevent such mortality, pairing corona to corona is normally avoided.

Breeding foreign finches

Exotic finches can be kept and bred in outdoor aviaries, or indoors in flights or box-type cages. Depending on the species, they may be kept as individual pairs or in colonies. Breeding exotic finches is not as photo-dependent as breeding birds from the temperate regions; breeding tends to be opportunistic, depending on local environmental conditions. Adequate warmth and a constant photoperiod (light to dark 12:12 to 14:10) will encourage most types of finch to breed throughout the year.

Nests built in the wild can be neat and compact, or untidy and straggly, and the chosen site ranges from ground level to tall trees. Several of the estrildid species build cock-nests. These are double nests: the first is where the cock bird roosts and through which the hen must pass to get to the second, inner nest where the eggs are laid.

In captivity, the majority of foreign finches are adaptable and can be encouraged to nest in boxes with holes, half-fronted boxes or enclosed wicker baskets. To make nest inspection easier, boxes are often mounted on the outside of the cage with lift-up lids.

Some species, such as the Zebra Finch, require little encouragement to nest; they become sexually mature at 3–4 months of age and produce clutches of up to eight eggs almost constantly. Other species are more problematic. Mimicking the results of recent rainfall by providing extra protein either in the form of livefood or eggfood or as seeding grasses will often encourage nesting. The added stimulus of providing a nest box and nesting material, and giving the birds extra bathing opportunities, will also encourage breeding.

Fostering

To minimize chick loss and maximize breeding potential, fostering of both eggs and chicks is often practised.

In clutches where only one chick hatches, parent birds often lose interest in feeding. Cross-fostering of a single chick to another nest allows the original parents to nest again. Fostering may also be done with mule and hybrid chicks by giving them to a reliable Canary to rear, in the hope of preventing losses.

Many breeders of exotic finches keep pairs of Bengalese Finches (see below) to act as foster parents. This involves synchronizing the breeding of the Bengalese foster parents with that of the other finches. Whilst it may increase the number of young reared, cross-species fostering also increases the potential for the spread of disease between species; and young fostered by an alien species are often less inclined to breed with their own species. The loss of innate parenthood is also exacerbated.

Bengalese Finch

The Bengalese or Society Finch is a domesticated species and has no wild counterpart. Its ancestry is not altogether clear, but it is probably a domesticated variety of the Striated or Chinese White-rumped Munia. Hybridization with other munias may have taken place during its domestication, which is credited to the Chinese several hundred years ago. The Bengalese Finch comes in many colour varieties, and is a popular show bird in its own right, but possibly its biggest avicultural merit is its willingness and ability to hatch and rear chicks from other species. Indeed, such is the keenness of this little bird to rear young that a 'pair' of male birds can be successfully used as foster parents.

Breeding and management of softbills

Very few softbills are kept as house pets. The Greater Indian Hill Mynah and the Java Hill Mynah used to be commonly kept as cage pets but are no longer freely available and their popularity has declined.

Most softbills are kept in outdoor planted aviaries or, in the case of less hardy species, environmentally controlled conservatory-type aviaries. Many species will happily live in mixed collections with finches and doves and with other softbills of a similar size, provided that they are given sufficient space.

Breeding

During the breeding season many softbills become very territorial and readily attack other aviary inhabitants. They are also renowned nest robbers, stealing both eggs and chicks. If breeding is to be seriously considered, most species are best housed as individual pairs.

Pair compatibility is much more of a problem with softbills than with finches. A pair of birds that have peaceably shared an aviary in the non-breeding season may, as the breeding season approaches, suddenly start fighting and need to be separated to prevent serious injury. Some species, such as members of the starling family, which are cooperative breeders, can be bred on a colony basis.

Softbills build a variety of nest types. Many are hole-nesters; others build typical cup-shaped nests lined with leaves, mud or feathers. Large quantities of live food are usually required to encourage breeding and for the successful rearing of young.

Colour mutations

Colour mutations (Figure 4.5) occur naturally within any population of birds. Many more colour mutations are present in wild birds in a heterozygous recessive form, with the birds appearing phenotypically normal. In exotic birds the majority of colour mutations are autosomal recessives and inbreeding will soon bring these mutations to the surface. With domestication, artificial selection and aviculture, many of these 'hidden' colours have been revealed and colour mutation strains of many species have become established.

Many cage bird species have lent themselves to the establishment of new colour forms, especially the Australian finches. Unusually the Gouldian Finch from Australia's Northern Territory (where it is under severe threat of extinction) exists naturally in three colour forms. The most common is the black-headed, a sex-linked recessive mutation; the red-headed is a sex-linked dominant mutation; and the least common, the yellow- or orange-headed, is an autosomal recessive mutation. Different coloured backs, bibs, fronts and feather types have been developed to go with these (and other) head colours.

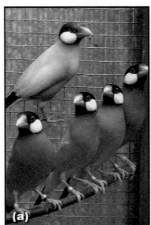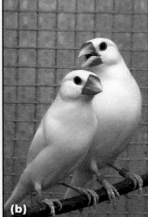

4.5 Colour mutations in Java Sparrows: **(a)** one fawn and four normal colour; **(b)** white. (© S. Nesbitt)

In European birds, the Greenfinch has both base (melanin) and pigment (bio-chrome) colour variations and structural feather mutations resulting in examples of lutino, cinnamon, pied, pastel, satinette and other colour forms. Similar colour mutations are found in the Blackbird.

Colour mutations play a valuable role in aviculture. Novel and unusually coloured or feathered birds command a high price and many aviculturalists dedicate their time and efforts to breeding and improving these strains of birds into self-sustaining populations. The normal-coloured birds have, to a greater degree, become less of a commodity, placing less demand on wild-caught stock. The irony is that many 'normal' birds are becoming less available in captivity and also increasingly scarce in their natural habitat. The common grey Java Sparrow, for example, was once plentiful in the wild but is now officially designated as endangered. Similarly, its avicultural value was superseded by a range of colour variants and moves are now in place to re-establish the 'normal' colour form.

It is important for veterinary surgeons to be able to separate true colour mutations from abnormal feather coloration resulting from pathological metabolic disorders.

Mules and hybrids

Hybridization between different species has been recorded as occurring naturally in wild populations. Creation of avian hybrids is largely deemed to serve little worthwhile purpose in captive husbandry where the sole merit of propagation of a species is in its pure form, but hybridization between different species of European finches, and between finches and Canaries (the latter hybrids being commonly referred to as mules), is a popular branch of aviculture. The purpose of hybrid and mule breeding is to produce a quality bird for showing or as a singing bird. Only male birds are shown, as they present the best coloration.

Both hybrids and mules are sterile and their merit is purely in their showing quality – with one very notable exception. Hybridization between the now critically endangered Red Siskin of South America and the domesticated Canary produces a fertile F1 generation. The Red Siskin's ability to impart its colouring, the 'red factor', to the Canary has led to the development of the coloured Canary.

Show training

The majority of bird shows in Europe take place between September and January. Shows can be for a range of birds, for a single species or for a particular breed, and are divided into classes for age, sex and colour. The standard of feather quality, body shape, general demeanour and presentation are judged. Fanciers usually have a show 'team'; they exhibit a number of birds at different shows as each bird comes into prime condition. Exhibiting birds is referred to as 'benching'.

Juveniles hatched in the current year undergo a partial moult prior to the show season, losing the majority of their contour feathering but maintaining their flight feathers (primaries), which are not replaced until the following year's moult. This gives rise to the terms 'unflighted' and 'flighted' to differentiate between those bred in the current year and older birds, and is important for classification on the show bench.

Birds are generally exhibited singly in small cages, each breed having its own specification for cage design. Young birds are trained to become accustomed to the show cage: either it is fastened to the door of the stock cage and the young birds are encouraged to 'run' in and out, or the birds are caught up and placed in the show cage for short periods of time.

References and further reading

Lander P (1981) *British Birds in Aviculture.* Saiga Publishing
Carr V (1980) *Cage Bird Hybrids.* Saiga Publishing
Lint K and Lint A (1988) *Feeding Cage Birds: A Manual of Diets for Aviculture.* Blandford Press
Restall R (1996) *Munias and Mannikins.* Russel Friedman Books
Vince M (1996) *Softbills – Care, Breeding and Conservation.* Hancock House

Useful periodicals

Aviculture Magazine (quarterly magazine of the Aviculture Society)
Cage and Aviary Birds (weekly newspaper of the Fancy)

Useful websites

Australian Finch Society: www.the-australian-finch-society.co.uk
Aviculture Society: www.avisoc.co.uk
British Bird Council: www.britishbirdcouncil.com
Canary Council: www.netcomuk.co.uk/~ncabirds/CANARY
National Council for Aviculture: www.netcomuk.co.uk/~ncabirds/NCA1
Sturnids: www.riverbanks.org/subsite/pact/sturnids.pdf (*The Sturnidae Husbandry Manual and Resource Guide*)
Waxbill Finch Society: www.waxbillfinchsociety.org.uk
Zebra Finch Society: www.zebrafinchsociety.co.uk

5

Anatomy and physiology

Ruth Maria Hirschberg

Integument

The integument is a complex organ which mediates between an organism and its environment. In birds, the most obvious roles of the skin are protection from harmful environmental influences and thermoregulation, both of which are achieved by various degrees of cornification or pigmentation and through the development of specialized integumentary accessory organs, such as the feathers that cover most parts of the body and are thus the most eye-catching feature of the avian integument. The feathers form an insulating and protective body cover; a contiguous coat of feathers enables streamlining and flight; additionally, feathers play a role in behaviour and communication.

Specific localized skin modifications enable other particular functions: the modified micro-anatomy of the oral or nasal openings (i.e. different types of bills) facilitates specific feeding habits, and different forms of digital extremities (claws, talons or falculae) enable specific locomotory modes in different environments, as well as grasping capacities (for example, in birds of prey or tree-climbing birds).

Feather patterning

Generally, the skin of the body can be subdivided into distinct feather tracts (pterylae) and featherless regions (apteriae). In both of these regularly alternating areas the integumental layers are comparatively thin, because the feather coat itself is protective (the apteriae are protected by the contour feathers of the pterylae). In contrast, the skin of the lower tarsus and feet is generally covered by reptile-like scaly skin.

This general feather patterning can vary according to environmental conditions or specific behavioural characteristics. Most owls and a few diurnal raptors have feather-covered tarsometatarsi, for thermoregulatory reasons, and some owls living in cold climates even have feathered digits. Vultures are characterized by their sparse (plumes only) or complete lack of feathering on the head and neck area, presumably related to their feeding habits.

Skin layers

The epidermis, as the outermost layer of the integument, is particularly adapted to withstand various mechanical forces and hence produces a resistant cornified superficial layer. This can contain either soft or hard keratin, resulting from two different keratinization procedures. Integumentary structures exposed to high local mechanical stress, such as bills and claws, undergo hard keratinization.

The two connective tissue layers of the skin are the dermis, a predominantly connective tissue layer with dense vascular and nerve networks, and the subcutis, a more loosely arranged connective tissue layer that may contain adipose tissue and is connected to the adjacent outer fascial layer of the body. The feathers (hard cornified structures) are the product of a close dermo-epidermal interaction. Whereas dermis and epidermis form the feather follicle, which generates the form and structure of the feather itself, the dermis and more particularly the subcutis form a very complex modified dermo-subcutaneous apparatus for anchoring and controlling individual feathers or feather groups, respectively (Homberger and de Silva, 2003). Feather coordination during flight is enabled by specific dermal and subcutaneous muscles, the latter forming the patagia of the wings.

Skin glands

The avian skin in general does not contain sebaceous or sweat glands. Nevertheless, specific modified skin glands may be found in specific locations, such as the uropygial gland at the dorsal aspect of the base of the tail (particularly well developed in birds living in aquatic surroundings, but missing in some pigeons), within the outer auditory canal, or the ventral glands of the cloaca. The uropygial or preen gland is a bilobed holocrine gland producing a lipid secretion employed for feather maintenance. The sebaceous function for the whole skin is ensured by specific sebokeratinocytes that are an integral part of the avian epidermal layers and prevent dehydration of the skin surface. The missing thermoregulatory function of sweat glands is mostly compensated for by heat loss via the respiratory tract and, in part, via the feet. The skin of the feet, depending on the respective species' environmental circumstances and habits, may consequently feature specific vascular modifications such as an increased number of arteriovenous anastomoses and sphincteric arteries, thus enabling adaptation to climate conditions.

Skin modifications

Scaly skin of the legs

The distal portion of the leg is covered by scaly skin. Like feathers, the scales represent dermo-epidermal modifications. While the epidermis of the scales features increased (mostly hard) keratinization and cornification, the supporting connective tissue layers attach the scales to the adjacent substratum such as bones, tendons and joints of the foot, allowing for firm grasp and ground contact. With regard to size and shape, there are scutate (dorsal aspect) as well as scutellate and reticulate (lateral and palmar aspect) scales (see Figure 5.2).

Claw and toe pads

The avian claw comprises the modified skin covering the tip of the distal phalanx. It is developed for protection of the phalanx and, species-specifically, as an organ for grasping (birds of prey), digging, climbing and/or defence. Accordingly, the falculae of raptors are curved sharply pointed claws or talons, in contrast to the blunter and more compact claws of pigeons. Ospreys have long sharply curved talons that resemble fish hooks – appropriate for catching their main prey, fish – whereas vultures have only slightly curved talons that enable a sure grip and secure balance while feeding on larger carcasses.

The epidermis produces the strongly cornified claw capsule, while the connective tissue layers (dermis and subcutis) of the claw provide specific anchorage and force-transmitting structures as well as the clinically important neurovascular supply of the claw (Figure 5.1). The cornified claw capsule can be subdivided into a hard 'claw plate' and a softer 'solear' part. Some species, such as owls and nightjars, have pectinate middle claws with scales that resemble the teeth of a comb and these are used to preen and straighten feathers. A few species display rudimentary claws at the tips of the wings, including Bat Hawks, Golden Eagles, most vultures, Secretary Birds, Ospreys, Caracaras and Gyrfalcons and possibly also (though very small) harriers and Black-winged Kites.

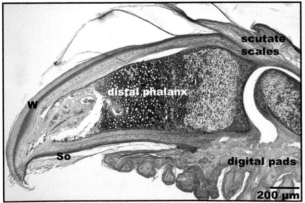

5.1 Cross-section of a developing avian claw, displaying the distal phalanx encased in the heavily cornifying modified skin of the claw that thus forms the cornified claw capsule with wall (W) and solear (So) aspects. Also note the distal scutate scales and the digital pads. (Trichrome stain.)

The toe pads (tori, pulvini) are specialized circumscript local skin modifications on the palmar aspect of the toes, featuring a particularly well developed connective tissue layer that cushions ground contact (Figure 5.2). Like the scales, the digital pads are closely attached to the underlying bone

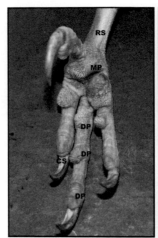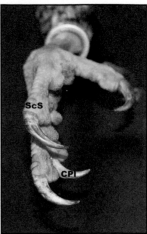

5.2 Plantar and medial view of the digits of a falcon. Note the opposed position of the first digit and the typically shaped claws, i.e. the talons or falculae. The dorsal aspect of the toes and tarsometatarsus is covered by scutate scales (ScS), while the side and plantar aspects are covered by small reticulate scales (RS). The metatarsal (MP) and digital (DP) pads feature prominent surface modifications that enable a better grasp. The claws comprise the hard (and in this case distinctly pointed) claw plate (CPl) and the softer claw sole (CS).

structures via retinacular ligaments. In bird-catching and some fish-catching raptors (like the Osprey), the toe pads have wart-like projections – the spiculae – which produce a sandpaper-like surface and thus enable a surer grip on agile or slippery prey.

Bill

The bill, or rhamphotheca, represents the oronasal opening and comprises the two beaks, i.e. the heavily cornified skin covering the upper and lower jaws. The nasal opening and the junction area towards the feathered skin of the head are often modified. For example, in pigeons there is a waxy covering (operculum) on the nares; and the Cinclidae (dippers) have a membrane for closing their slit-like nares. The base of the beak of raptors is covered by a waxy membrane that reaches up to the nares; also called the cere, this is often hard and yellow. A characteristic of falcons is the bilateral so-called 'falcon-tooth' or 'tomial tooth' of the upper beak (see Figure 5.12) with a corresponding notch within the lower beak, enabling the typical neck- or head-bite. A similar beak-tooth is developed in predatory passerine species such as the shrikes (Laniidae).

Brood patch

The brood patch in raptors, pigeons and passerine birds is located at the caudal half of the ventral apterium. Controlled by breeding hormones, the skin of the brood patch may lose all the feathers and become highly vascularized prior to laying. As the skin is also densely innervated and contains many thermoreceptors, the bird is able to control incubation when pressing the brood patch against the eggs. In pigeons, both males and females develop brood patches, while in raptors and most passerine species brood patches occur only in the females. Re-feathering of the brood patch is achieved with the next moult.

Feathers

According to its different functions in different species, the feather coat may contain different types of feathers (pennae and plumae) in varying density and distribution. All feather types comprise a dermo-epidermal intracutaneous part and a cornified extracutaneous part. The complex three-dimensional architecture of the cornified cells of the feather can be detected not only in the penna (contour feather; Figure 5.3) but also in the less complex pluma (down feather). The shaft is the central support of the feather, continued by the vane with its barbs, barbules and barbicles. The barbicles stabilize the vane of the penna by interdigitation with the barbules of the next barb.

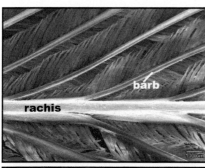
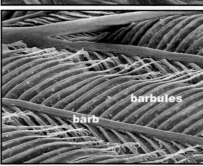
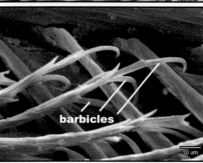

5.3 Scanning electron micrographs displaying the structure of the feather vane of contour feathers. The rachis gives rise to the lateral branches (barbs, rami) that then ramify into proximal and distal barbules (radii). The proximal and distal barbules of adjacent barbs overlap and are stabilized by barbicles (hamuli). (© H. Bragulla)

Feather types

Feather types are illustrated in Figure 5.4.

Pennae: Contour feathers (pennae) form the majority of the plumage and are characterized by a distinct shaft and feather vane. There are different types of pennae for different locations and functions:

- *Tectrices* (proper contour or cover feathers) covering most other types of feather
- *Remiges* (flight feathers) at the caudal aspect of the wing
- *Retrices* (tail feathers) at the base of the tail, enabling navigation
- *Ornamentrices* (ornamental feathers) in some birds only (e.g. some pigeons).

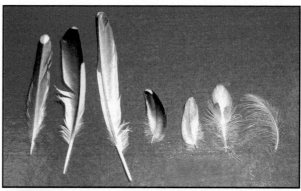

5.4 Feather types (European Goldfinch). From left to right: rectrix (tail feather), dorsal view; remex (flight feather), dorsal view; remex, ventral view; tectrix (contour feather), dorsal view; tectrix, ventral view; semiplume; plume.

Plumae and setae:

- *Down feathers* (plumae) are characterized by a short or missing shaft and long soft barbs. They are found under the contour feathers and form an insulating undercoat, while semiplumes combine both types of feathers (pluma and penna): they are downy at the base and have the characteristics of contour feathers at the top.
- *Powder down feathers* (pulviplumae) are continually growing feathers whose apical barb cells decay and thus form a fine white dust, coating the whole bird. These are particularly well developed and numerous in pigeons, causing the 'waxy' appearance of their plumage.
- *Filoplumes* are assumed to be sensory detectors in close contact with Herbst corpuscles. Because they occur in close association with contour feathers, they are presumed to assess strains and movements of the pennae during flight.
- *Bristle feathers* (setae) are protective feathers comparable to the mammalian vibrissae and occur around the eye, nares and ear.

Plumage colour

Variations in plumage colour provide camouflage and sexual dimorphism as well as juvenile or adult characteristics. Plumage coloration is accomplished in several ways.

- Melanocytes produce brown, yellow and black melanins that are dispensed to adjacent epidermal cells of the feather.
- Reds and yellows are synthesized from dietary carotinoid pigments that are then dissolved in fat globules within the feather cells.
- White and blue are so-called structural colours due to reflection and refraction of light through airspaces and specialized cornified cells within unpigmented or semi-pigmented feathers.

Moulting

As feathers tend to wear out, and because neonatal, juvenile and adult plumages are usually different in both colour and shape, the feathers are replaced at regular intervals (see Chapter 24).

Musculoskeletal system

The skeletal system of birds (Figure 5.5) is character-ized by weight reduction in order to facilitate flight and, in compensation, by strengthening structural features. For example, the medullary cavity of partic-ular bones (e.g. humerus (excepting oscine passer-ines), femur (birds of prey) and some vertebrae) is replaced by air-filled projections of the air sacs (see 'Respiratory system', below) in mature birds and thus becomes *pneumatized*. The *mineral content* of avian bones is higher than mammalian bones, which explains why avian bones under stress tend to split, rather than break as in mammals.

The term *medullary bone* describes a phenom-enon of labile bone normally occurring in female birds during the reproductive phase. Its formation is controlled by oestrogens and androgens and physio-logically it serves as a calcium repository for egg shell production; thus phases of formation and destruction alternate during the laying cycle. For further details, see Chapters 11 and 21.

Skull

The upper jaw is formed by the premaxillary, maxillary and nasal bones and, due to a craniofacial elastic zone, it can be moved relative to the rest of the skull via the 'leverage' system formed by the bones of the palatal and zygomatic skeleton. The lower jaw consists of two fused mandibles that do not articulate directly with the skull. Upper and lower jaws may thus move in different directions relative to each other. Together with a species-specific muscular system, this enables the bird to use the beak as a multi-purpose tool adapted to its particular feeding habits and other behaviour.

Because of the wide visual field of birds the orbit dominates the skull, while the neurocranium is less prominent. The orbit and the upper jaw accommodate the paranasal sinus system of birds, i.e. the infraorbital sinus (see 'Respiratory system', below).

Vertebral column, thorax, thoracic girdle and pelvis

Vertebrae

In most birds the existence of numerous and highly mobile cervical vertebrae results in a very flexible neck. In contrast, the vertebrae of the trunk are inflexible and mostly fused, thus enabling flight and the bird's bipedal posture. The cranial thoracic vertebrae form the *notarium*; the caudal thoracic, lumbar and sacral bones fuse completely to form the *synsacrum* (Figure 5.5). The coccygeal vertebrae form the *pygostyle* and thus support the tail feathers.

Thorax

The very stable thorax sustains the cranial part of the body cavity and comprises the thoracic verte-brae (notarium), the ribs and the well developed sternum. Each avian *rib* contains two parts, the costovertebral and the costosternal bone, and the ribcage is additionally reinforced by the uncinate processes. Because the main flight muscles origin-ate from it, the *sternum* features the *carina*, a high ventral crest typical in flying birds (Figure 5.5). The cranial visceral aspect of the sternum features a pneumatic *foramen* through which it is pneumatized by processes of the clavicular air sac (particularly distinct in raptors).

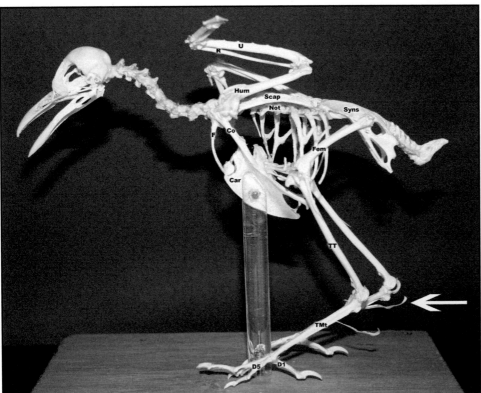

5.5

Mounted skeleton of the Eurasian Blackbird (lateral view). Note the ossified flexor tendon elements of the lower legs (arrow).
Car = carina;
Co = coracoid; F = furcula (fused clavicles);
Fem = femur;
Hum = humerus;
Not = notarium;
R = radius;
Scap = scapula;
Syns = synsacrum;
TMt = tarsometatarsus;
TT = tibiotarsus; U = ulna.

Thoracic girdle

The thoracic girdle is supported by the sternum and consists of the matched *scapulae*, the *clavicles* (generally fused, thus forming the *furcula* (excepting some pigeons)) and the *coracoid* bones (see Figure 5.5). The coracoids act as struts, holding the shoulder at a constant distance from the sternum. The scapulae lie closely adjacent to the rib cage. The furcula acts as a spring and stores energy when compressed during the down-beat flight movement. All three bones of the thoracic girdle articulate with the head of the humerus, where their joined articular surfaces form the triosseal foramen through which the tendons of the supracoracoid and deep pectoral muscles pass.

Pelvis

The matched pelvic bones of flight birds generally do not fuse to form a complete pelvic girdle, but fuse with the synsacrum in order to stabilize the trunk, and thus form the os innominatum. Together with the synsacrum, the iliac bones form deep osseous recesses (renal fossae) protecting the adjacent kidneys, nerves and blood vessels. The caudodorsal aspect of the acetabulum (socket of the hip joint) features the so-called *antitrochanter* abutting the femoral trochanter and thus preventing abduction of the limb when the bird is in a normal standing position. The pubic bone remains in part separate from the ileal and ischiadic bones.

Thoracic, abdominal and caudal muscles

The ribcage and the abdomen are supported by thoracic and abdominal muscles that mainly act as respiratory muscles (see 'Respiratory system'). The caudal muscles direct the position and movement of the pygostyle and thus assist the tail feathers during flight.

Wing

The wing comprises the humerus, the antebrachial bones (radius and ulna) and the bones of the manus, which are fused to form a three-fingered 'hand'. While radial and ulnar carpal bones remain separate, the distal carpals and metacarpals fuse to form the carpometacarpal bone. The first (alular) digit is quite mobile, but the second (major) and third (minor) digits again fuse to form an osseous clasp.

The wing as a whole is very mobile when flexed. When extended it tends to move at the shoulder joint and otherwise resists dorsal and ventral forces. The shafts of the flight feathers are deeply anchored within the dorsal aspect of the ulna (secondary flight feathers) and manus (primary flight feathers) (Figure 5.6).

Flight muscles

Wing movement during flight is achieved by contraction of the pectoral muscle system (Figure 5.7). The supracoracoid muscle, assisted by the major and minor deltoid muscles, achieves lifting of the wing due to the course of its tendons through the triosseal foramen and insertion on the dorsocranial edge of the humerus. Thus, contraction of these muscles rotates the humerus, causing the elevation of the wing's leading edge. This allows the bird to maintain its position in the air between down-strokes. The

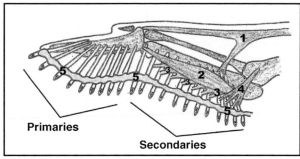

5.6 Schematic drawing of the wing, displaying primary and secondary flight feathers and the relevant musculoelastic elements of the wing (modified after Nickel *et al.*, 1977). 1 = propatagial tensor muscle; 2 = flexor carpi ulnaris muscle, and 3 = its elastic ligament; 4 = secondary extensor muscle; 5 = elastic inter-remigial ligament.

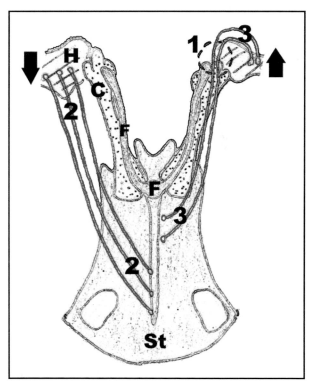

5.7 Schematic drawing displaying insertion and action of the flight muscles (modified after Nickel *et al.*, 1977). The pectoral muscles (2) achieve downward movement of the wing, whereas the supracoracoid muscles (3) achieve lifting of the wing due to diversion of fibres via the triosseous foramen (1). H = humerus; C = coracoid; F = furcula (fused clavicles); St = sternum, with prominent carina.

superficial pectoral muscle, in turn, has to achieve the down-stroke of the wing during flight and is therefore massively developed, representing approximately 15–20% of the body weight of the bird. During slow flight and take-off, the dorsal muscles of the shoulder girdle elevate the wing.

The *patagia* are specifically modified portions of the skin spanning the area between the bones of the forelimb that support flight movement. They are supported by specific patagial muscles acting in synergy with the extensor muscles, and by elastic tendons that maintain the aerofoil shape of the wing.

Most important is the *propatagium*, ranging from the shoulder via the elbow to the carpus. While the elbow displays a wide range of movements when flexed, the radius and ulna allow pronation and supination.

Wing shape

The shape and length of the wings are characteristically adapted to species-specific flight and hunting patterns. Species that extensively use rising air currents for soaring, like most eagles and buzzards, have broad wings. Hawk eagles and most hawks are described as shortwings and display fast and very manoeuvrable flight modes. Falcons with high speed and long-distance flight patterns have comparatively long wings.

Leg

The leg is comprised of the femur, the tibiotarsus (fused tibial and proximal tarsal bones), remnants of the proximal fibula, the tarsometatarsus (fused middle and distal tarsal bones together with the fused metatarsal bones), the separate primary metatarsal bone and the digital bones (see Figure 5.5).

Depending on locomotion, stance and feeding habits, the digits display a specific alignment. With the so-called *anisodactyl* position in pigeons, passerines and raptors the first digit or *hallux* (displaying the biggest claw) faces caudally, while digits II, III and IV face cranially. The opposition of the first digit with regard to the remaining digits allows a firm grasp and perching position, even on thin branches. The Osprey, like owls, is able to move the fourth digit into a caudal, opposed position (i.e. *zygodactyl*), which enables a firm grasp on its slippery, wriggling prey as well as 'aerodynamic' prey transport during flight.

The length of the tarsometatarsus and the toe length are related to the typical hunting behaviour of respective raptor species. For example, members of the accipiter family (woodland birds preying on other birds) feature long toes that may easily slip under the plumage to grip their prey, and equally long and slender tarsometatarsi to thrust their feet deeply into thick brush where their prey is hiding. Other raptors with different hunting techniques (e.g. Peregrine Falcon) also feature long toes for gripping prey but have comparatively short tarsometatarsi. Thus lengths of toes and tarsometarsi are a means to distinguish different raptor species.

A typical passerine feature is the enlarged opposible and independently mobile hallux together with an evolutionary loss of most of the small muscles of the forward toes that together enable a balanced grip while displaying a marked simplicity and thus economy in digital structure.

Leg muscles

The main muscle mass of the leg is positioned close to the body and so many muscles have long insertion tendons. The locking mechanism between the flexor tendons and their sheaths maintains grip with a minimum of muscle activity when the toes are flexed. This flexor tendon mechanism is also engaged in tightening the grip of the toes of raptors in order to hold their prey securely. The digital pads of these species contain numerous mechanoreceptors that presumably trigger contraction of the flexor tendons after the first prey contact.

In some species (raptors; passerines such as woodcreepers), many leg tendons are converted into ossified bony rods. This conversion occurs almost exclusively in muscles that flex the leg and the toes. It is therefore suggested that these tendon ossifications are an adaptation to prevent stretching of the flexor tendons in those birds that feature heavy and prolonged loading during either (vertical) climbing (Bledsoe *et al.*, 1993) like woodcreepers, or catching and transport of heavy prey as in some raptors. In the latter, some antebrachial and tarsal ligaments and cartilaginous structures are likewise ossified, thus forming sesamoid bodies. (For a detailed description of the pelvic limb anatomy in raptors, see Harcourt-Brown, 2000; Einoder and Richardson, 2006.)

Body cavity

Birds do not have a diaphragm, and thus the thoracic and abdominal cavities merge.

The *pleural cavities* are created during early development, but due to the high dorsal position of the avian lungs the visceral aspect of the lungs and the parietal body wall fuse, so that the dorsal and lateral aspects of the lungs are directly connected to the body wall whereas the ventral aspect fuses with the so-called horizontal septum.

The *peritoneal cavity* is further subdivided into four separate hepatic cavities and the intestinal cavity (Figure 5.8). Structures that divide the originally unitary peritoneal cavity are the hepatic ligament and the dorsal mesentery. The intestinal peritoneal cavity contains the gastrointestinal tract from stomach to rectum, the gonads and the spleen. The kidneys and reproductive tract lie within the extraperitoneal space, whereas the gizzard is situated retroperitoneally. There is a *pericardial cavity* encircling the heart. In addition to these 'classic' serosal cavities are the *air sacs*, derived from bronchial projections. These air-filled cavities are connected to the respiratory system (see later).

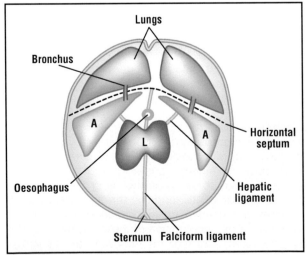

5.8 Schematic drawing of the body cavity. A = air sacs; L = liver.

Digestive system

The avian digestive system shows a great diversity according to different feeding and dietary habits. The morphological variations include gross anatomical differences such as form, size and length of the different regions of the digestive tract. In particular, a relation between length of intestines and type of food consumed is detectable (diet high in vegetable fibre: long intestines; protein-based diet: short intestines). The form of the stomach, especially the relation of proventriculus and gizzard, also seems to depend on feeding habits.

Thus, species living mainly on hard vegetable fibres such as seeds (e.g. pigeons and many passerine birds) have developed specifically adapted modifications of the oesophagus (crop, extensive mucus glands, etc.) and stomach (e.g. a well developed gizzard), have longer intestines and often, but not always, have distinct caeca for microbial digestion (Figure 5.9). Species living mainly on fruits, which have easily accessible nutrients, display less differentiated stomachs, shorter intestines and mostly rudimentary caeca. Raptors, living on meat- or fish-only diets, generally have a well developed proventriculus and only rudimentary gizzard but a well developed pancreas (for protein digestion), medium-length to short intestines and generally only rudimentary caeca.

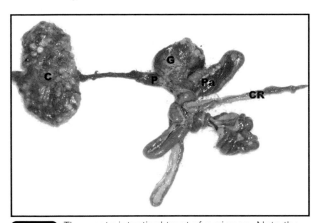

5.9 The gastrointestinal tract of a pigeon. Note the complex arrangement of the jejunoileum. C = crop; CR = colorectum; G = gizzard; P = proventriculus; Pa = pancreas within the duodenal loop.

The relation between caecal length, or caecal differentiation, and food preference is not always a direct one, as avian caeca also fulfil other functions than microbial digestion of vegetal fibres. Thus, at first glance surprisingly, the seed-eating pigeons and all passerines – even the distinct seed eaters among them – feature only comparatively small caeca. On the one hand, this may be compensated for by the otherwise very typical and thus very efficient characteristics of the 'seed-eater' gastrointestinal tract (well developed crop, distinct two-chambered stomach, long intestines). On the other hand, recent studies suggest that the small caeca of passerine birds may be non-functional in microbial fibre digestion but do play an important role in fluid and osmoregulation

due to their extensively enlarged mucosal surfaces (Reyes and Braun, 2005): this comparatively short caecum type is presumably involved in reabsorption of electrolytes and water from urine, which is transported in a retrograde direction from the cloaca to the colorectum and on to the caecum (see below). As the caeca are also important for absorption of proteins, it is not surprising that, for example, owls (regardless of their low-fibre diet) display comparatively well developed caeca.

Generally, passage of feed is very flexible and may be adapted to nutrient content and degree of intestinal filling. Thus, food may be soaked in proventricular gastric fluids and move in a retrograde direction to the crop, where the food is then pre-digested. Likewise, the direction of bowel movement may change from ortho- to retrograde (e.g. bypassing the caeca).

Oropharyngeal cavity

The oropharyngeal cavity has a wide opening towards the nasal cavity (palatopharyngeal choanae), the rostral part of which may be obstructed by the tongue during inspiration. The tongue has mainly extrinsic muscles and is specifically adapted (density of mucosal papillae, flexibility, etc.) to the species' feeding habits. The number of oral and adjacent salivary glands is likewise adapted to the diet; for example, fish eaters display less developed and fewer salivary glands than seed eaters.

Oesophagus and crop

The oesophagus is situated on the right side of the neck and may form a diverticulum, i.e. the crop or ingluvies (lacking in owls) (Figure 5.10). The mucosa (degree of cornification, formation of a papillary body, density of glands, distribution of muscular elements, etc.) varies, presumably according to the diet. For example, many raptors feature disseminated smooth muscle elements within the oesophagus and crop that may be related to regurgitation of pellets. These muscular elements are lacking in the Osprey, a species that very seldom forms pellets. The Peregrine

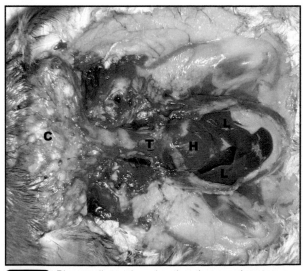

5.10 Pigeon dissection showing the prominent crop (C), the position of the heart (H) within the pericardium and the two liver lobes (L). T = trachea.

Falcon, a species that plucks and gorges on its prey and thus mainly feeds on comparatively lubricated meat chunks instead of whole fur- or feather-covered (and thus dry surfaced) prey, has no mucous glands within the cranial part of the oesophagus or within the crop. As raptors commonly have comparatively large salivary glands, the number and density of mucous glands within the oesophagus is generally reduced compared with passerine birds and pigeons.

The crop is dilatable and serves as storage space, either for transport or where the digestive tract is already full. As mentioned above, pre-digestion may occur within the crop due to saturation of food with gastric fluids after retrograde oesophageal movement. In pigeons, the involvement of cellulolytic crop microflora in the degradation of dietary fibre has been suggested (Shetty *et al.*, 1990).

Pigeons have a well developed bilateral crop situated cranial to the thoracic opening. Most passerine birds have a unilateral crop that may be situated at any location within the cervical part of the oesophagus but in most species lies to the right and close to the cranial thoracic aperture. Many raptors have a unilateral crop that is only distinct when filled and it may be situated either close to the cranial thoracic opening or further proximal within the cervical part of the oesophagus.

By storing food within the crop, pigeons may postpone a major part of digestion until late in the night and use the extra heat from digestion-related thermogenesis for heat that otherwise would have to be generated by active (and extra energy-consuming) thermoregulation via shivering.

Crop milk

The pigeon crop has another unique role. Under the influence of prolactin, desquamated epithelial cells of the crop are employed as a nestling food, described as 'crop milk', produced by both the male and the female parent. Chicks are fed on pure crop milk during the first week or so of life. Thereafter it is mixed with, and then replaced by, predigested adult food.

Stomach

The stomach is subdivided into a proventriculus (pars glandularis, producing hydrochloric acid and pepsinogens), an intermediate zone or gastric isthmus (mucous glands), the gizzard (pars muscularis) and the pyloric part (mucous glands, gastrohormonal cells). As noted above, the differentiation of proventriculus and gizzard depends on dietary habits.

- *Seed and foliage eaters* display a distinct division between the proventriculus and a well developed gizzard. The muscular tunic of the gizzard is highly developed in order to allow a grinding movement. The grinding surface of the gizzard is formed by the koilin layer, a hard keratin-like layer covering the mucosal surface, which is only so pronounced in birds with a high-fibre diet (see Chapter 9). The koilin is produced by a secretion from the gizzard tubular and surface glands that hardens in contact with hydrochloric acid from the proventriculus. The counterpart for the grinding of seeds is formed by uptake of small stones ('grit') that are pulverized over time and use.
- *Birds with a high-protein diet* (raptors, including carnivores, fish eaters and insectivores) have a rudimentary gizzard with thin muscular tunic and nearly no koilin layer.
- The stomach of *seasonal fruit eaters* (some passerine birds) has structural characteristics that fall between those of the seed eaters and the protein eaters.

Raptors, and some passerine birds such as crows, regurgitate casts or pellets (residuals of prey material) that are formed within the gizzard. In contrast to those of owls, raptor pellets contain almost no bony material.

Intestines

The length of the intestines and particularly the characteristics of the caeca are closely related to feed type. In general, the intestines are proportionately shorter than in mammals and are continuously villous. Distinctions of intestinal sections are defined according to their blood supply, the aperture of the bile in relation to pancreatic ducts and the location of the Meckel diverticulum (residuary of the omphalic sack).

The *duodenum* is U-shaped and receives the opening of the bile and pancreatic ducts localized within its ascending part. The *jejunoileum* allows digestion under the influence of bile and pancreatic enzymes and is thus the longest part of the intestines. It is longest in seed eaters (pigeons, passerine birds) and thus is arranged in varying folds and loops. Pigeons have a complex arrangement of the jejunoileum, with a turban-like coiled part and a shorter 'classical' supraduodenal loop. Most raptors have a double-coiled ileojejunal loop.

The matched *caeca* flank the ileum and are connected via the iliocaecal ligament. They are comparatively small in pigeons and passerines, and vestigial in most raptors (excepting owls), and may incorporate lymphatic tissue. The *colorectum* (Figure 5.11) is very short and runs straight towards the coprodeal part of the cloaca.

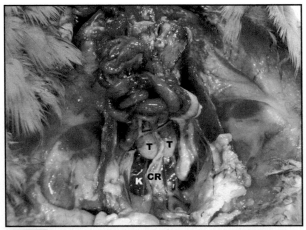

5.11 Pigeon dissection showing the loops of the small intestines tilted cranially, thus revealing the course of the colorectum (CR), and the position of the testes (T) and the caudal division of the kidneys (K).

Pancreas

The pancreas produces digestive enzymes (exocrine part: amylases, lipases, proteases) and metabolic hormones (endocrine part: insulin, glucagons, somatostatin). It features three lobes: the dorsal and ventral lobes are situated within the mesentery of the duodenal loop, while a small lienal (splenic) lobe runs from the cranial part of the pancreas towards the spleen. Each lobe has its own excretory duct opening into the ascending part of the duodenum. The splenic lobe contains most of the endocrine pancreatic tissue.

Liver

The liver is a bilobed parenchymal organ that lies adjacent to the sternum, ribcage, pericardium and lungs as well as the stomach and upper intestinal loops (see Figure 5.10). The liver is the main metabolic organ of the body and additionally produces the bile that enables digestive fat emulsion. Each liver lobe is drained by a bile duct that reaches the ascending duodenal loop. The right bile duct may dilate to form the *gall bladder* (lacking in pigeons and some passerine species but particularly well developed in most carnivorous and fish-eating raptors). The avian liver receives blood via two hepatic arteries and two portal veins.

Respiratory system

Upper respiratory tract

The upper respiratory tract (nares, nasal cavity, paranasal sinus) provides a 'strainer system' for the respiratory air intake. While the nares act as mechanical filters, the increased surface of the mucosa covering the nasal conchae and paranasal sinus acts as a micro-filter system that also warms and moistens the air.

Nares

The rather large osseous nasal openings are reduced in size via the often slit-like nares of the upper beak. Protective structures of the nostrils are setae (Turdidae, Muscicapidae, corvids), waxy membranes (raptors, Cinclidae) and cartilaginous opercula (pigeons). The nostrils of falcons contain a specific baffle that presumably regulates the amount of air entering the nasal cavity during high-speed flight (Figure 5.12). It has also been suggested that, in an as yet undetermined way, this cone or central tubercle extending from the nasal septum is used in olfaction, or as an indicator of air speed by sensing changes in pressure or temperature produced by different external airstream velocities.

Nasal cavity

Within the nasal cavity, generally three rostrocaudally arranged nasal *conchae* are developed: the rostral, the middle and the caudal conchae, but the latter is lacking in pigeons and many raptors. The rostral concha is generally covered by cutaneous mucosa, receives secretions of the nasal gland and therefore is responsible for filtering, warming and moistening the respiratory air. The middle concha has a

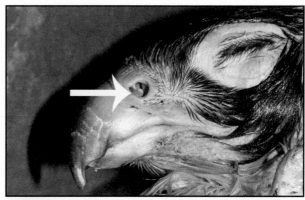

5.12 Head of a falcon. Note the prominent cone or tubercle (arrowed) within the nostrils that acts as a baffle during high-speed flight. The bill displays the species-specific shape, with the characteristic 'tomial tooth' of the upper beak. The proximal part of the upper bill forms the yellow waxy membrane of the ceres.

mucociliary epithelial covering as well as lymphatic tissue and is mostly responsible for defence. The caudal concha is covered by olfactory epithelium, which, in those species lacking this concha, is situated within the nasal fundus.

Paranasal sinus

The connection of nasal cavity and paranasal sinus is situated in the caudal aspect of the nose, mostly hidden by the caudal concha. The avian paranasal sinus is represented by the *infraorbital sinus*. It is defined by the maxillary and nasal bones (osseous part of the sinus) as well as by a membranous part under the eye globe within the orbita. Thus, the eyeball 'rests' on an air-filled cushion.

Lower respiratory tract

The air then passes through the wide *choanae* (palatopharyngeal opening) to the larynx. The avian *larynx* displays a less refined construction than that of mammals: while it can open and shut during deglutition, it is not employed in sound creation. It opens into the windpipe or trachea, which in turn is stabilized by complete cartilaginous rings (which may calcify). The trachea ends at the bifurcation, which is situated at the thoracic opening, quite a distance away from the dorsally situated lungs.

Syrinx

The structures of the bifurcation form the syrinx (Figure 5.13), a movable structure responsible for sound creation that is particularly well developed in passerine birds and pigeons. The skeletal elements of the syrinx comprise the caudal tracheal rings (*tracheal syringeal cartilages*) and the first cartilaginous elements of the two main bronchi (*bronchial syringeal cartilages*) as well as a middle cartilaginous 'partition wall', the *pessulus* (lacking in larks), between the openings of both bronchi.

The tracheal syringeal cartilages are modified to form the so-called *tympanum*. The space between the last tracheal and the first bronchial cartilage is spanned by a membrane-like connective-tissue structure, the *lateral tympaniform membrane*. Likewise, the space

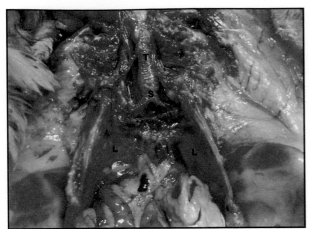

5.13 Pigeon dissection showing the syrinx. Note the trachea (T) and its bifurcation, and the dorsal position of the relatively small lungs (L). The specifically shaped tracheobronchial junction forms the syrinx (S).

between the pessulus and the respective first medial bronchial structure is spanned by a membrane, the *medial tympaniform membrane*. The tension of both membranes is regulated via intrinsic and extrinsic syringeal muscles. Thus, similar to the tension regulation of the laryngeal vocal folds in mammals, sound or voice may be modulated in the avian syrinx. In pigeons and passerines the tympanum may be specifically modified and display both complete and incomplete tracheal rings. The system of tracheo-syringeal muscles is most derived in oscine passerines while suboscines, and even more so pigeons, show a less complex vocal organ. While mockingbirds and Wood Thrushes, for example, have seven to nine pairs of syringeal muscles, pigeons have only one pair.

Bronchi, air sacs and lung

Behind the syrinx, the two principal or primary bronchi enter the left and right lungs, which are situated within the dorsal aspect of the ribcage and closely connected to the thoracic wall and the horizontal septum. The primary bronchi cross the lung and then open into the major air sac, i.e. the abdominal air sac (Figure 5.14). During lung passage, numerous secondary bronchi arise from the primary bronchi, giving rise to smaller and smaller airways (the *parabronchi* or tertiary bronchi) (Figure 5.15), all of which are variously interconnected but finally pass though the lung and again into major bronchi that then empty into the air sacs.

Besides the abdominal air sac, there are cervical, clavicular, cranial thoracic and caudal thoracic air sacs (Figure 5.14). Each air sac originally develops in a pair, but the cervical and clavicular air sacs fuse during early development and thus become unpaired in the mature stage. In passerine birds, the cranial thoracic sacs may even fuse with the clavicular sac. The cervical and clavicular air sacs enter the vertebrae, humerus (excepting oscine passerine birds), sternum (particularly in raptors) and other soft tissue structures situated in the neck and shoulder region (e.g. the axillary air sac diverticulum). The two paired thoracic and the two paired abdominal sacs are situated caudoventral to the lung and 'push' between the body wall and the peritoneal sacs.

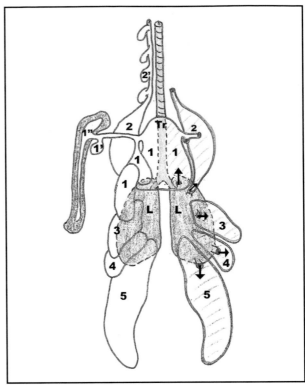

5.14 System of air sacs (modified after King and McLelland, 1984). The right side displays opening of the major bronchi supplying the respective air sacs. The colours indicate functional grouping into caudal (blue) and cranial (green) compartments. 1 = unpaired clavicular air sac with axillary diverticle (1') and the recess pneumatizing the humeral bone (1''); 2 = cervical air sac with vertebral recesses (2') pneumatizing the cervical vertebrae; 3 = cranial thoracic air sac; 4 = caudal thoracic air sac; 5 = abdominal air sac; L = lungs; Tr = trachea.

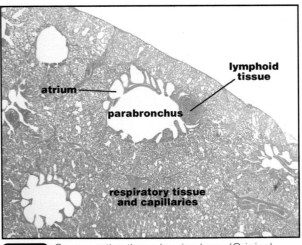

5.15 Cross-section through avian lung. (Original magnification × 25; H&E.)

Because the air sacs develop from bronchial processes and thus contain smooth muscle within their lateral walls (i.e. adjacent to the body wall), and due to their respective positions close to the thoracic and abdominal wall or wing, they act as bellows to pull air through the lungs. The respiratory movements of the body wall elevate and depress the sternum and also expand and contract the rib cage. These movements, or the neck and wing movement, respectively, expand

and contract the air-filled sacs and thus cause circulation of the respiratory air, while the volume of the lungs is not influenced. Although there is no diaphragm, the movements caused by contraction of the inspiratory thoracic muscles and the shoulder girdle increase the internal volume of the bird, drawing air into the air sacs during inspiration, while expiration is caused by contraction of the expiratory thoracic and the abdominal muscles. These active respiratory muscle movements may be impaired in sternal, ventral or (even more so) dorsal recumbency during anaesthesia.

The complex system of airways – from the bronchi connected to the abdominal and caudal thoracic air sacs back to the secondary bronchi within the lung, then on to the cranial thoracic, clavicular and cervical air sacs and back into the lung – allows a unidirectional path through the majority of the lung tissue for the majority of the respiratory air (Figure 5.16).

Gas-exchange tissue

Final gaseous exchange takes place in the smallest section of the airway, the *air capillary*. Originating from a central parabronchus, the air capillaries of one pulmonary lobule arise from numerous atria and form an anastomosing three-dimensional network through which the air passes and finally again reaches a parabronchus. Between the air capillaries, blood capillaries form a matching network, thus allowing for a close area of contact enabling gaseous exchange. The parabronchi contain cartilaginous shards and smooth muscle whereby airway size is controlled. Comparable to mammalian pulmonary alveoli, the air capillaries are covered by a phospholipid-containing surfactant. Because they are much smaller (3–10 μm, smallest in passerines) than their mammalian equivalent (35–50 μm), a greater oxygen diffusion gradient is encouraged and the risk for pulmonary oedema is decreased in the avian lung. Additionally, the blood–gas barrier is one-third thinner in birds than in mammals. As there are no blind-ending parts within the gas-exchanging tissue of the avian lung, there is no dead space (residual air volume) during the respiratory cycle and nearly all the air is involved in gaseous exchange. The avian lung also has a 20% greater volume of capillary blood per gram organ weight than the mammalian lung.

5.16 Movement of air through the lung of a bird. Inspiratory movements increase air sac volumes and expiratory movements decrease them. The volume and shape of the lung remains the same. Because of the arrangement of the parabronchi and the possible presence of an aerodynamic valve, the air is moved unidirectionally through the parabronchi and therefore through the area of gaseous exchange. (© Nigel Harcourt-Brown)

All the features of the avian respiratory system make gaseous exchange in birds far more effective than in mammals and allow 'full-blooded' flight under conditions (e.g. at great heights with low oxygen pressure) that would result in extreme hypoxia in mammals.

Urogenital system

Urinary tract

The kidneys (Figure 5.17) lie in the renal fossae formed by the synsacrum and the iliac bone and are thus well protected. Each kidney is divided into a cranial, middle and caudal division (or 'lobe') by blood vessels passing the kidneys (Figure 5.18). As in mammals, the kidneys are responsible for maintaining the water and salt content of the body and dispose of metabolic waste products via ultra-filtration of the blood. The organ has a distinct outer cortical and an inner medullar layer and is subdivided into lobules. Birds have no renal pelvis but instead display branches of the ureter.

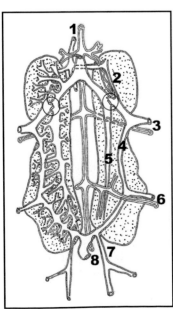

5.17 Pigeon dissection showing the position of the kidneys (K), the adjacent testes (T) and the ureter and the spermatic duct running towards the urodeum of the cloaca (C). L = lung

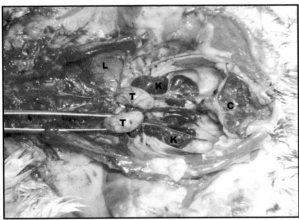

5.18 Schematic drawing displaying the vascular system of the kidney (modified after Baumel, 1993). The encircled areas show the localization of the renal valve that enables redirection of venous return. 1 = descending aorta and cranial vena cava; 2 = cranial portal vein; 3 = external iliac artery and vein; 4 = caudal portal vein; 5 = caudal renal vein; 6 = ischiadic artery and vein; 7 = internal iliac vein; 8 = median sacral artery and caudal mesenteric vein.

Nephrons

The nephron is the functional unit of the kidney. It consists of a capillary glomerulus (Figure 5.19) that forces the primary urine into the Bowman's capsule and on into the nephronal tubule system, where water and salts are exchanged according to a counter-current system with the concomitant peritubular capillary system of the kidney. Two different types of nephron can be found in the avian kidney: the 'avian' or medullar type (as described above) located within the medulla; and the 'reptilian' or cortical type located within the cortex and containing a less-developed glomerulus and no nephronal loop. The latter type is unable to concentrate salts in the tubular system.

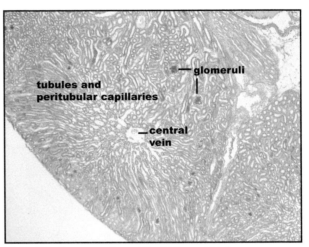

5.19 Cross-section of the kidney at high magnification, displaying one lobule. (Original magnification × 50; H&E.)

Uric acid

The end product of avian nitrogen metabolism is uric acid (rather than urea as in mammals). Uric acid is formed in the liver and excreted via both glomerular filtration and tubular secretion. Mixed with salts, uric acid forms spheres that in combination with mucus become a colloidal solution within the ureter, thus preventing the insoluble urates from precipitating within the body.

Renal portal system

The development of a renal portal system (see Figure 5.18) is another distinct feature of the avian kidney. Blood from an afferent venous system (i.e. the renal portal vein), as well as the blood of the efferent venous flow from the glomerulus, drains into the counterflow peritubular capillary plexus that surrounds the nephronal loop. Thus, the secretion efficiency of toxic metabolites via the tubular system is enhanced compared to mammals. Approximately two-thirds of the blood entering the kidneys is derived from the low-pressure venous system, whereas the high-pressure blood supply for glomerular filtration is achieved by input from the three renal arteries (cranial renal, external iliac, ischiadic). The renal portal vein collects blood from the external iliac, ischiadic, internal iliac and caudal mesenteric veins via a ring-like portal system. The venous blood thus collected from the hind leg and the caudal parts of the body and body cavity then drains via the portal vein into the peritubular capillary system, allowing excretion of urates from the caudal part of the body. A valve within the portal ring is able to shunt the venous blood either away from or through the whole kidney or only parts of the kidney. The smooth muscles within the shunt are innervated by adrenergic (relaxation) and cholinergic (contraction) nerve fibres, and it has been suggested that in times of exertion, such as during flight, the valve is open and blood from the hind limbs is directed to the central circulation (Burrows *et al.*, 1983). A clinical implication of this renal shunt system is that injection of drugs into the legs may therefore lead to toxic levels within the renal tissue, or even to direct excretion of the drug without achieving working dosages in other parts of the body (see Chapter 8).

Urine

The urine of birds is comparatively viscous, due to its high mucus content and the colloid dispersion of uric acid crystals. It flows through the ureter towards the urogenital division of the cloaca: the *urodeum*. Via retrograde peristaltic movement, the urine may then be transferred into the coprodeum and even into the colorectum and the caecum, where it may be stored until defecation and further concentrated due to water and salt reabsorption in the bowel (particularly in birds living in arid or semi-arid surroundings).

Genital tract

Male

In contrast to mammals, the avian male gonad remains at its site of origin, i.e. next to the adrenal gland and medial to the cranial division of the kidney (see Figure 5.17). The size of the *testes* may vary with sexual activity phases. Avian testes have no connective tissue capsule and are thus pliant and display a well developed superficial blood vessel system. Sperm, produced within the testicular seminiferous ducts, is moved via efferent ductuli to the caput epididymidis, which is situated medial to the gonad.

It is difficult to identify separately the *epididymis* and *ductus deferens* (as in mammals) of the spermatic duct, because the whole sperm-transporting convoluted duct then runs in one direction. Generally, the part situated immediately alongside the gonad is termed the epididymis and the remaining descending part is called the ductus deferens. The caudal part of the spermatic duct enlarges distally to form the *sperm receptacle* or *seminal glomerulus*. The latter is particularly well developed and convoluted in passerine species. The duct opens into the urodeum. The external projection caused by the seminal glomerulus during the nuptial phase is called the *cloacal promontory*, and enables male passerine birds to be sexed. Copulation and insemination are achieved via a *vestigial non-protruding phallus* when the cloacae of the male and female are pressed together in the mating process. After copulation, sperm are stored within mucosal folds of the female genital tract (see below).

Female

In most female birds, only the left side of the reproductive tract is fully and functionally developed. Rudiments of the right oviduct may occur in the form of fluid-containing cysts originating from the urodeum.

In certain falconiform birds the female may possess paired ovaries and reproductive tracts. Paired ovaries and genital tracts, whereby the right-side organs sometimes appear to be only vestigial, have been reported for the genera *Accipiter*, *Circus*, *Falco*, *Buteo* and *Aquila*. Paired ovaries may also occur in pigeons and some passerine birds but are considered less frequent and therefore 'abnormalities' in these species. The condition may lead to mis-sexing by mistaking paired ovaries for testes.

Ovary: The ovary is closely attached to the body wall via a short and heavily vascularized mesovary and (like the testis) lies next to the adrenal gland and medial to the cranial division of the ipsilateral kidney. It is also in close contact with the adjacent abdominal air sac.

Prior to and particularly during the mating season, the surface of the ovary is covered with many *follicles*. These are small in immature birds and are enlarged by incorporation of yolk material in adult mating birds. The follicle comprises a thin epithelial covering suspended on a stalk of blood vessels, nerves, smooth muscle and connective tissue fibres, and the large *oocyte* (egg cell) containing the characteristic yolk material. Because the follicle cover displays a thin non-vascularized 'equator' line (i.e. the *stigma*), it opens at this weak spot and releases the oocyte during ovulation. The oocyte is then 'grasped' by the capacious cranial opening (*infundibulum*) of the oviduct. Oocytes that have not been grasped by the infundibulum are generally reabsorbed.

The emptied follicle tissue, or *calyx*, regresses after ovulation and an avian *post-ovulatory follicle* develops rather than a corpus luteum. Vertebrate groups in which viviparity has not evolved (as with birds) generally exhibit a predominantly pre-ovulatory pattern of progesterone production (Callard *et al.*, 1992), while the post-ovulatory follicle is suggested to contain relaxin-like peptides (Brackett *et al.*, 1997). The regression of the avian post-ovulatory follicle is extremely rapid; for example, in pigeons all post-ovulatory follicles have disappeared at the beginning of the next laying cycle (e.g. after 25–30 days).

Oviduct: The oviduct is responsible for egg-cell impregnation as well as for the production of the numerous layers ensheathing the egg cell that collectively form the avian egg. The 'classical' morphological subdivision of the female genital tract into oviduct proper (tube), uterus and vagina is applied and defined by the particular egg layer produced in each division (Figure 5.20). The oviduct is suspended from dorsal and ventral ligaments that maintain the extensive oviduct vasculature, and its size depends on seasonal sexual activity. The avian oviduct has a highly regulated size–function relationship consistent with the high maintenance energy cost of this organ. Accordingly, the oviduct regresses during late

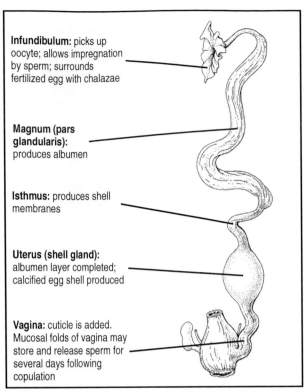

Infundibulum: picks up oocyte; allows impregnation by sperm; surrounds fertilized egg with chalazae

Magnum (pars glandularis): produces albumen

Isthmus: produces shell membranes

Uterus (shell gland): albumen layer completed; calcified egg shell produced

Vagina: cuticle is added. Mucosal folds of vagina may store and release sperm for several days following copulation

5.20 Schematic drawing of the female genital tract (modified after Nickel *et al.*, 1977).

oviposition 'from the top down' as soon as the more proximal regions have completed their function while the distal regions still retain an oviductal egg (Williams and Ames, 2004).

Cloaca

The cloaca is the terminal portion of both the urogenital tract and the alimentary tract, each of which forms a compartment of the cloaca: the urodeum and the coprodeum, respectively. The outermost compartment of the cloaca is the proctodeum, which, together with the dorsal and ventral vental labia, forms the vent, i.e. the opening for urogenital and alimentary tracts.

- The *coprodeum* is the cranial cloacal compartment and is generally not distinctly delineated from the rectum. Delineation from the adjacent urodeum is achieved by a distinct muscular fold that 'shields' the urodeum and proctodeum from faecal contamination in healthy birds: if the coprodeum is full of faeces, eversion of the copro-urodeal fold through the urodeum to the outside enables defecation. During egg-laying, the copro-urodeal fold is contracted and thus prevents contamination.
- The *urodeum* contains the openings of the genital tract and the urinary tract. While the ureter opens dorsally into the urodeum, the papilliform opening of either vagina or ductus deferens is situated ventrolaterally. Delineation from the last compartment of the cloaca is again achieved via a contractible uro-proctodeal fold.

- The *proctodeum* contains the dorsal access to the cloacal bursa (see 'Lymphatic system', below) and can contain a variety of tumescent mucosal structures, including the already mentioned vestigial non-prudent phallus. The dorsal and ventral vental labia may contain mucous glands, and form the outer opening.

Cardiovascular system

Birds have to be able to sustain sudden and prolonged high levels of muscular activity. Thus, the avian heart is relatively larger and beats faster (200–800 beats/min) than that of mammals of equal size. Birds have a high cardiac output combined with a higher arterial blood pressure (180/140 mmHg).

The four-chambered heart lies ventral to the lung and cranial to the liver (see Figure 5.10). It is surrounded by the pericardium, which is attached to the sternum via sternopericardiac ligaments and the hepatic peritoneal sacs. The right atrioventricular valve is a muscular flap on the free wall of the ventricle; all the other valves are similar to those of mammals.

The arteries and veins are broadly similar in distribution to those of mammals. Two venous anastomoses are distinct:

- A jugular anastomosis at the head–neck border allowing the blood in the left jugular vein to be shunted to the much larger right jugular vein
- An anastomosis between the femoral and ischiadic veins allowing the femoral vein to be the main venous return of the leg (Figure 5.21).

Birds have a right and a left cranial caval vein while the caudal caval vein reaches only up to the cranial renal divison. There is no azygous vein within the thorax. Passerine birds feature only the left carotid artery.

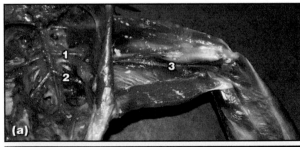

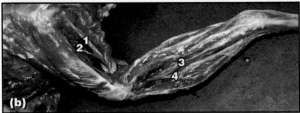

5.21 Dissected hindlimb of a falcon to show superficial and deep vascular structures, with associated nerves, on the medial aspect. **(a)** 1 = external iliac artery and vein; 2 = ischiadic artery and vein; 3 = medial femoral vein. **(b)** 1 = ischiadic artery and nerve; 2 = ischiadic vein; 3 = caudal tibial artery and lateral plantar nerve (tibialis nerve); 4 = cranial tibial artery and right profundus fibularis nerve. (continues) ▶

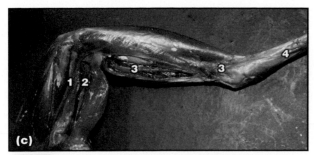

5.21 (continued) Dissected hindlimb of a falcon to show superficial and deep vascular structures, with associated nerves, on the medial aspect. **(c)** 1 = medial femoral vein; 2 = ischiadic vein; 3 = caudal tibial vein; 4 = superficial plantar metatarsal vein.

Details of renal circulation have been described above. At times of maximum energy demand, the blood can even bypass the kidney altogether.

Blood cells are illustrated in Chapter 9.

Lymphatic system

The central lymphatic organs of birds are the bone marrow and the thymus, and also the cloacal bursa (which is unique to birds). Peripheral lymphatic tissue can be found within the spleen and within the walls of the respiratory and gastrointestinal tracts (aggregated mucosal lymph nodules known as *organ 'tonsils'* are found within, for example, the caeca, stomach and lung). Macroscopic lymph nodes are generally not developed.

The *thymus* can be found along the length of the neck, lying directly beneath the skin, and may be lobated. It is the source of T-lymphocytes. The *cloacal bursa* is situated in the dorsal wall of the proctodeal division of the cloaca, from which it can be probed. It is the source of B-lymphocytes. Both the thymus and cloacal bursa undergo fatty involution with the onset of sexual maturity.

The *spleen* lies within the dorsal mesentery between the proventriculus and the gizzard. Apart from its lymphatic function, the spleen may also be responsible for recycling of aged erythrocytes, though this is mainly achieved in the liver in birds.

The lymphatic ducts drain into the caval veins. Within the trunk, they usually accompany the major arteries, whereas within limb and neck regions they follow the major veins.

Endocrine system

The *hypophyseal* and the *epiphyseal glands* are similar to those of mammals. They are responsible for controlling seasonal or diurnal cycles and affect subordinate hormone glands. Light is the most powerful stimulus and can affect the system via three different pathways in birds: the eyes, the pineal gland and the extra-retinal photoreceptors located in the brain, which in turn communicate via rhythmic synthesis and release of the hormone melatonin. The matched *thyroid glands* are situated close to the trachea at the level of the coracoid bones. The *parathyroids* and the

ultimobranchial body can be found in close proximity. The *adrenal glands* are medio-cranial to the cranial kidney division. Corticosteroid-producing (interrenal) cells (cortical in mammals) and adrenal cells (medullary in mammals) are intermixed in birds. For the pancreas, see 'Digestive system' and Figure 5.9 above; for the gonads, see 'Urogenital system' above.

Nervous system

The avian *central nervous system* is similar to that of mammals, although the brain is not as large as in mammals of comparable size.

While the cortical cortex is poorly developed, the optic lobe is huge, and the total cross-sectional area of the optic nerves is greater than that of the cervical spinal cord, as can be expected in macrophthalmic animals. The olfactory region, on the other hand, is generally poorly developed.

Passerine birds are characterized by their comparatively large brain size, advanced capacity for learning and overall behavioural plasticity and therefore display appropriate anatomical features of the nervous system. For example, oscine passerines (i.e. 'typical' songbirds) feature characteristic oestrogen receptor-bearing cell areas in the forebrain that are presumably related to the steroid-dependent differentiation of vocal control areas (Gahr *et al.*, 1993). Food-storing passerine species display an enlarged hippocampal complex, i.e. the area of the brain that enables a map-like representation of environmental landmarks used for navigation, as an adaptation associated with the use of a specialized memory capacity (Krebs *et al.*, 1989). Pigeons, particularly the homing pigeon, likewise feature specific function-related characteristics. Two conflicting hypotheses compete to explain how a homing pigeon can return to its loft over great distances (Mora *et al.*, 2004; Gagliardo *et al.*, 2006): one suggests the perception of atmospheric odours (via the olfactory branch of the trigeminal nerve) and the other the perception of the Earth's magnetic field (via superparamagnetic magnetite crystals within the afferent trigeminal nerve terminals of the upper beak and the ophthalmic branch of the trigeminal nerve) as mediators for homing.

Structural features of the avian spinal cord are comparable to those in mammals. Typical avian peculiarities are that the length of the spinal cord equals that of the vertebral column (i.e. there is no cauda equina) and that there are marginal nuclei within the peripheral white matter that are likely to be ventral commissural neurons projecting information across the cord. The so-called glycogen body within the lumbosacral cord is thought to regulate vascular reflexes and to secrete neuropeptides.

Both brain and spinal cord are ensheathed in the *meninges*. The epidural space is filled with a gelatinous rather than a liquid substance.

Special characteristics of the avian lumbosacral spinal cord (i.e. enlargement around the large glycogen body and a system of lumbosacral meningeal canals that look like and may function in a similar manner to the semicircular canals in the inner ear) have recently been interpreted as a sense organ for equilibrium that matures rapidly after hatching in semi-precocial birds such as the pigeon and is assumed to play a role in the control of locomotion on the ground (Necker, 2005).

Cervicothoracic and lumbosacral swellings of the cord represent the origins of the *brachial* and *lumbosacral plexus* for the spinal nerves supplying wing and leg. Nerves from the lumbosacral plexus run between the kidneys and the pelvis before reaching the leg.

The *autonomic nervous system* is comparable to that of mammals. A typical avian characteristic is the structure of the cervical part of the sympathetic nerve system: the vertebral nerve (running along the cervical vertebral column) that carries sympathetic nerve fibres to the neck region contains numerous segmental cervical ganglia in birds and thus forms a 'neck division' of the sympathetic trunk.

Senses

Vision is a bird's most important sense and only the eye is discussed here in detail.

The eye and vision

In most birds, the weight of the eye exceeds or at least equals that of the brain.

The structure of the avian eye (Figure 5.22) is adapted to the bird's need for three-dimensional orientation during flight and to behavioural peculiarities. The eye has small rostral chambers (the *anterior* and the *posterior chamber* in anatomical terms) and the *cornea* is thinner than in mammals. The caudal portion of the eye (the vitreous chamber, containing the *vitreous body*) is much larger and is species-specifically shaped.

- Slender-headed day-active birds (e.g. pigeons) have a discus-like flat posterior chamber, with a resulting short eye axis.
- Day-active bird species with broader heads (e.g. day-active raptors; many passerine birds, such

as sparrows) have a conically shaped posterior chamber, allowing the retina to have all-round visual acuity (rather than a single region of acute vision as in mammals).
- Night-active raptors, such as owls, have a tube-like posterior chamber with a distinctly concave middle region.

In all bird species, the optical axis of both cornea and lens converge towards the middle of the eye, in order to support binocular vision.

The bulb of the eye and its internal muscles are stabilized by osseous *scleral platelets* that adhere to the cornea. The *ciliary body* suspends the lens and contains two striated muscles. Thus, birds have conscious control over the iris.

The *lens* is softer than in mammals, enabling quick accommodation, and it is also transparent to ultraviolet light. The lens accommodation is controlled by a sclerocorneal muscle that forces the ciliary body against the lens, increasing the curvature of the lens. The shape of the lens is related to behaviour of the species. The insertion area of the ciliary body is shaped as an annular pad that is particularly well developed in day-active raptors, such as hawks, and reduced in night-active species. The anterior face of the bi-concave lens is much flatter in day-active birds compared with night-active species.

The avian *retina* is comparatively thick and avascular. Density and distribution of cones and rods is again related to habit: day-active birds display more cones than rods, and *vice versa* in night-active species. Each cone has its own ganglion and the brain receives a one-to-one signal, thus enabling excellent visual acuity. In contrast, several rods are synapsed to a single ganglion, allowing even small amounts of light to trigger an impulse and thus enhancing night vision. The retinal area with the greatest density of rods (area centralis) represents the centre of maximum optical resolution. It may contain a slight concavity, the fovea centralis. The structure of this *central fovea* is characteristic in different bird species.

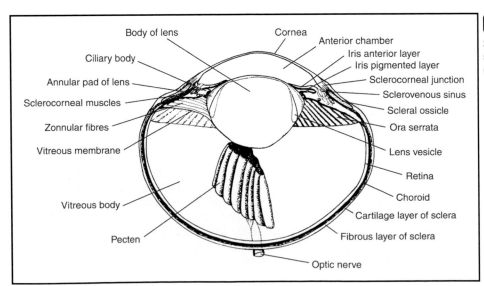

5.22 Schematic drawing of the structures of the eye. (© Nigel Harcourt-Brown)

Body of lens
Cornea
Anterior chamber
Iris anterior layer
Iris pigmented layer
Ciliary body
Sclerocorneal junction
Annular pad of lens
Sclerovenous sinus
Sclerocorneal muscles
Scleral ossicle
Zonnular fibres
Ora serrata
Vitreous membrane
Lens vesicle
Retina
Choroid
Vitreous body
Cartilage layer of sclera
Pecten
Fibrous layer of sclera
Optic nerve

- Seed-eating birds possess a single, round central fovea near the optical axis of the eye. This presumably allows the bird to concentrate firmly on an object and its position.
- Bird species living in spacious surroundings possess a horizontal area centralis with a single fovea. Presumably this allows for using the position of the horizon as an optical reference point.
- Day-active raptors possess a pair of central foveae: one close to the optical axis, the other on the temporal aspect of the eye. This allows precise assessment of distance (environmental landmarks) and relative velocity of moving objects (prey) during flight. The temporal fovea is sited in such a way that the image is projected to both the left and the right eye. Thus, these species presumably have stereoscopic binocular vision.

The eyes of diurnal birds of prey possess more sensory cells in the upper hemisphere (which perceives images from the ground) than in the lower hemisphere (which perceives images from the sky). Thus these birds tend to invert their heads either near the belly or over the back when they want a better overhead view (Brown, 1997).

The *pecten oculi* is a thin pleated structure within the vitreous chamber that is associated with the optic disc and the optic nerve. The pecten is a densely vascularized and heavily pigmented structure with many melanocytes. It may function as an intraocular 'shade' against glistening sunlight and is probably involved in supplying nutrients and oxygen to the relatively avascular posterior segment of the eye.

The cornea is protected by the upper and lower *eyelids* (which may have setae) as well as a predominantly transparent (particularly in day-active birds) nictitating membrane (i.e. the third eyelid). Eyelid movement, achieved by palpebral muscles, spreads the secretion of the lacrimal gland of the third eyelid; it is then drained by the tear duct originating at the nasal angle of the eye. By way of eye protection, many raptors close the nictitating membrane prior to striking their prey. Falcons use their third eyelid as an ocular protective layer during stoop flight, comparable to the osprey closing the third eyelid under water. Pigeons employ all three eyelids to blink.

References and further reading

Baumel JJ (1993) *Handbook of Avian Anatomy: Nomina Anatomica Avium. 2nd edn.* Nuttall Ornithological Club, Harvard University, Massachusetts

Bledsoe AH, Raikow RJ and Glasgow AG (1993) Evolution and functional significance of tendon ossification in woodcreepers. *Journal of Morphology* **215**, 289–300

Brackett KH, Fields PA, Dubois W *et al.* (1997) Relaxin: an ovarian hormone in an avian species (*Gallus domesticus*). *General and Comparative Endocrinology* **105**, 155–163

Bragulla H, Hirschberg RM and Heidbrink S (2003) Vergleichende funktionelle Anatomie des Verdauungstraktes verschiedener Greifvögel in Bezug zum Nahrungsspektrum (Comparative functional anatomy of the gastrointestinal tract in different raptors with regard to dietary habits). In: *Zoonosen. Bericht des 25. Kongresses der Deutschen Veterinärmedizinischen Gesellschaft e. V., Berlin (Proceedings of the 25th Congress of the German Veterinary Association).* DVG-Verlag, Gießen, pp. 142–150

Brown L (1997) *Birds of Prey.* Chancellor Press, London

Burkhard S (1992) Vorkommen und Ausbildung der Fingerkrallen bei rezenten Vögeln (Occurrence and expression of claws on fingers of recent birds). *Journal of Ornithology* **133**, 251–277

Burrows ME, Braun EJ and Duckles SP (1983) Avian renal portal valve: a re-examination of its innervation. *American Journal of Physiology: Heart and Circulation Physiology* **245**, H628–H634

Callard IP, Fileti LA, Perez LE *et al.* (1992) Role of the corpus luteum and progesterone in the evolution of vertebrate viviparity. *American Zoologist* **32**, 264–275

Einoder L and Richardson A (2006) An ecomorphological study of the raptorial digital tendon locking mechanism. *Ibis* **148**, 515–525

Gagliardo A, Iaolae P, Savini M and Wild JM (2006) Having the nerve to home: trigeminal magnetoreceptor versus olfactory mediation of homing in pigeons. *Journal of Experimental Biology* **209**, 2888–2892

Gahr M, Guttinger HR and Kroodsma DE (1993) Estrogen receptors in the avian brain: survey reveals general distribution and forebrain areas unique to songbirds. *Journal of Comparative Neurology* **327**, 112–122

Harcourt-Brown N (2002) Avian anatomy and physiology. In: *BSAVA Manual of Exotic Pets 4th edn,* ed. A Meredith and S Redrobe. BSAVA, Gloucester

Harcourt-Brown N (2000) *Birds of Prey: Anatomy, Radiology and Clinical Conditions of the Pelvic Limb.* Zoological Education Network, Florida

Hirschberg, RM, Bragulla H and Heidbrink S (2001) Comparative morphology of the gastrointestinal tract of raptor birds. *Journal of Morphology* **248**, 209

Hodges RD (1974) *The Histology of the Fowl.* Academic Press, London

Homberger DG and de Silva KN (2003) The role of mechanical forces on the patterning of the avian feather-bearing skin: a biomechanical analysis of the integumentary musculature in birds. *Journal of Experimental Zoology B: Molecular Development and Evolution* **298**, 123–139

King AS and McLelland J (1984) *Birds: Their Structure and Function, 2nd edn.* Baillière Tindall, London

Kinsky FC (1971) The consistent presence of paired ovaries in the Kiwi (Apteryx) with some discussion of this condition in other birds. *Journal of Ornithology* **112**, 334–357

Krebs JR, Sherry DF, Healy SD, Perry VH and Vaccarino AL (1989) Hippocampal specialization of food-storing birds. *Proceedings of the National Academy of Sciences USA* **86**, 1388–1392

Laurila M, Hohtola W, Saarela S and Rashotte ME (2003) Adaptive timing of digestion and digestion-related thermogenesis in the pigeon. *Physiology and Behaviour* **78**, 441–448

McLelland J (1990) *A Colour Atlas of Avian Anatomy.* Wolfe Publishing, Aylesbury

Mora CV, Davison M, Wild JM and Walker MM (2004) Magnetoreception and its trigeminal mediation in the homing pigeon. *Nature* **432**, 508–511

Necker R (2005) The structure and development of avian lumbosacral specializations of the vertebral canal and the spinal cord with special reference to a possible function as a sense organ of equilibrium. *Anatomy and Embryology* **210**, 59–74

Nickel R, Schummer A and Seiferle S (1977) *Anatomy of the Domestic Birds.* Verlag Paul Parey, Berlin

Quinn TH and Baumel JJ (1990) The digital tendon locking mechanism of the avian foot (Aves). *Zoomorphology* **109**, 281–293

Raikow RJ and Blesoe AH (2000) Phylogeny and evolution of the passerine birds. *BioScience* **50**, 487–499

Rashotte ME, Saarela S, Henderson RP and Hohtola E (1999) Shivering and digestion-related thermogenesis in pigeons during dark phase. *American Journal of Physiology* **277**, R1579–R1587

Reyes L and Braun EJ (2005) The functional morphology of the English sparrow cecum. *Comparative Biochemistry and Physiology A: Molecular Integrated Physiology* **141**, 292–297

Shetty S, Sridhar KR, Shenoy KB and Hegde SN (1990) Observations on bacteria associated with pigeon crop. *Folia Microbiologica (Praha)* **35**, 240–244

White CM (1969) Functional gonads in peregrines. *The Wilson Bulletin* **81**, 339–340

Whittow GC (2000) *Sturkie's Avian Physiology, 5th edn.* Academic Press, San Diego

Williams TD and Ames CE (2004) Top-down regression of the avian oviduct during late oviposition in a small passerine bird. *Journal of Experimental Biology* **207**, 263–268

6

Handling and transport

Aidan Raftery

Capture

Basic equipment for capturing and handling birds includes:

- *Towels*: paper or cloth
  - Paper best (disposable) but only useful for small birds
  - Towels need to be washed and autoclaved between uses
- *Gloves*: avoid if possible (with exception of raptors, where only one glove is needed) as they reduce dexterity; more likely to result in injury to patient and handler
- *Hoods*: if used, should be provided by the falconer (difficult to sterilize)
- *Nets*:
  - Need to be of appropriate size and mesh diameter for each patient
  - Must be easy to sterilize
  - Should have padded rim, flexible on at least one side.

Good organization is essential: prolonged attempts to capture a bird will cause additional stress (this is especially crucial for smaller and more critically ill birds, which more easily go into shock); and incorrect or clumsy attempts at restraint will put both bird and handler at risk of injury.

Capture therefore needs to be planned in advance and executed smoothly, with a calm approach that generates the minimum of stress. Ideally the bird should not realize the handler's intentions until it is in their grasp.

- If the bird is to be captured from a cage in a consulting room, all windows and doors need to be closed securely in case the bird escapes into the room.
- Similarly there should be no possibility of escape from an aviary during capture attempts. Double-door systems with doors opening inwards are strongly recommended; otherwise there is a high risk of escape when entering or leaving the aviary. Hanging cloth or plastic strips at the entrance is not an effective alternative to double doors.
- A suitable transport cage should be ready for the bird after it has been captured.

Capturing raptors

Raptors are often kept in aviaries. Hunting falconry birds are usually kept on a perch or block (see Chapter 2). Trained birds are easily captured by their handler. The recommended capture method is the least traumatic possible for the bird in its situation.

Perches and blocks

To facilitate capture, falcons are often hooded first. Birds kept on a perch or block can be asked to step on to a gloved hand by grasping the leash or jesses and placing the gloved hand either in front of or behind the bird. Once on the glove the bird can be cast with a towel by an assistant.

Aviaries

A trained raptor loose in an aviary may step on to a gloved hand, or sometimes the feet can be grasped and then the bird is secured in a towel.

Towels: Capture may sometimes be achieved by simply throwing a towel over and then wrapping the bird with it. All raptors (including owls, but not vultures) may flip on their backs to defend themselves, in which case:

1. Using one hand, dangle a towel towards the bird's legs.
2. The bird will grasp the towel and can be lifted into the air.
3. With the other hand (which needs to be gloved) grab the bird's feet, turn it around and secure its wings.

Nets: If a capture net is necessary (and this should be only as a last resort), the approach should be calm. The lighting should be reduced for diurnal species; conversely, increased lighting may help in capturing nocturnal species. The net must be deep enough to contain the bird if it is used to push the raptor to the ground; or, if being used for trapping, it needs to be deep enough to be flipped 180 degrees to close the net. The mesh should be of a size that avoids the bird's limbs or digits becoming entwined. Once in the net, the bird is immediately secured by placing a towel round its body to prevent it from flapping its wings and injuring itself or breaking feathers.

Capturing pigeons

Exotic pigeon and dove species kept in aviculture are usually calm birds that readily become tame, but some aviary species will panic and shed feathers, especially if capture attempts are prolonged. Similar principles as described below for passerine birds apply. Free-flying exhibition varieties and racing pigeons are usually easily caught by their keeper when in the loft.

Capturing passerine birds

Passerine birds are usually kept in either an aviary or a cage.

Aviaries

Catching birds in an aviary can be very difficult. If possible, the lighting should be reduced and then the bird should be calmly driven away from its co-inhabitants into a separate area or ideally into a trap. The capture needs to be quick and smooth.

- *Capture traps*, built into the aviary, are areas into which the birds can be corralled and which can then be closed off from the main body of the aviary. Sometimes they can then be detached and function as a transport cage.
- *Towels* are often used as visual barriers to enable corralling or capture.
- *Hand nets* (Figure 6.1) may also be used. The net should be small (rim 15 cm in diameter for finches) and its mesh, ideally nylon, must be the correct size for the species, both to prevent escape and to prevent limbs becoming entangled. Risk of injury in small birds is reduced if the rim is padded and flexible. The net must be deep enough to contain the bird and able to be flipped through 180 degrees to 'bag' it.
- *Mist nets* may be needed in large heavily planted aviaries if there is no built-in capture trap. Mist netting is much more stressful to the birds, which can be critical for those already in poor health.

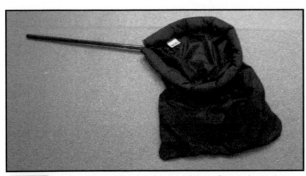

6.1 A good quality bird net, with soft mesh and a padded rim. (© John Chitty)

Cages

The lighting should be reduced and most of the cage furniture should be removed. Capture is best achieved with the aid of a disposable paper towel, or for larger birds a cotton towel. With very small birds, however, the towel may impede safe restraint. For most passerine species the use of gloves is unnecessary and is more likely to injure the bird.

Transport

Transport methods depend on the species, the bird's size and its training. In general it is best to assume that travelling is a stressful experience and attempts should be made to reduce the stress as much as possible. This will have the greatest effect on the smallest species, especially if they are ill.

The journey should be planned so that the bird's time spent in an unfamiliar container and in travelling is minimized. Thus the bird should be transported as soon as it is placed in the container and arrangements should be made to ensure that facilities at the end of the journey (be that a new enclosure or provision of veterinary care) are ready for the bird as soon as it arrives.

It is best to transport diurnal species at night, and nocturnal species during the day, when they will be inactive. Travelling at night in the summer months may also result in a more favourable ambient temperature. Large fluctuations in temperature during transport should be avoided and the container should be kept darkened and protected from direct sunlight, and should be well ventilated. Precautions should be taken to ensure that the bird is not breathing in engine fumes or other noxious gases during the journey and that it is protected from any startling loud noises.

All containers need to be secure. If a container is to be reused for other birds, the best material is plastic as it is impervious to water and is easily cleaned, disinfected and dried. Cleaning is very important: faeces and food contamination can act as fomites as well as supporting fungal growth to produce fungal spores and other dust that may be inhaled.

Transport of raptors

Raptors should always travel individually, in closed darkened boxes with plenty of ventilation (Figure 6.2). The box should be constructed of plastic or some other material impervious to water. Traditional wooden boxes can get damp and go mouldy, which results in spore formation as the box dries out, leaving the next bird at risk of inhaling fungal spores.

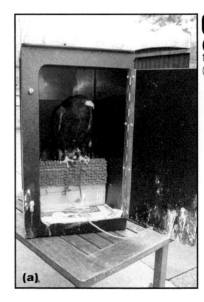

6.2

(a) Harris' Hawk in a travelling box. (continues) ▶

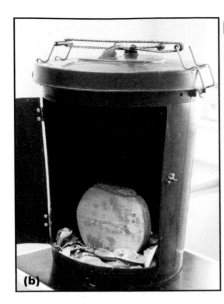

6.2
(continued)
(b) Raptor transport boxes can be fashioned out of anything. The important issues are that they are easily cleaned and disinfected, have a perch, are secure and dark, and the tether can be secured on the outside.
(b, © John Chitty)

Container design

- The bird should not be touching the top or sides of the box and it is important to ensure that there is no risk of damage to feathers, especially wing tips and tails, from contact with the floor or sides.
- A *tail guard* is recommended to protect the tail feathers. This can be made from X-ray film or cardboard and fixed to the tail with tape that comes off easily without damaging the feathers (Figure 6.3). Alternatively a rubber band can be used to keep the tail feathers together so that they protect and support each other.
- A *perch* is usually provided for trained birds, but untrained and wild birds travel best without a perch as they will sometimes lie down. Where a perch is provided it must be of a suitable size and provide an adequate grip.
- The *floor* should be of a non-slip material, preferably with a soft surface (e.g. carpet, which gives a good grip and can be removed for cleaning).
- If possible the *walls* should be also be lined with removable carpet or other padding.

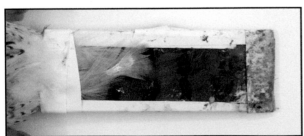

6.3 Tail guards may be fitted to travelling raptors to prevent damage to the deck feathers.
(© Michael Lierz)

Management for transport

- Spraying with water before transport will calm some nervous birds.
- For the transport of healthy raptors for less than 36 hours, food and water are not required (with the exception of areas where ambient temperatures are above 25°C, when water should be provided during the journey).
- In most cases, birds that are fitted with jesses will have the leash attached to make it easier to capture them. However, hooded falcons are often transported without a leash to avoid trapping themselves.
- Trained falconry birds are often transported hooded and simply perched in a car on a cadge (Figure 6.4).

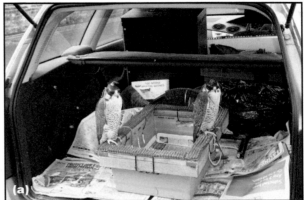

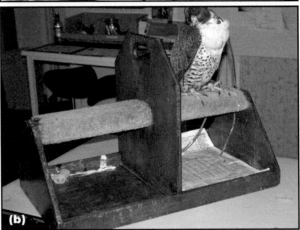

6.4 **(a)** Use of a cadge to transport hooded falcons. The leash length and spacing between the birds should be such that, if the hood comes off one of the birds, it will not be able to reach and attack other birds. **(b)** Smaller carrying cadge. Hooding is an effective means of calming travelling raptors. (b, © John Chitty)

Transport of pigeons

Most show and racing pigeons are relatively calm birds and there are fewer problems in transporting them. Specialized transport containers are available commercially (Figure 6.5). Alternatively, for short journeys and following the principles set out above, many containers (e.g. disposable cardboard boxes) can be utilized as improvised transport boxes. In summary the container needs to be secure, darkened, well ventilated, with enough room to stand up and something to grip on the floor (perches are not provided in pigeon transport boxes). There should not be enough room to flap wings as this makes injury, especially feather damage, more likely.

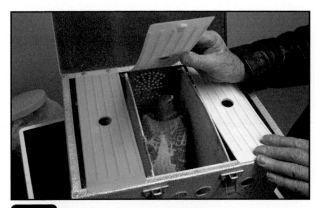

6.5 Pigeon in travelling box. (© John Chitty)

Transport of passerine birds

Passerine birds are usually transported either in small cardboard boxes or in specially designed transport cages (Figure 6.6).

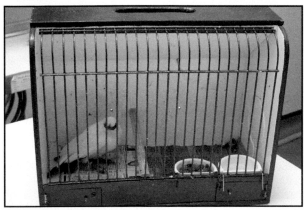

6.6 Bali Starling brought to the clinic in a travelling/ show cage. (© John Chitty)

- *Cardboard boxes* are satisfactory if the journey is to be a short one, but species with sharp strong beaks will need the security of a transport cage even for short journeys.
- *Transport cages* for passerine birds usually contain a small perch and the opening is often very small, designed so that a normal-sized hand can fit in without leaving any big gaps for the bird to escape through during the capture. This is problematic for those with big hands or when a towel is used for the capture.

Container design

- Provision of perches will make birds more comfortable and will keep the tail feathers from being soiled and damaged.
- There should not be enough space to allow flight within the container, as this would greatly increase the chances of injury during transport.
- For highly strung species, the top of the container should be padded.

Management for transport

- The inside of the container should be as dark as possible but with enough light so that the birds

can find food or water if they are being transported during the day.
- Food can be scattered on the floor and water is best provided as pieces of fruit or as moist sponges.
- It can often be less stressful if breeding pairs are transported together.
- Small birds of the same species can be transported in groups, but only compatible birds that will not fight should travel together. Each bird should have enough space to be able to assume normal posture and to groom itself unimpeded by other birds.

Handling

It is essential that the veterinary team is proficient in handling the species that are being accepted as patients. Familiarity and proficiency with handling techniques will reduce stress for the patient and reduce the risk of injury to both bird and veterinary staff. Skilled handling will instil the owner with confidence in the veterinary clinician, resulting in a mutually beneficial client–clinician relationship. Additionally, good handling skills are essential if a good clinical examination is to be completed.

Handling raptors

In all raptors and owls the feet are dangerous; vultures (Figure 6.7), eagles, owls and falcons will also bite. In general it is safest to regard both bill and feet as dangerous and properly restrain both.

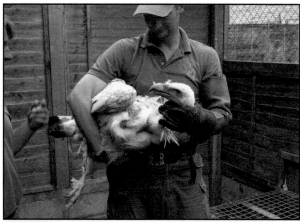

6.7 Restraint of a large vulture requires control of the head primarily, as these species can inflict a nasty bite. The handler is wearing an eagle sleeve in addition to a glove. In *Gyps* species, as here, the feet are not a significant threat, but in some (e.g. *Torgos* spp.) the feet are dangerous too and therefore at least two handlers are always needed. (© John Chitty)

Trained raptors will usually be presented to the veterinary surgeon on the glove, with the falconer holding the leash short, i.e. 'on the fist'. From this position the bird can be cast using a towel (Figure 6.8). The bird is approached from behind and grasped with a towel large enough to control the wings adequately. Effective restraint of the wings is especially important to prevent damage to them, which in a falconry bird may end its usefulness to its owner.

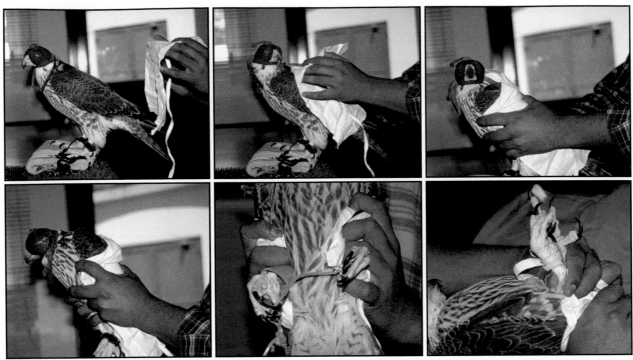

6.8 Casting a hooded falcon. The bird is approached from behind with a towel which is placed around the body restraining the wings. The feet are controlled simultaneously between the small and ring fingers. The bird is then positioned to facilitate examination. (© Michael Lierz)

The bird is held with its back towards the handler's chest. The feet should be also held, either one in each hand or, preferably, both feet in one hand with a finger between the legs. Those with small hands may find it difficult to restrain larger birds safely.

It is possible to restrain smaller species by holding wing and tail feathers and feet in one hand, with the second hand securing the head and neck. However, raptors in this situation will often damage their own tail feathers by grasping them. Some falconers will be unhappy with this restraint method and it should be avoided.

Hooded birds are much easier to restrain. The hood will only be removed to allow clinical examination of the head.

Risks to the handler
- *Hawks* and *falcons* may inflict wounds with both their beaks and talons.
- *Vultures* (which also have dangerous beaks) may regurgitate foul-smelling stomach contents. The regurgitation is a stress response, often before handling, and is not desirable. Therefore ideally handling should be planned around feeding times.
- *Pigeons* may defecate during handling.
- *Passerine birds* may stab or bite with the beak. Ability to cause injury depends on beak type and size.

Removal from container
Aviary raptors are often presented in a transport box with a side door. They should be restrained with a towel as described above. A cardboard box opening at the top is the most common improvised transport container. In this case the room lighting should be turned down (except in the case of owls) and the bird is captured from the box by placing a large towel over the opening and collapsing it on to the bird (Figure 6.9). The feet and wings can then be controlled through the towel. Gaining control of the feet is very important before attempting to lift out the bird. Sometimes a gloved assistant may be needed to reach beneath the towel to capture the feet so that the bird can be safely lifted from the container, with the primary handler controlling the wings. Alternatively, with a large bird, the primary handler grasps a leg in each hand and the assistant holds the bird's head.

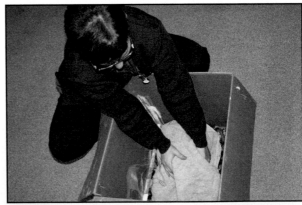

6.9 Using a towel to capture a Red-tailed Hawk from an improvised transporter (a cardboard box).

Occasionally a bird will lie on its back and defend itself with its feet, making capture and restraint more difficult. In this case the feet should be grabbed with a gloved hand and then the bird is supported upright whilst an assistant uses a towel to cast it, simultaneously controlling and protecting the wings.

Releasing a raptor's grip

If a handler is impaled by the talons of a raptor, the bird should be released. (This is one of those occasions that proves the importance of proper preparation and securing of windows and doors before attempting capture, so that the bird cannot escape from the room.) If the bird struggles, its grasp will tighten and an assistant will be needed to release the grip. The first task is to straighten the bird's leg to relax the tendon-tightening mechanism. Forcible disengagement from the grip of a large raptor such as a Golden Eagle is extremely difficult.

Handling pigeons

Pigeons are submissive and do not peck or scratch. They can be held in a similar fashion as recommended below for passerine birds, with the head projecting between the thumb and the index finger, with or without the use of a towel. More commonly these birds are held with the legs extended backwards between the middle and index fingers, with the thumb controlling the tail feathers and the wing tips (Figure 6.10). The other hand should be cupped to support the front of the body. Racing pigeons are used to being handled and their owners often prefer to catch and restrain the bird themselves. If necessary they are often capable of holding the bird for clinical examination.

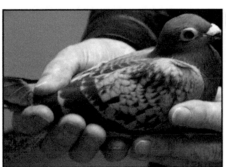

6.10

Restraint of a racing pigeon. (© John Chitty)

Handling passerine birds

Passerine birds vary in size but the most commonly presented species weigh less than 50 g. The most common holding technique is to control the head by having it projecting between the thumb and the index finger. The bird's back lies against the palm of the hand, with the remaining fingers controlling one wing and the other wing controlled by folding in the base of the thumb (Figure 6.11a). The other hand is used to control the legs which, being longer and thinner, are much more prone to iatrogenic damage than psittacine legs. The two feet should not be held against one another but kept separate, to avoid trauma caused by rubbing together if the bird struggles (Figure 6.11b).

An alternative holding method is to have the head projecting between the index and middle fingers, which leaves the thumb free to control one wing and the remaining fingers to control the opposite wing (Figure 6.11c).

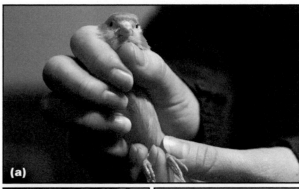

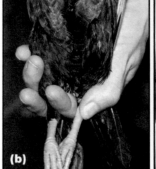

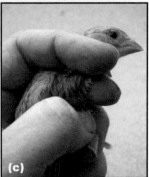

6.11 **(a)** Canary held using the most common grip. **(b)** The correct method of securing the feet, with a finger separating the legs. **(c)** The 'ringer's grip', demonstrated on a Greenfinch. (c, © John Chitty)

Use of a small towel (preferably a disposable paper towel) will help to control the wings and for the tame bird is less likely to make it fearful of the handler's hands. Positioning of fingers is similar whether a towel is used or not. Larger birds will be more easily caught and held with a towel (Figure 6.12).

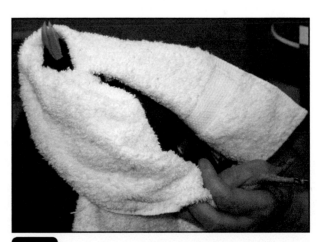

6.12 Restraining a Greater Hill Mynah using a towel.

Most birds will not struggle if held firmly but gently, but they should not be held across the sternum (if movement of the sternum is restricted the bird will be prevented from breathing). These methods of restraint facilitate a good clinical examination, with most areas that need to be examined being accessible.

7

Examination, triage and hospitalization

Romain Pizzi

Accepting an avian case

Signs that may not be an emergency when described in a dog or cat could well be so in an avian patient. Simple written guidelines are the best means of ensuring that urgent cases are correctly prioritized, especially in large practices with several reception staff. Attempts should always be made in avian cases, with the possible exception of chronic or ongoing problems, to see birds within 24 hours. As a guideline for receptionists, birds with signs listed in Figure 7.1 should be seen as soon as possible.

- Any change in breathing pattern
- Noisy breathing, 'whistling' sounds when breathing, change in voice
- Unsteady on feet or collapse
- Nervous signs, twitching, or seizures
- Acute injuries, or bleeding
- Depression, appearing fluffed-up, change in normal behaviour (Figure 7.2)
- Suspected egg-binding or cloacal prolapse
- Changes in the appearance of mutes (faeces/urine in raptors) or droppings (faeces/urine in pigeons and passerine birds)
- Failure to turn the crop over (empty) or changes in casting time/appearance (raptors) (Figure 7.3)
- Anorexia

7.1 Emergencies that receptionists must schedule to be seen as soon as possible.

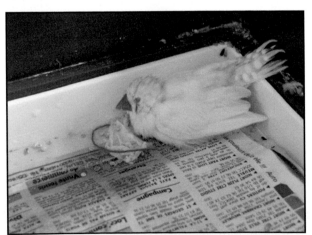

7.2 Egg-bound Zebra Finch. Note closed eyes and fluffed feathers and the fact that the bird is on the floor of the cage. This bird is severely ill and such a presentation should be considered an emergency. (© John Chitty)

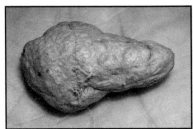

7.3 A falcon's normal fresh casting, consisting of fur and feathers.

It is important for staff and clients to recognize that birds will normally hide signs of ill health as an anti-predator response. Disease may be far progressed or of a life-threatening nature, even if the owner has only noticed mild or acute-onset clinical signs. If in any doubt the rule should be to check with the veterinary surgeon who normally sees avian cases in the practice.

Receptionists also need simple guidelines on how owners should best transport their bird to the surgery (see Chapter 6) and what owners should bring with them.

- For *raptors* a mute (faecal) sample, travel box and a falconry glove should be brought in with the bird. While the practice should have its own basic falconry equipment, such as bow and block perches for overnight stays and longer periods of hospitalization, leather falconry gloves are more difficult to disinfect adequately and it is often best to use the owner's own glove when hospitalizing a raptor.
- *Pigeons* should be brought in a transport box, with a fresh pooled faecal sample from the loft, as well as a sample of the feed in a clear plastic bag and any supplements given. Pigeon keepers should also be encouraged to bring any antiparasitic treatments and other medications they may be using, so that the active ingredients (rather than trade names) can be confirmed. Photographs of the lofts are helpful in assessing the husbandry and hygiene of the flock.
- *Passerine birds* are best brought in their normal cage, which should not be cleaned out (to allow a gross examination of the droppings). If the birds are kept in an outdoor aviary, a pooled faecal sample should be brought. While suitable for parasitology, this unfortunately will not preserve the gross appearance of the droppings, which can yield useful additional information (see later).

It is wise for receptionists to enquire on arrival if an avian case is judged to be an emergency. If there is any doubt, a veterinary nurse can perform a quick assessment if the veterinary surgeon is busy. This will prevent the scenario of a patient dying in the waiting room while waiting to see the veterinary surgeon because no-one was aware that it was an urgent case.

History and assessment of husbandry

When presented with a sick bird, there is an immediate inclination to perform a clinical examination. Triage is clearly the priority, but once any life-saving interventions have been performed, it is essential that a comprehensive history be taken.

The history is an essential part of any health assessment and in less urgent cases it can often largely be completed in the reception area by means of a questionnaire (Figure 7.4), while the veterinary surgeon is occupied with other clients.

Confirmation bias is best avoided by taking as complete a history as possible before performing a clinical examination. This will prevent unintentional leading questions that will appear to confirm or reinforce a premature presumptive diagnosis that may be incorrect.

Clinical examination

The clinical examination of any bird presented to a veterinary surgeon is the most important part of any diagnostic work performed. No amount of time or money spent on other diagnostic tests such as ultrasonography, radiography, haematology and biochemistry or endoscopy can compensate for an incomplete or poorly performed examination, as all other work should be based on its findings. While some aspects of avian behaviour and anatomy can make examination different or more difficult, the basic principles remain the same as for any other animal.

Raptor History Form

Please fill this in while you are waiting to see the veterinary surgeon

Date: _____ Surname: _____

Species: _____ Age: _____

Gender: _____ Length of time owned: _____

Source of bird (captive bred/wild caught): _____ Hand or parent reared: _____

Flying weight: _____ Moulting weight: _____

Current activity: _____ Flight performance: _____

Aviary type: _____

Perching (block/bow/indoors/free flight): _____

Perch surface material: _____ Disinfection frequency and agent: _____

Mutes and casting appearance: _____

Other birds kept: _____

Type of quarry bird is flown at: _____

How often bird is flown: _____

Diet (chicks/quail/rats/other): _____

Diet storage (freezer): _____

How is frozen food defrosted (air thaw/water/overnight)? _____

Supplements given: _____

What is the problem you are seeing the vet for today? _____

When did you first notice signs? _____

Has the bird had any treatments at home for this? _____

Previous illness in this bird: _____

Other health problems in other birds this year: _____

Any other questions you would like to ask: _____

_____

7.4 Examples of history forms for raptors, pigeons and passerine birds. (continues) ▶

Pigeon History Form

Please fill this in while you are waiting to see the veterinary surgeon

Date: _____ Surname: _____

Age (squab/young bird/adult): _____ Length of time owned: _____

Source of bird (bred/bought in): _____ Type of bird (breeder, racer, show): _____

Flight performance if racer: _____

Loft types (stock/racing/widowhood/young bird): _____

Floor space: _____

Number of birds in loft: _____ Perch number: _____

Stocking density (if known): _____

Flooring (slats/mesh/litter/scraped): _____

Disinfection frequency and agent: _____

Other birds kept: _____

Diet (please describe): _____

Any supplements given: _____

Routine vaccinations and other drugs: _____

What is the problem you are seeing the vet for today? _____

Is this an individual bird or a flock problem? _____

When did you first notice any signs? _____

Has the bird had any other treatments at home for this? _____

Any other health problems in other birds this year: _____

Any other questions you would like to ask: _____

_____

Passerine Bird History Form

Please fill this in while you are waiting to see the veterinary surgeon

Date: _____ Surname: _____

Age: _____ Species/breed: _____

Purpose of stock (display/breeding/showing): _____ Length of time owned: _____

Source of bird (bred/bought in): _____

Enclosure (cage or aviary): _____ Enclosure size: _____

Site (indoor/outdoor): _____ Contact with wild birds: _____

Perch type: _____ Number of perches: _____

Flooring type (soil/litter/concrete): _____

Other enclosures: _____

Disinfection frequency and agent: _____

Bird species and numbers kept: _____

Diet (please describe): _____

Any supplements given: _____

What is the problem you are seeing the vet for today? _____

Is this an individual bird or a flock problem? _____

When did you first notice any signs? _____

Have the birds had any treatments at home for this? _____

Any other health problems in other birds this year: _____

Any other questions you would like to ask: _____

_____

7.4 Examples of history forms for raptors, pigeons and passerine birds.

The purpose for which a bird is kept (racing, showing, hunting, working, breeding) must always be kept in mind when the examination is performed. Falconry birds that are kept only for breeding, need different levels of performance and hence physical perfection compared to the same species used for hunting. The financial value of the bird must also be taken into account. While the decision making as to levels of treatment is the owner's to make and not the veterinary surgeon's, care must be taken not to limit treatment options offered on presumed cost. Falconers may have a very strong bond with a bird, even if it is not particularly valuable in financial terms. Racing pigeons can be surprisingly valuable; and owners of show canaries may also highly value a particular individual and be quite prepared to pay for extensive diagnostics and treatment. In contrast, some working falconry birds are worthless to their owner if not totally fit for their purpose and may have a relatively low replacement cost, mitigating against protracted treatment.

Remote observation

A remote examination of the bird's behaviour is useful, and of course easiest using binoculars if making a site visit. Birds have excellent eyesight and will alter their behaviour if they are aware of being watched, as an anti-predator response.

In the surgery, looking through the keyhole in the consulting room door or via a peephole can help. An alert raptor may revert to looking fluffed up and sleepy once left alone in the room, or may even been seen to droop a wing or favour one of its legs on the perch.

With a group of passerine birds in a cage, remote observation through the keyhole may help to show whether all the birds are showing signs of ill health when the owner has only noticed the most severely affected bird. Fluffed-up sleepy birds, a bird being bullied by healthy cage mates or sitting on the cage floor, and even slight dyspnoea may all become apparent when the birds are unaware that they are being observed.

Weight and body condition

Determining body weight is not just important for calculating drug dosages but is an essential part of the clinical examination. This should always be coupled with body condition scoring, judged by the pectoral musculature and prominence of the carina of the sternal keel. Symmetrical thin pectoral muscles and a prominent keel may indicate that the owner has been starving birds too much, or flying birds too light. In contrast, asymmetry of the pectoral muscles (while uncommonly seen) generally indicates a chronic injury.

- *Falconers* normally weigh their birds at least once a day and have a flying weight for a particular bird. This is a weight at which a bird is sufficiently hungry to hunt, but it can be misleading and is only appropriate after a few seasons. Too low a weight in small raptors, particularly males, can lead to hypoglycaemia, manifesting as weakness and collapse. During a flying season a bird's flying weight may change and falconers may not

notice that a bird is gradually losing body condition until this affects its performance.
- *Pigeon keepers* may be aware of small changes in a bird's body condition, as they associate the pectoral muscle mass with the bird's performance; many check condition when they handle any birds.
- Few keepers of *passerine birds* will check body condition and they may be unaware that a bird is emaciated, as the body feathers will hide this.

Sexual dimorphism

- Size sexual dimorphism is marked in many *falcons*, with some small tiercels weighing almost half that of the largest females. Other species show less size dimorphism but have dimorphic plumage in adults. Short-wings (*hawks*) often have an overlap in weights of males and females, with sexual dimorphism only obvious at extremes. DNA sex determination (or laparoscopic examination of the gonads, see Chapter 13) may be needed.
- *Pigeons* are generally sexually monomorphic, with gender determination based on behaviour, although experienced fanciers may sex birds based on the male's often rounded or bolder head. In some cases males may have a hypertrophied cere (Figure 7.5).
- In *Canaries* during the breeding season males have a cloacal promontory, caused by the swollen end of the ductus deferens (the seminal glomerulus) pushing against the cloacal walls. The cloaca points in a direction perpendicular to the tail. In contrast the females have a flatter vent, with the cloaca pointing in the same direction as the tail. However, this is only easily distinguished by the experienced keeper or breeder. Other elements of the history (e.g. a tendency to more developed or complicated song) may indicate that the bird is a male.

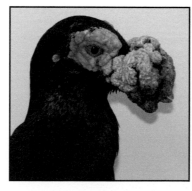

7.5

Know the normal! This cere hypertrophy can be normal in a male pigeon. While it will restrict vision and affect flying ability, it is deemed desirable in some show breeds. It also enables easy visual sexing. (Courtesy of Aidan Raftery)

Physical examination

The safe and effective handling of any bird is essential to the ability to perform a full clinical examination (see Chapter 6). It is also an opportunity to demonstrate to an owner one's knowledge and ability to deal with these patients. The same applies to the knowledge and use of falconry and pigeon racing terminology (see Chapters 2 and 3).

Ophthalmic examination

This is described in Chapter 25. Figure 7.6 shows a normal pigeon eye.

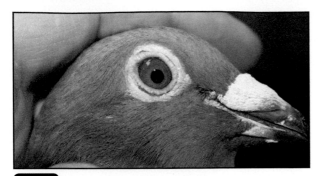

7.6 Normal pigeon eye. (Courtesy of Alistair Lawrie)

In cases of conjunctivitis, so-called 'one-eye colds', and rhinitis in pigeons, owners should be warned of possible *Chlamydophila* infection and its zoonotic potential. Chlamydophilosis can manifest with a variety of clinical signs, or in conjunction with other disease, and should always be a consideration. In contrast, *Mycoplasma* species are a common cause of conjunctivitis and upper respiratory tract disease in finches and canaries.

Upper respiratory tract

Nostrils and the periocular sinuses should be examined and palpated to differentiate chronic sinusitis from ocular disease. Raptors have an operculum in their nostrils (see Chapter 5) that should not be confused with a rhinolith. Diagnostic sinus flushing with physiological 0.9% saline or needle aspiration may be performed (see Chapter 20). The choanal slit on the dorsal aspect of the mouth should be examined for any discharges that may also indicate upper respiratory tract disease.

Beak and oral cavity

- Overlong and untrimmed beaks in *falconry* birds may be predisposed to chips and cracks. They may also be an indication of chronic illness and deranged metabolism, or inadequate nutrition. Injuries to the cere may also lead to weaknesses and splits in the beak. Falcons normally have a tomial tooth and notch bilaterally in the lateral rhamphotheca (upper beak); this helps with gripping and tearing food and should not be removed by overzealous trimming.
- *Pigeon* squabs normally have a relatively soft pliable beak, which should not be confused with a fracture or metabolic bone disease.
- Misshapen beaks may be seen in *passerine birds* that survive polyomavirus infection as fledglings.

Trichomoniasis and nematodes

Thick caseous plaques in the mouth or pharynx of pigeons are most commonly due to trichomoniasis (*Trichomonas gallinae*), referred to by keepers as 'canker'. Confirmation of the diagnosis is best performed by examination of very fresh saline wet preparations under microscopy for motile protozoa.

Examination of rapid-stained air-dried smears is useful in eliminating other causes, such as *Candida albicans*. Trichomonads may be difficult to visualize in chronic cases, and treatment may need to be presumptive.

Trichomoniasis is particularly common in falconry birds fed or hunting pigeons, such as Peregrine Falcons, and is referred to as 'frounce' by falconers. Oral trichomoniasis lesions may also be reflective of more extensive lesions extending lower down in the gastrointestinal tract.

Parasites such *Capillaria* and *Syngamus* nematodes may also be apparent in the pharynx or larynx (see Chapter 18). Some raptors may show an open mouth gape when cast for examination, which should not be confused with dyspnoea. Breathing should be checked for any audible clicks or other abnormal sounds that may indicate respiratory tract infections or parasites, with an *Aspergillus* air sacculitis always being of particular concern in raptors (see 'Cardio-respiratory system', below).

Ear

Examination of the external ear can help to detect birds (particularly owls) that have experienced cranial trauma (Figure 7.7). The posterior aspects of the scleral ossicles are apparent in the ears of most owls. Occasionally bacterial infections or trichomoniasis may affect the ear.

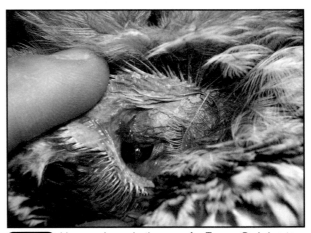

7.7 Haemorrhage in the ear of a Tawny Owl due to cranial trauma.

Gastrointestinal tract

Palpation of the crop should be considered in conjunction with the owner's history of when a bird has last been fed. Owls do not have a crop.

The crop should empty completely within a few hours of feeding, or crop hypomotility/stasis should be suspected, with resultant sour crop. This often manifests with a sour or rotten oral smell. This is most often a secondary problem, and the underlying cause must be determined. Thickening of the crop usually indicates an ingluvitis.

Pigeons with squabs will normally have a thickened crop wall due to their production of crop milk, which consists of lipid-laden desquamated epithelial cells. This occurs in both males and females and should not be confused with an ingluvitis.

The abdomen should be palpated. Masses, as well as gizzard fill (in raptors), may be evident.

'Black spot' caused by circovirus in Canaries results in abdominal distension and a swollen gall bladder visible through the skin in nestlings. Hepatomegaly may be visible through the skin in young Canaries suffering from atoxoplasmosis. *Macrorhabdus ornithogaster* can also result in the liver being visible due to proventricular dilatation.

Regurgitation generally does not occur normal in passerines.

The cloaca should be assessed for soiling of surrounding feathers and prolapses. An otoscope or endoscope can be used to examine the cloaca of anaesthetized birds (see Chapter 13).

Cardiorespiratory system

In assessing the cardiorespiratory system particular attention should be paid to rate and rhythm. A neonatal stethoscope is particularly useful. Dysrhythmias may be difficult to detect due to the rapid heart rate of birds. These may be due to numerous causes, primary cardiac disease, or systemic disease such as septicaemia or shock. The heart rate (Figure 7.8) can be very variable in the same bird, due to factors such as stress or exercise and training, and it can be difficult to assess during the clinical examination, because of the unnatural surroundings and stress caused by handling. Murmurs are occasionally discernible in birds, but their significance can be difficult to determine. Changes in the viscosity of the blood, due to anaemia, can also cause a physiological murmur.

Body weight	Resting heart rate	Restrained bird heart rate
25 g	274	500–600
100 g	206	400–600
300 g	163	250–400
500 g	147	160–350
1 kg	127	150–300
2 kg	110	110–180

7.8 Guide to approximate normal avian heart rates (beats per minute).

Careful auscultation of the respiratory system is essential. The avian lung has a rigid, faveolar structure, in contrast to the mammalian alveolar structure. This means that abnormal sounds heard on auscultation need different interpretation to those in mammals. For example, not having alveoli, birds do not develop crackles, but birds with an air sacculitis may demonstrate a clicking sound on auscultation due to adherence or friction of the inflamed air sac surfaces.

The syrinx is found at the tracheal bifurcation at the base of the heart. Voice or song changes can indicate tracheal parasites such as *Sternostoma tracheacolum* or *Syngamus trachea*, foreign bodies, or *Aspergillus* granulomas. These may lead to acute respiratory distress, and should be treated as a life-threatening emergency.

Chlamydophila infection should always be a consideration in birds showing signs of respiratory disease, especially in pigeons.

Musculoskeletal system

Careful palpation of the bones and joints of the wing and leg are important, as well as checking for normal range of joint flexion and extension, and that this is symmetrical in both wings and legs. The shoulders should be palpated for symmetry. While the humerus, clavicle and scapula are all easily palpable, the coracoid lies deeper within the pectoral musculature. Extending and releasing the wings also helps in assessing passive recoil and elasticity. Fractures may not be easily palpable, with only loss of symmetry and function causing one to suspect these important fractures, which may hold a guarded prognosis even in valuable birds. Radiography will often be needed to confirm coracoid fractures. The junction between the notarium (fused thoracic vertebrae) and synsacrum should also be palpated for any signs of pain or instability.

Examination of the feet is important in raptors. The plantar surface of both feet should be examined for signs of bumblefoot (see Chapter 16). The plantar foot surface is easily examined by using a wire speculum, such as that used for opening parrots' beaks, to keep the toes extended while the plantar surface is examined. The plantar base of each talon should be carefully checked for swelling or injuries, as this is the site of flexor tendon attachment.

Feathers

The condition of any bird's feathers is of paramount importance, and note should be made of broken feathers and whether these are associated with so-called fret marks (Figure 7.9). They may indicate low nutritional status, stress, or other underlying systemic disease.

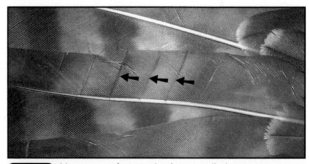

7.9 Numerous fret marks (arrowed) due to poor nutritional status.

Most raptors have relatively long tails, and distal damage to all the remiges (tail feathers) may indicate that a bird has been spending time on the ground rather than perching.

Examination of droppings

Examination of droppings (known as mutes in falconry) is a useful source of additional clinical information (Figures 7.10 and 7.11). The droppings voided from the cloaca consist of three separate parts: faeces, urates and urine.

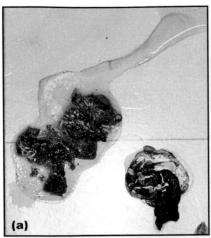
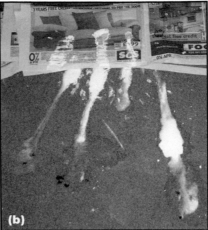
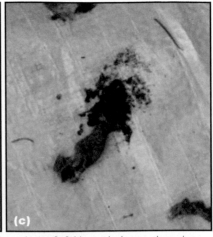

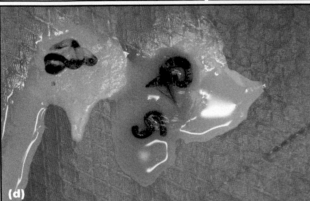

7.10 Normal droppings. **(a)** Normal pigeon droppings (right) consist of a semi-solid greenish faeces part and a white urate part attached; abnormal loose faeces (left) can be caused by polyuria or diarrhoea, but differentiation between the two conditions is difficult. **(b)** Normal hawk mutes: note the shape; this is known as 'slicing' and the distance and shape of the slice can be taken as a measure of good health. **(c)** Normal softbill dropping, much softer and looser than a raptor mute. **(d)** Normal raptor mutes: note that the presence of some fluid and colour is not always abnormal. (a, courtesy of M. Pees; b, © John Chitty; c, courtesy of Geoff Masson)

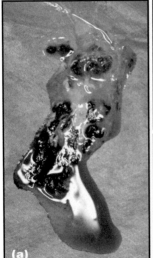
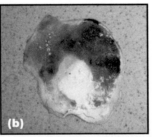
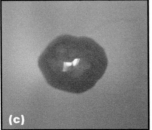

7.11 Abnormal droppings. **(a)** Mild enteritis in a raptor. **(b)** Malabsorption after treatment for *Pseudomonas* infection. **(c)** Reddish orange mute seen 10 minutes after the bird had received a multi-vitamin injection. (a, © Michael Lierz; b, courtesy of Tom Bailey; c, courtesy of Chris Lloyd)

While parasitological examination is of obvious importance (see Chapters 18 and 31), the macroscopic appearance of the droppings themselves, though not diagnostic, can give some further clues to underlying disease and disorders. The faeces may also give an indication of what the bird is actually eating and whether this differs from what the owner claims to be feeding.

Urates

The urates should be moist and a clean white in colour. Birds on high-protein diets, such as raptors, produce a larger urate portion in the droppings than do seed-eating passerine birds.

- Dry chalky urates are often an indication of dehydration.
- Green-stained urates (Figure 7.12a) are due to biliverdin leaching out of the faeces and are an indication that bile pigments are not being resorbed from the intestinal tract and reused by the liver. This is seen in starvation (Figure 7.12b) or aspergillosis in raptors.
- In pigeons, biliverdinuria is often seen with *Chlamydophila* infection.

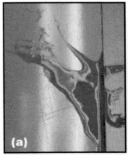
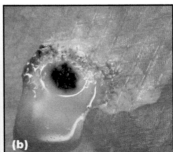

7.12 Green droppings. **(a)** Biliverdinuria from a falcon with lymphoma; this may be seen in many cases with severe liver damage. **(b)** Anorexia or an empty gut will produce a dark green faecal portion and some colour in the urine (a, © John Chitty; b, © Michael Lierz)

- Bacterial hepatitis can cause green urates in passerine birds.
- Pink discoloured urates are associated with blood or haemoglobin loss via the kidneys. This may indicate renal disease or haemolysis.

Urine

Polyuria (Figure 7.13) is a common, relatively non-specific finding, but may occur with heavy metal toxicities such as ingested lead in raptors or in renal disease.

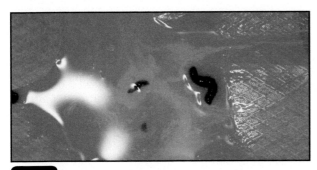

7.13 Polyuria. (© Michael Lierz)

Dry droppings without a urine portion (anurea) may indicate severe dehydration or renal disease, or a functional obstruction, such as egg binding.

Faeces

- Melaena, just as in mammals, indicates haemorrhage in the cranial gastrointestinal tract (Figure 7.14a,b). Fresh blood in the faeces (Figure 7.14c,d) is usually indicative of bleeding from the cloaca or uterus, or anticoagulant rodenticide toxicity.
- Raptor faeces are often malodorous, which is normal and not an indication of enteritis. In passerine birds, malodorous faeces or diarrhoea (to be differentiated from polyuria, Figure 7.15) may indicate bacterial enteritis.
- In pigeons, voluminous soft green faeces with watery urates and excess urine can be seen with coccidiosis in young pigeons, as well as with trichomoniasis and pigeon paramyxovirus (Figure 7.16). Haemorrhagic diarrhoea is occasionally seen in salmonellosis or severe nematode infection.

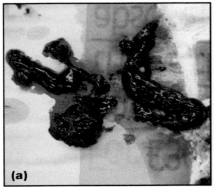
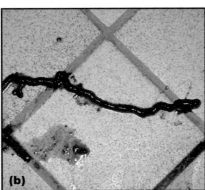
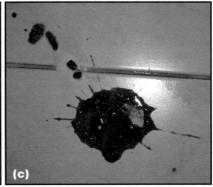

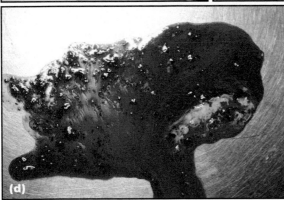

7.14 **(a)** Melaena in a falcon, resulting from gastric ulceration. Contrast with fresh red blood in the urine, where the blood is evenly distributed through the urinary portion, generally indicating renal blood loss. The presence of blood clots in the urine (much more common) indicates cloacal or uterine damage or may be seen in coagulopathies (e.g. rodenticide toxicity, see (d)). **(b)** Fibrinous haemorrhagic faeces, indicating coccidiosis in a falcon. **(c)** Haemorrhagic enteritis: fresh blood in the faecal sample often indicates clostridial enterotoxaemia. **(d)** Haematuria in a raptor. The presence of clots (in contrast to the lack of clots in (c)) shows that the blood comes from 'below' the kidneys, most probably from the cloaca or uterus. This is typically seen in coumarol toxicity. (a, © John Chitty; b,d, © Michael Lierz; c, courtesy of Tom Bailey)

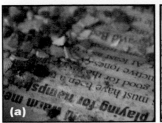
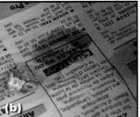

7.15 Abnormal passerine droppings. **(a)** Diarrhoea in a Greenfinch. **(b)** Polyuria in a Zebra Finch; compare the normal and abnormal droppings on the paper. (© John Chitty)

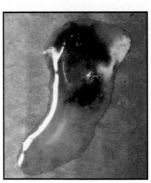

7.16

Pigeon paramyxovirus infection indicated by a pool of urine surrounding a core of dark green/black material. (Courtesy of Tom Pennycott)

- Undigested seeds in the faeces may be seen with *Macrorhabdus ornithogaster* infection and has been reported in nestling finches with *Cochlosoma* flagellate infections.
- Aerated stools, described as having a popcorn appearance, are reportedly seen in birds with enteritis due to a *Giardia* infection.

Triage and emergency medicine

Preparation for the arrival of a critical avian patient can save crucial time. It can also minimize handling and thus stress to the bird.

Before the bird's arrival a warmed oxygen enclosure should be prepared. Warmed fluids, intravenous catheters and an air sac tube should also be prepared, to limit handling time and stress.

Avian emergencies should be seen immediately, in a quiet area away from predatory animals such as dogs and cats. An initial rapid triage assessment should be performed and any life-threatening conditions such as severe haemorrhage attended to.

Triage is the initial assessment of a patient's condition, and the identification and treatment of life-threatening conditions. While the basic principles of triage apply to all animals, there are some obvious differences in the management of birds to that of domestic mammals. The 'ABC' of triage and emergency stabilization (airways, breathing, and circulation) (Figure 7.17) is just as useful as in other animals, but in birds it is important to remember that simultaneous cardiorespiratory arrest is common.

A	Airways	ET or air sac tube placement
B	Breathing	Oxygen supplementation Manual ventilation 1 breath per 4–5 seconds if intubated/air sac tube placed Doxapram 10–20 mg/kg i.v. (or sublingual)
C	Circulation	Intravenous catheterization and fluid administration (see Figure 7.19) Adrenaline 1 mg/kg i.v., sublingual or intratracheal Cardiac massage

7.17 Triage priorities.

A – Airways

In birds with dyspnoea due to tracheal trauma, foreign body inhalation or tracheal parasites, placement of an air sac tube (see Chapter 10) will help to stabilize the patient before the primary problem can be safely addressed. The patient is best briefly anaesthetized with isoflurane/sevoflurane for tube placement, as this provides oxygen as well as limiting stress. Once the tube is placed, birds will lighten in anaesthetic depth and may awake unless the anaesthetic system is connected to the air sac tube. Gaseous exchange, and hence anaesthetic agent uptake, is primarily in a caudal to cranial direction in the avian lung (see Chapter 5).

B – Breathing

Clinically dyspnoeic or collapsed birds may be placed in an oxygen enclosure while treatment is instituted. Care should be taken to monitor birds when removing them from oxygen enclosures once stabilized, as some can rapidly become dyspnoeic again.

In contrast to mammals, simultaneous cardio-respiratory arrest is common in birds and so respiratory rate and rhythm should be monitored carefully. In cases of respiratory arrest, positive pressure ventilation is instituted via an endotracheal or air sac tube, either manually by closing the valve and compression of the T-piece bag, or via a mechanical ventilator. Unlike in mammals, the rigid faveolar avian lung structure is not damaged by over-inflation, as the air sacs are inflated instead. These are much more resistant to damage, but can be ruptured if markedly over-inflated. Ventilation should be performed at one breath every 4–5 seconds (see Chapter 10).

Doxapram can be administered intravenously (or sublingually if intravenous access is not possible) at 10–20 mg/kg to stimulate respiration. It is most often of very limited application except in cases of anaesthetic overdose.

C – Circulation

Maintenance of cardiac output and circulatory volume is essential to ensure adequate tissue oxygenation. The mainstay of this is fluid therapy (see below). For routes and administration techniques, see Chapter 8. Control of haemorrhage is an important component of maintaining circulatory volume. Shock can also result in a reduced effective circulatory volume and poor peripheral vascular perfusion. The latter may be evaluated by the ulnar vein filling time (after occlusion). A filling time of >0.5 seconds is indicative of poor peripheral vascular perfusion, usually accompanied by decreased turgor of the vein. Other signs may be tachycardia, tachypnoea and either pale mucous membranes or injected mucous membranes of the mouth, conjunctiva and cloaca in cases of septic shock. These birds are usually extremely lethargic or depressed, even moribund, and need immediate intravenous fluids and broad-spectrum antibiosis.

Chronic infections, toxicities or nutritional deficiencies may result in birds presenting with anaemia. This will result in clinical signs similar to those seen in shock, such as oral and cloacal mucous membrane pallor, and in more severe cases lethargy, tachycardia and tachypnoea. Determining the packed cell volume (PCV) before instituting fluid therapy is essential in evaluating prognosis and response to therapy. In extremely anaemic birds care should be taken not to be overzealous with crystalloid intravenous fluid administration, as this can cause haemodilution, critically reducing the oxygen-carrying capacity even further. Extremely anaemic birds are best placed in an oxygen enclosure and more cautious intravenous fluid rates selected.

Emergency medication

Figure 7.18 lists emergency drugs and medication that should be ready to hand in any avian clinic, along with suitable dosages and routes.

Drug	Dose and route	Notes
Adrenaline	1 mg/kg i.v., sublingual	Cardiac arrest
Allopurinol	10 mg/kg oral q12h	Use in gout is highly controversial in raptors (see text), and maintenance of hydration is essential
Amoxicillin/clavulanate	150 mg/kg i.m., i.v.	
Atropine	0.2–0.5 mg/kg	
Butorphanol	0.1–4.0 mg/kg q6–12h	Good analgesia
Carprofen	2–5 mg/kg oral, i.m. q24h	Care in dehydration and renal dysfunction
Dexamethasone	2–6 mg/kg i.m., i.v.	Cranial trauma, but should be used with extreme care due to immunosuppression
Diazepam	0.25–1 mg i.m., i.v.	Control of seizures. Low dose once daily for 2–3 days can be used as appetite stimulant in raptors
Doxapram	10–20 mg/kg	Anaesthetic overdose
Edetate calcium disodium	35–50 mg/kg s.c., i.m. q12h	Lead and other heavy metal toxicity
Enrofloxacin	15 mg/kg i.m. q12h	Irritant injection, can cause significant pectoral muscle damage (care in working/racing birds). Can cause regurgitation
Furosemide	0.1–6 mg/kg oral, s.c., i.m., i.v. q6–24h	Some species very sensitive – ensure birds are not dehydrated or hyperuricaemic
Hyaluronidase	100 IU/litre	Speeds absorption of subcutaneous fluids (if intravenous not possible)
Kaolin/pectin	15 ml/kg oral	
Marbofloxacin	10 mg/kg i.m., i.v. q24h	
Meloxicam	0.1–0.2 mg/kg q24h	Analgesia and reduction of inflammation
Metoclopramide	0.3 mg/kg oral, i.m., i.v.	Sour crop/GIT hypomotility
Prednisolone sodium succinate	10–20 mg/kg i.v., i.m.	Acute head trauma, if used give within 4 hours of injury
Vitamin K	0.2–2.5 mg/kg oral, i.m. q6–24h	Anticoagulant toxicity

7.18 Emergency drugs and medication to be kept in the avian clinic.

Fluid therapy

Dehydration is less obvious on clinical examination in birds, but an assumption that presenting sick birds are likely to be 5–10% dehydrated is reasonable. PCV and total protein (TP) are useful for a rapid assessment and for monitoring the response to fluid therapy.

Hyperuricaemia is important, as it can rapidly result in precipitation of uric acid tophi in the renal tubules and to acute tubular necrosis. The use of allopurinol, a xanthine oxidase inhibitor, is highly controversial in the treatment of hyperuricaemia (on initial biochemistry) and the prevention or treatment of gout. A dosage of 50 mg/kg used in healthy Red-tailed Hawks led to a severe hyperuricaemia and induction of renal uric acid tophi deposition (renal gout) (Lumeij et al., 1998). When a dose of 25 mg/kg was used in the same species there was no nephrotoxicity, but also no significant effect on plasma uric acid levels (Poffers et al., 2002). If allopurinol is to be used, lower dosages are recommended and maintenance of hydration, preferably via an intravenous or intraosseous route, is essential. This author prefers not to use allopurinol in raptors at all, relying instead on intravenous fluid administration as the basis of prevention.

Intravenous, intraosseous, subcutaneous and oral routes (see Chapter 8 for techniques) are all useful, depending on the severity of dehydration, the species and the underlying pathology present. Suggested fluid administration rates are set out in Figure 7.19; Figure 7.20 gives a 'Quick guide' for critical patients.

Crystalloids and colloids

Some authors recommend intravenous boluses of crystalloids up to 30 ml/kg given over one minute, followed by shock rates of up to 90 ml/kg/h. While useful in rapidly expanding the circulatory volume, care is needed with these rates in anaemic birds or in birds suffering haemorrhagic shock. A rapid decrease in oxygen-carrying capacity due to haemodilution could further destabilize a bird. Initial bolus administration of colloids (e.g. Haemaccel, Hetastarch), followed by infusion of crystalloids is recommended and reduces the crystalloid requirements by 40–60%.

Isotonic crystalloids		
Initial intravenous bolus administration	10–30 ml/kg	Slowly over at least 1 minute
Shock rate	Up to 90 ml/kg/h	First hour only
Rehydration	Fluid deficit (ml) = estimated dehydration (%/100) × body weight (g)	Given over 6–12 hours
Maintenance requirements	50 ml/kg/day	
Other fluids		
50% dextrose	1 ml/kg	Slowly
Colloids (Haemaccel, Hetastarch)	5–15 ml/kg	Slowly, q8h up to 4X; hypoproteinaemia, decrease fluids to 1/3 to 1/2 maintenance
Oxyglobin	10–15 ml/kg	Significant blood loss
Heparin	0.25 ml/10 ml blood	Add to whole blood for transfusions

7.19 Intravenous fluid administration rates.

It is always best to weigh patients accurately and calculate fluid volumes carefully. However, there will be emergencies when time will be of the essence. These very rough guidelines are given for such emergencies, but the author cannot be held responsible for any losses incurred.

For a critical raptor
These rates are suggested for a Harris' Hawk weighing approximately 800 g.

- Give an initial 4–8 ml of a colloid mixed with 10–20 ml of a crystalloid, preferably via a syringe driver over the first hour, otherwise by a slow bolus injection over several minutes. Continue crystalloids at a rate of 8–10 ml/h for the following 8–12 hours. Colloids can be repeated every 8 hours if needed.
- Alternatively, 0.5–0.8 ml of 50% hypertonic dextrose can be given initially in hypoglycaemic birds. Dextrose must be strictly intravenous, and must not be used if the electrolyte status is not known. This is followed by intravenous crystalloids at a rate of 10–20 ml for the first hour, then reduced to 8 ml/h for a further 12 hours. If no colloids or dextrose are given, crystalloid rates can be up to 40–60 ml for the first hour.
- If subcutaneous fluids are used, give 40 ml of an isotonic crystalloid split between four sites.
- If oral fluids are given, 20 ml should be administered in anorexic or critical patients, and up to 40 ml in stable patients.

For pigeons

- If intravenous access is possible, administer 2–4 ml of a colloid mixed with 4–12 ml crystalloids given as a slow bolus over several minutes or infused over the first hour by syringe driver, followed by an infusion of 4–6 ml/h for 12 hours of a crystalloid fluid.
- Otherwise either an oral bolus of 5–20 ml of 5% dextrose solution by crop tube, or subcutaneous injections of 5–20 ml of warmed 0.9% NaCl, not exceeding 5 ml in one site, can be used.

For passerine birds

- Oral and subcutaneous fluids are usually the most practical in passerine birds.
- Give sick Canaries 1–2 ml of 5% dextrose orally on admission.
- Never give dextrose subcutaneously.
- Use isotonic fluids such as lactated Ringer's solution or 0.9% NaCl saline subcutaneously. Try not to exceed 0.5 ml in one site for a Canary.
- If giving irritant drugs (e.g. enrofloxacin) subcutaneously, diluting the drug in the fluids will help to limit irritation.
- The jugular can be used for intravenous bolus administration of 0.5–1 ml of isotonic fluids in the most severe cases.

7.20 Quick guide to fluid volumes for critical patients.

While the majority of authors report administration of colloids as intravenous boluses at 5–15 ml/kg, avian blood has a lower TP than mammalian blood and hence a lower colloidal osmotic pressure. In pigeons this is 8.1 mmHg, compared with about 25 mmHg in mammals. Commercial colloid solutions generally have an osmotic pressure of 20–25 mmHg and so it may make more physiological sense to administer colloids mixed with crystalloids via a syringe driver more slowly over the first hour (Gunkel and Lafortune, 2005).

Dextrose
Hypertonic 50% dextrose solution can be useful, especially in hypoglycaemic raptors, but it can worsen a bird's condition dramatically in the light of electrolyte disturbances. Many raptors appear to present as alkalotic (McKinney, 2003), with an associated hypokalaemia. Hypokalaemia may also be seen with gastrointestinal or renal disease (see Chapters 23 and 31). Intravenous dextrose will cause insulin release from the pancreas, which will shift potassium from the extracellular to intracellular compartment, exacerbating any existing hypokalaemia. Electrolytes should be measured before administration of intravenous hypertonic dextrose, and potassium chloride can be added to fluids to correct deficits (0.1–0.3 mEq/kg). Hypertonic dextrose should not be administered subcutaneously.

Blood transfusion and haemoglobin colloid

These are needed in cases of significant blood loss. The most common cause of acute blood loss is trauma. Birds are more resistant to circulatory volume loss than are mammals, and this is particularly so in athletic flying species such as falcons and pigeons. In one study some pigeons were able to survive blood loss equivalent to 9% of their body weight (Kovach *et al.*, 1969). While Jenkins (1997) believed this to be equivalent to their entire circulatory volume based on Sturkie's avian physiology (1986), and hence their survival being due to redistribution of fluid from the intracellular compartment, other authors have reported the circulatory volume in racing pigeons to be higher, at 16.3% of body weight (Campbell, 1993). Whichever authority is to be believed, this still illustrates athletic bird species' remarkable innate resistance to haemorrhagic hypovolaemia. Birds with an acute drop in PCV to below 20%, however, do need urgent circulatory volume and oxygen transportation support.

Oxyglobin: Oxyglobin is a purified polymerized bovine haemoglobin solution that has colloidal properties as well as the ability to transport oxygen. It has been used successfully in birds with crystalloid administration, as a bolus over several minutes.

Blood transfusions: Whole blood transfusions are limited by the availability of donors. In raptors it has also been demonstrated that in heterologous transfusions, such as from pigeons, the erythrocytes may unfortunately be relatively short-lived (Sandmeier, 1994), so blood should be collected from the same species (homologous transfusions) or from species that are as closely related as possible. Blood types have not yet been described in birds, limiting the application of cross-matching before transfusions (Gunkel and Lafortune, 2005), though there have been reported attempts at rough cross-matching by mixing donor erythrocytes with recipient serum and observing for any signs of gross haemolysis or agglutination.

Subcutaneous fluids

Subcutaneous fluid administration is often a viable option, especially in small passerine birds with gastro-intestinal disease. Absorption in less than 30 minutes is reported in small birds. Volumes up to 50 ml/kg can be given, and 10–15 ml/kg can be given in a single site, though some sources advocate up to 25 ml/kg in a single site such as the precrural fold. Hyaluron-idase can be added to enhance absorption.

One advantage of administering subcutaneous fluids is that irritant drugs such as enrofloxacin and edetate calcium disodium can be diluted in them, or even injected into an existing subcutaneous fluid pocket to reduce tissue irritation.

Oral fluids

Oral fluids are well tolerated and absorbed in all but the most critical cases, or those suffering severe gastrointestinal tract disease. An excellent choice is 5% dextrose, as it is absorbed rapidly from the gastro-intestinal tract without creating an influx of fluid into the intestinal tract, which would cause exacerbation of the dehydration. It is also helpful in correcting hypo-glycaemia. Isotonic crystalloids are also suitable. Rates of up to 50 ml/kg are reported, but lower rates should always be used in critical patients. Rates of 10–20 ml/kg are used except in owls, where a lower rate of 8 ml/kg given more frequently may be more suitable, due to their lack of a crop.

Stabilization and further examination

Care after fluid therapy

After fluid therapy has been initiated, the bird may be placed in a warmed oxygen enclosure and kept dark and quiet, with regular checks every 10–15 minutes to monitor treatment response (Figure 7.21).

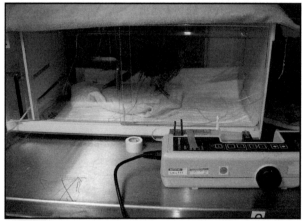

7.21 A Common Kestrel kept in a darkened oxygen enclosure.

Cranial trauma cases

The exceptions to keeping birds warm are cranial trauma cases. These birds should be kept in quiet, dark surroundings at a moderate to cool temperature, as keeping them warm will cause cerebral vasodilatation, with a resultant increase in intracranial pressure. While steroids have been given in cases of acute cranial trauma, their use remains controversial. If steroids are used, care should be taken due to the risks of immunosuppression, and only short-acting drugs such as prednisolone sodium succinate should be chosen. It is also prudent to use prophylactic antibiotics as well as itraconazole to help to prevent aspergillosis, a particular concern in sick, stressed and immunocompromised raptors.

Stabilization period

If a bird is already sufficiently stable it is advisable to take blood and at least perform a blood smear evaluation and PCV, and if possible some biochemistry tests (see Chapter 9), *before* initiating fluid therapy. The blood smear will help to demonstrate more marked inflammatory responses and blood parasites. These initial test results will also allow assessment of the bird's response to treatment.

If instigating treatment of a pigeon with a fluoro-quinolone or tetracycline, it is prudent if possible to store some faeces for later *Chlamydophila* poly-merase chain reaction (PCR) testing, as these drugs rapidly halt the shedding of elementary bodies and may lead to false-negative test results.

Once the bird has been initially stabilized to a degree, a more thorough physical examination and further diagnostic procedures may be performed. Brief anaesthesia and radiography may be indicated even if a bird is not entirely stable, for example in a collapsed bird, or a bird demonstrating seizures that are suspicious for lead toxicity from the history. In contrast, fractures are usually perceived as an emergency by owners, but apart from analgesia and some initial immobilization, these can usually wait until the bird is as stable as possible before there is a need for radiographs and any attempts at fracture repair. An exception is open fractures, which must be covered with sterile dressings and broad-spectrum antibiosis started to prevent the development of osteomyelitis.

As emergency avian patients will already be immunosuppressed, it is advisable to consider starting antibiosis during the stabilization period. In the case of susceptible raptor species it is also advisable to institute prophylaxis for aspergillosis with itraconazole at 10 mg/kg once daily.

Cardiorespiratory resuscitation

In the case of cardiorespiratory arrest, once an endotracheal tube or air sac tube is in place to establish an airway (A), the bird should be manually ventilated at 1 breath per 5 seconds (B), and adrenaline administered either intravenously or, if this is not possible, sublingually, while 'circulatory pumping' (C) is performed. Even a Canary can be intubated by using a intravenous catheter, attached to a cut-down 2 ml syringe barrel, and a connector. If this is not possible, a mask and cardiac massage may be sufficient.

Many texts describe cardiac massage with chest compressions over the sternum as the technique of choice, but in the author's experience, and considering the anatomy of the avian chest, this is rarely beneficial. In fact, many biologists use chest compression as a euthanasia technique in small passerine birds in the field. Instead, once adrenaline has been administered, venous return may be induced by placing the bird in dorsal recumbency and rapidly pumping the bird's legs cranially and caudally, holding the tibiotarsi. With this technique the author has been successful in resuscitating numerous birds, from small passerine species to large raptors. Another succesful method is to perform cardiac massage by inserting a finger below the sternum into the chest cavity.

Monitoring

Pulse oximetry
Pulse oximetry has limitations in the monitoring of critical avian patients. Cardiac and respiratory arrest are most often simultaneous in birds, and by the time changes are noticed via the pulse oximeter it may be too late. As well as encouraging retrospective rather than proactive monitoring, using a pulse oximeter can distract one from monitoring vital signs properly, and high heart rates and poor contact can mean that most of the time is spent adjusting the probe rather than actually monitoring the patient.

ECG monitoring
Electrocardiographic monitoring may be more useful in critical cases, or when anaesthetizing emergencies for procedures such as radiography or endoscopy. It should be remembered that the mean electrical axis of ventricular depolarization, the (Q)RS complex, is negative in birds due to depolarization starting subepicardially, in contrast to mammals (see Chapter 10). There is controversy about whether birds have a Q wave, and the entire ventricular depolarization complex's appearance is variable between different avian species, which means that different species cannot be compared.

Hospitalization

All of the species discussed in this Manual should preferably be hospitalized out of sight and sound of predatory animals such as dogs and cats, and, in the case of pigeons and passerines, out of sight of raptors as well. Although many working raptors are well used to dogs, it helps to limit stress and further immunosuppression of sick birds if they are kept in a quieter environment.

It is also wise to keep predatory birds (raptors) away from small mammals such as rabbits. Besides stress to the small mammals, there is also the risk of the raptor flying at the perceived quarry and potentially injuring itself in the cage. Furthermore, hospitalized rabbits are provided with hay and occasionally straw, and while the risk is small if changed daily, these could act as a source of *Aspergillus* spores for inhalation by an immunosuppressed raptor.

Wooden perches should preferably not be used for raptors. These are difficult to clean and disinfect adequately, and when moist (after cleaning) can encourage fungal growth, with the risk of an *Aspergillus* air sacculitis developing in already immunosuppressed birds. Leather-bound perches as used by many falconers are also difficult to disinfect adequately between birds. While Astroturf-covered perches are good for the prevention of bumblefoot in debilitated birds, these too can sometimes be difficult to scrub clean adequately between different birds. A solution is to make these Astroturf strips easy to remove (by using cable ties) and soak them in disinfectant between different patients.

Normal kennels may be used for raptors, but the front should be covered with cloth to decrease stress and prevent birds from injuring themselves if startled. Perspex-fronted kennels are better than bar-fronted kennels, in which a bird's limbs can become injured. If admitting falconry birds briefly as day-patients for diagnostic or clinical procedures, the use of the owner's own transport box or bow perch is often best and poses the least stress and disease risks to the bird.

Being perching birds, most raptors have relatively long tails. If not kept perched, or if they are ill, birds spending time on the ground will rapidly soil and break their remiges (tail feathers), which is clearly an important concern in these performance birds. It is essential to apply a tail guard in any raptor hospitalized for more than the briefest period (see Chapter 6).

Hygiene and warmth

Good hygiene and daily cleaning of cages is essential in debilitated and hence immunosuppressed birds. Between birds, disinfection is needed not only of cages and the furniture, such as perches, but also of crop tubes, specula and any other equipment used for more than one bird.

Natural branches can be used for perching passerine birds and simply disposed of after hospitalization rather than being reused.

If a dedicated avian ward is available, warming the entire room significantly is often best. If this is not possible, a source of warmth is needed. Commercial hospitalization units or incubators will keep small birds warm and also help to isolate individuals, preventing the spread of infectious agents to other birds in the ward. Orthodox metal wire bird cages will not keep sick birds warm or isolated, and will allow the spread of diseases such as chlamydophilosis in the hospital. Perspex oxygen cages are a simple alternative: they are easy to clean and disinfect and will isolate individuals, as well as being usable as an oxygen cage if needed.

Feeding and nutrition

There may be a temptation to feed a critically ill raptor on admission, but in many cases mild dehydration and reduced gastrointestinal motility may rapidly lead to crop stasis and 'sour crop'. Feeding should only be instituted once a bird's dehydration has been addressed. Even if birds do eat on their own, sick birds or those recovering from trauma have increased energy requirements and may need supplementary tube feeding.

Hill's a/d diet is useful for feeding debilitated raptors and has an energy concentration of 1.1 kcal/ml. This is obviously reduced if the diet is mixed with water for ease of tube feeding. In the absence of a commercial avian enteral formula, vegetable baby foods may be tube-fed to pigeons and passerine birds in practice.

> **All birds should be weighed once or twice daily to check that no weight loss has occurred.**

Volume and frequency of feeding

The basal metabolic rate (BMR) of birds is the minimum amount of energy needed for daily maintenance.

- BMR (kcal) = 78 × (weight (kg))$^{0.75}$ in non-passerine birds (raptors and pigeons).
- BMR (kcal) = 129 × (weight (kg))$^{0.75}$ in passerine birds.

Maintenance energy requirement (MER) is the BMR plus the energy needed for normal physical activity, digestion and absorption. In healthy birds MER is approximately 1.5 × BMR. In addition, birds recovering from trauma or disease have higher energy requirements, approximately 1.5–2 × normal MER. These formulae may be used to calculate the quantities and frequencies needed for feeding a hospitalized bird. Figures 7.22 and 7.23 give some rough limits for the volumes and frequencies of feeding possible.

	Healthy bird	Severe illness/trauma
Harris' Hawk	10%	15–20%
Pigeon	15%	20–30%
Canary	25%	40–50%

7.22 Guide to daily feeding requirements as a percentage of body weight.

Species	Volume (ml)	Minimum frequency
Harris' Hawk	20–45	q8–12h
Peregrine Falcon	20–60	q8–12h
Racing pigeon	1.5–8	q6–12h
Finch	0.2–0.5	q4–6h
Canary	0.3–1	q4–8h

7.23 Guide to tube-feeding volumes (data from Quesenberry and Hillyer, 1994). In debilitated starved birds, the frequency should be higher.

References and further reading

Carpenter JW (2005) *Exotic Animal Formulary*. Elsevier Saunders, St Louis

Doneley B, Harrison GJ and Lightfoot TL (2006) Maximising information from the physical examination. In: *Clinical Avian Medicine*, ed. GJ Harrison and TL Lightfoot, pp. 153–212. Spix Publishing, Palm Beach, FL

Gunkel C and Lafortune M (2005) Current techniques in avian anaesthesia. *Seminars in Avian and Exotic Pet Medicine* **14**(4), 263–276

Harrison GJ and Lightfoot TL (2006) Emergency and critical care. In: *Clinical Avian Medicine*, ed. GL Harrison and TL Lightfoot, pp. 213–232. Spix Publishing, Palm Beach, FL

Jenkins JR (1997) Avian critical care and emergency medicine. In: *Avian Medicine and Surgery*, ed. RB Altman, SL Clubb, GM Dorrestein and K Quesenberry, pp. 839–863. WB Saunders, Philadelphia

Kovach AGB, Szasz E and Mayer NPL (1969) Mortality of various avian and mammalian species following blood loss. *Acta Physiologica Academia Scientifica Hungarica* **35**, 109

Lichtenberger M (2005) Determination of indirect blood pressure in the companion bird. *Seminars in Avian and Exotic Pet Medicine* **14**(2), 149–152

Lumeij JT, Sprang EPM and Redig PT (1998) Further studies on allopurinol induced hyperuricaemia and visceral gout in red-tailed hawks (*Buteo jamaicensis*). *Avian Pathology* **27**, 390–393

McKinney P (2003) Clinical applications of the i-stat blood analyser in avian practice. In: *Proceedings 7th European AAV Conference, Loro Parque, Tenerife, Apr. 23–26*, pp. 347–352

Poffers J, Lumeij JT and Redig PT (2002) Further studies on the use of allopurinol to reduce plasma uric acid concentrations in the red-tailed hawk (*Buteo jamaicensis*) hyperuricaemic model. *Avian Pathology* **31**, 567–572

Quesenberry KE and Hillyer EV (1994) Supportive care and emergency therapy. In: *Avian Medicine: Principles and Application*, ed. BW Ritchie, GJ Harrison and LR Harrison, pp. 382–416. Wingers, Lake Worth, FL

Ritchie BW, Harrison GJ and Harrison LR (1994) *Avian Medicine: Principles and Application*. Wingers Publishing, Lake Worth, FL

Sandmeier P, Stauber EH, Wardrop KJ and Washizuka A (1994) Survival of pigeon red blood cells after transfusion into selected raptors. *Journal of the Avian Veterinary Medicine Association* **3**, 427–429

Whittow GC (2000) *Sturkie's Avian Physiology*, p. 685. Academic Press, San Diego

8

Basic techniques

John Chitty

Injection techniques

The following sections apply to all raptors, pigeons and passerine birds unless specifically stated otherwise.

Intramuscular injection

This is the most common route by which injectable drugs are given to captive birds. In general injections are given into the pectoral muscle mass rather than the leg because:

- The pectoral muscle mass is larger
- There are concerns over the presence of a renal portal venous system resulting in effects on the drug pharmacokinetics.

The smallest gauge of needle should be used with respect to the viscosity of the drug and size of bird. In general needles of 23 gauge or smaller are used, though 21 gauge needles may be used in larger birds when injecting viscous drugs and 25 gauge needles may be more appropriate when injecting non-viscous substances in passerine birds.

1. The feathers should be parted and the skin cleansed.
2. The needle is inserted into the mid to caudal portion of the muscle (Figure 8.1) and the substance is injected into the *middle* of the mass, i.e. passing caudal-to-cranial parallel with the sternum.

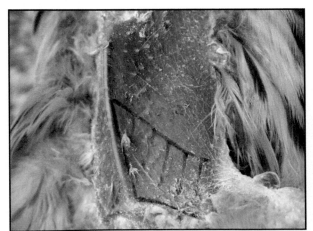

8.1 Pectoral muscle mass (in an emaciated Hobby). The shading shows the area favoured for injections and for microchips. (© John Chitty)

3. Prior to injection the operator should draw back to ensure that the substance is not being inadvertently injected into a blood vessel. It is especially important to avoid the venous plexus between the muscle layers.

Care should be taken with irritant substances and volume.

- *Irritant substances*. Certain drugs, e.g. enrofloxacin and certain long-acting oxytetracycline preparations, may be extremely irritant. Post-mortem examination of birds that have received multiple intramuscular injections of these compounds may show extensive areas of bruising. In the live bird, high levels of plasma creatinine kinase may be seen following even a single injection of an irritant drug.
- *Volume*. Injection of 0.1 ml into a 500 g bird is equivalent (on a weight-to-weight basis) to a single injection of 14 ml in a 70 kg human. Although this argument is extremely simplistic and the pectoral muscle mass is comparatively much larger than any in humans, care should be taken with injecting large volumes as this may be a source of pain in an already sick bird.

Therefore, repeated injections of irritant drugs should preferably be avoided and the oral route should be used as soon as practicable, especially in falconers' birds or racing pigeons (to avoid potential effects on performance). If this is not possible, or if it is felt that oral absorption would not be reliable, the intramuscular route should be used but injection sites should be varied. In these cases, and where injection volumes are small, use of leg muscles is acceptable. The cranial tibial muscle should be used (Figure 8.2).

Large volumes of drugs (>1 ml/500 g) should be split between sites or placed subcutaneously if possible.

Microchip placement

This is an effective means of identifying the individual bird in a way that is difficult for bird or person to modify or damage.

The microchip should be inserted into the left pectoral muscle mass (see Figure 8.1) as per British Veterinary Zoological Society recommendations. This may be done with the bird conscious or anaesthetized; the author recommends that all birds <200 g should be anaesthetized for this procedure.

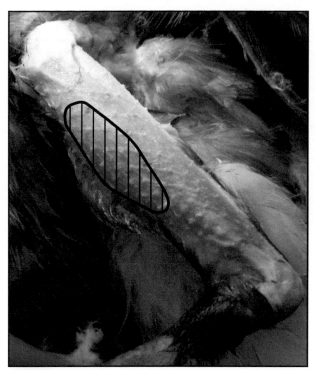

8.2 Caudal tibial muscle mass (Eurasian Buzzard). The shaded area is used for intramuscular injection. (© John Chitty)

It should be noted that *microchipping may be inappropriate for very small passerine birds*, due to the difficulties in placing a large chip in a very small muscle mass without causing damage. Subcutaneous placement may cause less damage (though skin closure will be required); however, it is easy to find and remove microchips placed subcutaneously.

Prior to insertion the bird should be scanned in case it is already microchipped. There have been many guidelines issued by different authorities in different countries on implantation sites. As a result, microchips may have been implanted in the right pectoral muscle, the base of the neck or either thigh. The *whole* bird should be scanned before concluding that it is not already microchipped. If in doubt the whole bird should be radiographed, as this is the only way to prove conclusively that there is no microchip present.

1. The feathers are parted and the skin is prepared aseptically.
2. The needle is inserted in the caudal third of the muscle mass and directed cranially so that the microchip is placed in the approximate middle of the mass between superficial and deep pectoral muscles. It is extremely important not to place the microchip too far cranially, so as to avoid a large plexus of nerves and blood vessels in this region. Placement of microchips too deep into the muscle mass has been associated with reports of microchip migration and subsequent interference with the tendons of the shoulder.
3. Occasionally, haemorrhage may be a problem. This may be avoided by stretching the skin to one side so that the holes in skin and muscle are not aligned. The skin hole may be closed with a suture or with tissue glue.
4. Digital pressure should be placed on tissue overlying the needle as it is withdrawn, to reduce the chance of the microchip being withdrawn with the needle.

> Implanted microchips should be read whenever the bird is examined. If the chip cannot be detected, the bird should be radiographed.

Subcutaneous injection

This is a very useful route for fluid therapy and large-volume drugs. However, irritant drugs should not be injected subcutaneously instead of intramuscularly as there is a risk of skin necrosis, especially where large volumes are given.

Absorption from these sites is rapid and large volumes of fluid (up to 20 ml/kg) may be absorbed within 15 minutes. This absorption rate may be increased by adding hyaluronidase at 150 units/litre.

The injection site is prepared as described above, the ideal site being the large precrural fold (Figure 8.3).

Care should be taken not to enter the body cavity inadvertently while injecting.

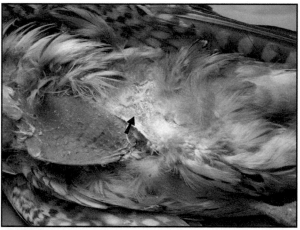

8.3 Precrural fold (arrowed) in a Hobby. The area has been plucked. (© John Chitty)

Intravenous injection and blood collection

Intravenous injection and blood collection sites are shown in Figures 8.4 to 8.9.

Wetting the skin with a spirit-soaked swab improves visualization. Wetting the feathers will keep them out of the way, but care must be taken not to overdo this as hypothermia may result. In passerine birds care must be taken not to cause toxicity, as the birds will preen their feathers immediately afterwards.

In most cases, two operators are required for bleeding or injecting conscious birds, apart from very small passerine birds (where the simple one-handed holding technique described in Chapter 6 greatly facilitates the procedure).

Site	Restraint	Pros	Cons	Tips
Right jugular vein (Figure 8.5a)	Bird should be restrained or anaesthetized and neck extended. Parting of feathers reveals the vein running under a large apterium. Placement of digit at base of neck raises the vein	Easy. Large volumes can be taken. Haemostasis relatively simple. Restraint may be stressful to sensitive or dyspnoeic birds	Very difficult for left-handed operators, though left jugular may be utilized in larger species. Handling may be difficult in larger species (eagles, vultures) or in large falcons (e.g. female Gyrfalcons) whose muscular neck can be hard to extend. Struggling birds may cause laceration of the vein and fatal subcutaneous haemorrhage; general anaesthesia may therefore be appropriate	Anaesthesia may be recommended for this technique. Gentle digital pressure applied afterwards to avoid haematoma formation
Superficial ulnar/basilic vein (Figure 8.5b)	Bird is restrained or anaesthetized and placed on its back. One wing is extended and the vein visualized. Operator raises vein with free hand	Easier for left-handed operators. Restraint relatively simple, especially in larger species	Fragile vein and may be hard to draw large volumes, especially in smaller birds. Haemostasis can be hard to achieve and bird should be released to allow it to calm down and its blood pressure to drop. This is preferable to prolonged handling. Unlike jugular venepuncture, this haemorrhage is unlikely to be fatal and at least is readily visible; however, small losses may cause a lot of mess and distress to owners. Occasionally a haematoma may form along with a slight wing drop that may last a day or two	To facilitate haemostasis a drop of tissue glue may be helpful
Superficial plantar metatarsal/ caudal tibial vein (Figure 8.5c)	Bird is restrained and leg extended. Operator can raise the vein with free hand. Chicks can be left in 'sitting' position with feet in front of them. Restraint is normally minimal, but in adults the leg must be fixed to avoid operator injury	Superficial, simple to visualize and raise. Restraint easy, especially in juveniles/chicks. In chicks, excellent site for catheter placement	Haemostasis difficult	Tissue glue may facilitate haemostasis or a light temporary dressing may be applied
Toe clip			Inappropriate in raptors, where damage to talons is undesirable and lack of access to other veins unlikely	

8.4 Venepuncture sites in raptors.

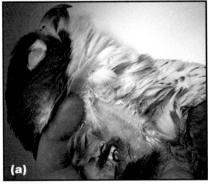 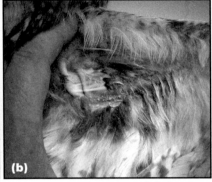 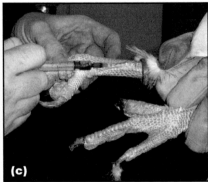

8.5 Intravenous injection and blood collection sites in raptors. **(a)** Jugular vein (Peregrine Falcon, anaesthetized). **(b)** Ulnar vein (Tawny Owl). **(c)** Venepuncture of the caudal tibial vein (White-headed Vulture). (a,b, © John Chitty; c, courtesy of the Hawk Conservancy Trust)

Site	Restraint	Pros	Cons	Tips
Right jugular vein (Figure 8.7a)			Vein does not lie under an apterium and is very hard to visualize (even after feather removal) as skin is so thick, therefore rarely used	
Superficial ulnar/basilic vein (Figure 8.7b)	Bird is restrained or anaesthetized and placed on its back. One wing is extended and the vein visualized. Operator raises vein with free hand	Restraint simple	Fragile vein and may be hard to draw large volumes. Haemostasis can be hard to achieve and bird should be replaced in carrier to allow it to calm down and blood pressure to drop. This is preferable to prolonged handling. This haemorrhage is unlikely to be fatal and at least is readily visible; however, small losses may cause a lot of mess and distress to owners	To facilitate haemostasis a drop of tissue glue may be helpful. Bending the needle prior to venepuncture greatly facilitates the technique

8.6 Venepuncture sites in pigeons. (continues) ▶

Site	Restraint	Pros	Cons	Tips
Superficial plantar metatarsal/ caudal tibial vein (Figure 8.7c)	Bird is restrained and leg extended. Operator can raise vein with free hand	Superficial, simple to find and raise. Easily visualized. Restraint is easy	Very fragile and only possible to draw small volumes. Haemostasis difficult	Only of use where other veins damaged or where very small volumes of blood required. Tissue glue may facilitate haemostasis
Toe clip (Figure 8.7d)	Bird is restrained and a nail cut short enough that the nail bed is penetrated. To increase bleeding, nail should be cut in opposite manner to that described for nail trim (see later)	Easy	Unsuitable for collection for biochemistry/ haematology due to contamination from tissue fluid or from urates/faeces on claw. Impossible to collect large volumes. Technique may cause pain. Haemostasis important, as is risk of introducing infection	Only of use when collecting very small volumes or single drops. Vein should be cauterized afterwards; silver nitrate or potassium permanganate are appropriate. Attention should be paid to welfare aspects of this technique

8.6 (continued) Venepuncture sites in pigeons.

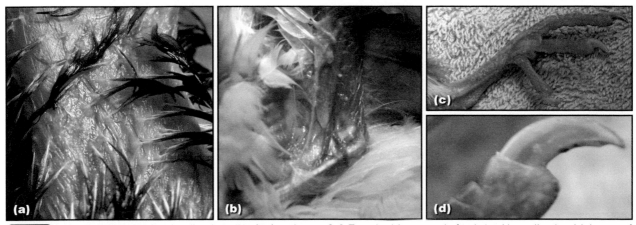

8.7 Intravenous and blood collection sites in the pigeon. **(a)** Even in this sparsely feathered juvenile, the thickness of the skin hinders finding the jugular despite wetting the skin. **(b)** Ulnar/basilic vein. **(c)** Caudal tibial vein. **(d)** Nail: the 'quick' is clearly visible. (© John Chitty)

Site	Restraint	Pros	Cons	Tips
Right jugular vein (Figure 8.9a)	Bird should be restrained using one-handed ringer's grip and the neck extended. Parting of feathers reveals the vein running under a large apterium. Placement of digit at base of neck raises the vein	Easy. Relatively large volumes can be taken. Haemostasis relatively simple (< 150 g). Restraint may be stressful to sensitive or dyspnoeic birds – these should be anaesthetized	Very difficult for left-handed operators. Struggling birds may cause laceration of the vein and fatal subcutaneous haemorrhage; general anaesthesia may therefore be appropriate. Some operator experience is necessary	Gentle digital pressure applied afterwards to avoid haematoma formation
Superficial ulnar/ basilic vein (Figure 8.9b)	Bird is restrained or anaesthetized and placed on its back. One wing is extended and the vein visualized. Operator raises the vein with free hand	Easier for left-handed operators. Restraint relatively simple	Vein far too small to be of practical value in smaller species, can only really be utilized in larger passerines	In small finches, a drop of blood may be obtained for smear by needle prick of ulnar vein
Superficial plantar metatarsal/ caudal tibial vein (Figure 8.9c)			Too small to allow taking of a full sample in these species	Needle prick allows collection of drop or two for blood smear etc.

8.8 Venepuncture sites in passerine birds. (continues) ▶

Site	Restraint	Pros	Cons	Tips
Toe clip	Bird is restrained and a nail cut short enough to penetrate nail bed. To increase bleeding, nail should be cut in opposite manner to that described for nail trim (see later)	Easy	Unsuitable for collection for biochemistry/haematology due to contamination from tissue fluid or from urates/faeces on claw. Impossible to collect large volumes. Technique may cause pain. Haemostasis important, as is risk of introducing infection	May be of use when collecting very small volumes (e.g. for sexing) or for obtaining single drop for blood smear (e.g. screening for atoxoplasmosis). Vein should be cauterized afterwards; silver nitrate or potassium permanganate are appropriate. Attention should be paid to welfare aspects of this technique

8.8 (continued) Venepuncture sites in passerine birds.

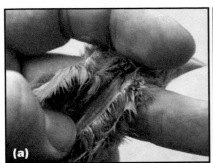 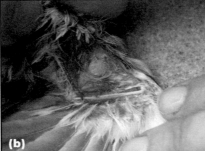 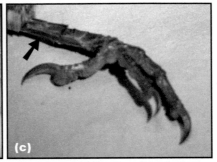

8.9 Intravenous injection and blood collection sites in a Greenfinch. **(a)** A modified ringer's grip allows access to the jugular vein. **(b)** Ulnar/basilic vein. **(c)** Caudal tibial vein. (© John Chitty)

The size of needle and syringe used for collecting blood will vary depending on size of bird (e.g. 2.5 ml syringe and 23 gauge 5/8" needle for blood collection from the jugular vein of a 1 kg Harris' Hawk; 1 ml syringe and 25 gauge 5/8" needle for collection from a pigeon's ulnar vein; 0.5 ml insulin syringe with 27 gauge needle for collection from a Canary's jugular vein). For haematology collection the largest needle size that can be used safely should be selected where possible, so that damage to blood cells is avoided.

As with mammals, blood up to approximately 1% body weight may be safely removed (e.g. up to 10 ml from a 1000 g Harris' Hawk; up to 0.2 ml from a 20 g finch). It is important to note that this figure is based on healthy birds; the proportion should be slightly reduced for sick or dehydrated birds.

Injected drugs should be given slowly to avoid embolic effects.

Intravenous catheter placement

In some cases, placement of an intravenous catheter may be considered either for continuous or bolus fluid therapy, or where repeated use of intravenous drugs is required. Either the right jugular or basilic vein may be used, but the former may be more difficult to maintain without extensive dressings and the latter is preferred in birds larger than 300 g. In raptors (especially chicks and juveniles) the caudal tibial vein may be used (Figure 8.10). Most passerine birds are too small for this technique to be attempted with any degree of ease.

The catheter can be taped or sutured in place. When placed in the basilic vein, extensions can be

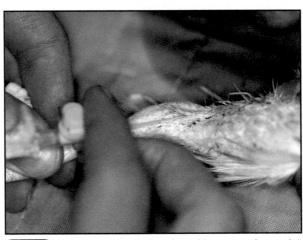

8.10 Intravenous catheter placed in a raptor's caudal tibial vein. (© Michael Lierz)

used allowing an injection port to be positioned on the dorsum of the wing, giving easier access. Where repeated access is to be used the catheter should be heparinized at the start and finish of the dosing.

Intraosseous injection

This is an alternative route for continuous or bolus fluid therapy. Fluids are injected into the medullary cavity of either the ulna or the tibiotarsus (the pneumatized humerus must *not* be used!). Uptake into the main circulation is virtually instantaneous, due to the central venous sinus.

In each case the bird should be anaesthetized (unless extreme urgency is required) and the site should be prepared aseptically.

A needle is introduced into the bone. This can either be a specialized bone needle (Cook UK, Letchworth) or a standard injection needle (18 gauge 1.5" for birds > 700 g; 21 gauge 1" for birds between 200 and 700 g; 23 gauge 1" for birds < 200 g). The technique is more tricky in small passerine birds (< 100 g) and there is a greater risk of iatrogenic bone fracture, but with care it can be accomplished using a 25 gauge 5/8" needle.

- *Ulna*. The dorsal condyle just proximal to the carpus should be identified. With the carpus flexed, the needle is driven through this proximally into the medullary cavity where it can be 'felt' *in situ*. To confirm correct positioning, a small volume of fluid may be injected while watching the basilic vein, where the fluid bolus may be seen. Alternatively, radiography may be used to confirm needle position (Figure 8.11).
- *Tibiotarsus*. The cranial cnemial crest is identified just distal to the stifle and the needle is inserted through this distally into the medullary cavity. As the 'tibial plateau' on the lateral side is wider than the medullary cavity, the needle should be inserted from the craniomedial aspect of the proximal tibiotarsus. This route may appear to be simpler than the other, but it is more difficult to confirm that the needle is in place other than 'feeling' it within the bony cavity.

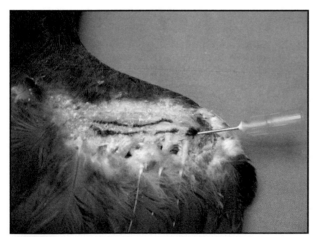

8.11 Plucked wing of a Hobby. The positions of the radius and ulna are marked. The needle is inserted through the dorsal tuberosity of the ulna. (© John Chitty)

In either case the needle is finally taped or bandaged in place.

In this author's opinion these sites are easier to access and maintain than the intravenous route. However, as the fluid needs to be given under pressure some specialized equipment is required; this may be either a syringe pump or 'Flowline' apparatus (Arnolds, UK). Alternatively the needle may be capped and bolus fluids given at intervals.

Care should be taken when placing this equipment in osteoporotic birds as iatrogenic fractures may result. It is advised that it should not be left in place for more than 3 days as there is some risk of osteomyelitis.

Crop tubing

This is a simple and effective means of providing oral drugs or fluids, or for feeding sick birds (Figure 8.12). Plastic or metal tubes may be used. Metal tubes (straight or curved) are available commercially in a range of sizes suitable for birds from small finches to large raptors. They should be used with care, as oesophageal perforation is possible with rigid tubes. Compared with parrots, there is much less chance of any of the species in this Manual (with the exception of large eagles and vultures, in which a metal tube should always be used) chewing and breaking the tube. Therefore, a number of different tubes commonly found in veterinary practice may be used or adapted for this purpose (Figure 8.13). Metal Spreull needles used for ear flushing in dogs and cats also make excellent crop tubes for small raptors, pigeons and larger passerine birds.

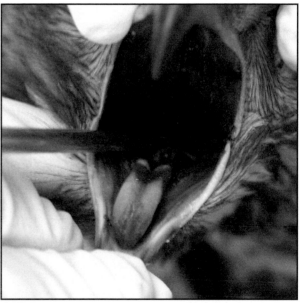

8.12 Crop tubing a raptor. Note the extension of the head and the position of the tube over the glottis and along the right side of the mouth. (© John Chitty)

Species	Tube
Raptor	Dog urinary catheters ideal Tubes of a variety of lengths should be kept, allowing use in a range of species It is vital that the cut end is filed and heated to make a smooth edge – cut edges can cause a lot of damage
Pigeon	Jackson cat catheters are ideal in their normal shape (minus stylet!) or with the end removed and smoothed (as above) Alternatively a dog catheter may be cut and smoothed as above
Passerine birds	Jackson cat catheters may be used for larger species (e.g. mynah bird). Lachrymal cannulae excellent for smaller species but should be used with some care as they are more rigid than other plastic tubes

8.13 Crop tubes used in practice for raptors, pigeons and passerine birds.

As a general rule, the largest tube size possible should be used to help to avoid glottal insertion.

1. The bird should be restrained in a towel and the bill opened using the thumb and index finger placed in the commissures of the beak. In very large raptors (eagles or large vultures) a mouth gag may be used.
2. The neck is extended and the tube is passed on the right side lateral and dorsal to the glottis. This is much easier than in parrots as none of these species have such a large fleshy tongue. Should resistance be encountered or the bird become distressed, the tube should be withdrawn and the process attempted again.
3. Prior to administering the fluid bolus, the tube should be felt within the crop.
4. Fluids should be pre-warmed and given slowly to avoid regurgitation. The volume should not exceed 20 ml/kg in each dose, but the process may be repeated as soon as the crop empties.

Greater care should always be taken with owls. They do not have a crop; therefore the tube is placed into the distal oesophagus and a smaller volume of fluid should be given (up to 12 ml/kg) as a bolus. Gentle palpation of the abdomen may indicate if the bird can tolerate a bolus of fluid. Similarly it is more difficult to assess whether or not the tube is in the oesophagus, not the trachea. The neck should always be palpated prior to the injection of any fluid. This should permit the finding of two tubes: the trachea (having complete rings) *and* the stomach tube. If in doubt the stomach tube may be gently moved so it can be felt more easily.

Anaesthetized birds should be allowed to recover fully before being given fluids or medication by crop tube.

The above technique may also be used to obtain a diagnostic crop washing. The tube should be inserted and warmed isotonic saline passed into the crop. A small volume is aspirated and submitted for cytology, culture/sensitivity, etc.

Beak trimming

Pigeons and passerine birds

It is very rare for pigeons to require beak trimming. Occasionally congenital deformities or injuries may result in displacement and misalignment of the beak. In these cases the soft beak is easily trimmed or maintained using small nail clippers.

It is also relatively unusual for passerine birds to require beak trimming. Misalignment may occur, as in pigeons, but it is rarely necessary to do more than trim back the tips of the beaks with a sharp set of clippers. In larger passerine birds a small Dremel grinder may be useful for reshaping a beak.

In the event of over-trimming, bleeding tissue may be cauterized using heat or chemicals (e.g. potassium permanganate).

Raptors

Trimming (or coping) of the beak is frequently performed in raptors.

As in other species, the principal natural means of maintenance of beak shape are:

- Its own action (wear of upper against lower beak)
- Grinding of the beak against substrate or against bones etc. in prey.

Overgrowths in raptors may occur due to:

- Malformation in young birds (rare)
- Damage to beak and/or cere such that beak growth is affected or permanent deficits in beak tissues result. This may be from trauma or disease (e.g. bacterial or parasitic infection)
- Iatrogenic. Unnecessary or badly done beak trims may damage sensitive tissues, resulting in worsening of the problem
- Abnormal keratin metabolism (e.g. malnutrition or liver disease). It is important to make a thorough assessment of any adult bird presenting with an overgrown beak (Figure 8.14). Malnutrition, resulting in lack of sulphur-containing essential amino acids, is rare in birds being fed whole carcasses, but it may be possible that some birds do suffer from inability to process these compounds. If such deficiencies are suspected, methionine may given as a supplement and the effects assessed
- Lack of bone in the diet. Some falconers feel that this may result in inadequate wear of the beak. However, this is rarely proven and beak changes may reflect dietary imbalance more than a simple lack of solid material.

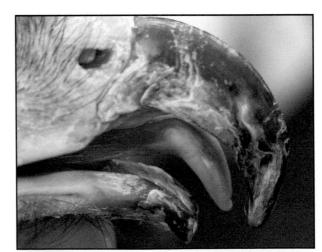

8.14 Beak dystrophy in a Harris' Hawk. Note the smoother newer beak growth near the cere, reflecting some response to an essential amino acid supplement. The beak is elongated, reflecting abnormal wear between the two beaks. (© John Chitty)

As in parrots, the principal aim is not just to trim the beak but to reshape it with the ultimate aim that the beak will be able to 'maintain itself'. With this in mind it is essential that the normal anatomy of the beak is known for that species, before undertaking the procedure (Figure 8.15).

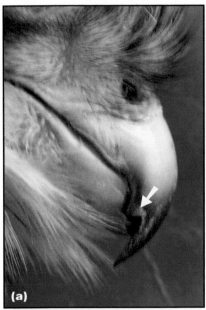

8.15

(a) Normal falcon beak (Common Kestrel). Note the tomial 'tooth', which must be left intact when coping the beak. (b) Normal hawk beak (Eurasian Buzzard), which lacks the 'tooth'. (© John Chitty)

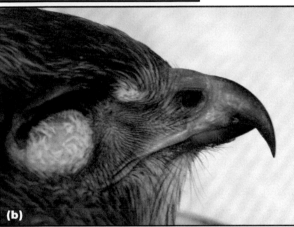

It is rare that the reshaping can be done using clippers alone. Many experienced falconers will undertake this procedure themselves using small clippers and a set of files. Either good quality files (those used for sharpening dental instruments are excellent (S Girling, 2004, personal communication)) or low-torque, low-speed grinding tools (e.g. Dremel Minimite) are ideal for beak shaping. Grinding pieces in a range of different sizes and shapes make the job much easier.

Many falconry birds can be coped conscious while cast. However, general anaesthesia is indicated where extensive reshaping is required or where the bird is not calm and easily handled.

Beak layers should be taken back carefully and slowly to avoid entering the sensitive underlying tissues. If haemorrhage is encountered, the area should be cauterized with potassium permanganate or silver nitrate and no further tissue should be removed in this region.

Nail/talon trimming

> In all cases, any underlying causes for nail overgrowth should be identified and corrected.

Pigeons and passerine birds

It is very unusual for pigeons to be presented with overgrown nails for trimming.

Finches are frequently presented with very overgrown (sometimes curling) nails. The reasons for this include:

- Perches. Perch width should be appropriate to the bird's size and individual preference. Overgrown nails may be seen in conjunction with pressure lesions on the feet
- Failure to perch properly (e.g. due to arthritis)
- Malnutriton or liver disease. Abnormal keratin metabolism may result in an adult bird suddenly developing overgrown nails.

Raptors

While it may seem perverse to consider trimming talons as long sharp talons would seem essential for successful hunting, raptors are sometimes presented for trimming.

- In some 'handling' or display birds the falconer may request the tips of the talons to be removed and blunted to reduce the chances of injury to inexperienced handlers.
- In other cases, it may be felt that overlong talons may be contributory to self-injury and bumblefoot (though these theories are largely discredited).
- Some falconers may request blunting of talons in young birds that are too aggressive when grabbing at the lure; they feel that these may be predisposed to self-injury.
- Some cases may be due to malnutrition or liver disease, as described above.
- It is also possible that, following injury, a talon may grow back abnormally and so not wear down correctly.

Equipment and method

In this section the word 'nail' is used for both nail and talon, for ease of reading.

In general, specialist bird-nail clippers or very small cat-nail clippers may be used. In raptors a grinding tool (e.g. Dremel Minimite on high speed) can be very useful. In the latter case the nail can be shaped using the grinder but care must be taken not to damage the skin of the foot. Haemorrhage is less likely, as the heat from the grinder will aid in cauterizing the nail (Figure 8.16).

Where clippers are used the nail should be cut from side to side (Figure 8.17). This results in the nail being squeezed over the artery and haemorrhage being reduced. It will also reduce the chances of the nail splitting.

The artery is often found near the end of the nail. It is easy to see and avoid in white nails but less so in black nails. Therefore small amounts should be taken off each nail until either a desired length is reached or bleeding starts. There is no 'set length' to achieve when clipping nails but each case should be judged individually.

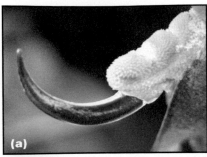
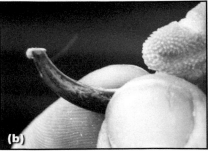
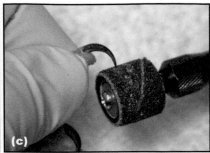

8.16 Nail cutting in falcons. Some falconers like very long talons **(a)** to be 'blunted' at the end of the flying season, as in this Harris' Hawk **(b)**. The talon is not drastically shortened but merely blunted. **(c)** A grinding tool is excellent for this purpose (here being used on the talon of a Hobby). (© John Chitty)

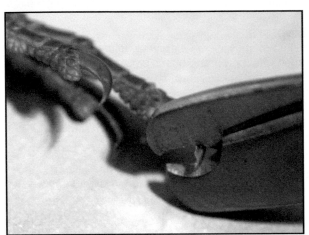

8.17 Clipping a finch's claw. Note the side-to-side squeeze so that bleeding is minimized should the blood vessel be cut accidentally. If a blood sample is required, the clippers should be applied 'top to bottom'. (© John Chitty)

There is usually no need to perform this procedure under general anaesthesia, unless the nails are grossly overgrown and haemorrhage will be unavoidable in bringing the nails back to a normal length. In these cases anaesthesia avoids the need for prolonged restraint.

Haemorrhage may be stopped by use of silver nitrate powder/sticks or potassium permanganate powder/crystals. Some practitioners advocate pressing the end of the talon into a bar of soap in order to seal the blood vessel and cleanse the lesion. The bird should be closely monitored until bleeding stops.

Just as in dogs, there is no set time for a re-clip, which should be done as required. Many birds will never need a clip.

Ring removal

A variety of identification rings may be attached to birds' legs. Damage to these rings by the bird's beak is very unlikely in these species and longer metatarsal bones than in parrots means that ring problems are less common. However, where a ring of inappropriate size has been placed an underlying pressure necrosis of the skin may result; this can progress to a deep infection or abscess. Other external causes, swelling or crusting of the underlying skin or movement of a ring into an inappropriate place (e.g. over the intertarsal joint) may result in constriction of and damage to underlying tissues. Further swelling results in increased constriction and severe damage to underlying structures, which can cause loss of the foot unless the ring is removed.

It is important that the legal consequences of removing an identification ring are considered and that appropriate action (e.g. placement of a microchip) is taken where this is necessary (see Chapter 37). Any removed ring should be retained and returned to the owner. Where possible, cutting should take place away from the engraved area so that the identification remains clear. It is also vital to keep accurate records of the procedure, signalment of the bird, and the number of the removed ring.

Removal of a ring, even in finches where light rings are used, is not always simple. Heavier rings on large eagles can be extremely difficult to remove. Routine equipment found in clinics may not be appropriate, as many clippers, cutters and saws will damage underlying tissues directly or by causing twisting of the ring during cutting. The latter may be the most common cause of iatrogenic fractures during this procedure. The risk is greatest in finches, where thin rings are easily cut using conventional nail clippers, but injury is common when the use of inappropriate tools causes ring twisting and leg fracture.

It is recommended that practices seeing birds invest in specialist ring cutters (e.g. from Veterinary Instrumentation, Sheffield, UK, or Veterinary Speciality Products, Boca Raton, Florida) and a Dremel tool with cutting burs for removing tougher rings. When using a cutting bur it is vital to avoid heat damage to the underlying tissues. The ring should be surrounded with wet swabs and regularly checked for overheating. If it feels hot, cutting should be stopped and the ring cooled with water before recommencing.

Small pliers, narrow-jawed bulldog clamps or old artery forceps may be used to grip and bend the cut ring away from the leg. Where specialist cutting equipment cannot be obtained a small hacksaw blade may be used to cut steel rings, but it should be noted that this technique is extremely difficult to perform without damaging underlying tissues.

To reduce patient struggling, it is recommended that ring removal is always carried out under general anaesthesia.

Imping

This technique is used to replace rectrices and remiges damaged during hunting. It has been used for many centuries in falconry, especially for accipiters, which frequently damage these feathers when crashing through hedges and bushes during hunting. It can also be used in feather-chewing raptors that have damaged the remiges such that they can no longer fly. It is rarely, if ever, performed on pigeons or passerine birds.

The technique is simple but fiddly (Lierz, 2000). Trained and hooded falconry birds will often be imped while conscious, as they are calm and still. Less experienced veterinary surgeons may prefer to anaesthetize the bird, or may approach an experienced falconer for help.

The best source of new feathers is from the same bird and falconers should always be advised to keep moulted remiges as they may come in useful later (it is often a mark of the experience of the falconer if they already do this). Failing this, feathers from the same species should be used. However, there is a disease risk in imping feathers from one bird to another. Feathers can be sterilized using ethylene oxide or they can be frozen prior to use in order to reduce contamination.

If desperate, feathers from a different but similarly sized species may be used.

1. The stump of the damaged feather is trimmed so that the exposed end is smooth.
2. The replacement feather is trimmed to 'fit' on to the end of the old calamus, creating a new feather of the same length as the original. For this reason the equivalent feather must be used if possible (i.e. P1 to P1, P2 to P2, etc.).
3. The replacement is grafted on to the old.
   i. A plastic or dowelling rod (or small-diameter knitting needle or kebab skewer) is trimmed or whittled so that it fits snugly into the base feather at one end.
   ii. The other end is similarly trimmed to fit into the calamus of the new feather.

iii. Cyanoacrylate (tissue) glue is applied to each end and the rod is inserted into the calami. This stage must be done quickly before the glue dries. It is extremely important that the apposition of the old and new feathers is exact and that the replacement feather is oriented correctly (Figure 8.18).

Surprisingly, these grafted feathers can be very strong and quite capable of allowing flight.

Broken blood feather

This is a common problem and should be the primary differential for any bird presented with profuse bleeding.

It is important that the bleeding is controlled in the correct manner. While ligation of or application of haemostatic compounds to the affected feather may be effective in the short term, these feathers frequently bleed again and often become infected. This may trigger feather chewing (in susceptible species) and in some cases dystrophy or cyst formation.

The feather should therefore be removed as soon as possible. It is generally done with the bird conscious. The damaged blood feather is grasped and pulled out slowly while slightly twisting the feather. Any residual bleeding from the follicle is controlled by gently squeezing the follicle for a few seconds. This technique stops haemorrhage by twisting and stretching the artery that enters via the base of the feather. It also stimulates the development of a new feather.

It should be noted that there are distinct regional preferences in approaching this problem. For example, falconers in Germany are opposed to removal of bleeding feathers and prefer to leave the damaged feather in situ. Hyaluronidase is injected into the base of the feather to stimulate detachment and thus replacement. This illustrates the importance of inexperienced veterinary surgeons conversing with falconers and reading falconry texts when beginning to deal with these species: traditions are very strong and falconers can be very sensitive.

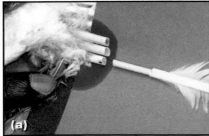
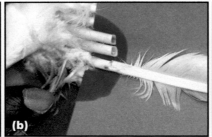
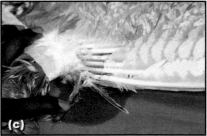
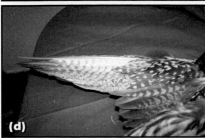

8.18 Imping. **(a)** A bamboo stick is glued into the new feather shaft using two-component glue. **(b)** The bamboo stick is now inserted into the old feather shaft. Note the paper below the feathers to avoid glue spoilage onto underlaying feathers. **(c)** All feathers to be imped are inserted. The glue needs about 5 minutes to harden, which allows the feathers to be rotated into the correct positions. **(d)** A correctly imped wing; the repair is not noticeable. (© Michael Lierz)

Euthanasia

Euthanasia of the sick bird is an option for the clinician where therapy is not possible, practicable or affordable and the bird is suffering.

Whatever the indication, euthanasia must be carried out in a humane manner and the decision taken with sensitivity for the owner. The human–bird bond is rarely as intense as with parrots and their owners, but many falconers are very close to their birds.

- *Ideally euthanasia should be by intravenous injection of pentobarbital.* It may be useful to induce anaesthesia prior to this injection. If owners are to be present, it may be prudent to consider health and safety aspects of waste anaesthetic gases. Sedation using intramuscular ketamine may also be used.
- Where the body is required for post-mortem examination, euthanasia may be achieved by overdosage of the volatile anaesthetic agent.
- Intracoelomic injection of pentobarbital cannot be recommended. It may result in rapid death, but it often does not and these injections may be associated with considerable pain to the bird. They may also disrupt internal anatomy, thus affecting necropsy findings.
- Intracardiac injection of pentobarbital may be achieved in smaller passerine birds, but inadvertent intrapulmonary injection may cause unnecessary distress to the bird.

In the field situation, such as severe injury to a hunting raptor, other methods may be considered. In these cases a physical means of euthanasia may be more appropriate to reduce bird suffering than transporting it for injection.

- Cervical dislocation is rarely easy in larger raptors, but a sharp hard blow to the head will render the bird unconscious or dead very quickly.
- Passerine birds and pigeons may be easily and quickly euthanased using cervical dislocation.

Reference

Lierz M. (2000) Imping feathers in birds of prey. *Exotic DVM* **1**(6), 13–15

9

Clinical pathology and post-mortem examination

Gerry M. Dorrestein

Haematology

Sample collection

Sites and techniques for venepuncture are illustrated in Chapter 8. When a live bird is presented for euthanasia and post-mortem examination it is a good habit to collect as much blood as possible from the right jugular vein: this will provide haematological and biochemical values in addition to the necropsy findings and it is useful to practise collection technique, especially in small birds. Heart puncture is mentioned in the literature but this may lead to organ damage and obscure pathological changes in the heart muscle or pericardium.

Many passerine species are extremely small and only tiny amounts of blood may be safely obtained. Obtaining a few drops of blood from the jugular vein means that a smear can be made; the rest may be collected into one or two heparinized capillary tubes. These may be spun and a PCV obtained. The buffy coat thickness may also be assessed. The tube may then be broken to obtain plasma for measurement of total solids and one or two biochemical tests. Some practices have machines that are able to perform a large number of tests on a single drop of blood.

Blood smears

Blood smears should be made with fresh non-heparinized blood as heparin interferes with staining. Fresh blood can be obtained either from a needle used to obtain the sample or from blood collected directly into a non-heparinized microhaematocrit tube. EDTA-treated blood can also be used (Figure 9.1). The smear is made using the standard two-slide wedge technique or by using the slide and cover glass method (see *BSAVA Manual of Clinical Pathology*). After spreading the blood the smear is air-dried.

Tests

A general blood examination includes a complete blood count (CBC) and plasma uric acid, bile acid, calcium, enzyme activities (Figure 9.2) and protein electrophoresis (Figure 9.3). Electrophoresis may not be available from all laboratories or may take several days. If such tests are not available or are not practicable, levels of total protein, albumin and globulin (and albumin:globulin ratio) may be obtained by other means. The CBC includes packed cell volume (PCV), red cell parameters (counts, size, haemoglobin measurements), white blood cell count (WBC) and the percentages of heterophils, lymphocytes and monocytes (Figure 9.4). Laboratory reference ranges for biochemical and haematological parameters are given in Appendix 3.

Additional tests are selected based on the clinical findings and the results of the general screening and other laboratory tests. If there is uncertainty about sample type and handling, the laboratory performing the analysis should be contacted. This is especially true for the analysis of toxic agents, where the choice of the container (zinc) and anticoagulant (lead) may significantly influence the values.

Heparinized blood	EDTA and clotted blood
Smaller sample required as it gives more plasma	Large sample required
Total protein is higher	Less serum available Fibrinogen absent
Separate immediately*, as cells break down, releasing enzymes and electrolytes	Allow to clot for an hour at room temperature and centrifuge in a gel tube
Can post. Plasma should be separated	Can post
Potentially poor cytology, so prepare air-dried smears	Good cytology

9.1 Comparison of heparinized and EDTA-treated blood for histology and biochemistry. * Unless requiring haematology and biochemistry from same sample (main changes affect electrolytes; these should always be tested patient-side or on separated posted samples).

Plasma proteins	
NB Heparin raises protein by approx 5 g/l due to presence of fibrinogen	
Albumin	Synthesized in the liver. Decreased in chronic disease, liver failure, starvation
Globulins	Increased in chronic hepatitis, acute/chronic infections
Enzymes	
Alanine aminotransferase (ALT)	Present in many tissues. Elevated by non-specific cell damage; non-specific
Alkaline phosphatase (ALP)	Present in duodenum and kidney; low hepatic activity; tissue-specific isoenzymes. Increased by cellular activity; elevation normal in juveniles and during egg-laying
Aspartate aminotransferase (AST)	Present in liver, heart, kidney, skeletal muscle, brain. Increased in liver/muscle disease, vitamin E/selenium deficiency. Increased by haemolysis. Last to elevate and last to recover in liver disease. Combine interpretation with other tests, e.g. CK.
Gamma-glutamyl transferase (GGT)	Present in biliary and renal tubular epithelium. Increased by hepatocellular damage, some renal disease. In most species: <5 IU/l = normal; 5–10 IU/l = questionable; >10 IU/l = abnormal. Combine interpretation with other tests.
Lactate dehydrogenase (LDH)	Present in skeletal/cardiac muscle, liver, bone, kidney; tissue-specific isoenzymes. Increased in hepatic necrosis, haemolysis, muscle damage. Non-specific. In liver disease levels rise and fall more quickly than AST.
Other indicators of liver disease	
Bile acids	Rapid, sensitive increase and decrease in liver disease. Fasting may affect levels. In most species: <75 µmol/l = normal; 75–100 µmol/l = questionable; >100 µmol/l = abnormal.
Bilirubin	Many species cannot convert biliverdin to bilirubin. <10 µmol/l = normal. <5 µmol/l = colourless serum. Carotenoids can mimic jaundice

9.2 Biochemistry interpretations.

Change in fraction	Associated with
Decreased albumin	Decreased production (such as liver insufficiency), increased (gastrointestinal) loss (such as enteritis), or increased use (such as chronic inflammation)
Elevated α-globulins	Acute inflammation or infection, reproductively active female
Elevated β-globulins	Acute inflammation or infection
Elevated γ-globulins	More chronic inflammation or infection

9.3 Common abnormalities on plasma protein electrophoresis.

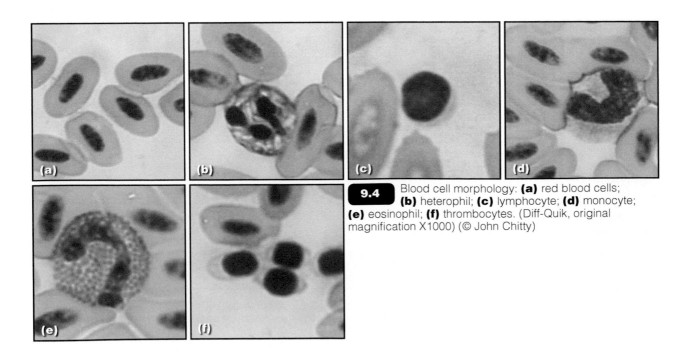

9.4 Blood cell morphology: **(a)** red blood cells; **(b)** heterophil; **(c)** lymphocyte; **(d)** monocyte; **(e)** eosinophil; **(f)** thrombocytes. (Diff-Quik, original magnification X1000) (© John Chitty)

Cytology

Cytological evaluation is always an adjunct to other diagnostic procedures. In the clinic a cytological examination of swellings, discharges from eyes, nostrils and wounds, fluids, mouth and cloacal swabs, and faecal smears can give much additional information about the nature and the aetiology of a process or sign. At PME, cytology is an invaluable tool for defining the presumptive diagnosis and for starting treatment in a flock situation. It is an indispensable tool for a rapid investigation of possible bacterial, mycotic or yeast infections (Figure 9.5) or even viral disease. The diagnosis of many protozoal infections depends on demonstrating the organisms in impression smears of a selection of organs. Cytology is also useful for a quick differentiation between tumour and inflammation. However, the veterinary surgeon should be aware of the limitations of diagnostic cytology: it does not always provide a definitive diagnosis; it does not give information concerning the architecture of the tissue (cells in the same smear may have originated from different areas of the organ or lesion), the size of the lesion, or the invasiveness of a malignant lesion; the cells observed may not necessarily represent the true nature of the lesion (e.g. an impression smear of the ulcerated surface of a neoplastic mass will reveal only inflammation and infection). Cytopathology should not compete with histopathology; the two should complement each other in achieving the final diagnosis. It is important to note that occasionally one is unable to characterize the cells in a specimen and that a repeat smear or biopsy and histopathological evaluation may be required to define the lesion.

A successful cytological examination is only possible if four conditions are achieved:

- Representative sample
- Good quality smear
- Good staining technique
- Correct evaluation of the cytological findings.

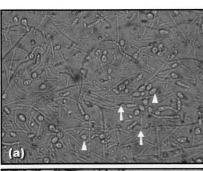
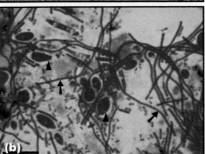

9.5

Gouldian finch with yeast-related enteropathy: **(a)** wet mount; **(b)** stained with Hemacolor®. Arrows point to bacteria; arrowheads point to yeasts. (Original magnification: (a) X40; (b) X100)

Sample collection

- Abdominocentesis, tissue and bone marrow biopsy, crop wash, nasal flush, sinus aspiration, tracheal wash, air-sac wash and urine collection are possible collection methods.
- It is important that cytological specimens are taken from fresh sources, since cells degenerate rapidly following the death of the patient or removal of the tissue.
- Cytological samples of the alimentary tract of live birds can be using a cotton swab or crop aspiration. Postmortem samples of the alimentary tract are obtained by scraping any lesions with a cotton swab or spatula blade. The material can also be used for microbiological culture and microscopic examination.

Fine-needle aspiration

Fine-needle aspiration often provides a good sample for a rapid presumptive diagnosis without radical tissue removal, and this can be performed in the examination room.

Direct smears

Direct smears can be made from aspirated fluids, e.g. ascites or cyst contents. They can be made using the wedge method or the coverslip method commonly used for making blood smears. A 'squash-prep' procedure should be used to make smears from thick tenacious fluid or from fluid that contains solid tissue fragments. Fluids that have low cellularity require concentration methods to increase the smear cellularity. Sediment smears made after slow-speed centrifugation (500 rpm for 5 minutes) of the fluid or smears made with cytocentrifuge equipment will usually provide adequate cytological specimens.

Contact smears

Impressions of organs should be made from a freshly cut surface, which should be fairly dry and free of blood. This can be achieved by gently blotting the surface on a clean paper towel. Impression smears can then be made by gently touching the microscope slide against the surface of the mass. It is important not to use too much pressure and to air-dry the slide quickly. Several imprints of the same organ should be made on each slide. If the imprints show poor cellularity, more cells may be obtained by scraping the mass with a scalpel blade to improve exfoliation of the cells. The impression procedure can be repeated, or more smears can be made from the material remaining on the scalpel blade. When a mycotic process is suspected, this is the only technique to use to ensure that fungal hyphae will be present on the cytology slide.

In a standard PME, impression smears are made from the cut surfaces of liver, spleen and lungs, and also from rectal scrapings. Extra impressions are made from macroscopically altered organs.

Fixation and staining

Once a sample has been collected and a smear made, the specimen must be properly fixed to the slide. If smears are to be sent to a diagnostic laboratory, they must be air-dried, properly packed (broken slides are fairly common) and accompanied by a distinct identification and case history.

The method of fixation depends on which staining procedure is to be used. Fresh air-dried blood smears and cytology slides are adequate for Romanowsky stains (e.g. Giemsa) and many rapid stains. Two or more slides should always be made, leaving at least one unstained in case special staining is needed.

Cytologists use a variety of stains and staining methods including: Giemsa – for cells; Gram – for bacteria; acid-fast – for *Mycobacterium*; modified Giminez – for *Chlamydophila*; Stamp – for *Chlamydophila*; Prussian blue – for haemosiderosis or iron storage; and Sudan III – for fat globules. Proper fixation must be applied if specific stains are used. To obtain this information the diagnostic service should be contacted.

The cytological descriptions in this chapter are based primarily on slides stained with a modified rapid Wright's stain (Hemacolor®, Merck). The great advantage of rapid stains is a short staining time (usually 20 seconds), which allows quick examination of the specimen and provides satisfactory staining quality. These stains are suitable for use in veterinary practice where a simple staining procedure is desirable. Many rapid stains also provide permanent reference smears for comparison with other cytological specimens

Although there are many different recommendations for parasite handling, storage and fixation, the author recommends that all parasites should be collected in glycerine alcohol (9 parts 70% ethanol and 1 part glycerine).

Microscopic examination

Once smears have been stained and dried they are ready for microscopic examination. For a reliable evaluation of haematological or cytological changes it is often necessary to consult a haematologist or cytopathologist. The recognition of many aetiological agents is often easy, however, and can give a presumptive diagnosis.

Scanning and low magnifications (X100 or X250) are used initially to obtain a general impression of the smear's quality. At these magnifications, the examiner is able to estimate the smear's cellularity, to identify tissue structures or large infectious agents (e.g. microfilariae, fungal elements) and to determine the best locations for higher-power examination. Oil immersion (X1000 magnification) is used to examine cell structure, bacteria and other small objects.

In addition to viewing cellular structure, the cytologist should determine background characteristics (e.g. iron granules), the amount of peripheral blood or stain precipitation present, the thickness of different areas in the smear, and the distribution of the cells.

- The background characteristics may be useful in defining the nature of the material being examined. Protein aggregates create a granular background with the rapid stains. Bacteria, crystals, nuclear material from ruptured cells and exogenous material (e.g. plant fibres, pollen and talcum or starch crystals from examination gloves) may be seen in the non-cellular background of the smear.

- Excessive peripheral blood contamination of a specimen will dilute and mask diagnostic cells; this will make interpretation difficult.

- Stain precipitate on the smear should not be confused with bacteria or cellular inclusions. Stain precipitate varies in size and shape and will be more refractive than bacteria or most cellular inclusions.

- The thickness of the smear will affect the appearance of the cells and the quality of the smear. Thick areas do not allow the cells to expand on the slide, so they appear smaller and denser when compared with the same cell type on thinner areas of the smear. Therefore, examination of the cells in thick smears should be avoided. The cellular distribution should also be noted.

Microbiological culture

Frequently avian veterinary surgeons are requested to collect samples from multiple-organ systems for microbiological culture. Choanal cleft and cloacal aerobic cultures are often included in routine laboratory screening for birds, but any tissue or fluid can potentially be sampled. It is most important that the sample is taken only from the intended site, as cleanly as possible.

A sterile swab of appropriate size should be used, moistened with sterile water or non-bacteriostatic saline. Biopsy or necropsy tissue and fluids may require different sampling and handling, depending on the material. A routine rapid stain of tissue from the sample area will give an indication of which microorganism can be expected and will help in selecting the proper culture media. In an in-house laboratory, but also after receiving back the results from a reference laboratory, the stained smear can be used for interpretation of the findings. Cultures must be interpreted carefully, and the significance of a given organism's growth should be based on clinical history, physical examination, and other supporting diagnostic tests.

Collection and culture media should be appropriate for the suspected microorganism. For routine aerobic and anaerobic bacterial cultures, commercially available sterile swabs and appropriate transport media should be used. Blood agar (Figure 9.6) and MacConkey agar plates are standard media for most in-house aerobic bacterial cultures. The blood agar plate should be inoculated first, as MacConkey agar inhibits most non-enteric Gram-negative rods (except *Pseudomonas*) and all Gram-positive microorganisms. Most Gram-negative enteric bacteria (e.g. *Escherichia coli*, *Klebsiella*, *Salmonella*) grow well on MacConkey agar.

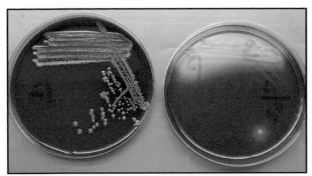

9.6 Growth of *Escherichia coli*) on blood agar and selective brilliant green phenol agar.

Viruses, certain bacterial organisms (e.g. *Chlamydophila*, *Mycobacterium*, *Mycoplasma*), many fungi and protozoal organisms require special culture media and the reference laboratory should be contacted for specific collection, handling and transport instructions. In general, if there is uncertainty about the need for special culturing techniques, fluid and tissue samples can be frozen. For longer storage an ultrafreezer at −70°C can be found at many diagnostic laboratories. With the exception of most dermatophytes and *Malassezia* sp., all medically important fungi (including *Aspergillus* and *Candida*) will grow on blood agar incubated aerobically at 37°C. Sabouraud's and malt dextrose agar are used specifically to inhibit most bacterial proliferation and to promote fungal growth (Figure 9.7).

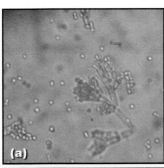

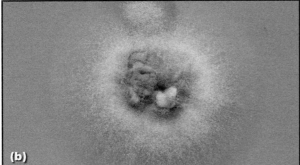

9.7

Aspergillus fumigatus: **(a)** conidia on conidiophores in wet mount; **(b)** growth on malt agar after 48 hours.

Diagnostic tests for infectious diseases

Chlamydophilosis

Most birds with clinical signs of *Chlamydophila psittaci* infection suffer from an acute hepatitis. In pigeons and captive raptors, however, chlamydophilosis can be endemic without much in the way of clinical signs, but occasional fatalities. Plasma chemistry can demonstrate elevated liver enzymes in clinical cases and a decreased albumin:globulin ratio due to hyperglobulinaemia on plasma protein electrophoresis. CBC shows leucocytosis.

In-house test procedures for *C. psittaci* involve cytological staining or specific antigen detection. These tests detect shedding of *C. psittaci* in swabs from the conjunctiva, choana or cloaca. In an impression smear of the swab, the organisms stain red with Stamp's or Machiavello's stain (modified Ziehl–Neelsen).

Commercially available enzyme-linked immunosorbent assays (ELISAs) can detect *Chlamydophila* antigen in the swab sample. Most were originally developed for the detection of human *Chlamydia trachomatis* and *C. pneumoniae*, but are also suitable for *Chlamydophila psittaci*. Immunofluorescence (IF) tests are also available.

The disadvantage of cytological staining and antigen detection tests is that they only detect organisms that have been shed. False-negative results can occur due to intermittent shedding, or inhibition of shedding by antibiotic treatment. Specialized laboratories provide polymerase chain reaction (PCR) tests for *C. psittaci* DNA. Serological tests measuring antibodies against *C. psittaci* are also available. Serology is not useful for immediate diagnosis in an individual bird, though high antibody titres are an indication that *Chlamydophila* is present. When using serology, paired sera are mandatory to diagnose an ongoing *C. psittaci* infection.

As chlamydophilosis represents a significant zoonotic risk, it is recommended that at PME, after opening the body cavity, an examination is made for the presence of this infection before proceeding further. In many cases there are visible lesions at PME, such as pericarditis, air sacculitis and hepatitis (hepatomegaly, often with serofibrinous deposits over the surface). In some cases, however, no such lesions are apparent. The spleen, or the yellow material at the affected air sacs when present, is the organ of choice when testing for chlamydophilosis. An impression is made, air-dried and stained by modified Ziehl–Neelsen and examined under a high-power (X100) objective. *Chlamydophila* organisms appear as clusters of tiny magenta bodies within the blue-green staining cytoplasm of the host cells. The traditional confirmatory test has been culture examination, but this has been largely replaced by the PCR test.

Circovirus infection

A PCR is available for the detection of DNA from pigeon circovirus. The assay is performed with liver tissue fixed in 70% alcohol. A positive PCR in a dead nestling confirms that circovirus may be the causative agent of mortality. If an adult bird without clinical signs tests positive on PCR, it is possible that this is due to a transient infection. The virus can be seen using electron microscopy but cannot be cultured.

At PME juveniles demonstrate hepatic necrosis and often secondary infections such as bacteraemia or an acute aspergillosis. Bursa, bone marrow and liver samples should always be taken at PME; some of each tissue should be frozen, some of each fixed in buffered formalin and some fixed in 70% alcohol to be sent for PCR. If there is a financial constraint, bone marrow samples should be tested by PCR first. On histology, basophilic inclusion bodies are seen in the bursa.

In Canaries and finches, specific circoviruses are found that are related more to psittacine circoviruses than to the pigeon circovirus. In Canaries, the typical basophilic inclusions can also be found in the intestinal muscles. The extent of distribution of these circoviruses amongst passerine birds is not yet known.

Polyomavirus infection

Avian polyomavirus (APV) infection has been found in birds of prey and passerine species, including Canaries, but not in pigeons thus far. APV can be detected with a PCR. Viraemia can be seen in blood samples and the virus can also be found in cloacal swabs. After the virus is no longer present in the blood, it can still be shed in the cloaca for up to several weeks; however, such shedding is intermittent and DNA can thus can be missed. If a bird dies from APV infection, PME will demonstrate haemorrhages and hepatic necrosis. In young birds the bursa can sometimes be enlarged (Figure 9.8). Intranuclear inclusion bodies are found in different organs, but mostly in the spleen and the glomerulus epithelial cells of the kidneys. These two organs should always be collected at PME, but especially when APV infection is suspected.

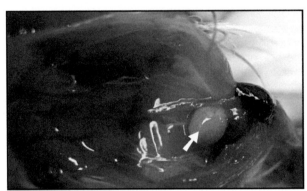

9.8 Enlarged bursa of Fabricius (arrowed) in a Canary with polyomavirus. (Courtesy of Peter Coutteel)

Tests for specific conditions in raptors

Polyuria/polydipsia (PU/PD)

Primary polyuria is directly related to renal disease. Systemic disorders such as diabetes mellitus, stress, liver disease, hypercalcaemia or psychogenic polydipsia can cause secondary polyuria. Targeting laboratory examination of these patients includes urine analysis (Figure 9.9), CBC and plasma biochemistry. Further differentiation between primary and secondary causes of polyuria requires blood examination. For an accurate diagnosis of the cause of PU/PD, additional diagnostic procedures such as radiography, endoscopy and biopsy are often necessary.

Parameter	Normal value in parrots
Specific gravity	1.005–1.020
pH	6.0–8.0
Protein	Trace amounts
Glucose	Negative or trace
Ketones	Absent
Bilirubin	Absent
Urobilinogen	0.0–0.1
Blood	Negative or trace

9.9 Normal urine parameters. *NB These values are for parrots as data are unavailable for other species. It is likely that other species will have similar normal parameters, but caution should always be exercised when extrapolating from one family of birds to another.*

The urine of a bird with polyuria can easily be collected from a fresh dropping on a non-absorbent surface. Standard urine-stick tests can be used for the detection of glucose, haemoglobin and protein.

- The avian glomerulus is impermeable to most proteins, including albumin. Therefore no protein, or only a trace of protein, should be present in avian urine. Glomerulonephritis can result in marked protein loss. Tubular damage can induce a mild proteinuria.
- In the normal avian kidney, all glucose is resorbed in the proximal tubule. Therefore tubular diseases can cause distinct glucosuria. Glucosuria can also occur when hyperglycaemia is present and the absorption capacity of the tubules is exceeded.
- Haematuria may be present with inflammatory or neoplastic diseases of the kidney, ureter or cloaca.

Uric acid and urea

Uric acid, the major nitrogenous waste product of birds, can be measured to evaluate renal function (blood creatinine concentrations are not reliable in birds). Approximately 90% of uric acid is secreted through the proximal tubules; only a small portion is filtered by the glomeruli. It is believed that, as in mammals, the avian kidney has substantial excess capacity. Elevated plasma uric acid levels in the raptor can be related to postprandial high levels, to damage of more than 50% of the proximal tubules or to severe dehydration.

Determination of plasma urea may be beneficial in differentiating kidney disease from dehydration. Urea, synthesized by the liver, is excreted by glomerular filtration, and reabsorption increases with dehydration. Increased plasma uric acid with normal plasma urea is likely to be indicative of renal disease. Elevation of both plasma uric acid and urea indicates dehydration, but renal disease may still be present.

Glucose

Plasma glucose can be measured to investigate other possible causes of PU/PD. If the sample will be stored for longer than several hours, it is advisable to separate plasma and blood cells to prevent lowering of glucose levels.

Occasionally birds demonstrate transient hyperglycaemia; therefore birds with hyperglycaemia should be tested again after 2 days. Often, stress hyperglycaemia cannot be distinguished from diabetes mellitus (DM), but repeated measurements of glucose levels >55 mmol/l are likely to be associated with DM. Determination of blood glucagon and insulin may also be important in diagnosing DM, but tests for these hormones are not routinely available. Histology of the pancreas showing atrophy or inflammation of the pancreatic islets confirms DM; thus, endoscopic or surgical biopsy may be a more important means of confirming diagnosis.

Calcium

PU/PD due to hypercalcaemia can be caused by egg laying, excess of dietary calcium or vitamin D3, or malignancies. When performing a PME on a bird with hypercalcaemia, attention should be paid to the status of the ovary and oviduct. Oversupplementation with calcium and vitamin D3 can lead to dystrophic calcification of the renal tubules. PME of these patients should also focus on hyperplasia or neoplasia of the parathyroid glands.

It is important to note that total plasma protein levels markedly influence plasma calcium concentrations. Total plasma calcium measured in most laboratories consists of an ionized fraction and a protein-bound fraction. About one-third of total plasma calcium is protein-bound and biologically inactive; therefore, elevated protein concentrations can falsely increase total calcium while the biologically active calcium concentration remains normal.

Green/yellow urine

Green to yellow urine can indicate anorexia or liver disease. Biliverdin is the most important bile pigment in birds. Anorexia leads to a higher concentration of faecal biliverdin and thus to a greenish discoloration of the faeces (see Figure 7.12); diffusion of biliverdin pigments from the faeces may result in green discoloration of the urine. Over 90% of bile is resorbed in the jejunum and ileum and enters the enterohepatic cycle. In birds with impaired clearing capacity of the liver, increased excretion of biliverdin results in a green staining of urates and urine.

Determination of avian plasma enzymes can give information on current liver damage (see Figure 9.2). Elevations in plasma enzyme activities are related to leakage of enzymes from damaged liver cells, but do not necessarily indicate impaired liver function. Damage of liver cells is usually related to hepatitis or liver neoplasia. On the other hand, chronic liver fibrosis or lipidosis produce little acute hepatocellular leakage and damage. Plasma enzymes useful in the detection of liver cell damage include aspartate aminotransferase (AST), gamma-glutamyl transferase (GGT), and glutamate dehydrogenase (GLDH).

- Plasma AST is a very sensitive indicator of liver cell damage. However, specificity of this enzyme is low, because AST is also present in muscle tissue. Trauma, injections or rough handling can also lead to elevation of plasma AST. To differentiate between liver and muscle damage, plasma creatine kinase (CK) can be measured. CK has a high sensitivity and specificity for muscle damage. If both AST and CK are elevated, muscle damage is present and liver disease is not proven.
- Although GGT is a specific indicator of liver damage, avian GGT activity is low.
- GLDH is the most liver-specific enzyme, but its sensitivity is low. GLDH is located within the mitochondria of the liver cells. Elevated plasma GLDH activity indicates severe liver cell damage and necrosis, which can occur with viral, bacterial or mycotic hepatitis.

Determination of plasma bile acid concentration provides information on the clearing capacity for bile acids by the liver. Impaired liver function with elevated plasma bile acids can be caused by pathological changes such as liver fibrosis or lipidosis. It should be emphasized that in these severe liver diseases, normal plasma liver enzyme activities can be measured if no acutely damaged liver cells are present. Radiography, ultrasonography and endoscopy can be helpful in liver disease, but biopsy is essential to establish a definitive diagnosis.

The dyspnoeic bird

CBC and biochemistry alone cannot reveal specific respiratory diseases but can add information to other tests such as radiography, tracheoscopy and endoscopy. Acute and chronic inflammation of the respiratory system can lead to leucocytosis and changes in plasma protein electrophoresis (see Figure 9.3).

Heterophilia is the first haematological change seen in inflammatory disease, followed by lymphocytosis and/or monocytosis in more chronic stages of disease. Stress responses can also induce heterophilia. Therefore, the WBC should be reviewed carefully against the recent history. An increase in the heterophil:lymphocyte ratio may be a measure of physiological stress. On plasma protein electrophoresis, birds with aspergillosis often demonstrate elevation of globulin fractions, which causes a decrease in the albumin:globulin ratio. It must be emphasized that elevation of globulins represents non-specific inflammation or viral, bacterial, parasitic or fungal infection. In some cases of dyspnoea, especially in older birds, no abnormalities are found with routine diagnostic procedures except for an elevated PCV. If other causes for high PCV are ruled out, it is possible that the bird has lung atrophy; in such cases PCVs of 60% and higher are found repeatedly. The diagnosis can only be confirmed with lung biopsy or on PME.

Gastrointestinal problems

Blood panels do not specifically identify gastrointestinal diseases, though inflammation may be detected with CBC and plasma protein electrophoresis. Biochemistry may reveal underlying diseases of other organs.

Faecal assessment should be part of every avian clinical examination and is mandatory in the bird with gastrointestinal disease (see Chapter 18). Parasites can be detected in fresh faeces using direct saline smears and flotation. Cytology may indicate abnormal bacterial flora and yeast infection. Bacterial and fungal culture can identify the causative pathogen.

In the regurgitating avian patient, a crop swab should be obtained. A direct smear, cytology and culture can be performed to detect flagellates, bacteria or yeasts.

Determination of plasma amylase and lipase may be helpful in the assessment of pancreatitis, and pancreatic necrosis or carcinoma but pancreatic biopsy is necessary to diagnose pancreatic disorders.

The ADR raptor

The 'Ain't doin' right' bird might be presented for one or more of the following problems observed by the falconer:

- The bird is not flying at its usual performance level given its appetite, weight and condition
- It tires easily
- It does not gain weight in spite of increased feeding
- It is losing body condition/weight.

Clinical examination will confirm whether body condition is as the falconer describes and whether it is or is not appropriate for that stage of the season. The differentials for this type of presentation are many and a thorough investigation is required, including clinical examination, radiography and endoscopy. Laboratory work is also of vital importance. While some tests will be dictated by the results of other tests, the following are recommended as part of a minimum database:

- CBC, protein electrophoresis, AST, CK, uric acid (often best performed after starvation for 12–24 hours), sodium, potassium, calcium (total and ionized), GLDH, bile acids
- Faecal parasitology (ideally on a pooled sample collected over 3 days).

In some cases there will be minimal changes on blood tests. In these cases it may be necessary to perform repeated tests at 5–7-day intervals to assess progress of any pathological condition.

Post-mortem examination

A complete PME is often the best method for evaluating and understanding a disease process. The ultimate goal is to take that information and experience and to apply it to living patients. In addition to the obvious goal of determining a cause of death, a PME can thus provide the clinician with valuable information concerning case management and therapy. In some cases a PME is essential due to potential legal actions. To obtain the maximum value from a PME,

consultation with a pathologist and histopathology are necessary. In an ideal situation with no economical restraints, clinicians would be able to submit whole birds to the pathologist for PME and histopathology. In many cases the clinician will have to do the PME and select tissues for submission. If so, the procedure must be carried out in a safe fashion respecting relevant legislation and good practice. To make a diagnosis the pathologist uses the clinical history (including haematology, blood chemistry, morphological techniques, therapeutic measurements), the gross description of the lesions, culture results and other data, as well as the cytological and histological appearance of the lesions. Absence of any of these or incorrect submission of tissues will hamper this process. The quality of information received from examination of the samples is directly proportional to the quality and choice of the specimens submitted and the information that accompanies them.

Where a bird has been euthanased, an indication should be given as to how this was performed. Injections of barbiturate euthanasia solutions can create extensive lesions; the best method of euthanasia is an overdose of an inhalant anaesthetic gas as this leaves the least amount of artificial changes to the body.

- The PME should be performed as soon as possible after death.
- To promote rapid cooling of the carcass, thoroughly soak the plumage in cold water to which a small amount of soap or detergent has been added to aid complete wetting of the plumage and skin. It also prevents spreading of spreading of infectious material by feather dust.
- If the carcass is going to be sent to a pathological laboratory, place it in a plastic bag, squeeze out all excess air, seal or tie the bag, refrigerate, and contact the laboratory for further instructions.
- If the carcass has been cooled immediately upon death and can be submitted to the laboratory within 72–96 hours it should be refrigerated (*not* frozen) and packed with sufficient ice or cool packs to keep it cold until arrival at the laboratory.
- If delivery to the laboratory is expected to be delayed beyond 96 hours, the carcass should be frozen immediately, rather than simply refrigerated. Frozen tissue specimens or carcasses must be packed with ice packs (or other frozen coolants) to keep them frozen until arrival at the laboratory. Freezing will leave artefacts and is suboptimal for histopathological examination; it also decreases the likelihood of success in isolating some bacteria (e.g. mycoplasmas) or demonstrating some parasites stadia.
- If the carcass is extremely small (e.g. embryos, nestlings or very small adult birds) the entire carcass may be submitted for histological examination. This is best accomplished by opening the body cavity, gently separating the viscera, injecting some formalin into the duodenum and fixing the entire carcass in formalin.

Whether the practitioner is performing the PME or simply collecting diagnostic material, preparation must be systematic. The correct selection of material for further examination and correct method of sampling, storage and shipping of material will increase the quality of results tremendously. When adequate time to do a proper PME or adequate facilities to carry out the procedure correctly and safely are not available, it is likely that mistakes will be made, systems missed or hygiene and safety compromised. In that case it may be preferable to submit the carcass to a specialist pathology laboratory.

A written report of the PME findings helps the clinician to keep track of the disease status of a bird collection.

Preparation

To perform the PME, it is advisable to use a well lit, well ventilated area (preferably under a fume hood) in a designated room and to wear adequate protective clothing and gloves. Aerosols from feathers, faeces and exudates can be infectious. If there is any possibility of a zoonotic disease (e.g. chlamydophilosis, mycobacteriosis) a mask and possibly more extensive protection should be worn. It is also important to contain the feather dander and faeces in cases of avian polyomavirus, circovirus and other viral infections, so as not to contaminate the premises, clothing or adjacent birds.

Disinfectant solutions should be readily available for cleaning up after the PME, but neither these solutions nor their fumes should come in contact with tissues being collected, as they may lyse cells and destroy microorganisms needed for culture. Tissues that are to be cultured and blood or tissue cytological smears should not be exposed to formalin fumes, as this could severely distort staining and interpretation.

Equipment

It is helpful to have two sets of instruments designated for PME and not used around living birds. Both sets should be thoroughly cleaned and sterilized after use. One set is used for opening the bird and the other to collect internal organ samples for culture and viral diagnostics. Each instrument pack should include: two scalpel blades and handles (one for cutting, one for burning organ surfaces before taking a microbiology sample); thumb forceps; and scissors. In one set there should also be a rongeur-type instrument for cutting bone and removing the brain. A set of ophthalmic instruments and a head loupe are invaluable for small birds, neonates or dead-in-shell embryos. Other useful equipment includes a gram scale, a hand-lens or dissecting microscope, and absorbent paper tissues. In addition to the instruments, there should be to hand:

- 10 % neutral buffered formalin (= 4% formaldehyde)
- 70% ethyl alcohol for wetting and disinfecting the feathers and skin and for collecting samples for PCR

- 70% ethyl alcohol mixed with 10% glycerine for collecting parasitological specimens
- A bottle with saline (0.9% NaCl) with a pipette (for parasitological examination) and
- Appropriate containers.

Other equipment for ancillary diagnostic procedures includes:

- Syringes and needles to obtain samples for serology, haematology or cytology
- Clean glass slides for impression smears
- A stain set for cytology (e.g. rapid stains and Stamp or Macchiavello)
- Clean glass slides and coverslips for wet mounts (parasitology)
- Burner for heating and sterilizing wire loops and one scalpel blade before taking a sample for microbiology
- Sterile swabs or culture tubes with appropriate transport media for bacterial or fungal culture
- Transport media or material for PCR of *Chlamydophila*, mycobacteria and viruses
- Petri dishes or freezer-proof tubes or small zipper bags for submission of tissues for viral isolation.

Figure 9.10 suggests equipment layouts for PME. Before the PME, glass slides, sealable bags and formalin jars should be labelled with the case number or owner's name and details of the tissues enclosed, in an effort to save time and prevent interruptions in the flow of the PME.

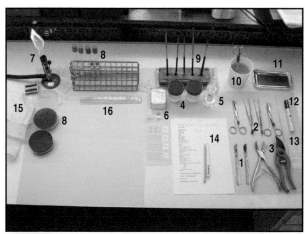

9.10 Lay-out material and instruments for a PME: (1) two scalpel blades and handles; (2) one pair anatomical and one pair surgical forceps and two pair scissors; (3) bone-cutting forceps; (4) containers with 10% buffered formalin; (5) saline with pipette for wet mounts; (6) clean marked glass slides for cytology and wet mounts (parasitology); (7) burner for heating and sterilizing a scalpel blade and wire loop for culturing; (8) culture media for bacteriology and mycology; (9) wire loops for microbiological sampling; (10) container with disinfectant for the instruments; (11) aluminium foil plates for holding small organs or tissues; (12) waterproof marker; (13) preprinted labels; (14) copy of PME work-form and checklist; (15) paper towels for cleaning in between; (16) ruler.

Record keeping: A digital camera might be useful for documentation of gross lesions or where litigation is possible. In the latter case, there should always be a label showing the bird's laboratory reference number and the date. Blue or green paper should be used as a background for the carcass or organs, and a plastic ruler or disposable paper measuring tape provides a scale. Generally it is better to take photographs during the PME, ideally having an assistant to help rather than having to remove gloves before using the camera. In many cases it is possible to perform most of the PME using forceps and scissors, without touching the carcass.

To record findings during the PME, scribbling paper can be used that can be discarded with the carcass after finishing the examination and writing the final report.

PME protocol

The particular routine used for gross PME of birds can vary, but what remains the same is that all organs are examined. The use of a checklist will ensure this. All findings should be documented and this checklist should become part of the medical record.

Impression smears are a useful adjunct to a complete PME. In the author's protocol two sets of impression smears are made from liver, spleen, lung and rectum. Organs with pathological changes are automatically added. The choice of tissues for histopathology can be determined by several philosophies:

- *Economic reasons.* This is a poor rationale. It is better to collect samples of everything (all organs, the grossly normal and abnormal) and, after consulting the pathologist, send in the selected tissues and keep the others 'just in case'. Then, at the very least, the diagnosis does not get cremated with the carcass
- *Completeness.* This is especially valid for a scientific research. All tissues listed in Figure 9.11 should be collected

Standard selection for routine examination	Additional tissues (depending on gross lesions observed at necropsy)
Lung	Skin, including feather follicles
Heart	Trachea
Kidneys	Air sac
Proventriculus	Thyroid glands
Ventriculus	Parathyroid glands
Duodenum	Adrenal glands
Spleen	Oesophagus
Liver	Crop
Pancreas	Small intestine
	Rectum
	Caeca and cloaca
	Gall bladder
	Gonads
	Pectoral muscle
	Bone marrow
	Cloacal bursa
	Thymus
	Brain
	Ischiadic (sciatic) nerve

9.11 Tissues routinely collected on PME for histopathology.

- A *standard selection* (first column in Figure 9.11) completed with a choice based on the PME findings. This list is practical and will in most cases lead to sufficient diagnostic support.

The priority is to collect tissues from organ systems that appear to be involved in the problem, based on clinical signs and gross lesions. When lesions are present, the sample should include some normal tissue as well.

Normally selected tissues are fixed in an adequate amount of 10% neutral-buffered formalin (volume 1 to 10) for histopathological examination. The best method is to fix the tissues or organs in large pots so that they can fix in a large quantity of formalin. Before viscera are posted (after 12–24 hours fixation) they should be drained off and the fixed tissues placed in a bag or container, which is wrapped in formalin-soaked tissue paper. This method gives good fixation for a large volume and is cheaper on postage. Any specimen must be <5 mm thick for good fixation. Formalin will not penetrate well into the brain through the unopened calvarium or into the marrow of bone unless the bone has been cracked. Wet formalin-fixed tissue may be conveniently stored and shipped in plastic heat- or glue-sealed bags.

Tissues for histopathology should *not* be frozen, but tissues for toxicological analysis (Figure 9.12) *should* be frozen.

- Collect liver, pancreas, kidney, brain, muscle and fat and freeze individual samples separately.
- Also collect crop or proventriculus or ventriculus samples and freeze.
- If needed, other gastrointestinal areas should be collected in separate non-metal containers; they may be frozen at −20°C after being wrapped in aluminium foil.

Toxicological testing requires some idea of what toxin is being considered. This information often comes from the history and histopathological findings. It is essential to check with the toxicology laboratory for submission of the most appropriate tissues and amounts.

- The most common toxins tested are *heavy metals*, such as lead and zinc. Usually liver and kidney are required for this analysis, though zinc accumulates in the pancreas preferentially.
- *Poisonous plants* can be found in the digestive tract and submitted to a botanist or to a university botany department for identification.
- *Polytetrafluorethylene* (Teflon) and other toxic inhalation products are rarely detectable in tissues and the diagnosis is usually made with history of exposure, the presence of pulmonary oedema and haemorrhage, and exclusion of other causes of death.
- *Mycotoxins* may be implicated in the case of multiple birds suffering liver damage.
- *Aflatoxins* can be detected in foodstuffs, but usually by the time chronic liver damage is evident the offending foodstuff is often no longer available.
- In cases of *acute toxicosis*, freeze samples of the feed along with liver and kidney, pending further investigation.

9.12 Toxicology.

- Freezing for virus isolation is best done at −70°C. If this cannot be accomplished, the tissues for viral isolation should be placed in sterile containers on wet ice and sent by rapid mail.

Pending the diagnostic work-up, most commercial laboratories can hold tissues frozen at −70°C if asked.

History

Before starting the PME itself, it is important to make a differential list of clinical diagnoses and be aware of the affected organ systems based on clinical signs and laboratory findings. This list will help determine what samples are needed for supporting or confirming a particular diagnosis. Most clinical signs are not visible in a dead bird. For example, torticollis, which is essential for the differential diagnosis of PMV infection in pigeons or passerines and which would indicate that the pancreas should be collected for histology. The most relevant data should be summarized on the PME work sheet. The differential list should identify the most important organ systems involved.

When an owner comes in with a dead bird, the same information and history about the case should be taken as for a live patient coming into the practice. This includes: identification (species, age or purchase date, leg ring or microchip details); information about housing, feeding and any environmental changes; observed clinical signs; medical history; and pertinent laboratory data (when available).

In many cases a bird is presented dead with a history of sudden death. This history should be evaluated in light of the gross changes seen, so that tissues can be selected properly:

- If there are changes suggestive of chronicity, the gastrointestinal tract and liver may be the primary problems
- If the bird appears to be in good condition and there are no gross changes, organs such as the heart, respiratory system, brain and endocrine glands need to be examined, as disease of these organs is often the cause of acute death
- In the absence of any clinical or gross indication of which organs to select and if there are limitations due to economical considerations, liver and spleen are recommended, as these organs are involved in many systemic disease problems

- In birds under a year old it is essential that the bursa of Fabricius be examined, as it is an indicator of the condition of the bird's immune system and is often involved in viral infections (see Figure 9.7). This organ often contains specific viral inclusion bodies of circovirus not seen in other organs
- The cage or packing material should be inspected for the presence of parasites or other relevant information.

In cases where litigation is possible and the PME is done in the clinic:

- Document everything seen thoroughly
- Save leg band(s) and microchips
- Take photographic evidence of all stages of the PME, even if no changes are seen
- Collect many different samples
- Store the carcass afterwards in the freezer until the case is closed
- Send a complete set of tissues to the laboratory and save a duplicate set
- Save material for possible toxicological analysis
- Do any other ancillary tests indicated, such as microbial studies and PCRs.

External examination of the carcass

1. Record the identification details (band number, microchip).
2. Palpate for obvious swellings or fractures and confirm that all joints are fully mobile.
3. Check for proper bone mineralization by attempting to bend a long bone. In females, radiography is useful for assessing medullary bone.
4. Record information about general body condition, weight, muscle mass, joints, integument (including beak and nails), plumage (for defects, ectoparasites, faeces), body orifices (eyes, ears, nostrils and vent), uropygial gland (absent in some species), trauma and abnormalities (Figure 9.13).

    Be aware that abnormal plumage results in extreme energy loss because of the lack of insulation.

    Judge the feeding status by checking the muscles on the keel and assessing the filling of the crop and intestines.
5. Take survey radiographs when heavy metals are suspected (e.g. rifle bullets or ingested lead).

Finding	Diagnosis	Tests
Broken or frayed feathers (Ra,Pi,Pa)	Housing problems, feather picking, delayed moult, mites. Differentials: handling problems	History, information diet
Fret marks (Ra,Pi,Ra)	In wing and tail primaries	
Blood feathers, plucked and in the follicle, along with any skin lesions		Collect and place in formalin for histology
Changes of the skin and nares (Pa,Ra,Pi)	Cnemidocoptes infestation, yeast infection	Wet mount, cytology, culture, histology

9.13 Examples of alterations found at external examination in raptors (Ra), pigeons (Pi) and passerine birds (Pa). (continues) ▶

Finding	Diagnosis	Tests
Bruising (Ra,Pi,Pa)	Trauma	n/a
Skin haemorrhages (Pa)	In juveniles related to polyomavirus infection	Histology of spleen and kidney
Thickening of the joints (arthritis) of the wings	Salmonellosis	Cytology, culture, histology
The unfeathered portion of the legs and the feet (Ra,Pi,Pa)	Avipox lesions, bumblefoot, herpesvirus pododermatitis, ectoparasites and self-mutilation	Wet mounts, cytology, histology of abnormal tissues
Examine the site of the uropygial gland at the base of the tail (in some species absent) (Ra,Pi,Pa)	Often a site of chronic inflammation and neoplasia	Cytology, culture and histology
Conjunctivitis and sinusitis(Ra,Pi,Pa)	Chlamydiosis, bacterial or fungal infection (For chlamydophilosis see liver lesions)	Stamp stain, cytology, bacterial or fungal culture
Conjunctivitis (Ra,Pi,Pa)	Avipox lesions	Cytology, histology and culture
Lens cataract or panophthalmy	Toxoplasmosis	Cytology, histology
Abdominal or other swellings (Ra,Pi,Pa)	Tumours, egg-related peritonitis	PME

9.13 (continued) Examples of alterations found at external examination in raptors (Ra), pigeons (Pi) and passerine birds (Pa).

Preparation of the bird

Small birds are wetted and plucked; all other birds should be wetted with 70% alcohol before the PME. This is done to allow for better visualization of the skin, to part the feathers to permit incision of the skin and to prevent loose feathers from irritating or harming the prosector (from zoonosis) and contaminating the viscera.

The bird is positioned on its back. In small birds the wings and legs are pinned to a dissecting board with nails or needles; large birds are fixed on a metal tray with pieces of rope. A useful tip is to pin or bind the legs over the wingtip; this keeps the feathers out of the way.

The bird should be transferred to the safety cabinet if one is available.

The necropsy

General considerations are as follows:

- Post-mortem tissue changes must be distinguished from true ante-mortem lesions. The amount of time between death and PME, and the ambient temperature, are factors that must be considered. Post-mortem changes can affect subsequent histological examination of tissues
- A relative lack or excess of blood contributes to the size, colour and consistency of any organ. Colour changes may occur before or after death. The differences will be noted with experience
- The consistency of an organ may be affected by ante-mortem conditions and by the amount of time between death and the PME.
- Tissue loss may lead to symmetrical or asymmetrical changes in organ size and weight. Loss can indicate necrosis or atrophy and excess tissue may be due to hypertrophy, hyperplasia or neoplasia

- Ornithologists and biologists weigh the bird and organs, and take standard ornithology measurements: beak to tail (if plumage is good), chordal or tibial length. Weighing should be done before the carcass is wetted. They also score condition. In pet birds, condition is based only on the amount of pectoral muscle present – cachectic (absence of muscle) to fully trained muscle (and some stages in between) – and the amount of body fat.

General procedures for conducting a thorough PME include the following:

- Use a gram scale for measuring body weight and weighing organs
- Open all tube-like structures
- Cut all parenchymatous organs in slices of 1.5–2 mm to find small focal lesions
- Keep tissue for formalin fixation at least 3–5 mm in thickness (10 mm maximum)
- Keep ratio of tissue to formalin at 1:10
- Collect tissue samples continuously during the PME to prevent desiccation – do not wait until the gross examination is finished
- Remember to collect and submit specimens from a broad spectrum of organs and systems
- Routinely collect heart, lung, liver, spleen, kidney, gonad and adrenal, proventriculus and a piece of intestine (duodenum and pancreas) for histopathology
- When suspecting a viral problem, freeze the tissue as soon as possible at –70°C (or temporarily to –20°C) or collect tissue on wet ice until shipment.

Step 1. Subcutis

1. Make a midline incision in the skin along the sternum from the mandible to the cloaca. Take care to avoid the oesophagus and crop.

2. Reflect the skin using rat-tooth forceps and a scalpel to expose the subcutis and fat, crop, pectoral muscles, keel, abdominal wall, and medial aspect of the legs.
3. Note: colour of the muscles; fat deposits; abdominal volume and liver size; subcutaneous haemorrhages; oedema; abscesses; bruising or evidence of injections in the pectoral muscle; and parasites in the subcutis or pectoral muscle. Especially when the bird has been force-fed, look for signs of regurgitation (air sac) or feeding via the trachea, crop perforation or crop burnings. Judge the amount of food in the crop.

Examples of breast muscle and abdominal pathology are given in Figure 9.14.

Finding	Diagnosis	Tests
Wasted muscles	Chronic undernourishment. Differentials: gastric bleeding (Figure 9.15), aspergillosis	History and other pathological findings
Pale parallel stripes in leg muscle or breast muscle	*Leucocytozoon* spp. or sarcosporidiosis (sarcocystis)	Cytology stripe reveals the bradyzoites
A large dark spot distal to the keel at the right side in the abdomen	Swollen liver	Diagnosis: see later
Swollen abdomen	Hydrops ascites, liver leucosis, liver amyloidosis (Figure 9.16), distended intestines	Diagnosis during continuation of the PME

9.14 Breast muscle and abdomen: examples of pathology.

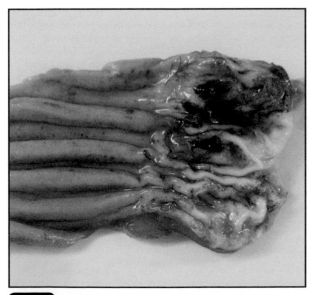

9.15 Haemorrhages in the gizzard of a falcon.

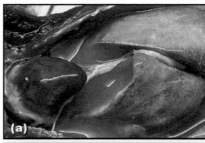

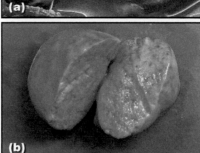
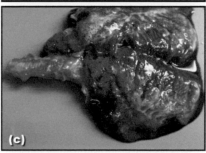
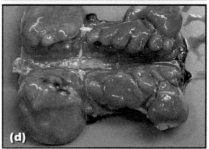

9.16
Amyloidosis and hydrops ascites in a Gyrfalcon x Lanner falcon: **(a)** liver amyloidosis and hydrops *in situ*. **(b)** spleen amyloidosis; **(c)** lungs with severe oedema **(d)** kidney amyloidosis.

Step 2. Body cavity *(in situ)*

1. Starting at the level of the coracoid bone, make a longitudinal incision through the pectoral muscle down either side of the thorax.
2. Grasp the sternum with thumb forceps and slightly elevate, maintaining tension on the abdominal wall.
3. Using a scalpel blade, make a transverse incision just caudal to the edge of the sternum, being careful not to lacerate the liver.
4. Remove the keel and pectoral muscle in one piece by cutting with heavy rongeurs, scissors or poultry shears through the ribs, coracoid bones and clavicle, and notice the air sacs that are now being exposed. Be careful not to cut the brachiocephalic arteries, particularly in freshly dead birds, or blood will enter the lungs via the thoracic air sacs.
5. The exposed organs should now be examined visually *in situ* (and a picture taken) before they are any further disturbed.

Because chlamydophilosis represents a significant zoonotic risk, it is recommended that at this point an examination is made for the presence of this infection before proceeding further:

- If the bird has a history or lesions suggesting *Chlamydophila psittaci* infection, microscopic examination (impressions of spleen or air sac, stained with a modified Ziehl–Neelsen) should be performed before proceeding further with the PME
- If the smear proves positive for *Chlamydophila* it is questionable whether one can justify completing the PME in a clinical setting. The carcass should be wrapped up in disinfectant-soaked paper towels and transferred to a polythene bag for safe disposal or storage in the freezer for confirmation by a referral laboratory.

6. Compare the *in situ* view with radiographs if available and confirm or reconsider the conclusions and abnormalities seen on them. Special attention should be paid to the situation of the air sacs when the diagnosis of (mycotic) air sacculitis (Figure 9.17) has been made: normal air sacs appear as glistening transparent membranes. This is also the time to verify clinical diagnoses relating to heart conditions, calcium

endocrinological diseases (parathyroid), thyroid gland and liver problems, and to note the pancreas in the duodenal loop, hydropic changes and severe gastrointestinal problems. Be aware of artefactual lesions caused by injection of barbiturates or other euthanates as brownish discoloration, often with crystalline deposits.

7. Take smears from any abnormal material or exudate, also from the air sacs when alterations are seen. If abdominal fluid is present, collect it with a sterile syringe for analysis and make a smear (cytospin).

Examples of air sac and pericardial pathology are given in Figure 9.18. For examples of liver pathology, see Step 6.

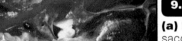

9.17

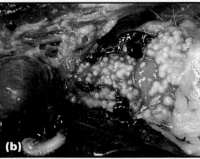

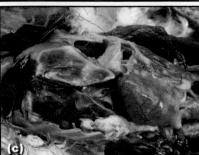

(a) Mycotic air sacculitis *in situ* due to aspergillosis in a Capuchinbird. (b) Subacute air sac aspergillosis in a Goshawk. (c) Subchronic air sac aspergillosis in a Goshawk.

Finding	Diagnosis	Tests
Opaque and wet air sac or with fibrin material	*Chlamydophila* infections	Cytology of collected material stained with modified ZN, IFT, PCR See also clinical findings and liver pathology
Opaque air sacs often with purulent deposits	Bacterial infection	Rods or cocci in cytology smear; culture and sensitivity test
Air sacs and/or pericardium covered with several white/yellow plaques	Fungal infection	Wet mount showing hyphae, scraping of the material as stained smear, culture (Sabouraud's medium)
Air sacs solid with white/yellow material	Chronic fungal infection, mostly aspergillosis	
Air sacs, especially cervical and prescapular, with small black dot occasionally seen in canaries and Gouldian finches	*Sternostoma tracheocolum* infestation	Magnifying-glass and wet mount
Air sacs filled with food	Forced feeding	Wet mount and histology
Suppurative pericarditis	Bacterial infection (including *Chlamydophila*)	Cytology of collected material stained with modified ZN, IFT, PCR See also clinical findings and liver pathology
Pericardial sac filled with fluid (hydropericardium)	Inanition, cachexia, polyomavirus (in juveniles)	Muscle wasting, oedema and gelatinous fat tissue, spleen and kidney histology
Pericardium and other serosae with white mucoid chalky deposits	Visceral gout (Figure 9.19)	Macroscopy, wet mount with crystals (polarized light); often in combination with nephritis See also clinical blood values if PU/PD
(Filarid) worms in air sac	*Serratospiculum* spp. (*Cyathostoma* spp.)	Macroscopy, wet mount Faecal examination Collect worms in 70% alcohol with 10% glycerine

9.18 Air sac and pericardium: examples of pathology.

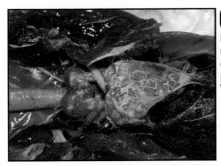

9.19
Deposition of uric acid crystals in the pericardium of a White Bellbird.

Step 3. Thyroid, parathyroid glands and thymus

1. Identify the thyroid and parathyroid glands located cranial to the heart and lateral to the trachea adjacent to the carotid arteries bilaterally and collect for histology. Normal parathyroids are barely visible.
2. Look for the thymus in juvenile birds laterally and at both sides of the neck, cranial to the thyroid gland, as multiple grey lobes, and collect for histology.

Examples of pathology of the thyroid, parathyroid glands and thymus are given in Figure 9.20.

Finding	Diagnosis	Tests
All species, especially juveniles, parathyroid hypertrophy	Metabolic bone disease	Macroscopy, histology
'Abscesses' next to trachea	*Salmonella*, *Escherichia coli* or other bacterial infections in thymic remnants	Rod-shaped bacteria in cytology, culture, histology

9.20 Parathyroid gland and thymus: examples of pathology.

Step 4. Spleen

1. The spleen can be found by grasping the gizzard with forceps, elevating and incising through the attached membrane/air sac and then rotating it towards the right side. This exposes the spleen in the angle between the proventriculus, gizzard and liver.
2. Evaluate the size, colour and shape and note any pale foci.
3. Remove and measure the spleen and divide it into samples: one each for virology, *Chlamydophila* diagnostics, bacteriology and histopathology. The normal form can be round to elongated, depending on the species (not congested; no blood reservoir in birds).
4. Make impression smears from a fresh cut surface after blotting to remove excess of blood.

Examples of pathology of the spleen are given in Figure 9.21.

Finding	Diagnosis	Tests
Swollen spleen together with air sac opacity	*Chlamydophila* infection	Cytology of collected material stained with modified ZN, IFT, PCR
Swollen spleen with white foci	Herpesvirus infection or *Sarcocystis*	Liver necrosis with intranuclear inclusion bodies or protozoa, cytology, histology, IFT, virus isolation
Normal sized totally necrotic spleen	Reovirus infection	Histology, PCR
Swollen and pale red spleen	(Bacterial) septicaemia	Cytology with bacteria, culture
Swollen and dark spleen	Atoxoplasmosis	Cytology, histology
Multiple irregular yellow foci in the spleen	Mycobacteriosis	Similar foci in other organs; on cytology non-staining rods; acid-fast staining positive Differentiation of avian-type, avian/mammalian-type or mammalian strains by culture or PCR
Large firm spleen	Neoplasia	Cytology, histology
Enlarged friable spleen with multiple miliary necrotic foci	Salmonellosis, yersiniosis (Figure 9.22)	Similar foci in the liver; cytology with rod-shaped bacteria; culture
Small grey spleen	Lymphoid depletion stress, viral infection	Cytology, histology, virus identification

9.21 Spleen: examples of pathology.

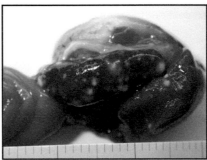

9.22
Splenomegaly with necrotic foci in a Canary with subacute pseudo-tuberculosis.

Step 5. Heart and large vessels

Special attention should be paid to the heart when clinical signs such as respiratory distress were obvious, the radiograph shows cardiomegaly or hepatomegaly or when a hydrops ascites was present. A normal heart shows coronary fat and no epicardial vascular congestion.

1. After noting the pericardial lesions, heart blood can be collected using a sterile syringe and needle for bacteriology.
2. Remove the heart and large vessels and cut across the apex to check for an 'open' lumen and to assess the thickness of the ventricular walls.

Finding	Diagnosis	Tests
Vessels		
Yellowish raised intimal plaques on the wall inside the large vessels; vessels stiff	Arteriosclerosis	Macroscopy, histology
Mineralization of large vessels	Renal disease or hypervitaminosis D	Clinical renal panel, kidney pathology
Heart		
Epi- or endocardial haemorrhages	Septicaemia or agonal event (polyoma, circovirus (passerines))	Continue PME
Gelatinous serous pericardial fat	Starvation, chronic illness	Continue PME
Pale foci or streaks in myocardium	Degenerative myopathy Related to vitamin E/selenium deficiency	Histology
Changes (inflammation, necrosis) in the myocardium	Myocarditis Caused by septicaemia or viral disease (e.g. West Nile virus) or toxoplasmosis	Cytology, histology, microbiological isolation, continue PME
Cardiomyopathy with muscle cysts	*Sarcocystis* or *Leucocytozoon*	Cytology, histology
Enlarged lumen of left ventricle and only little difference in thickness of ventricle walls	Heart failure	Congestion of the lungs and/or liver

9.23   Large vessels and heart: examples of pathology.

3. Open the heart and large vessels in the direction of the blood flow.
4. Look for thrombi, valvular endocarditis lesions and pale areas in the myocardium. Remember that the right atrioventricular valve in birds is a muscular structure.
5. Open the large vessels to look for atherosclerosis (mainly aorta, pulmonary artery or carotids).

Examples of pathology of the heart and large vessels are given in Figure 9.23.

Step 6. Liver

1. Evaluate the clinical pathological results for liver disease.
2. Separate liver from the viscera by holding the hepatic peritoneum in the forceps and cutting it with scissors.
3. In a freshly euthanased bird, blood spreading into the carcass after cutting the portal vein can hide many changes. In such cases it may be better to wait some hours before doing the PME, or remove the blood from the vein using a syringe.
4. Examine the liver for evidence of swelling, discoloration, inflammation, congestion and diffuse or focal lesions (Figure 9.24).

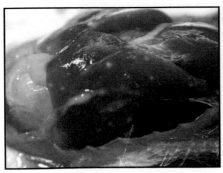

9.24

Liver with necrotic foci *in situ* in Canary with subacute pseudo-tuberculosis.

5. At this point, also aseptically collect liver samples: one sample each for bacteriology, virus isolation or DNA probe (PCR) testing, *Chlamydophila* testing and histopathology. Sear a small area of one lobe of the liver and take a sample using a wire loop or sterile Pasteur pipette for bacterial culture. If there are discrete lesions, try to take a sample through the edge of a lesion.
6. If there are no on-site culture facilities, remove one lobe of the liver, using a sterile scalpel blade and forceps, and transfer it directly into a sterile sample pot. Hold the sample in a refrigerator at 4°C until it can be posted, preferably with an ice pack in an insulated container together with the other samples (each in its own sample pot).
7. To make cytological preparations: hold a small part of the liver in forceps, blot off any excess blood using filter paper and make impression slides from the cut surface on to two or three microscope slides. Stain one with Hemacolor® and, when appropriate, one with modified Ziehl–Neelsen (for *Chlamydophila*). The third slide can be used for an extra staining or send to a laboratory for confirmation by immunostaining for *Chlamydophila*. Take a separate sample from abnormal foci.
8. Use any remaining tissue for toxicology, if indicated.

Examples of pathology of the liver are given in Figure 9.25.

Step 7: Gastrointestinal tract

With the heart and liver removed, the gastrointestinal tract is more accessible. The size and appearance of the crop, proventriculus, gizzard, duodenum and pancreas should be noted, but it is best to leave detailed examination of these organs until later.

Finding	Diagnosis	Tests	Comments
Enlarged red variegated liver with pale areas	Hepatitis	Cytology with many inflammatory cells; microbiology, material in freezer, histology	Elevated activity of liver enzymes
Enlarged liver with necrotic foci	Hepatitis from *Chlamydophila* infection, herpesvirus or adenovirus infection	Cytology, culture, histology	Often highly increased enzyme activity and yellow urates
Very extensive acute liver necrosis	Peracute or acute hepatitis caused by bacterial septicaemia, polyomavirus, herpesvirus	Macroscopy, cytology, histology, virology, culture	Often highly increased enzyme activity and yellow urates
Focal yellow proliferation with often central necrosis	Mycobacteriosis	Similar foci in other organs, in cytology non-staining rods, acid-fast staining	No increased enzyme activity or yellow urates
Small round necrotic foci	Salmonellosis or yersiniosis (Figure 9.25)	Cytology with rod-shaped bacteria; culture, histology	
Evenly enlarged (often variegated) pale liver	Leucosis, amyloidosis (see Figure 9.16)	Macroscopy; other organs often included; cytology and histology	
Evenly enlarged (often variegated) pale soft liver	Degeneration	Cytology, hepatocytes with vacuoles; histology	
Normal form but yellowish-pale liver	Anaemia	Cytology, histology	Look for trauma or blood mites
Enlarged orange-yellow liver	Fatty liver, lipidosis	Macroscopy, cytology, histology with Sudan III stain	Little increased enzyme activity
Small pale firm liver	Chronic liver fibrosis	Histology	No increased enzyme activity, but yellow urates

9.25 Liver: examples of pathology.

1. Sever the oesophagus where it passes between both bronchi and reflect the gastrointestinal tract to the right side of the bird, or caudally over the tail, to view the adrenals, gonads, kidneys, bursa and lungs. Do not cut the rectum.
2. If the intestines cannot be reflected because of peritoneal adhesions, check for a possible point of entry of infection, such as perforation of the gizzard or accidental damage to the intestine following laparoscopy.
3. In a case of egg peritonitis there will be masses of yellow inspissated yolk interspersed between adhering loops of intestine.

Step 8: Genitourinary system
The adrenals (orange to yellow) are often obscured by active gonadal tissue and so it is easier to collect the cranial division of the kidney with the adrenals and gonad(s) attached for histopathology.

1. Sex the bird visually. In most avian species, only the left ovary and oviduct develop in females, but in many raptors the right ovary and oviduct are developed at least during the first year of life. Both testes develop in male birds. The gonads may be pigmented.
2. Record the general size of the follicles and notice discoloured, inflamed or shrunken follicles. If these are found, sample for bacteriology, including selective media for *Salmonella* spp.
3. If the oviduct is hypertrophied, open it to look for exudate and tumours, and collect samples for cytology, bacteriology and histopathology as needed.

Examples of pathology of the genital tract are given in Figure 9.26.

Finding	Diagnosis	Tests
A swelling inside the oviduct	Egg binding, egg concrements	Open the oviduct
Irregular swellings related to kidney or gonads	Tumour	Macroscopy, cytology and histology

9.26 Common genital tract: examples of pathology.

The kidneys are nestled in the renal fossae of the synsacrum, with the lumbosacral nerves plexus lying deep to the caudal division of the kidney. The ureters run down the ventral surface of the kidney bilaterally.

1. Especially when clinically the uric acid concentration in the blood was elevated or when visceral gout was diagnosed on observation in situ, pay extra attention to the kidneys. Differentiate between renal pathology and dehydration: this is best done by viewing the

dorsal side (after removal of the kidneys) under a dissecting microscope and evaluating the amount and location of the urates in the tubuli.

2. In addition to kidney/adrenal/gonad tissue collected for histopathology, aseptically collect renal samples for virology (polyomavirus–paramyxovirus infection), toxicology (lead, zinc, herbicides) and bacteriology (if exudate is present).

3. After removal of the kidneys, evaluate the lumbosacral plexus, especially in cases of pelvic limb weakness or malfunction. Sample these nerves into formalin for histopathological evaluation.

Examples of pathology of the kidney are given in Figure 9.27.

Finding	Diagnosis	Tests
Pale normal sized kidneys with a fine reticular pattern of white urates over surface and in tubules (use magnifier or dissection microscope)	Urate congestion, dehydration. DDX: herbicide intoxication	Histology (fixation 100% alcohol, *not formalin* – uric acid crystals will dissolve)
Irregular pale swollen kidney with white foci often combined with visceral gout	'Renal gout', nephritis	Histology (fixation 100% alcohol)
Irregular swollen kidney with multifocal abscessation	Bacterial infection	Cytology, culture, histology
Enlarged hyperaemic kidneys	Acute nephritis	Histology
Pale swollen friable kidney	Kidney degeneration	Histology
White firm small kidneys	Chronic kidney fibrosis	Macroscopy; histology
Granulomas	*Aspergillus* spp.	Scraping of the cut surface of the granuloma Hemacolor®, culture (Sabouraud's agar), histology
Irregular swelling and growth	Tumour. Causing clinical leg paralysis by pressure on the sciatic nerves	Cytology and histology

9.27   Kidney: examples of pathology.

Step 9: Respiratory tract

Examine the lungs *in situ* before removing them. Pay especially careful attention to this organ system when clinically there was an obvious dyspnoea.

1. If the lungs appear congested or show discrete lesions, they should be cultured for bacteria and fungi. Samples are best taken with the lung *in situ* using a hot scalpel to sear the surface.

2. If a viral condition is suspected (e.g. paramyxovirus), place lung tissue plus a portion of the trachea in a sterile container and store at 4°C until posted to a reference laboratory with other sampled organ tissues (brain and duodenum with pancreas).

The lungs are fixed in place within the avian thoracic cavity and are not freely moveable. Removal requires gentle teasing of the lung tissue away from the ribs. In many cases lungs have changes in the dorsal part only and these can be missed if the lung is not removed. The avian lung is one tissue in which gross lesions may appear quite significant, but on histopathological evaluation turn out to be just passive congestion. Conversely, grossly normal lungs may contain significant histological lesions. Therefore, lung should always be included for histopathology; and because lesions can be focal or multifocal, it is best to include a large portion of at least one lung.

3. Cut through the lungs at intervals; make an impression smear of the lung (along with impressions from liver, spleen and a smear from the intestines). This impression of the lung is also used to evaluate the blood cells for pathological changes and blood parasites (*Plasmodium*, *Haemoproteus* (Figure 9.28) and *Toxoplasma* pseudocysts).

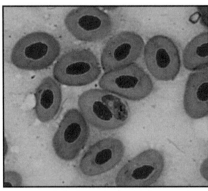

9.28   *Haemoproteus* in a blood smear from a Buzzard. Hemacolor®; original magnification X100.

4. At this point, open the bird's beak; insert a large pair of scissors into the oropharynx and cut through one side of the mouth.

5. Reflect the mandible and examine the oropharynx, including the choanae, the tongue and the glottis. Notice any large amount of mucous material and diphtheritic changes; e.g. pox lesions.

6. Insert a pair of sharp scissors into the glottis and cut down the trachea both dorsally and ventrally, dividing it into two longitudinal halves. It is important to do this carefully and cleanly, checking in particular for haemorrhage, exudate, foreign bodies, granulomas and parasites, items of inhaled food and also for white caseous fibrinous material adhering to the mucosa, in the syrinx or bronchi. Such material is usually mycotic and, if present, should be examined microscopically (stain crushed preparations) and cultured on Sabouraud's medium.

Examples of pathology of the lung and trachea are given in Figure 9.29.

Finding	Diagnosis	Tests
Lung		
Dark-coloured grey lungs	Lung oedema. Often the result of a chronic circulatory problem or acute cardiac failure	On cut surface transparent sero-hemorrhagic fluid, affected tissue sinks in water, cytology, histology
Dark-coloured wet red lungs	Lung congestion. Watch for congestion in other organs and acute alterations of the heart – DDX polytetrafluoroethylene (Teflon®) toxicosis, acute mycotic infection and *Sarcocystis* infection	From a cut surface only blood; Affected lungs float in water, the lungs are supple and evenly bright red, cytology, histology
Dark firm lungs often variegated and focal changes	Pneumonic foci, mycobacterial infection	Affected areas firm and sink in water, cut surface cytology (inflammatory cells); histology, culture
Diffuse pneumonia (in combination with tracheitis and bronchitis)	*Bordetella avium*	Culture (fastidious grower), histology
Dark, supple, collapsed, dry lung	Atelectasis	On cut surface only a dark colour of surface of lung and dried up
Scattered through the lungs white–yellow foci	Aspergillosis (Figure 9.30), mycobacteriosis	Wet mount with hyphae, acid-fast rods (in routine rapid staining, non-stained rods); culture, histology, PCR
Irregular scattered necropurulent pneumonic foci with a hyperaemic zone	Bacterial pneumonia e.g. *Salmonella* spp. or *Yersinia* spp. *Pasteurella* spp.	Cytology and culture
Trachea		
In the syrinx white caseous–fibrinous material	Syringal mycosis	Wet mount with hyphae, culture (Sabouraud's agar), histology
In the trachea red or white worms	*Syngamus* spp., *Cyathostoma* spp.	Microscopic examination of the material, histology
Black dots	*Sternostoma* mites	
Mucous and fibrin	Avipox	

See also examples in crop/intestines (e.g. trichomoniasis, avipox, candidiasis)
See also examples on external examination

9.29   Respiratory system: examples of pathology.

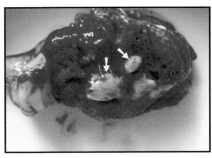

9.30
Mycotic processes (arrowed) in the lungs of a Capuchinbird with subacute aspergillosis.

Step 10: Gastrointestinal tract

1. Going back to the pharynx, extend the cut downwards for the length of the oesophagus and into the crop, looking for lacerations and punctures, peri-oesophageal abscesses, parasites (e.g. *Capillaria*) and other abnormalities. Note that in pigeons the crop is thickened during feeding of the nestlings (see Chapter 27); do not confuse this with any pathological changes.
2. When any abnormality is visible, take a mucosal scraping for a wet mount and for a stained smear.
3. The crop contents can be collected in a plastic bag and frozen, if there is any suggestion of a toxic ingestion.
4. At this point, the oesophagus distal to the crop can be transected. Caudal traction of the distal oesophagus and sharp dissection of the mesenteric attachments can be used to remove the entire gastrointestinal tract.
5. Continue the dissection to make a circular incision around the vent, leaving a margin of intact vent skin and the bursa of Fabricius attached to the tract. The bursa is present in young birds, usually less than 6–12 months of age, and is located dorsal to the cloaca (see Figure 9.8). The bursa should always be collected when it is present and divided in half for histology and freezer (PCR of circovirus or polyomavirus).
6. Open the distal oesophagus with scissors, continuing into the proventriculus and gizzard (with koilin layer; Figure 9.31).
7. Examine the wall (mucosa and serosa) for pathological changes and gastric worms and the contents for amount, foreign bodies and heavy metals.

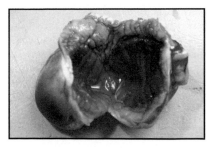

9.31
Gizzard with green koilin layer due to reflux of bile.

8. Collect and freeze the contents for possible toxicological analysis.
9. Rinse the mucosa with water and make wet mount and dried smears of mucus and/or mucosal scrapings.
10. Do not separate the proventriculus and gizzard. The isthmus is a common place for avian gastric yeast (*Macrorhabdus ornithogaster*) and gastric carcinoma. Collect a large specimen of proventriculus, isthmus and gizzard (all in one piece), containing at least one large serosal nerve and blood vessel, for histopathology.
11. Open the pylorus and proceed into the duodenal loop. The largest limb of the pancreas lies in the duodenal loop mesentery while the small splenic pancreatic lobe is located adjacent to the spleen.
12. Collect a transverse section through the duodenal loop with pancreas attached (Figure 9.32) in formalin (for lymphoplasmacytic pancreatitis (PMV), inclusion body pancreatitis (herpesvirus, adenovirus), pancreas necrosis (avian influenza, West Nile virus), vacuolar necrosis (zinc)) and one piece for toxicology (zinc, with liver and kidney).

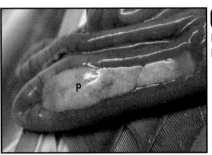

9.32
Duodenum with pancreas (P).

13. Continue opening the intestine through the jejunum and ileum to the rectum.
14. In neonates, the yolk sac and stalk should be evaluated for the degree of absorption. Collect a sterile sample of the yolk material for culture, make a stained smear and place the yolk sac membrane into formalin.
15. Collect opened untouched sections of intestine for histopathology.
16. Make wet mounts of intestinal contents (usually two different sides) and stained smear of mucosal scrapings for microscopic evaluation (parasites and ova, oocysts, cryptosporidia, flagellates (*Giardia*), yeast and motile bacteria) and bacterial culture (see Figure 9.6).
17. Open the cloaca to look for papillomatous lesions, cloacoliths, trauma and inflammatory lesions.

To summarize, intestinal samples should include: wet mounts (diluted with saline) from at least two different sites; smears for quick stain and possibly for acid-fast stain; contents for aerobic and possibly anaerobic (spores in cytology) or *Campylobacter* culture. Tissue and ingesta for virology (EM negative contrast, virus isolation, or PCR) should also be collected.

Examples of pathology of the gastrointestinal tract are illustrated and described in Figures 9.33 to 9.36.

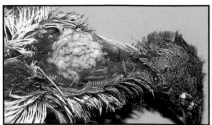

9.33
Candidiasis in a Gouldian finch.

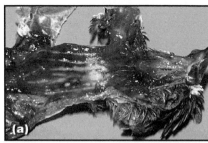

9.34
Trichomoniasis. **(a)** Gross lesion in a Bengalese finch. **(b)** *Trichomonas columbae* in a crop smear from a pigeon.

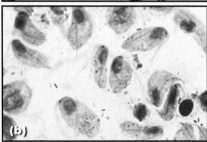

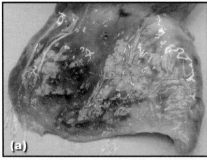

9.35
Tetrameres fissipina in a Wood Pigeon: **(a)** proventriculus – serosal side. **(b)** proventriculus – mucosal side; **(c)** worm egg (50–58 x 22–29 µm) in faecal sample.

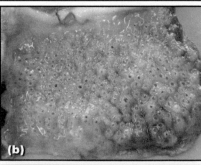

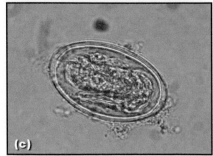

Finding	Diagnosis	Tests
Crop		
Thickened wall with white material (Turkish towel)	Yeast infection, candidiasis (see Figure 9.33) In juvenile birds	Wet mount smear, cytology, culture
Thickened wall with grey/yellow material	Trichomoniasis (= frounce (Ra)) Especially in juvenile birds, sometimes with trapped air bubbles. In adult birds flagellates can be present without changes	Wet mount, cytology (see Figure 9.34), and histology
Local red mucosal thickening	Papillomas	Histology
Stomach (proventriculus and gizzard)		
Empty proventriculus with excess of mucus, especially at isthmus region, often with petechiae	Avian gastric yeasts (*Macrorhabdus ornithogaster*)	Wet mount and cytology
Thickening of proventricular wall with red 'filling' in glandular lumen	*Tetrameres* (see Figure 9.35)	Wet mount, parasitology, histology
Irregular thickening of mucosa of proventriculus	Gastric worms (e.g. *Dispharynx nasuta*)	Wet mount, parasitology, histology
Irregular koilin layer that is difficult to remove from wall	Endoventricular mycosis	Deep scraping wet mount, cytology, culture
Empty stomach with black staining of the mucous	Gastric haemorrhage (see Figure 9.15)	Wet mount, cytology and histology
Intestines		
Haemorrhagic black contents in entire small intestine	Haemorrhagic diathesis (massive leakage of blood into intestine)	History (fasting for longer period), macroscopy
Thickened wall with or without blood in lumen	Enteritis	Wet mount and cytology; parasitology; microbiology
Thin wall with haemorrhagic contents or stuffed with worms	Ascaridiasis *Beware*: rarely *Ascaridia* in small seed-eating passerine birds	Demonstration of worms at gross PME or larvae in wet mount
Thickened areas of bowel or multifocal granulomas	Mycobacteriosis	In cytology non-staining rods, acid-fast staining positive, histology, culture or PCR
Intestines with part or whole seeds	Gastric problems, e.g. *Macrorhabdus*, yeast infection	Wet mount, cytology (also of the stomach), culture, histology
Haemorrhagic content	Lead intoxication, *Clostridium* infection, *Pseudomonas* infection, *Giardia* spp.	Lead in gizzard; lead analysis liver and kidneys; cytology, culture
Cloaca		
Congested swollen red mucosa	Papilloma	Histology
Pancreas		
Irregular pancreas with haemorrhages	Paramyxovirus pancreatitis Avian influenza Especially in finches with torticollis	Histology

9.36 Gastrointestinal tract: examples of pathology.

Step 11: Nasal and infraorbital sinuses

1. Check the nasal and infraorbital sinuses by cutting through the upper beak caudal to the nostrils and inspect the conchae for symmetry and presence of mucus or purulent material.
2. Collect material for culturing and compare the result with the findings in a stained smear from that material. It is impossible to collect uncontaminated samples from the sinuses, and so cultural examination is always of doubtful value.
3. Collect material for histological examination when there are pathological changes.

Example: The presence of turbid mucus suggests bacterial or mycotic sinusitis. Confirmatory tests would be wet mount cytology and culture.

Step 12: Neurological examination
The brain and spinal cord can be very important in the diagnosis of some diseases. It is always essential to open the skull when clinically neurological symptoms were found or in the history the bird could have flown into a window before being found dead.

1. After removing the skin, examine for evidence of traumatic injuries. Beware of areas of haemorrhage within the calvarium, which are common agonal changes and do not imply head trauma.
2. The dorsal calvarium should be carefully removed with rongeurs. Visualize the brain in situ for any obvious abnormalities, such as abscesses, which should be cultured, and intracranial or submeningeal haemorrhages.
3. Remove the brain by inverting the skull and transecting the ventral and cranial attachments. When this is difficult, especially in young or small birds, open the cranium and place the skull in fixative and send the brain in situ to the pathologist. When indicated, collect a portion of the forebrain for virology and toxicology, before fixing the rest in formalin.
4. To inspect and collect spinal cord, cut the vertebral column with cord in situ into several pieces and fix in formalin. This process will allow easier removal using rongeurs, with minimal damage to the less fragile fixed spinal cord.
5. In birds with a head tilt or neurological disease, fix a large portion of the petrous temporal bone containing the middle ear and send it to the pathologist.

Step 13: Musculoskeletal system
Bone marrow is most easily collected from the tibiotarsus for both cytology and histology.

1. Clean the bone and use rongeurs to break the bone.
2. After collecting bone marrow for a smear, fix the bone marrow *in situ* in formalin.
3. Once fixed, the previously fragile bone marrow can be dissected out and examined histologically. In bone marrow, leukaemic or aplastic processes and occasionally circovirus inclusions or TB lesions can be found. Bone marrow is also an excellent place to look for circovirus, especially in birds whose bursa has involved.
4. Samples of skeletal muscle should be collected for histopathology when changes are seen or suspected based on clinical biochemical indications (CK). Muscular lesions may include trauma, haemorrhage, degeneration, mineralization and injection or vaccine site reactions. Myositis, degenerative myopathy, and *Sarcocystic* infection can be diagnosed histologically.
5. In tropical finches, orange-coloured muscles are often seen; the cause is still unclear.
6. The muscles of the legs and ischiadic nerve running on the posterior surface of the femur should be examined, especially when clinical paralysis of the hind legs was seen.
7. Finally, check all the major limb joints. Any bone or joint lesion demonstrated radiographically should be opened and sampled for culture and histopathology. Be aware of the medullary bone changes in breeding females. The flexibility of bones (tibiotarsus, ribs, etc.) can be used to assess poor mineralization when calcium deficiency is very advanced. The rachitic 'rosary' at the costochondral or costovertebral junction and deformation of the keel or other long bones are obvious lesions of metabolic bone disease.
8. Other findings in the joints are nematodes (*Pelecitus*), bacterial arthritis (stained smear and culture), and articular gout (large deposits of urate crystals).

Final activities
This completes the gross PME and the remaining parts of the carcass can be placed in a plastic bag and frozen until diagnostic testing has been completed.

- Examine wet mounts as quickly as possible. Warming (maximal body temperature) before examination will help in detecting moving flagellates.
- Stain any exudates and impression smears collected.
- When chlamydophilosis is suspected, send a collection of liver, spleen and lung for *Chlamydophila* diagnostics (modified ZN, PCR and fluorescent antibody test).
- Send tissues, exudates or swabs for bacterial or fungal culture as indicated. With the exception of samples for *Campylobacter* (which does not survive freezing well), these samples can often be frozen if not sent for culture immediately.
- A pool of parenchymal tissues (liver, spleen, lung, kidney (inclduing adrenals and gonads) and brain) and a separate pool of intestinal contents should be refrigerated or frozen for possible virus isolation or DNA probe testing.
- Select a group of formalin-fixed tissues with lesions or a group of tissues that commonly contain histological lesions that could lead to diagnosis and submit them for histopathology. This often includes tissues such as heart, liver, kidney, spleen, lung, bursa (always when available), duodenum, pancreas and proventriculus/ventriculus. Save the remaining formalin-fixed tissues just in case the diagnosis is not made with the first set.
- Samples collected for ancillary diagnostics should be packed, labelled and stored properly until shipment. See that each sample is provided with the essential documentation.
- Make a detailed PME report (Figure 9.38), including establishing connections to the clinical findings, and use this to document the samples.

> **Try to establish a relationship between the clinical history and the post-mortem findings.**

PME Report Form and Checklist

1. Bird species, weight, age/leg band number, sex, and summarized history.

2. Date of PME, your name.

3. Macroscopy:

   External examination

   General body condition: muscle mass: robust, well muscled, moderately muscled, thin, emaciated, depot fat

   Feathers/integument/ectoparasites

   Palpation of skeleton

   Body openings/oral cavity

   Internal examination

   In situ description (take pictures)

   Fat/subcutis/body wall

   Body cavity (air sacs/pleura/peritoneum)

   (Para)thyroids, thymus

   Spleen (size, colour)

   Heart, aorta, other vessels

   Liver

   Reproductive system (gonads, reproductive tract)

   Respiratory tract (nasal/sinus, choanal, larynx, trachea, syrinx, air sacs, lungs)

   Urinary tract (kidneys, ureters) and adrenal glands

   Digestive tract (beak, tongue, oropharynx, oesophagus, crop, proventriculus, gizzard, duodenum and pancreas, small intestine, yolk sac, caeca, rectum (colorectum), cloaca, bursa of Fabricius, vent)

   Special senses (eyes, ears, nares)

   Musculoskeletal system: muscles, skeleton (sternum, ribs, vertebrae, long bones), bone marrow, joints

   Brain, pituitary, spinal cord, meninges, peripheral nerves

4. Wet mounts (crop, rectum, etc.)

5. Cytology (liver, spleen, lung, rectum)

6. *Chlamydophila* examination

7. Tentative (differential) diagnosis

8. Ancillary diagnostics: bacteriology, mycology, virology, parasitology, toxicology, others

9. Tissues saved:

10. Tissues submitted for histopathology:

11. Material for further examinations (tissues, tests):

    Bacteriology

    Virology

    PCR

9.38   PME report form and checklist.

References and further reading

Aguilar RF, Shawk DP, Dubey JP and Redig PT (1991) Sarcocystis-associated encephalitis in an immature northern goshawk. *Journal Zoo and Wildlife Medicine* **22**, 466–469

Campbell TW (1995) *Avian Hematology and Cytology, 2nd edn.* Iowa State University Press, Ames

Echols S (1999) Collecting diagnostic samples in avian patients. *Veterinary Clinics of North America: Exotic Animal Practice* **2**, 621–649

Echols S (2003) Practical gross necropsy of exotic animal species: Introduction. *Seminars in Avian and Exotic Pet Medicine* **12**, 57–58

Ferrer M, Garcia Rodrigues I, Carrillo JC and Castroviejo J (1987) Hematocrit and blood chemistry values in captive raptors (*Gyps fulvus, Buteo buteo, Milvus migrans, Aquila heliaca*). *Comparative Biochemistry and Physiology* **4**, 1123–1127

Fudge AM (2000) Laboratory reference ranges for selected avian, mammalian, and reptilian species. In: *Laboratory Medicine – Avian and Exotic Pets*, pp. 376–400. WB Saunders, Philadelphia

Gee GF, Carpenter JW and Hensler GI (1981) Species differences in hematological values of captive cranes, geese, raptors and quail. *Journal of Wildlife Management* **2**, 463–483

Gerlach C (1978) Grundlagen der Blutdiagnostik bei Greifvögeln. *Praktische Tierarzt* **59**, 642–650

Gylstorff I and Grimm F (1987) *Vogelkrankheiten*. Verlag Eugen Ulmer, Stuttgart

Hernandez M (1991) Blood chemistry in raptors. *Proceedings, Conference of the European Communion Association of Avian Veterinarians, Vienna*, pp. 411–419

Höfle U, Blanco JM, Spergser J, Johne R and Kaleta EF (2002) Mycoplasma and avian polyoma virus infection in captive Spanish imperial eagles (*Aquila adalberti*). *European Association of Zoo and Wildlife Veterinarians (EAZWV) 4th scientific meeting, joint with the annual meeting of the European Wildlife Disease Association (EWDA) May 8–12, 2002, Heidelberg, Germany* pp. 161–167

Lavin, S,Cuenca R, Marco I, Velarde R and Vinas L (1992) Hematology and blood chemistry of the Marsh Harrier (*Circus aeruginosus*). *Comparative Biochemistry and Physiology* **103**, 493–495

Lierz M (2002) Blood chemistry values of the Saker Falcon (*Falco cherrug*). *Tierärztliche Praxis*, **30**, 386–388

Lierz M (2003) Plasma chemistry reference values for gyrfalcons (*Falco rusticolus*). *Veterinary Record* **153**, 182–183

Lierz M (2005) Avian renal disease: pathogenesis, diagnosis and therapy. *Veterinary Clinics of North America: Exotic Animal Practice* **6**, 29–55

Lierz M and Hafez HM (2006) Plasma chemistry reference values in hybrid falcons in relation to their species of origin. Veterinary Record **159**, 79–82

Lumeij JT and Overduin LM (1990) Plasma chemistry reference values in psittaciformes. *Avian Pathology* **19**, 234–244

Lumeij JT, Remple JD, Remple CJ and Riddle KE (1998) Plasma chemistry in peregrine falcons (*Falco peregrinus*): reference values and physiological variations of importance for interpretation. *Avian Pathology* **27**, 129–132

Phenix KV, Weston JH, Ypelaar I *et al.* (2001) Nucleotide sequence analysis of a novel and its relationship to other members of the family Circoviridae. *Journal of General Virology* **82**, 2805–2809

Rae MA (2003) Practical avian necropsy. *Seminars in Avian and Exotic Pet Medicine* **12**, 62–70

Rampin T, Manarolla G, Pisoni G, Recordati C and Sironi G (2006) Circovirus inclusion bodies in intestinal muscle cells of a canary. *Avian Pathology* **36**, 277–279

Raue R, Schmidt V, Freick M *et al.* (2005) A disease complex associated with pigeon circovirus infection, young pigeon disease syndrome. *Avian Pathology* **34**, 418–425

Schmidt RE, Reavill DR and Phalen DN (2003) *Pathology of Pet and Aviary Birds*. Iowa State Press, Ames

Svobodová M (1996) Sarcocystis from goshawk (*Accipiter gentilis*) with great tit (*Parus major*) as intermediate host. *Acta Protozoologica* **35**, 223–226

Svobodová M, Voříšek P, Votýpka J and Weidinger K (2004) Heteroxenous coccidia (Apicomplexa: Sarcocystidae) in the populations of their final and intermediate hosts: European buzzard and small mammals. *Acta Protozoologica* **43**, 251–260

Todd D, Scott ANJ, Fringuelli E *et al.* (2007) Molecular characterization of novel circoviruses from finch and gull. *Avian Pathology* **36**, 75–81

Wernery U, Kinne J and Wernery R (2004) *Colour Atlas of Falcon Medicine*. Schlutersche, Hanover

Wittig W, Hoffmann K, Müller H and John R (2007) [Detection of DNA of the finch polyomavirus in diseases of various types of birds in the order Passeriformes]. *Berliner und Münchener Tierärztliche Wochenschrift* **120**, 113–119

10

Anaesthesia and analgesia

J. Jill Heatley

Anatomy and physiology

Avian respiratory and cardiovascular physiology is reviewed here only as it applies to anaesthesia and management of the anaesthetized avian patient. Chapter 5 gives a more comprehensive description.

- The trachea and glottis (Figure 10.1) are characterized by complete rings of cartilage and lack of an epiglottis.
- Mucus produced by the trachea is generally viscous and may be copious, becoming thickened and tenacious via drying of cold anaesthetic gases.
- The lack of epiglottis facilitates intubation but predisposes birds to aspiration upon efflux during and immediately after anaesthesia.
- Small birds (<100 g) are generally not intubated for anaesthesia because of an increased risk of mucous plugging the endotracheal tube.

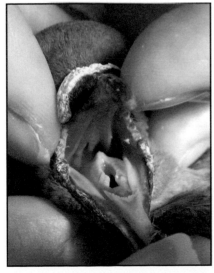

10.1

The glottis of a pigeon.

- Avian air sacs do not function in gas exchange but act as gas reservoirs. When the patient is placed in dorsal recumbency, the viscera may compress the caudal air sacs, resulting in reduced air sac volume and ventilation.
- Diverticulae of air sacs (pneumatization) in cervical vertebrae, vertebral ribs, sternum, humerus, pelvis and femur, can affect anaesthetic depth during repair of these areas.
- Surgery in areas of air sacs or diverticulae

during coelomic, soft tissue or orthopaedic surgery may result in escape of anaesthetic gases into the surgical field. Use of cautery, laser and radiosurgical devices should be limited in these cases.
- Both inspiration and expiration require active movement of the ribs and sternum via cervical thoracic and abdominal musculature. An absence of keel movement reflects a lack of gas exchange; thus it is preferable to position the bird so as to have least effect on respiration.
- Intermittent positive pressure ventilation (IPPV) during anaesthesia is almost always indicated during even the shortest anaesthetic episode. A rate of at least 2 breaths per minute is used to assist the spontaneously ventilating intubated bird, while a rate of 10–15 breaths per minute is recommended in the apnoeic bird (Paul-Murphy and Fialkowski, 2001). Common negative effects of controlled ventilation seen in mammals, such as decreased venous return and respiratory alkalosis, have not been reported in avian patients placed on a mechanical ventilator with an intact respiratory system.

Preanaesthetic assessment and examination

Preanaesthetic assessment of avian patients varies depending on species, clinical presentation and the clinician's preference and experience. In debilitated, anaemic or fractious patients, or those in respiratory distress, anaesthesia may be necessary, after a brief observational examination, to complete the physical examination and to facilitate the collection of samples for a minimum database. Avian patients with respiratory difficulty may actually be relieved from the stress of respiration and restraint via rapid anaesthetic induction with 100% oxygen.

The preanaesthetic assessment should include a risk assessment of anaesthesia in the patient, which may be modelled after standard American Society of Anesthesiologists guidelines. Anaesthetic risk should be communicated to the owner, preferably in writing, prior to anaesthetizing the bird. The owner should consent both verbally and in writing to anaesthesia and/or pain control for their bird. Clients should also be informed of any off-label use of drugs in their birds.

Restraint and handling

Appropriate handling and capture techniques (see Chapter 6) avoid injury to the handler and injury or death of the patient, and reduce patient stress by effecting a quick capture and anaesthetic induction.

Examination

The primary aim of the preanaesthetic examination is to determine the patient's cardiopulmonary status. Patient size and temperament will affect the ability to measure some parameters. Performance of the pre-anaesthetic examination one day prior to the anaes-thetic event facilitates patient acclimation to the hospital and may decrease stress, allowing the patient to show any additional signs of disease. Chapter 7 describes the examination.

Minimum database

Prior to anaesthesia or a planned prolonged anaes-thetic episode, collection of the minimum database is based on clinician preference, species, patient size and monetary limitations. The object of the mini-mum database is to assess the patient's ability to tolerate anaesthesia and anaesthetic drugs, espe-cially those that require liver or kidney action for removal from the patient. Often it may be foregone in lieu of a full diagnostic work-up during a brief anaesthetic event to facilitate venepuncture and radiography in the sick avian patient. It may also be foregone in very small or fractious species, or those with immediate life-threatening illness in need of surgical intervention.

Fasting

The decision to fast is based on many factors, including species, size, physiology, projected length of the anaesthetic event, type of procedure, diet and the patient's clinical condition. Water should con-tinue to be provided to the patient until 1–3 hours prior to the procedure. All ingestible non-food objects should be removed from the enclosure to avoid pre-anaesthetic ingestion.

Preanaesthetic fasting is indicated to avoid or decrease regurgitation reflux and subsequent aspir-ation and secondary asphyxiation or pneumonia. Fasting is also indicated to reduce the volume of the gastrointestinal tract to facilitate gas flow through the respiratory tract. Birds undergoing lengthy anaesthetic procedures may be more prone to passive reflux, which is facilitated by deep anaesthetic relaxation of smooth muscle.

Recommendations concerning preanaesthetic fasting extend beyond species size alone. Raptors, with the exception of vultures, produce a pellet or casting (see Chapter 16) generally once a day. Pellet egestion usually occurs at night in owls and in the early morning in diurnal birds of prey. Anaesthesia should be delayed until the raptor has cast or lacks casting material in the gastrointestinal tract. Thus raptors should either be fed a meal devoid of casting material prior to surgery, or be monitored and only taken to surgery after casting.

Food should be withheld from raptors for at least 6–12 hours. As casting may take as long as 16 hours in the larger species, this length of fasting, or more, is appropriate (Figure 10.2).

Pigeons tend to have extensive crops and regurgitate when stressed by handling. These species also tend to be heavy bodied when compared with raptors or passerine birds of similar mass and can tolerate a relatively longer fast.

Passerine birds are generally small; they have a relatively small crop and a high metabolic rate and they suffer rapid depletion of glycogen stores. Thus fasting for longer than a few hours is seldom recommended. They may also be more prone to hypoglycaemic shock and have a decreased ability to detoxify and eliminate anaesthetic agents. In anaesthesia of passerine species, preoperative and perioperative administration of glucose as well as monitoring blood glucose should be considered. In the bird with a critical condition and poor body condition, fasting may be entirely unnecessary.

Factor	Fast?	Duration of fast	Examples, comments
Species prone to regurgitation or with extensive crops	Yes	As long as possible based on body condition score and weight	Vultures, Barn Owl, other raptors; pigeons; crows, mynahs
Surgery of neck, cervical oesophagus or crop area	Yes	Until crop empties	Tracheal laceration, crop fistula, laceration repair
Body condition score 1/5	No	None	Stabilize prior to procedure
Body condition score 2/5	Yes	Short	Stable, eating well, gaining weight
Body condition score 3/5 or greater	Yes	As indicated based on body condition score, species and weight	
Body weight > 1 kg	Yes	12–48 hours	Red-tailed Hawk, Golden Eagle
Body weight 600–1000 g	Yes	6–12 hours	Small hawks
Body weight 400–600 g	Yes	4–6 hours	Pigeons, good body condition score
Body weight 200–400 g	Yes	2–4 hours	Pigeons; stable passerine birds
Body weight < 200 g, stable	Yes	1–2 hours	Small passerine birds
Body weight < 200 g, unstable	No	None	

10.2 Factors for consideration when determining appropriate preanaesthetic fasting.

In the face of crop stasis or inability to wait for crop emptying, the crop may be gavaged and the contents aspirated. However, this action may be limited by diet and temperament in some species. Should preanaesthetic fasting be desired but unattainable, or the fasting status of a bird uncertain but the anaesthetic event a certainty, precautions can be taken to avoid aspiration in the event of regurgitation or reflux (Redig, 1998):

- Intubate the patient
- Block the pharynx with gauze sponges of appropriate size
- Incline the patient's body with the head up
- Restrain the patient in a vertical position during recovery
- In vultures, apply digital pressure to the upper neck in the oesophageal region during mask induction to reduce regurgitation.

Approach to analgesia

Physiology, perception and recognition of pain

While the intensity and quality at which birds feel pain may be unclear, birds have similar nociceptive nervous system pathways to mammals and so are likely to experience similar pain sensations to mammals. Opioids and prostaglandins both modulate pain pathways in birds as in mammals, and birds have similar pain receptors.

It is incumbent upon the avian veterinary surgeon to recognize signs of pain in birds. Further, practitioners should assume that pain is present and alleviate pain when dealing with any condition expected to cause pain. Should the lesion, disease or procedure cause damage to tissue, cause pain in any species, or cause abnormal behaviour (including a lack of normal behaviour), analgesia should be provided. Examples of clear indications for use of analgesics in the avian patient include burns, fractures, luxations and lacerations. In addition to humane reasons, treatment of pain facilitates return to normal function and decreases healing and recovery time.

Behaviours associated with pain may be difficult to interpret, as they are affected by age, gender, species, breed, strain, individual and social behaviours, environment, the type (acute or chronic) and source of pain (visceral or somatic). Predatory species may be more likely to exhibit pain behaviours than prey species. The clinician should be familiar with normal and abnormal behaviour for the species and be aware that social dynamics may affect behaviour. In flocking species, the overt exhibition of behaviours associated with pain may result in expulsion from the flock or predation. Thus the flight-or-fight response along with stoicism, immobility or hiding pain, categorized as conservation/withdrawal responses, are natural behaviours for survival in many species. Immobility may provide a greater likelihood of escape from predation, decrease damage associated with pain and provide temporary analgesia when pain cannot be avoided or lessened through the bird's actions. Conservation/withdrawal responses are associated with chronic pain and are typified by the sick bird fluffed at the bottom of the cage.

Behavioural abnormalities associated with pain in birds range from increased activity, which is generally associated with acute pain, to subtly decreased activity occurring in response to chronic pain. While there is no reliable or universal indicator of pain in any species, clinical signs associated with pain in birds may include but are not limited to:

- Change in temperament, aggression or passivity
- Impaired, reduced or abnormal mobility, including immobility and lameness
- Abnormal posture, especially hunched or crouching and head pulled in towards the body; reluctance to assume normal posture, including standing and perching
- Wing flapping or clamping
- Escape reaction (jumping, foot lifting, wing flapping)
- Restlessness, anxiousness, struggling, excessive movement, insomnia
- Constipation, decreased food or water intake, reduced environmental pecking
- Increased respiratory rate, blood pressure
- Vocalizing, or reduced vocalization
- Chewing, biting or feather picking at the painful site
- Decreased activity including preening, beak wiping and head shaking
- Decreased interest in surroundings or conspecifics.

Pain control

Treatment of pain should include a variety of methods. While specific drug types and administration techniques are discussed below, these do not supersede or abolish the need to attend to the basic principles of pain management. There must be appropriate physical, environmental and behavioural management.

- The underlying source of pain should be determined and eliminated or ameliorated (e.g. stabilizing a fracture, luxation or open wound).
- Dehydrated, anaemic, hypoproteinaemic or emaciated patients should receive appropriate fluid and nutritional support.
- Appropriate environmental modifications to alleviate pain might include providing appropriate perch surfaces and locations and appropriate bedding, diet, environmental temperature and ambient noise for the species.
- Anxiolytics, tranquillizers and muscle relaxants may be administered to reduce fear, anxiety and muscle tension, thereby reducing central nervous system activity.

Preferred methods of pain control allow lowered drug dosages and inhalation anaesthetic to achieve better effect.

- Balanced or multimodal analgesia (use of multiple types of analgesic that affect different aspects of pain pathways simultaneously) provides more effective pain control than the use of a single analgesic (Hawkins, 2006).
- Analgesic synergy (the use of multiple analgesics to reduce the total necessary dose of each drug) reduces each analgesic drug dose and the risk of drug toxicity. For example, a centrally acting opioid might be combined with a peripherally acting non-steroidal anti-inflammatory drug to take advantage of this effect.
- Pre-emptive analgesia requires administration of analgesics prior to a noxious stimulus to prevent sensitization of the CNS, thereby reducing the potential for pain and inflammation during recovery (Hawkins, 2006). In pre-emptive analgesia, opiates, NSAIDs and local anaesthetics may be used in combination pre-, intra- and postoperatively. In pigeons undergoing orthopaedic surgery, those patients treated pre-emptively and postoperatively returned to normal behaviours more quickly than those only treated postoperatively.

Analgesics

Analgesics for use in raptors, pigeons and passerines, and a comparison of their mechanisms of action are included in Figure 10.3.

Opioids

Opioids mediate pain though receptors such as μ, κ and δ found in the central and peripheral nervous systems. They are indicated for alleviation of moderate to severe acute pain such as that induced by trauma or surgery. They have anaesthetic-sparing effects; they reduce the amount of gas anaesthetic necessary to induce or maintain general anaesthesia and are therefore indicated as premedicants for balanced or pre-emptive analgesia.

Opioids investigated or used clinically in birds include morphine, butorphanol, buprenorphine, fentanyl and codeine, but investigation has been limited primarily to Psittaciformes and the domestic fowl. Of these opioids, butorphanol is currently the analgesic drug of choice in birds, based on studies in Psittaciformes.

Drug Class *Mechanism of action*	Species	Dose (mg/kg) and route	Indication	Comment
Buprenorphine Opioid *Partial μ agonist,* *κ antagonist*	Raptors, pigeons [abc]	0.01–0.05 i.m. q8–12h	Pre-emptive anaesthesia, possibly 8–12 h duration	Anecdotally effective in pre-emptive pain control raptors and pigeons, not clinically effective in some other avian species [abcde]
Butorphanol Opioid *Mixed agonist/antagonist,* *weak μ antagonist and* *strong κ agonist*	Current drug of choice for alleviation of avian pain based on clinical studies and consistent neurophysiology in pigeons and pharmacokinetic studies in owls and hawks	0.5–4 i.m., i.v. q2–4h	Analgesia, pre- and postoperative, pre-emptive and balanced sedation	Reduces inhalant anaesthetic necessary to induce and maintain avian anaesthesia Dose-related respiratory depression may be less of a concern with butorphanol than with pure μ agonists [odefijklm]
	Raptors [fg]	0.5–0.2 most common		Hyperalgesia may be caused at doses of 6 mg/kg
	Raptor [h]	1–4 i.v., i.m., orally 0.3–1 i.m.		> 1 mg/kg dose may cause recumbency
Carprofen Proprionic NSAID *Weak COX-1/COX-2* *inhibitor*	Raptor [h]	1–2 q12h	Analgesia, anti-inflammatory	
	Birds [c]	1–4 s.c., orally, i.m. q12–24h	Analgesic	Short-term use, less than 7 days
Ketoprofen Proprionic NSAID *Potent COX-1 inhibitor*	Birds [c]	1–5 i.m. q8–12h	Analgesic	Dosing based on physiological action, analgesic effect has not been clinically assessed
	Raptors, pigeons, waterfowl [n]	1 i.m. q24h × 1–10 days	Analgesic	
Meloxicam Oxicam NSAID *Selective COX-2 inhibitor*	Birds [cl]	0.1–0.5 s.c., orally q24h	Analgesic	Long half-life in pigeons ~4 hours [o]
Piroxicam Oxicam NSAID *Selective COX-2 inhibitor*	Birds [l]	0.5 orally	Treatment of chronic osteoarthritis	Moderate improvement of lameness

10.3 Analgesics. ([a] Clyde, 1994; [b] Lawton, 1996; [c] Hawkins, 2006; [d] Paul-Murphy *et al.*, 1999; [e] Paul-Murphy *et al.*, 2004; [f] Paul-Murphy and Fialkowski, 2001; [g] Redig, 1998; [h] Huckabee, 2000; [i] Machin, 2005b; [j] Curro *et al.*, 1994; [k] Picker, 1994; [l] Paul-Murphy and Ludders, 2001; [m] Paul-Murphy, 2006; [n] Beynon, 1996; [o] Baert and DeBacker, 2003.)

Nalbuphine may also be of clinical use in birds in the near future (Hawkins, 2006). Tramadol is an orally administered opioid with few side effects that has shown promise for use in pigeons (Myers, 2005).

Clinical use and pharmacokinetic studies of standard opioid formulations in birds indicate a clinical effect of 2–4 hours. Side effects common to opioids include cardiac and respiratory depression, gastrointestinal tract slowing, constipation and sedation. Most opioid analgesics are administered parenterally, based on liver metabolism and subsequent poor oral bioavailability in mammals, but this effect has not been investigated in birds.

Opioids should be used cautiously in combination with isoflurane anaesthesia, based on the combined potential for respiratory depression. Many opioids may be reversed with antagonists but this will also result in cessation of analgesic effects.

Non-steroidal anti-inflammatory drugs

NSAIDs are commonly used for pre-emptive analgesia and relief of traumatic and post-surgical pain. Those used in birds include aspirin (acetylsalicylic acid), carprofen, celecoxib, dimethylsulfoxide, flunixin meglumine, ibuprofen, ketoprofen, meloxicam, piroxicam, phenylbutazone and tepoxalin.

NSAIDs cause analgesia and reduce inflammation via inhibition of cyclooxygenase (COX) enzyme isoforms, which prevent production of prostaglandin, a local mediator of inflammation. COX-1 and COX-2 isoforms both function in antinociception but COX-1 is constitutive, rather than inducible, and functions as a cytoprotectant throughout the body. While newer drugs focus on blocking solely the COX-2 enzymatic pathway rather than COX-1 or both pathways, the most efficacious analgesics may be mixed inhibitors, blocking both COX-1 and COX-2 pathways.

Flunixin, ketoprofen and carprofen are potent analgesics in avian species. The analgesic effects of flunixin and ketoprofen may last up to 12 hours (Machin, 2005a). However, flunixin meglumine causes a variety of toxic side effects in birds, including renal failure even at low doses, and has fallen out of favour (Paul-Murphy and Ludders, 2001). Other common side effects of NSAIDs include prolonged clotting time and gastrointestinal ulceration.

NSAIDs may be administered intramuscularly or orally. Few pharmacokinetic or analgesic studies have been performed with NSAIDs in birds and allometric scaling for drug dose determination appears inappropriate. All dosages should be interpreted and applied cautiously based on clinical judgement and response of the animal. NSAIDs should be used cautiously in birds as class, species, gender and temporal physiological state may cause differential toxicity, with possibly fatal consequences. For example, recent vulture population declines in Asia have been linked to ingestion of the NSAID diclofenac used in cattle. When feasible, assessment of perfusion, hydration and kidney function should occur prior to NSAID administration. All patients undergoing NSAID treatment should be monitored for renal output, hydration and faecal blood. Aspirin (acetylsalicylic acid), flunixin meglumine, phenylbutazone and ibuprofen will not be further discussed here as better alternatives exist based on lack of serious side effects and availability of easily administered formulations.

Carprofen and *ketoprofen* are analgesic, anti-inflammatory and antipyretic.

- Carprofen shows good anti-inflammatory activity and, perhaps because of weak COX inhibition, it has a wide margin of safety. It may be administered for short-term relief of pain in birds.
- Ketoprofen was only poorly bioavailable in quail when administered intramuscularly or orally and displayed a very short half-life (Graham *et al.*, 2005). In ducks, a decrease of inflammatory mediators persisted for 12 hours after ketoprofen administration (Machin and Livingston, 2002). Ketoprofen is available in topical gel, oral tablets and injectable formulations, but only injectable and oral formulations have been investigated for use in birds.

Celecoxib, *meloxicam* and *piroxicam* are selective COX-2 inhibitors.

- Piroxicam provides mild to moderate relief from pain associated with degenerative joint disease and may also be indicated in other chronic inflammatory conditions of birds.
- Meloxicam may have a greater margin of safety based on its COX-2 activity. This drug's pharmacokinetics have been investigated in a variety of avian species, including pigeons. Clinically, it is effective for treatment of pain associated with osteoarthritis in birds and is often used as an avian analgesic based on ease of administration and dosing. It is available as an oral suspension and in injectable form.

Dimethylsulfoxide (DMSO) has not been studied as a sole agent for analgesia and anti-inflammatory treatment in birds but is used clinically as an anti-inflammatory and as a carrier of other medications. It may be given topically or orally and may lack many of the undesirable side effects of other NSAIDs.

Local anaesthetics

Local anaesthetics used in avian species include bupivicaine, lidocaine and benzocaine and EMLA cream (eutectic mixture of 2.5% lidocaine and 2.5% prilocaine) (Figure 10.4). Information about local anaesthetic use in birds is sparse and anecdotal, with controlled scientific investigation of these drugs limited to domestic fowl and ducks.

These drugs block ion channels and prevent generation and conduction of nerve impulses. They are most often used in topical applications for minor procedures (catheter placement, endotracheal intubation), for local infiltration at the surgical site for pre-emptive analgesia (placement of air sac tubes, intraosseous catheters, laparotomy), or for local nerve blockade (nerve infiltration prior to transection decreases prevalence of phantom limb syndrome). Local anaesthetics control local pain but do not lessen the stress of handling or physical restraint.

Drug	Dose (mg/kg)	Route	Comments/indications
Lidocaine [abc]	<2.5	Local infiltration	Local anaesthetic, treatment of arrhythmias, duration unknown in birds, 60–120 min in mammals, preoperative. Dose >4 mg/kg may cause toxicity, seizures in raptors
Bupivicaine [bd]	≤2.0	Local infiltration	Combine with DMSO for topical application, 4-hour duration in domestic fowl
Prilocaine/ lidocaine (EMLA [e])	Unknown	Topical application	Avoid toxicity via prolonged contact time or application to open follicles, damaged skin or mucous membranes. Calculated dose should not exceed 2 mg/kg lidocaine topically
Benzocaine [f]	Unknown	Topical application	For small bird minor wound repair. Apply minimal amount to avoid likelihood of toxicosis
Microencapsulated ammonia [g]	Unknown	Topical application	Indicated in non-penetrating traumas, decreased risk of secondary infection

10.4 Local anaesthetics for use in avian patients. ([a] Ludders, 1994; [b] Hocking *et al.*, 1997; [c] Huckabee, 2000; [d] Glatz *et al.*, 1992; [e] Hawkins, 2006; [f] Clubb, 1998; [g] Harrison *et al.*, 2006)

The use of sedation or general anaesthesia should be considered for use in combination with local anaesthetics in the avian patient.

Based on pharmacodynamics and the physiology of the avian blood–brain barrier, the duration of action of local anaesthetics in birds may be less while the sensitivity to toxicity may be greater than in mammals (Hocking *et al.*, 1997). Signs of local anaesthetic toxicosis in birds include distress immediately after injection, recumbency with outstretched legs, drowsiness, depression, ataxia, nystagmus, muscle tremors, seizures, vomiting, hypotension, cardiac arrhythmia and arrest (Machin, 2005; Hawkins, 2006). Response to local anaesthetics may vary dramatically based on the individual, health status and species. Most commercially available local anaesthetic preparations are highly concentrated. To lessen the risk of toxicosis when administering local anaesthetics in birds, a variety of techniques, used in conjunction, are recommended:

- Calculate the total patient dose and administer no more than this amount
- If necessary, dilute the total patient dose to facilitate local administration
- Use insulin or skin-testing syringes with zero-volume hub attached needles to facilitate appropriate volume and dose administration in the desired region.

Preanaesthetics and sedatives

Administration of preanaesthetics may be foregone in many avian patients to avoid repeated capture and restraint and is generally unnecessary for most avian patients. However, preanaesthetic administration of sedatives, anxiolytics and pain control agents may be indicated in the fractious, anxious or excited bird.

Some preanaesthetic agents have an anaesthetic-sparing effect and thereby decrease negative cardiovascular effects of the primary anaesthetic agent, such as hypotension or incidence of arrhythmia. Commonly used classes of preanaesthetic agents in avian species include benzodiazepines and the opioids, but parasympatholytics are also occasionally indicated. Acepromazine is no longer in common use.

Parasympatholytics

Parasympatholytics (anticholinergics such as atropine) are not routinely indicated for avian anaesthesia. Useful properties include reduction of respiratory and salivary secretions, inhibition of gastrointestinal motility including the crop, and prevention of vagally induced bradyarrhythmia. Whether the reduction or further thickening of respiratory secretions in the avian respiratory tract is beneficial (due to reduced chance of endotracheal tube blockage) or detrimental (based on increased viscosity of tracheal secretions causing an increased chance of endotracheal tube blockage) remains controversial (Paul-Murphy and Fialkowski, 2001; Gunkel and LaFortune, 2005). Because of this concern, use of parasympatholytics as preanaesthetic agents is usually forgone in smaller avian patients, which usually have high resting heart rates. However, preanaesthetic or anaesthetic bradyarrhythmias or prevention of cardiac dysrhythmias stemming from the oculocardiac reflex of ophthalmic surgery are indications for anticholinergic administration. Prevention of reflex bradycardia may be difficult if the anticholinergic is administered as a preanaesthetic and is no longer active during the surgical procedure (Abou-Madi, 2001). Slight differences between drug activities exist; glycopyrrolate is a more selective anti-secretory agent that is more potent and of longer duration of action, but atropine is preferred for cardiac emergencies because of its fast onset, despite its shorter duration of effect (Heard, 2000).

Anaesthetics

Inhalation anaesthesia is preferred for use in birds, as it gives rapid induction and recovery, ease and rapidity of control of anaesthetic depth, recovery independent of organ transformation, and improved oxygenation due to administration of oxygen with anaesthetic gases. Cardiorespiratory depressant effects are less than those of most injectable drugs.

Injectable anaesthetics as a sole anaesthetic agent are generally reserved for field use or limited to certain procedural indications where gas anaesthesia is impractical or impossible to administer. Nonetheless, injectable anaesthetics, used alone or in conjunction with gas anaesthesia, are still routinely used in a variety of avian procedures and, rarely, may be preferable to the use of gas anaesthesia.

Injectable anaesthetics

Advantages of injectable anaesthetics (Figure 10.5) include low cost, ease of portability, availability, minimal necessary equipment, rapid administration and induction of anaesthesia, and the possibility of remote administration. Disadvantages include biotransformation and elimination dependent on organ function, narrow margin of safety, the need to obtain an accurate weight prior to drug administration, cardiopulmonary depression, prolonged or violent recovery, lack of adequate muscle relaxation, difficulty in maintaining an adequate plane of anaesthesia for surgery, problematic anaesthetic reversal and variation in individual, species or class response.

Historically a variety of anaesthetics have been used in birds, sometimes with serious untoward effects. Use of barbiturates, chloral hydrate, alphachloralose and phenothiazines will not be discussed here.

Drug	Species	Dosage (mg/kg), route	Comments/indications	Cautions
Atipamezole	Raptors[a]	5 × medetomidine dose i.m., i.v.	Alpha-2 adrenergic antagonist	
	Most birds	0.25–5.0 i.m.		
Atropine	Birds[bc]	0.02–0.08 i.m., s.c.	Preanaesthetic	
	Raptors[d]	0.2 i.m., sublingual, intratracheal	Pre- or intraoperative bradycardia	
	Birds[e]	0.04–0.1 i.m., i.v.	Premedication, bradycardia, gastrointestinal reflux, excessive salivation	
Diazepam	Raptors[f]	0.5–1.0 i.m., i.v. prn	Sedative	
	Birds[b]	0.2–0.5 i.m.	Preanaesthetic sedative	
	Pigeons, most avian species[c]	0.2–1.0 i.v.	Preanaesthetic sedative	
	Passerines[g]	0.5 orally	Anxiolysis and food acceptance in new captives	1 mg/ml oral suspension
Flumazenil	Birds[b]	0.05 i.v.	Reversal of benzodiazepines. Bolus or preferably titrate to effect	Make sure additional agents, such as ketamine, have dissipated prior to reversal
	Most birds, pigeons[c]	0.02–0.03 i.m. 0.05 i.v.		
	Quail, most birds[ch]	0.1 i.m.	Midazolam reversal 6 mg/kg	Average of 1.6 minutes recovery, no relapse sedation
Glycopyrrolate	Birds[bc]	0.01–0.02 i.m., i.v.	Premedication, to decrease respiratory secretions and prevent or alleviate bradycardia	Increased viscosity of tracheal secretions may predispose to endotracheal tube blockage
	Birds[e]	0.01–0.03 i.m., i.v.		
Propofol	Pigeon[i]	14 i.v.	Probably high-end dose, loss of voluntary reflexes occurs in 2–7 minutes	Cardiopulmonary depression common especially during bolus induction. Intubation, assisted ventilation, supplemental oxygen recommended. Propofol best suited to short field procedures or induction agent only. Prolonged recovery in Great Horned Owls and Red-tailed Hawks
	Red-tailed Hawk[j]	3.4–5.6 i.v.	Induction	
	Red-tailed Hawk[j]	0.4–0.5/min CRI		
	Great Horned Owl[j]	2.7–4.1 i.v.	Induction	
	Great Horned Owl[j]	0.4–0.7/min CRI		
	Barn Owl	4–12 i.v.	Induction, anaesthesia over 14 minutes	
	Barn Owl	0.5/min CRI		
	Raptor[e]	1.33–14 i.v.	Anaesthesia	
Ketamine/ xylazine[k]	Raptor	K 4.4, X 2.2 i.v.	Field anaestheic protocol; not superior to gas anaesthesia	Cardiac depressive effects and difficult recoveries
	Falcon, hawk	K 25–30, X 2 i.m.		
	Owl	K 10–15, X 2 i.m.		
	Turkey Vulture	K 10, X 0.5–1.0 i.m.		

10.5 Injectable preanaesthetics, anaesthetics, sedatives and reversal agents. Information included in this table includes anecdotal as well as nociceptive and pharmacokinetic data. Caution should be used when extrapolating drug dosages between species, as individual, gender, class and species differences exist, especially in patient reactions to opioid and non-steroidal inflammatory drug categories. Different levels of analgesia, toxicity or other adverse affects may occur in different individuals, genders, species or classes. ([a] Pollock *et al.*, 2005; [b] Abou-Madi, 2001; [c] Gunkel and LaFortune, 2005; [d] Redig, 1998; [e] Heard, 2000; [f] Huckabee, 2000; [g] Massey, 2003; [h] Day and Roge, 1996; [i] Fitzgerald and Cooper, 1990; [j] Hawkins *et al.*, 2003; [k] Carpenter, 2005; [l] Zenker *et al.*, 2000; [m] Kreeger *et al.*, 1993.) (continues)

Drug	Species	Dosage (mg/kg), route	Comments/indications	Cautions
Ketamine/ diazepam[k]	Eagles, Vultures	K 3–8, D 0.25 i.v.		
	Falcons	K 8–15, D 0.5–0.1 i.m.		
	Raptors	K 10–40 i.v., D 1.0–1.5 i.m., i.v.	Induction or surgical anaesthesia	Rapid bolus may cause apnoea, arrhythmia and risk of death
Ketamine/ medetomidine[k]	Pigeons	K 1.5–2.0, M 60–80 µg/kg i.m., i.v.		
	Raptors	K 2–5, M 25–100 µg/kg i.v. lower dose i.m. higher dose		
Midazolam	Quail[g]	2–6 i.m.	Sole sedative	Peak sedation at 10 minutes for highest dose. No cardiovascular effects seen at any dose
	Birds[b]	0.1–0.5 i.m.	Preanaesthetic sedative	
Telazol (tiletamine/ zolazepam)	European Buzzard[i]	40–80 orally	Immobilization after 30–60 minutes	Powdered form of the drug: immobilized by 30 minutes; birds given oral solution didn't reach immobilization until > 60 minutes
	Great Horned Owl, Screech Owl[m]	5–10 i.m.	Immobilization for 30 minutes, some decrease in heart rate at higher end of dose	Prolonged (4–5 h) recoveries with catalepsy, opisthotonus, ataxia
Xylazine	Raptors[f]	1–2.2 i.m., i.v.	Sedation, anaesthesia	Not for use in debilitated raptors based on cardiac depression
Yohimbine	Raptors[f]	0.2–0.2 i.m. i.v.	Reversal of xylazine	

10.5 (continued) Injectable preanaesthetics, anaesthetics, sedatives and reversal agents. Information included in this table includes anecdotal as well as nociceptive and pharmacokinetic data. Caution should be used when extrapolating drug dosages between species, as individual, gender, class and species differences exist, especially in patient reactions to opioid and non-steroidal inflammatory drug categories. Different levels of analgesia, toxicity or other adverse affects may occur in different individuals, genders, species or classes. ([a] Pollock *et al.*, 2005; [b] Abou-Madi, 2001; [c] Gunkel and LaFortune, 2005; [d] Redig, 1998; [e] Heard, 2000; [f] Huckabee, 2000; [g] Massey, 2003; [h] Day and Roge, 1996; [i] Fitzgerald and Cooper, 1990; [i] Hawkins *et al.*, 2003; [k] Carpenter, 2005; [l] Zenker *et al.*, 2000; [m] Kreeger *et al.*, 1993.)

Ketamine and ketamine combinations

Ketamine is a dissociative anaesthetic that also provides pre-emptive or postoperative analgesia of sharp superficial pain. As an *N*-methyl-D-aspartate antagonist, ketamine can prevent or abolish receptor-mediated nociceptive pathways in the central nervous system. As a sole agent ketamine is not adequate for laparotomy or orthopaedic surgery, because it does not control dull visceral pain. Further, ketamine as a sole anaesthetic agent in avian species may result in poor muscle relaxation and muscle tremors in the anaesthetic period, followed by recovery marked by incoordination, excitement, head shaking, wing flapping, myotonic contractions and muscle tremors.

Ketamine is generally administered in combination with an alpha-2 agonist or a benzodiazepine to improve muscular relaxation and depth of anaesthesia to palliate the excitatory effects of ketamine and to provide sedation and pain control in recovery.

Determination of a ketamine dose conforms to the principles of allometric scaling: larger birds (>1 kg) need a comparatively smaller dose (10–20 mg/kg) than smaller birds (<50 g) (70–80 mg/kg) to achieve similar anaesthetic effects. After intramuscular administration of ketamine, anaesthetic induction should occur in 5–10 minutes and anaesthesia should last 5–20 minutes, depending on the dose and size of the bird (Paul-Murphy and Fialkowski, 2001). Administration of ketamine to vultures should be avoided as they have been reported to show undesirable effects such as salivation, excitation and convulsions (Samour *et al.*, 1984).

Alpha-2 agonists

Alpha-2 agonists include *xylazine* and *medetomidine*. They are seldom used for avian anaesthesia but are occasionally indicated for field or remote immobilization. They have been used for anaesthesia in pigeons and a variety of raptors. These drugs are usually used in combination with other injectable drugs (dissociatives or benzodiazepines) in avian anaesthesia.

Alpha-2 agonists provide muscle relaxation, sedation and analgesia, which can smooth induction and recovery from anaesthesia. Specific antagonists are available to reverse the effects of alpha-2 agonists, allowing for rapid anaesthetic recovery. *Atipamezole* may be used to reverse effects of medetomidine, detomidine and xylazine. *Yohimbine* has been used to reverse the effects of xylazine in raptors (Degernes *et al.*, 1988; Freed and Baker, 1989). *Tolazoline* has also been used to reverse xylazine when used in combination with ketamine in vultures (Allen and Osterhuis, 1986).

Alpha-2 agonists have multiple negative effects in avian species that bar their use as a sole anaesthetic agent. All alpha-2 agonists are cardiopulmonary depressants. Decreases in heart rate, respiratory rate, blood pH, hypoxaemia and hypercarbia can result from xylazine or medetomidine administration (Samour *et al.*, 1984; Degernes *et al.*, 1988). Alpha-2 agonists can cause prolonged cardiac impulse intervals and cardiovascular arrhythmia and instability, which can lead to fatality when coupled with hypoventilation and hypercarbia (Paul-Murphy and Fialkowski, 2001).

In the avian patient, apprehension or excitement may override alpha-2 agonist sedative effects. Should an alpha-2 agent be chosen for preanaesthetic sedation or anaesthetic induction, it is essential that the bird is handled quietly, quickly and calmly with minimal struggling. Then the patient should be induced in a subdued environment for best results. Raptors may be hooded (if they are trained to accept the hood) if no induction chamber is available.

Medetomidine: Medetomidine alone appears to be an unacceptable sedative in avian patients. High doses of medetomidine in pigeons resulted in sedation without immobilization; high dose combinations of ketamine and medetomidine seemed adequate for surgical anaesthesia in pigeons but caused serious cardiovascular effects (Uzun *et al.*, 2003). Anaesthetic combinations of medetomidine/ketamine and ketamine/diazepam in pigeons also yielded unfavourable results: unreliable levels of anaesthesia and violent wing flapping resulted from the use of medetomidine with ketamine; and inadequate analgesia and prolonged recovery resulted from use of the ketamine/diazepam combination (Lumeij and Dennik, 2003).

Benzodiazepines

Benzodiazepines for use in raptors, pigeons and passerine birds include diazepam, midazolam and zolazepam. Benzodiazepines are characterized by anxiolytic, hyponotic/sedative, anticonvulsant, muscle relaxant, amnesic, hyperphagic and anaesthetic-sparing effects. They do not provide analgesia but minimal cardiovascular effects make them an option for use in birds with cardiovascular or other diseases. Other indications for use of benzodiazepines in birds include anxiolysis in wild-caught or newly introduced aviary birds, reduction of preanaesthetic anxiety and postanaesthetic recovery excitement, and facilitation of handling for brief non-painful procedures. Best effect is seen when these agents are administered 10–20 minutes prior to the procedure and the patient is not disturbed while the drugs take effect.

Diazepam is not water-soluble and causes pain and unpredictable results when given intramuscularly (Abou-Madi, 2001; Gunkel and LaFortune, 2005). Struggling, dysphoria, incoordination, ataxia and prolonged recovery can result from administration of diazepam and other benzodiazepines (Heard, 2000). The lower the dose of midazolam administered, the shorter is the duration of sedation. In wild passerines, anxiolysis and diet acceptance are improved with administration of an oral solution of diazepam (Massey, 2003).

Alfaxalone/alfadolone (Saffan) was formerly used successfully in raptors in field situations but is no longer available. The replacement alfaxalone preparation has not yet been fully evaluated in birds.

Reversal of benzodiazepines can be achieved with *flumazenil*, which is preferably titrated to effect to reduce negative excitatory or dysphoric effects while avoiding reversal of anxiolysis, sedation and muscle relaxation.

Telazol: Telazol, the combination of tiletamine (a dissociative anaesthetic) and zolazepam (a benzodiazepine), is no longer popular for use in birds with the advent of isoflurane anaesthesia. Advantages of telazol for use as an immobilizing agent include low cost, small delivery volume and the options of intramuscular or oral administration. It is a safe and effective immobilization agent in Great Horned Owls, Screech Owls and the Eurasian Buzzard. Disadvantages include prolonged (2–4 hours) sometimes agitated recoveries and a short surgical anaesthetic time; in Red-tailed Hawks administration fails to cause unconsciousness and causes increased salivation and cardiac and respiratory rates (Kreeger *et al.*, 1993). To the author's knowledge, telazol has not been investigated for use in pigeons or passerine birds.

Propofol

Propofol, the ultra-short-acting non-barbiturate isopropyl phenol, has been used for anaesthesia of several owl species, pigeons, Red-tailed Hawk and Common Buzzard.

Propofol provides a dose- and rate-dependent smooth, rapid onset induction in raptors, along with good muscle relaxation of short duration. Intravenous catheter placement is usually necessary for initial administration and continued infusion of this drug. Slow administration for induction may limit the onset of apnoea and respiratory depression typical of this drug (Hawkins *et al.*, 2003) and the slow infusion method requires continued vascular access, hence the intravenous catheter. To the author's knowledge, intraosseous injection of this drug for anaesthesia of birds has not been reported, but could theoretically be feasible in small birds, such as passerine species, when venous access is limited.

Properties of this anaesthetic that make it particularly suitable for field use include portability, low anaesthetic cost, and the lack of effect of ambient temperatures on drug properties. Propofol facilitates surgery of the respiratory tract when inhalant anaesthesia is unfeasible (Mama *et al.*, 1996). In some raptors a prolonged and difficult recovery characterized by head twitch, myoclonus and opisthotonus lasts for hours, though all birds recover without continued CNS abnormalities. Prolonged recoveries in Great Horned Owls and Red-tailed Hawks were attributed to low volume of distribution, differing hepatic metabolism of phenolic compounds and low clearance rates of phenolic compounds in these species (Hawkins *et al.*, 2003). In mammals, a balanced anaesthetic protocol that includes anxiolytics and pre-emptive analgesics is used to ameliorate excitatory effects and to provide a drug-sparing effect at induction and during continuous rate infusion, but a combined protocol has not been investigated in birds. The longer the constant rate infusion, the greater the likelihood that birds may suffer agitated recoveries. This characteristic, coupled with the relatively short induction and effect of propofol, may limit the drug's use in avian patients to induction or short procedures.

Some reflexive responses in raptors may differ slightly from the expected during the use of propofol. In one study, jaw tone and laryngeal reflex were immediately abolished upon induction with propofol, as was the response to feather pluck, but the third eyelid reflex was not lost during CRI. The pedal or toe pinch response was the last reflex to disappear, as expected.

Inhalation anaesthesia

The major disadvantage of inhalant anaesthetics remains the necessity for specialized equipment for delivery and scavenging of anaesthetic gas; however, small desktop units suitable for field use have been devised (Redig, 1998).

Halothane, methoxyflurane and nitrous oxide have been used in birds historically, but have been replaced by isoflurane and sevoflurane, which are safer for the staff and the patient, have fewer negative cardiovascular and pulmonary effects and have shorter induction and recovery times. Although isoflurane is currently the most commonly used inhalation anaesthetic in birds, sevoflurane is rapidly gaining in popularity and its use is only limited by cost and familiarity. The use of desflurane and enflurane may become more common in the future.

- *Isoflurane* is the preferred anaesthetic agent in avian species, on the basis of cost, rapid induction and recovery, the ability to change anaesthetic plane and minimal metabolism. Further, it does not sensitize the heart to catecholamine-induced arrhythmias.
- *Sevoflurane* has less solubility and therefore a shorter recovery time but requires a higher delivery percentage for induction, due to lower potency. Unlike desflurane and isoflurane, sevoflurane does not cause respiratory tract irritation, resulting in a less stressful induction.
- *Desflurane* provides a faster recovery time than sevoflurane or isoflurane but is unlikely to become widely used, because respiratory tract irritation and laryngospasm dictate the use of specialized equipment for delivery.

All anaesthetic gas exposure carries risk of genetic damage to those exposed (Hoerauf *et al.*, 1999). Therefore appropriate precautions should be taken, such as intubation or tight-fitting mask induction to minimize anaesthetic exposure, good ventilation to dilute anaesthetic gases and appropriate protective wear. Soaking systems (table, room) for the removal of waste gases are recommended. Pregnant women should avoid exposure to anaesthetic gases, either by avoiding anaesthetic events altogether or by wearing protective equipment.

Anaesthetic circuits and equipment

Choice of anaesthetic delivery system is based on bird size and includes non-rebreathing systems, paediatric circles and adult circle systems.

- For birds <2 kg, non-rebreathing systems (Ayre's T-piece, Bain coaxial circuit, Bain block) are used and require a minimum of 500 ml/minute for effective delivery of anaesthetic gas to the patient.
- For birds weighing 2–7 kg, non-rebreathing systems or a paediatric circle system may be used.
- For birds >7 kg (very large raptors), a standard adult circle system may be used.

These large systems require a gas flow of 1 l/minute for effective anaesthetic delivery. Therefore for most passerine, pigeon and raptor patients, a non-rebreathing system will be required. *Non-rebreathing systems* have the added benefits of reduced dead space, lessened resistance and ability to change the anaesthetic depth more quickly, because of the fast gas flow rate. The author prefers a Bain block, which allows use of a mechanical pop-off valve, assessment of pressure in the avian body during mechanical respiration and separation of the bag from the rest of the anaesthetic tubing to allow better visualization of bag movement during respiration.

Paediatric mechanical ventilators or those specially designed for the use of small exotic species (Vetronics, UK) are of advantage if used in birds. Mechanical ventilators provide consistent intermittent positive pressure ventilation to the patient and safe and effective anaesthetic delivery. Pressure-controlled ventilators deliver a certain pressure during each inspiration, while volume-controlled ventilators deliver a certain volume with each inspiration. Each type of system has advantages and disadvantages.

- Hypoventilation may result from a system leak or when the coelom is opened in a *volume-limited* ventilation system. Benefits of volume-limited systems are conservation of anaesthetic gas and alarms for endotracheal tube occlusion.
- Hypoventilation may occur with use of the *pressure-limited* system in cases of airway occlusion or lessened respiratory system compliance. Unfortunately, hypoventilation may be difficult to detect. Pressure-limited systems are preferred for use in the avian patient undergoing coelomic surgery, because this system controls anaesthetic depth by continuing to provide anaesthetic gas despite leakage into the surgical field.

Anaesthetic administration and induction

Anaesthetic induction with anaesthetic gas without other premedicants is commonplace in avian medicine. Birds may be induced in an induction chamber or, preferably, via facemask (Figure 10.6) to avoid excessive waste of anaesthetic gases to the environment. The mask should cover both nares and the mouth in passerine species, because the right and left paranasal sinuses do not communicate. In

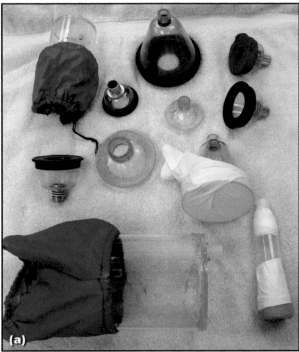

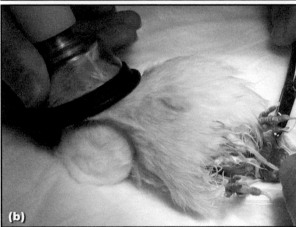

10.6	**(a)** A variety of facemasks, some with modification for use in avian anaesthesia.

(b) Mask anaesthetic maintenance is generally preferred for small birds in which endotracheal tubes may become occluded by thick tracheal secretions. Note the cotton ball placement for appropriate neck positioning to facilitate a patent airway.

- In the *low-to-high protocol*, birds are preoxygenated and then the anaesthetic gas percentage is increased incrementally over a few minutes until induction is obtained. This method reduces the risk of anaesthetic overdose but increases the risk of the excitatory phase of induction and slightly increases induction time. The low-to-high induction is recommended for use in birds which are already depressed or obtunded and very small species. These patients induce more quickly and, because of their physiology or illness, are less likely to undergo the excitatory phase. Further, these patients often induce and maintain a suitable anaesthetic plane prior to reaching the highest anaesthetic percentage setting on the vaporizer. Therefore this method allows the anaesthetist to titrate the lowest acceptable anaesthetic dose while avoiding apnoea in the critical patient.
- In the *high-to-low protocol*, the patient receives a high initial dose of anaesthetic until the first signs of induction occur (eyelid closure, relaxation of legs and wings, regular respiration). At this point, the vaporizer settings are reduced to a maintenance percentage. This method reduces struggling, lessens the time of induction and reduces the chance of the patient experiencing the excitatory phase. However, the possibility of overdose is greater and the anaesthetist must monitor induction closely to avoid apnoea. Additionally, while the likelihood of the excitatory phase is reduced, it can occur, especially in larger (>1 kg) species. Thus this method is generally reserved for the large, apparently healthy bird in good body condition but may be equally indicated for the fractious patient.

Intubation: In all but short non-invasive procedures lasting less than 20 minutes, and in patients > 100 g, *endotracheal intubation* should be performed. Intubation of patients <100 g may be performed with modified intravenous catheters or specially designed endotracheal tubes, but the risk of tube occlusion is greater in these diminutive patients.

Intubation for continued administration of anaesthetic gases to avian patients has several advantages. It allows control of respiration, rescue from apnoea and control of anaesthetic depth through IPPV; it reduces loss of anaesthetic gas to the environment, prevents aspiration of reflux and allows placement of monitoring devices for end-tidal CO_2 to determine the patient's ventilation status.

Intubation of the avian patient is made relatively easy by the lack of an epiglottis and teeth. To avoid damage to the complete tracheal rings of the avian trachea, intubation with an uncuffed endotracheal tube, or a cuffed endotracheal tube without inflation of the cuff, is preferred. Stability of the endotracheal tube within the trachea is also key to avoiding tracheal damage and inadvertent extubation during the anaesthetic episode. Use of stepped cole tubes or those that gradually increase in diameter may help to occlude the trachea at the glottis to avoid gas escape to the environment while also avoiding tracheal damage.

most situations the entire head of the patient can be introduced into the anaesthetic mask, which may require modification to fit the patient's neck properly and allow good visualization of the head. This whole-head method has the added benefit in some raptors and large-billed passerine species of neutralizing the bill as a weapon.

All anaesthetic gases should be adequately scrubbed by using systems that vent gases for appropriate disposal. Options include vacuum systems, soda-sorb canisters, or merely routing the waste anaesthetic tubing outside the building.

Preoxygenation is ideal but should be weighed against patient stress and struggling during restraint. The two main methods of facemask induction are the low-to-high protocol and the high-to-low protocol (Gunkel and LaFortune, 2005).

The tube is generally taped in place after intubation, thereby affixing it minimally to the maxillary beak or gnathotheca but also the rhamphotheca if necessary (Figure 10.7). Affixing the tube solely to the gnathotheca provides stability, while allowing for visualization of tube placement and the oral cavity for monitoring during the anaesthetic episode. Extubation is also facilitated by this method.

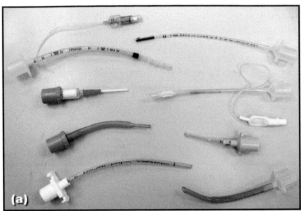

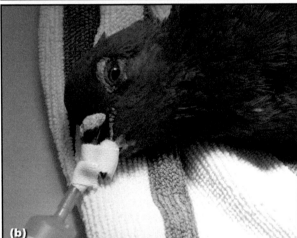

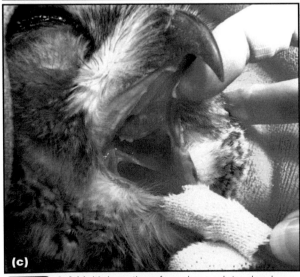

10.7 **(a)** Multiple options for avian endotracheal intubation. Cuffed tubes are not inflated; stepped tubes are inserted into the glottis until their wider part creates a partial seal. **(b)** An intubated pigeon. **(c)** Intubation of a Great Horned Owl, showing the endotracheal tube secured to the lower beak.

Air sac cannulation: This is an effective means of induction and maintenance of anaesthesia in passerine birds and pigeons. It allows escape of anaesthetic gas and can be used for resuscitation or ventilation in a bird with tracheal obstruction. Caudal thoracic air sac cannulation appears to be acceptable in all species.

1. The patient is induced via facemask and appropriate pain control via systemic routes and a local anaesthetic block at the incision site is provided.
2. With the bird in lateral recumbency, a central skin incision is made in the triangle created by the thigh musculature caudally, the ribs cranially and the ventralmost spinal musculature dorsally.
3. After the initial skin incision (which may be made with a cautery device), haemostats are bluntly and blindly introduced into the coelomic cavity. Care should be taken not to damage internal organs by overzealous introduction of the haemostats.
4. The tube is then placed in the coelomic cavity and a feather or thread may be placed near the tube aperture to visualize and confirm air flow of respiration though the tube.
5. The inflation of a cuffed endotracheal tube facilitates stabilization of the tube inside the coelom. Externally, the tube may be stabilized to the body wall with suture or a tape flange to the skin (Figure 10.8).
6. Anaesthetic gas may then be introduced via attachment of the anaesthetic circuit to this tube. The surgeon should beware anaesthetic gas escape from the trachea when this method is used.

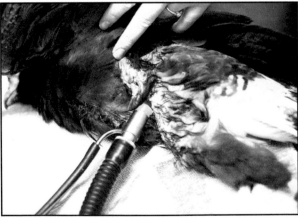

10.8 Air sac perfusion anaesthesia. The tube is inserted into the caudal abdominal/thoracic air sac cranial to the leg, then connected to a T-piece. (© John Chitty)

Patient support and monitoring

Adept and continuous monitoring is crucial for recovery and survival from the anaesthetic event. The most valuable 'equipment' in this respect is a dedicated anaesthetist to monitor the patient's vital signs, assess depth of anaesthesia and facilitate recovery. Attention directly to the patient, especially its respiratory quality, should be the primary concern rather than the variety of alarms created by equipment. Monitoring of pulse rate (and quality) and the quality of reflexes and muscle tone are also key in determining the patient's anaesthetic plane (Figure 10.9). Reflexes vary based on the species or anaesthetic used. Respiratory rate, depth and quality, as gauged by an anaesthetist, are the best single indicator of avian anaesthetic depth (Edling, 2006). Additional equipment commonly used for monitoring the patient undergoing anaesthesia includes the capnograph, the Doppler, the pulse oximeter, the electrocardiogram, the manometer (for determination of indirect blood pressure) and temperature probes.

Patient size	Monitoring
<100 g	Respiration observations, reflex observation, external stethoscope auscultation, intermittent Doppler, ECG
100–500 g	Above, plus capnograph, audible Doppler respiratory monitor
500–1000 g	Above, plus blood pressure determination (intermittent), pulse oximetry, oesophageal stethoscope
1–7 kg	All of the above

10.9 Recommendations for avian anaesthetic monitoring. Use of monitoring devices must be weighed against: application time; ease of application and monitoring; and acceptability to the patient. Devices should provide the ability to monitor vital signs. They should not cause undue harm to the patient nor interfere with anaesthesia or resuscitation attempts.

Thermal probes (thermometers with an appropriate range for avian species) are always indicated for monitoring body temperature of avian anaesthetic patients (40–44°C). Cloacally or thoracic oesophageally placed probes work equally well for determination of core body temperature, with the exception of birds with flaccid vents or those with large food-filled or otherwise flaccid crops.

Cardiovascular monitoring

Cardiovascular monitoring may be challenging, because of a high normal heart and pulse rate, small appendages, difficulty in accessing the thoracic oesophagus and the keel and pectoral musculature's hindrance of auscultation.

- Oesophageal or standard *stethoscopes* for auscultation of the heart beat can be useful in larger patients but it should be remembered that the heart beat may be the last indicator to become abnormal prior to death, providing little time for reaction and correction of anaesthetic issues.
- Similarly, an *electrocardiograph* may be used to monitor electrical activity and rhythm of the heart, but electrical activity of the heart will persist well past apnoea and possibly past patient death. Standard ECG clips may be replaced with sticky

patch leads or clips attached to needles subcutaneously inserted to avoid undue trauma to the patient and facilitate better readings.
- An 8 MHz *Doppler probe* placed over the tibiotarsal artery or radial artery can provide auditory recognition of the rate and quality of the pulse. Clips fashioned from tongue depressors, cotton wool balls and a rubber band may facilitate placement of this probe for continuous use during the anaesthetic episode (Figure 10.10).

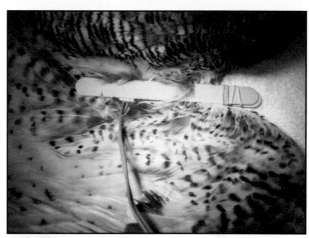

10.10 Close-up of Great Horned Owl with a Doppler probe held in place over the radial artery via a 'clip' created from tongue depressors, rubber band and a cotton ball.

Determination of blood pressure may also be performed during surgery and has been described in detail elsewhere (Lichtenberger, 2005). Briefly, the method for determination of non-invasive blood pressure in birds involves placement of the Doppler flow probe on the artery of an appendage distal to the placement of an inflatable cuff attached to a sphygmomanometer (Figure 10.11). The cuff is then gently inflated until the pulse is no longer audible. As the cuff is then slowly deflated, the point at which the pulse returns to audible is the systolic blood pressure. This measurement is generally repeated and an average taken over three to six measurements. Generally, avian systolic blood pressure should be maintained above 90 mmHg. Low blood pressure in the anaesthetized avian patient may be an indication for bolus fluid delivery to counteract poor organ perfusion during the anaesthetic episode.

Pulse oximetry may be used in birds, but can only provide trends of oxygenation, as no calibration curve taking into account the photometric behaviour of avian haemoglobin has been determined for birds; further, pulse oximetry monitors effectively in calm birds but readings fluctuate during surgery, dysrhythmia or blood loss (Schmitt *et al.*, 1998). Use of this monitoring technique is further limited by placement sites and the high avian heart rate. Hence pulse oximetry is best suited to short non-invasive anaesthetic procedures in healthy, large birds.

Capnography is a non-invasive method to determine the expired CO_2 as an estimate of appropriate ventilation in the anaesthetized bird (Edling *et al.*, 2001). This monitor provides values that estimate the

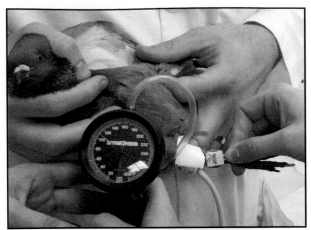

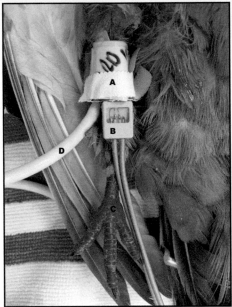

10.11 Determination of systolic blood pressure in a pigeon using a sphygmomanometer, with inflatable cuff (A) placed on the tibiotarsus, and a Doppler probe (B) placed on the dorsal metatarsal artery. C = foot; D = sphygmomanometer tube.

partial pressure of carbon dioxide and therefore the patient's ventilation. Estimation of appropriate ventilation is important, because birds do not have significant functional residual capacity and because inhalant anaesthetics used in birds at doses necessary for surgery cause substantial respiratory depression. End-tidal carbon dioxide should be maintained within the range of 20–40 mmHg via IPPV, mimicking that of the conscious bird. A capnograph used in combination with pulse oximetry is recommended in the critical avian anaesthetic patient.

Anaesthetic episode support
Every anaesthetized patient's plan should include consideration of fluid therapy (see Chapters 7 and 8), analgesia and sedation to provide a tranquil induction and recovery, and thermal support.

Thermal support
Thermal support should be provided to all avian patients undergoing an anaesthetic episode. Hypothermia of the anaesthetized patient may have severe

consequences and can result in patient death. Hyperthermia also can result in the death of an anaesthetized avian patient.

A number of factors may contribute to heat loss, including the large surface area in relation to body mass in small birds and the rapid flow of anaesthetic gases, especially with non-rebreathing circuits, through the respiratory system. In pigeons, the type of anaesthesia circuit used (Bain non-rebreathing, heated air ventilator, or unheated air ventilator) did not affect the core body temperature of the patient (Boedecker et al., 2005).

Surgical preparation, although necessary, contributes to patient heat loss because of the length of preparation, feather loss and the type of scrub used. Although the surgical field should be adequate, excessive removal of feathers should be avoided. Alcohol should not be used as a surgical skin preparation: it is irritating to tissue, can be toxic when absorbed though the skin, facilitates heat loss, and is flammable when used with some laser and electrosurgical units. Warmed water or saline and chlorhexidine scrubs are preferred in avian preparation.

To prevent heat loss or maintain core body temperature, two methods are used: passive insulation and active warming. *Passive insulators* commonly used in avian medicine include plastic bubble wrap, plastic drapes, or, in large patients, standard drapes or towels.

Active warming: Except in very short anaesthetic procedures in larger avian species, active warming is required in addition to passive warming techniques. Active warming devices include convective heating systems (forced-air warmers), radiant heating devices (infrared heat emitters and heat lamps) and conductive heating systems (warmed inspired gases, circulating-water blankets, heated surgical tables). These warming devices differ in their ability to maintain body temperature in the anaesthetized avian patient (Phalen et al., 1996):

- Devices that produce warmed inspiratory anaesthetic gases may be technically difficult to use in avian patients and do not contribute to the maintenance of core body temperature
- Radiant-heat energy sources maintain core body temperature more effectively than circulating-water heating pads
- External forced-air warming systems maintain core body temperature for longer (30 minutes) than circulating-water blankets or infrared heat emitters
- Core avian body temperature drops in the anaesthetized patient after 30 minutes, independently of the thermal support system used, with the exception of a radiant-heat energy source in one study
- Death has been caused by a heat lamp that produced point heat of 120°F (48.9°C) at the table interface (Hofmeister and Hernandez-Divers, 2005).

In practice, multiple methods of thermal support are generally applied while simultaneously monitoring body temperature.

Anaesthetic plane	Reflexes present	Reflexes absent	Expected physiological parameters	Comments
I Induction	All Palpebral, pedal, cere, voluntary movement of third eyelid	None	Sedate, lethargic, eyelids droop. Breathing deep or shallow, rapid and irregular based on patient excitement	
II	All	None, eyes closed	Feathers ruffled, head hangs down, arousable but does not resist handling. Increased third eyelid movement	Excitatory phase may occur here; more likely in large birds
III Light	Palpebral, pedal and cere present but slow. Corneal, withdrawal, pain on feather pluck	Lack of voluntary movement, no response to postural changes	Rapid, regular, deep respirations, no response to sound. Some jaw tone present	Preferred plane for minor non-painful procedures
IV Medium Surgical	Corneal present but sluggish	Palpebral, pedal, cere withdrawal, pain of feather pluck	Good muscular relaxation, slow deep regular respirations. Little jaw tone.	Preferred plane for surgery
V Deep	None, lack of corneal	All	Respirations slow and shallow to intermittent. Pupillary dilation	Death ensues, emergency pending

10.12 Stages of avian anaesthesia based on monitoring of physiological parameters, including reflexes.

Recovery

Recovery should be carefully monitored. The patient may be allowed to awaken in a quiet warm padded area or may be held bundled in a towel. Whatever method is chosen, the patient needs to be monitored for ventilatory depth, quality and rate. Thus lateral or ventrodorsal recumbency are generally preferred for recovery; these positions also facilitate ventilation. Generally, extubation is recommended when the patient begins to move the head, swallows, or has adequate neck tone. Reflexes and general muscle tone will also guide the extubation decision, based on the anaesthetic plane (Figure 10.12).

Common problems in the recovery period include hypothermia, endotracheal tube occlusion and regurgitation. Appropriate patient and equipment preparation, patient support and monitoring throughout the anaesthetic period and during recovery should avoid or lessen the likelihood of encountering these problems.

Management of anaesthetic emergencies

An overview of the expected clinical signs and appropriate clinical response and prognosis for each type of anaesthetic emergency is given in Figure 10.13.

Emergency	Clinical signs	Treatment	Prognosis
Apnoea	Lack of respiration based on keel movement	Confirm apnoea, intubate. Confirm level of anaesthesia by checking muscle tone and reflexes. Turn off anaesthetic gas or reverse anaesthetics. Give IPPV. Confirm pulse and heart beat. Administer dopram, repeat in 2 minutes if no appropriate response occurs. Consider administration of adrenaline and atropine after 2 minutes	Good if appropriate action is taken in a timely manner
Endotracheal tube blockage	Difficult, slow or non-existent expiration Slow recovery Duration of expiration prolonged Upon mechanical sigh or inspiration, air sacs fill normally but during expiration air sacs empty slowly or not at all	Remove endotracheal tube and replace if necessary. Provide 100% oxygen and reduce anaesthetic gas amount if recovery is feasible. Use of pre-emptive anticholinergics is controversial	Fair to good if appropriate actions are taken in a timely manner
Hypovolaemia	Loss of blood and fluid, poor perfusion as evidenced by thready or weak pulses	Volume replacement with warmed isotonic fluids, colloids or blood as indicated, preferably i.v. or intraosseous	Fair dependent upon volume lost Birds may lose up to 30% of their blood volume before experiencing shock
Vomiting, regurgitation	Liquid from mouth, in anaesthetic mask or, worse, in endotracheal tube	Hold head downward to drain liquid, clean oral cavity with gauze sponges or cotton-tipped applicators. Ensure choana is completely cleared of debris. Suction endotracheal tube and consider replacement of tube after oral cavity is cleaned	Fair to guarded Bird should be monitored for signs of aspiration pneumonia Antibiotic treatment may be considered
Hypothermia	Body temp below 38°C (100°F)	Thermal support, monitoring	Good to guarded
Cardiac arrest	ECG flatline, lack of pulse, extremity pallor	Intubate and give 100% oxygen and IPPV, discontinue or reverse anaesthetics. Alternate keel compression and caudal coelomic compression to simulate normal respiratory rate. Administer atropine, adrenaline and doxopram and dexamethasone i.v. or intratracheally	Guarded to grave

10.13 Common avian anaesthetic and perianaesthetic emergencies and appropriate clinical response and prognosis (Wheler, 1993; Ludders, 2001).

Drug	Species	Dosage (mg/kg)	Route	Indication
Adrenaline (1:1000)	Birds	0.5–1.0 mg/kg	i.m., i.v., intraosseous, intratracheal	Cardiac arrest
Atropine	Birds	0.5	i.m., i.v., intraosseous, intratracheal	CPR
Dexamethasone	Birds	2–6	i.m., i.v.	Shock
Doxapram	Birds, raptors	5–20	i.m., i.v., intraosseous, intratracheal	Respiratory arrest, apnoea, CPR, respiratory depression
Prednisolone sodium succinate	Birds, raptors	10–30 q15min prn	i.m., i.v.	CPR

10.14 Emergency resuscitation drugs (Pollock *et al.*, 2005).

With the advent of safe and effective inhalant anaesthetics for use in birds, anaesthetic emergencies are now less common. Typical perianaesthetic emergencies include apnoea, endotracheal tube blockage, hypothermia, regurgitation, hypovolaemia due to intraoperative haemorrhage or fluid loss, and cardiac arrest. Emergencies are preferably avoided by appropriate planning and availability of materials, equipment and drugs.

- Endotracheal tubes of appropriate length and diameter for the patient should be prepared prior to induction of any patient, irrespective of the expected anaesthetic episode length or route of induction.
- Oxygen and calibrated delivery equipment should also be immediately available.
- Appropriate anaesthetic emergency drug doses should be determined for the patient and written down, and also preferably be drawn up in appropriate syringes ready for immediate use.
- There should be an avian emergency kit, where all necessary drugs, syringes, dosages based on weight, and endotracheal tubes, which can be brightly coloured, are kept in the same place.

Avian cardiopulmonary resuscitation

Cardiopulmonary resuscitation may be challenging and is often hampered by the bird's small size and the keel bone, which restricts access to the heart for auscultation, injection or cardiac massage. The standard principles used in mammals are applied.

- In the event of respiratory or cardiac arrest an airway is established.
- While apnoea is common in the anaesthetized avian patient, cardiac arrest is not and generally signals the death of the patient.
- If the patient is already intubated, airway patency should be ensured.
- IPPV is begun at a rate consistent with that taken from the bird prior to anaesthesia.
- After breathing is initiated, the cardiovascular status is assessed and keel compressions and alternate compressions of the body cavity can be used to promote proper circulation.
- Vascular access, if not already obtained, should occur and then emergency drugs may be administered, based on the arresting system (Figure 10.14).
- If vascular access is not already obtained, some drugs may be administered intramuscularly or intratracheally.

References and further reading

Abou-Madi N (2001) Avian anesthesia. *Veterinary Clinics of North America: Exotic Animal Practice* **4**(1), 147–167

Allen J and Osterhuis JE (1986) Effects of tolazoline on xylazine ketamine anesthesia in the turkey vulture. *Journal of the American Veterinary Medical Association* **189**, 1011–1012

Baert K and DeBacker P (2003) Comparative pharmacokinetics of 3 nonsteroidal antiinflammatory drugs in 5 bird species. *Compendium of Biochemistry and Physiology C Toxicology Pharmacology* **134**, 24–33

Boedecker NC, Carpenter JW *et al.* (2005) Comparison of body temperatures of pigeons (*Columba livia*) anesthetized by three different anesthetic delivery systems. *Journal of Avian Medicine and Surgery* **19**(1), 1–6

Carpenter JW (2005) *Exotic Animal Formulary*. WB Saunders, Philadelphia

Clubb S (1998) Round table discussion; pain management in clinical practice. *Journal of Avian Medicine and Surgery* **12**(4), 276–278

Clubb SL and Meyer MJ (2006) *Clinical Management of Psittacine Birds Affected with Proventricular Dilatation Disease*. Association of Avian Veterinarians Conference and Expo, San Antonio, Texas

Curro TG, Brunson D *et al.* (1994) Determination of the ED50 for isoflurane and evaluation of the isoflurane sparing effects of butorphanol in cockatoos. *Veterinary Surgery* **23**, 429–433

Day TK and Roge CK (1996) Evaluation of sedation in quail induced by use of midazolam and reversed by use of flumazenil. *Journal of the American Veterinary Medical Association* **209**(5), 969–971

Degernes LA, Kreeger T *et al.* (1988) Ketamine xylazine anesthesia in red-tailed hawks with antagonism by yohimbine. *Journal of Wildlife Diseases* **24**(2), 322–326

Edling TM (2006) Update on anesthesia and monitoring in the avian patient. *Clinical Avian Medicine and Surgery*, ed. T Lightfoot and G Harrison. Spix, Palm Beach, FL

Edling TM, Degernes LA *et al.* (2001) Capnographic monitoring of anesthetized African grey parrots receiving intermittent positive pressure ventilation. *Journal of the American Veterinary Medical Association* **219**(12), 1714–1718

Fitzgerald G and Cooper JE (1990) Preliminary studies on the use of propofol in the domestic pigeon (*Columbia livia*). *Research in Veterinary Science* **49**, 334–338

Freed D and Baker B (1989) Antagonism of xylazine hydrochloride sedation in raptors by yohimbine hydrochloride. *Journal of Wildlife Diseases* **25**(1), 136–138

Glatz P, Murphy L *et al.* (1992) Analgesic therapy of beak trimmed chickens. *Australian Veterinary Journal* **69**(18), 18

Graham J, Kollias-Baker C *et al.* (2005) Pharmacokinetics of ketoprofen in Japanese quail (*Coturnix japonica*). *Journal of Veterinary Pharmacology and Therapeutics* **28**, 399–402

Gunkel C and LaFortune M (2005) Current topics in avian anesthesia. *Seminars in Avian and Exotic Pet Medicine* **14**(4), 263–276

Harrison G, Lightfoot T *et al.* (2006) Emergency and critical care. In: *Clinical Avian Medicine*, ed. G Harrison and T Lightfoot, pp. 213–232. Spix, Palm Beach, FL

Hawkins MG (2006) The use of analgesics in birds, reptiles and small exotic mammals. *Journal of Exotic Pet Medicine* **15**(3), 177–192

Hawkins MG, Wright BD *et al.* (2003) Pharmacokinetics and anesthetic and cardiopulmonary effects of propofol in red-tailed hawks *(Buteo jamaicensis)* and great-horned owls (*Bubo virginianus*). *American Journal of Veterinary Research* **64**(6), 677–683

Heard DJ (1997) Avian respiratory anatomy and physiology. *Seminars in Avian and Exotic Pet Medicine* **6**(4), 172–179

Heard DJ (2000) Avian anesthesia. In: *Manual of Avian Medicine*, ed. G.H Olsen and SE Orosz, pp. 464–492. Mosby, Philadelphia

Heatley JJ, Marks SL *et al.* (2001) Raptor emergency and critical care: assessment and examination. *Compendium on Continuing Education for the Practicing Veterinarian* **23**(5), 442–450

Hocking P, Gentle M *et al.* (1997) Evaluation of a protocol for determining the effectiveness of pretreatment with local analgesics for reducing experimentally induced articular pain in domestic fowl. *Research in Veterinary Science* **63**, 263–267

Hoerauf K, Lierz M *et al.* (1999) Genetic damage to operating room personnel exposed to isoflurane and nitrous oxide. *Occupational and Environmental Medicine* **56**, 433–437

Hofmeister EH and Hernandez-Divers SJ (2005) Anesthesia case of the month: hyperthermia and death in a Sun Conure. *Journal of the American Veterinary Medical Association* **227**(5), 718–720

Huckabee JR (2000) Raptor therapeutics. *Veterinary Clinics of North America: Exotic Animal Practice* **3**(1), 91–116

Jaensch SM, Cullen L *et al.* (2002) Air sac functional anatomy of the Sulphur Crested Cockatoo *(Cacatua galerita)* during isoflurane anesthesia. *Journal of Avian Medicine and Surgery* **16**(1), 2–9

Kreeger TJ, Degernes LA *et al.* (1993) Immobilization of raptors with tiletamine and zolazepam (Telazol). In: *Raptor Biomedicine*, ed. PT Redig, JE Cooper, JD Remple and DB Hunter, pp. 141–144. University of Minnesota Press, Minneapolis

Lawton MP (1996) Anaesthesia. In: *Manual of Raptors, Pigeons and Waterfowl*, ed. PH Beynon *et al.*, pp. 79–88. BSAVA Publications, Cheltenham

Lichtenberger M (2005) Determination of indirect blood pressure in the companion bird. *Seminars in Avian and Exotic Pet Medicine* **14**(2), 149–152

Ludders J (2001) Inhaled anesthesia for birds. In: *Recent Advances in Veterinary Anesthesia and Analgesia*, ed. R Gleed and J Ludders. International Veterinary Information Service, Ithaca, NY

Ludders JW (1995) Inhalant anesthetics and inspired oxygen: implications for anesthesia in birds. *Journal of the American Animal Hospital Association* **31**, 38–41

Lumeij J and Dennik J (2003) Medetomidine-ketamine and diazepam-ketamine anesthesia in racing pigeons (*Columbia livia domestica*) – a comparative study. *Journal of Avian Medicine and Surgery* **17**(4), 191–196

Machin KL (2005a) Avian pain: physiology and evaluation. *Compendium on Continuing Education for the Practicing Veterinarian* **27**(2), 98–109

Machin KL (2005b) Controlling avian pain. *Compendium on Continuing Education for the Practicing Veterinarian* **27**(4), 299–309

Machin KL and Caulkett NA (2000) Evaluation of isoflurane and propofol anesthesia for intraabdominal transmitter placement in nesting female Canvasback ducks. *Journal of Wildlife Diseases* **36**(2), 324–334

Machin KL and Livingston A (2002) Assessment of the analgesic effects of ketoprofen in ducks anesthetized with isoflurane. *American Journal of Veterinary Research* **63**, 821–826

Mama K, Phillips L *et al.* (1996) *Journal of Zoo & Wildlife Medicine* **27**, 397–401

Massey JG (2003) Diseases and medical management of wild Passeriformes. *Seminars in Avian and Exotic Pet Medicine* **12**(1), 29–36

Mulcahy DH, Tuomi P *et al.* (2003) Differential mortality of male Spectacled Eiders *(Somateria fischeri)* and King Eiders *(Somateria spectabilis)* subsequent to anesthesia with propofol, bupivicaine, and ketoprofen. *Journal of Avian Medicine and Surgery* **17**(3), 117–123

Myers D (2005) Therapeutic review. *Seminars in Avian and Exotic Pet Medicine* **13**(4), 284–287

Nilson PC, Teramitsu I *et al.* (2005) Caudal air sac cannulation in zebra finches for isoflurane anesthesia. *Journal of Neuroscience Methods* **143**, 107–115

Paul-Murphy J (2006) Pain management. In: *Clinical Avian Medicine*, ed. G Harrison and T Lightfoot, p. 233–239. Spix, Palm Beach, FL

Paul-Murphy J, Brunson D *et al.* (1999) Analgesic effects of butorphanol and buprenorphine in conscious African grey parrots (*Psittacus eritheus eritheus* and *Psittacus eritheus timneh*). *American Journal of Veterinary Research* **60**(10), 1218–1221

Paul-Murphy J and Fialkowski J (2001) Injectable anesthesia and analgesia of birds. In: *Recent Advances in Veterinary Anesthesia and Analgesia: Companion Animals*, ed. R Gleed and J Ludders. International Veterinary Information Service, Ithaca, NY

Paul-Murphy J, Hess J *et al.* (2004) Pharmacokinetic properties of a single intramuscular dose of buprenorphine in African grey parrots (*Psittacus erithacus erithacus*). *Journal of Avian Medicine and Surgery* **18**, 224–228

Paul-Murphy J and Ludders JW (2001) Avian analgesia. *Veterinary Clinics of North America: Exotic Animal Practice* **4**(1), 35–45

Pettifer GR, Cornick-Seahorn J *et al.* (2002) The comparative cardiopulmonary effects of spontaneous and controlled ventilation by using Hallowell EMC anesthesia workstation in Hispaniolan Amazon Parrots (*Amazona ventralis*). *Journal of Avian Medicine and Surgery* **16**(4), 268–276

Phalen DN, Mitchell ME *et al.* (1996) Evaluation of three heat sources for their ability to maintain core body temperature in the anesthetized avian patient. *Journal of Avian Medicine and Surgery* **13**(3), 174–178

Picker M (1994) Kappa agonist and antagonist properties of pigeons. *Journal of Pharmacologic Experimental Therapy* **268**, 1190–1198

Pollock CG, Carpenter JW *et al.* (2005) Table 34 Agents used in birds emergencies. *Exotic Animal Formulary*, ed. JW Carpenter. Saunders, Philadelphia

Redig PT (1998) Recommendations for anesthesia in raptors with comments on Trumpeter Swans. *Seminars in Avian and Exotic Pet Medicine* **7**(1), 22–29

Rembert MS, Smith JA *et al.* (2001) Comparison of traditional thermal support devices with the forced air warmer system in anesthetized Hispaniolan Amazon Parrots *(Amazona ventralis)*. *Journal of Avian Medicine and Surgery* **15**(3), 187–193

Samour J, Jones DM, *et al.* (1984) Comparative studies on the use of some injectable anesthetic agents in birds. *Veterinary Record* **115**, 6–11

Sandmeier P and Coutteel P (2006) Management of canaries, finches and mynahs. In: *Clinical Avian Medicine*, ed. G. Harrison and T. Lightfoot, pp. 879–914. Spix, Palm Beach, FL

Schmitt P, Gobel T *et al.* (1998) Evaluation of pulse oximetry as a monitoring method in avian anesthesia. *Journal of Avian Medicine and Surgery* **12**(2), 91–99

Sladky KK, Krugner-Higby L *et al.* (2006) Serum concentrations and analgesic effects of liposome-encapsulated and standard butorphanol tartrate in parrots. *American Journal of Veterinary Research* **67**(5), 781

Touzot-Jourde G, Hernandez-Divers SJ *et al.* (2005) Cardiopulmonary effects of controlled versus spontaneous ventilation in pigeons anesthetized for celioscopy. *Journal of the American Veterinary Medical Association* **227**(9), 1424–1428

Uzun M, Gultekin A *et al.* (2003) Effects of medetomidine-ketamine combination anaesthesia on electrocardiographic findings, body temperature, and heart and respiratory rates in domestic pigeons. *Turkish Journal of Veterinary Animal Science* **27**, 377–382

Wheler C (1993) Avian anesthetics, analgesics, and tranquilizers. *Seminars in Avian and Exotic Pet Medicine* **2**(1), 7–12

Wilson G, Hernandez-Divers SJ *et al.* (2004) Pharmacokinetics and use of meloxicam in psittacine birds. *Association of Avian Veterinarians Conference and Expo, Monterey*

Zenker W, Janovsky M *et al.* (2000) Immobilization of the Eurasian Buzzard (*Buteo buteo*) with oral tiletamine/zolazepam. In: *Raptor Biomedicine III*, ed. J Lumeij *et al.*, pp. 295–303. Zoological Education Network, Lake Worth, FL

11

Radiography

Michael Pees

General considerations

Radiography is an important and well described diagnostic technique in birds. It provides useful information about the size, shape and radiodensity of the inner organs. Due to the air sac system, most of the organs are outlined against each other (air as a negative contrast medium), facilitating radiographic assessment. Therefore radiography is one of the most often used imaging techniques in birds. Indications for radiological examinations are widespread and include cases of skeletal abnormalities, soft tissue swelling, dyspnoea and diarrhoea as well as poor performance and weight loss.

A radiographic examination is quickly done and assessment of the radiographs can be made after the examination without stress for the bird. A standard radiographic examination with two views can be performed within two minutes, causing no more stress than would an induction of anaesthesia. However, due to the necessary restraint of the patient (especially in dorsal recumbency), there might be an increased risk of circulatory problems in birds that are very sensitive to handling and fixation. In these cases anaesthesia might be indicated. For most other cases, radiography can be performed without anaesthesia, either with manual fixation or with special fixation devices. These devices are regularly used in countries such as the UK, where non-manual restraint of the bird for radiography is practised whenever possible under the guidance of a radiation protection adviser (RPA).

There is also an increased risk of circulatory collapse in birds with clinical signs of severe dyspnoea and/or swollen abdomen, and the indication for the radiographic examination should be considered carefully. In these cases, stabilization of the bird (fluids, heat, oxygen) before taking the radiographs is recommended.

In general, equipment necessary for the radiographic examination should be prepared in advance, in order to reduce the time for the examination as much as possible.

Equipment

Requirements for the X-ray machine are high. Due to the small size of most pet birds, it is necessary to use lower kilovoltage (kV) to achieve a good contrast. A high milliamperage (mA) is useful to allow short exposure times and therefore reduce movement artefacts. For most pet birds 40–45 kV is adequate, and exposure times should be not more than 0.05 seconds in the conscious bird. The recommended focal–film distance is between 80 and 100 cm. Grids should not be used.

The screens used for avian radiology should provide as much detail as possible, but at the same time allow short exposure times. For this purpose, high-definition screen–film combinations have proved most useful. Single emulsion films can provide more details but need longer exposure times and are therefore of limited value in birds. Modern mammography films can combine high detail resolution and acceptable exposure times. It might be necessary to check whether the automatic processors used in the practice are suitable for development of these films.

With ongoing technical development, the use of digital radiography will become more important and affordable. An important advantage is the possibility of post processing of the recorded images. High-definition digital radiology is currently used mainly for human mammography and there is considerable potential for its use in veterinary medicine – especially avian medicine – though there are huge quality differences between the machines that are available. (Dental machines for very small birds are not recommended, as results appear poor in comparison.)

It must be always be remembered that original data are necessary for assessment of the results, particularly with referrals where enhanced digital images have been submitted. Editing and magnifying techniques cannot replace poor equipment and examination techniques.

Positioning and views

In order to achieve good diagnostic results, one of the most important requirements is the correct positioning of the bird. Poor positioning can lead to worthless or even misleading radiographs. The patient's body should be as stretched as possible to reduce overlapping of different structures.

There are three important standard views: the ventrodorsal view, the lateral view and the caudocranial view of the wings. For skull radiography, special projections might be necessary. The bird can be restrained either manually or using a commercially available fixation plate.

Manual fixation is the most commonly used method of restraint outside the UK (Figure 11.1). A disadvantage is the radiation exposure for the veterinary surgeon, making it necessary to narrow the examination field as much as possible. This is a limiting problem, especially in small birds such as the Canary. The use of lead gloves or plates for protection of the hands is always necessary. For restraint the bird is fixed at the head with one hand, while the other hand holds the legs as distally as possible.

Acrylic *fixation plates* to restrain the bird in dorsal or lateral recumbency allow whole-body radiographs as well as the examination of the head and the toes, which is difficult with manual restraint (Figure 11.2). Several devices are available commercially. They are all based on a system of collars of different sizes for the fixation of the bird's neck, and laces for the fixation of the legs.

Ventrodorsal view

For this projection, the bird is placed in dorsal recumbency, and the legs are stretched as much as possible (Figures 11.3 to 11.5). This is difficult especially in large, healthy birds since they normally try to pull their legs to the body. The aim should always be to superimpose the keel over the vertebral column. With this position the right and the left parts of the body are displayed symmetrically. Improper positioning complicates the assessment of the organ sizes, especially of the liver, the heart and the proventriculus.

> The ventrodorsal projection is of special value for the assessment of the skeletal system (pectoral girdle, wing bones, hip joints, legs), the abdominal air sacs, the liver and the cardiac silhouette.

11.1 Radiographic examination in a raptor, manual fixation, ventrodorsal direction. NB. The holder should be equipped with suitable PPE; the gloves have been removed here merely to show the hold more clearly. The legs should be pulled as distally as possible. Ideally the keel should be superimposed on the vertebral column. The wings can be spread using lead plates or lead gloves.

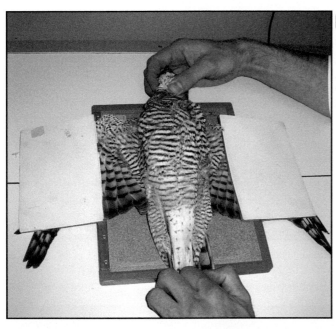

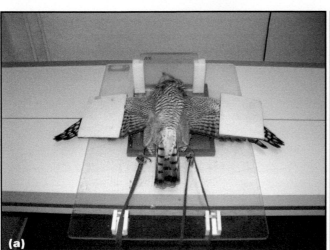

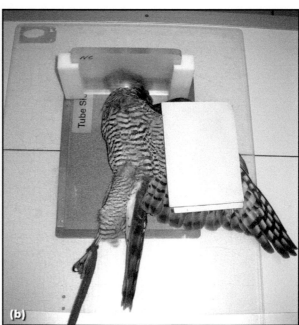

11.2 Radiographic examination in a raptor using a fixation plate. **(a)** For the ventrodorsal view the bird is placed on its back, with the legs pulled distally. **(b)** For the lateral view, the bird is turned 90 degrees and the wings stretched dorsally.

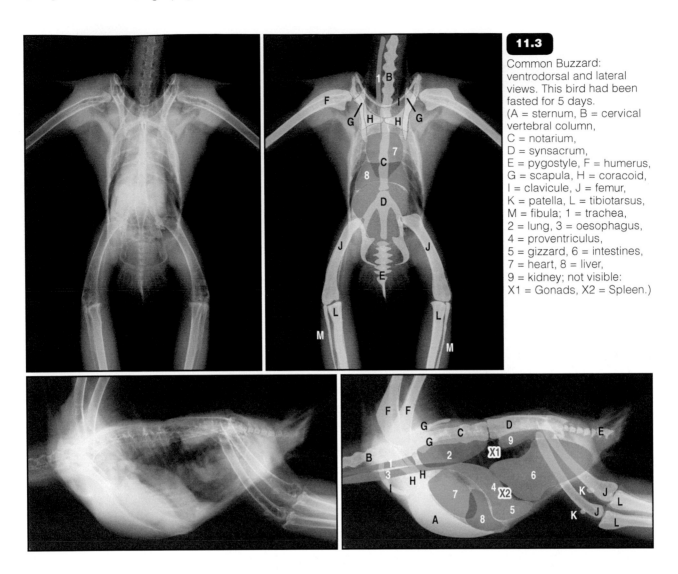

11.3
Common Buzzard: ventrodorsal and lateral views. This bird had been fasted for 5 days. (A = sternum, B = cervical vertebral column, C = notarium, D = synsacrum, E = pygostyle, F = humerus, G = scapula, H = coracoid, I = clavicule, J = femur, K = patella, L = tibiotarsus, M = fibula; 1 = trachea, 2 = lung, 3 = oesophagus, 4 = proventriculus, 5 = gizzard, 6 = intestines, 7 = heart, 8 = liver, 9 = kidney; not visible: X1 = Gonads, X2 = Spleen.)

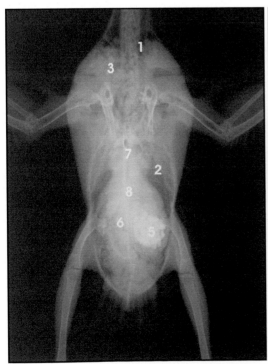

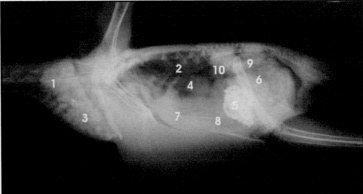

11.4 Racing pigeon: ventrodorsal and lateral views. This bird was fed only hours ago. Note the full crop and distended abdominal shadow. (1 = trachea, 2 = lung, 3 = crop, 4 = proventriculus, 5 = gizzard with grit, 6 = intestines, 7 = heart, 8 = liver, 9 = kidney, 10 = gonads.)

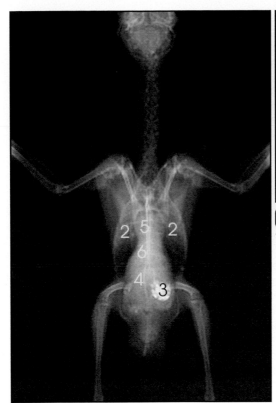

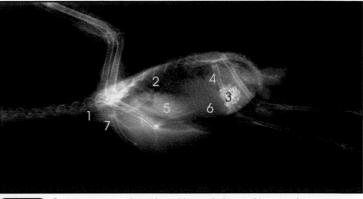

11.5 Canary: ventrodorsal and lateral views. (1 = trachea, 2 = lung, 3 = gizzard, 4 = intestine, 5 = heart, 6 = liver, 7 = crop.)

Lateral view

This view (Figures 11.3 to 11.6) is best obtained directly after the ventrodorsal radiograph. The bird is turned through 90 degrees by an assistant, with the same fixation as for the first view. The wings are carefully stretched dorsally and placed under the forearm of the holding person (manual restraint) or placed under some lead plates/sandbags (fixation plate). For this view, the aim is that both hip joints and coracoids should be superimposed. Insufficiently stretched legs can make this view impossible to interpret.

> The lateral projection is important for the assessment of the skeletal system (skull, spinal column, ribs, sternum, synsacrum), the gastrointestinal tract, the lungs, the air sacs, the cardiac silhouette and large vessels, the spleen, the kidneys and the gonads.

Caudocranial view

This view displays a second plane for the assessment of the wings (Figure 11.7). The bird is held manually in an upside-down position directly over the edge of the table. The wing is placed over the screen in maximum extension, with the cranial part as close to the screen as possible. Afterwards the wing position is adjusted to achieve a caudocranial projection through the bones.

> The caudodorsal view is important for the assessment of the wing bones and joints.

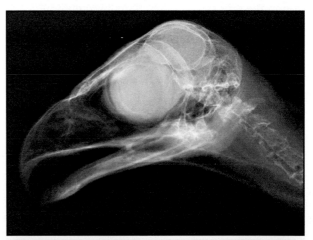

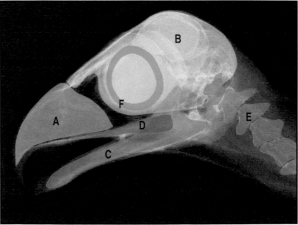

11.6 The head of a Goshawk, lateral view. (A = maxilla, B = cranium, C = palate, D = mandible, E = vertebral column, F = scleral ring.)

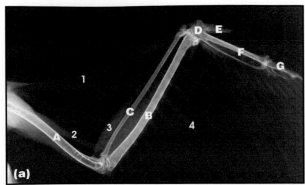

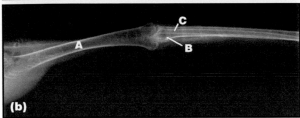

11.7 The wing of a Common Buzzard:
(a) ventrodorsal and **(b)** caudocranial view.
(A = humerus, B = ulna, C = radius,
D/E/F = carpometacarpus (D, Radial carpal bone; E, alar
digit; F, major metacarpal bone), G = phalanx;
1 = propatagium, 2/3 = muscles, 4 = feathers.)

Assessment and interpretation

Due to the size of the patients, most radiographs are
whole-body radiographs. The ventrodorsal and the
lateral view are commonly used for a general overview and normally provide sufficient information.
Assessment is according to guidelines published for
mammals. The author prefers to start with assessment of the skeletal system, followed by the respiratory tract and then the digestive, urogenital and
cardiovascular systems.

For correct interpretation, an adequate knowledge
of avian anatomy is essential. The basic anatomy is
similar in most birds but there are peculiarities in
many species (e.g. an angled trachea in the Indian
Hill Mynah; an extended intestinal tract in pigeons)
and of course huge variations in the dimensions of
the skeletal system.

Skeletal system and joints

For the assessment of the skeletal system, both
standard views should be used. Due to superimposi-
tion of different structures, assessment of the pectoral
girdle might be challenging. In cases of alteration of
the wing bones, an additional caudocranial projection
is strongly recommended in order to have a second
plane for radiological assessment. In every case of a
suspected alteration of the skeletal system, a comparison with the contralateral bone might be helpful.

- The normal bone is presented with a thin smooth
  cortex and less radiodense inner structures,
  depending on the pneumatization. This
  pneumatization varies between species. Bones
  with bone marrow (e.g. tibiotarsus, radius, ulna)
  appear more radiodense than bones connected
  to the air sac system (e.g. humerus).

- As a physiological condition, medullar bone can
  be present in sexually active females. In these
  cases, some bones (especially the humerus,
  femur and tibiotarsus) are presented with a
  radiodense content caused by additional
  calcium storage.

Common pathological findings are old and new
fractures, osteomyelitis, osteoarthritis and bone
deformations. Neoplasia is uncommon but possible.
Luxations are common after trauma.

- *Osteomyelitis* can arise from the medullary cavity
  of the bones. It is often the result of an open
  fracture, and can lead to osteolysis. In birds with
  osteomyelitis, an increased medullary bone
  density is commonly found in the area of
  infection. The surface of the bone often becomes
  roughened. If osteolysis is present radiolucent
  areas can be observed. If the joints are affected
  by the infection, there is often a soft tissue
  swelling visible, and examination of joint fluid can
  be helpful to secure the diagnosis.
- *Bone infection* can also be caused by
  Mycobacterium (tuberculosis) and might result in
  focal decalcification and hyperostosis in the large
  bones, especially the humerus, radius/ulna,
  femur and tibiotarsus.
- *Bone deformations* and pathological fractures are
  commonly the result of improper husbandry and
  are diagnosed mainly in nestlings.
  Osteodystrophy in adult birds is usually caused
  by malnutrition. In both cases, the cortical bone is
  thinned and/or less radiodense.
- In *fractured* bones, callus formation can be
  observed radiologically after approximately 14
  days. There is normally a massive periosteal
  reaction, depending on the dislocation of the
  fractured bone parts.

Respiratory system

- The cartilaginous/ossified rings of the *trachea*
  can be seen especially in older birds. The *syrinx*
  can be assessed in the cranial thoracic region
  and is most visible in the lateral view.
  Assessment of stenosis within the trachea or
  syrinx (e.g. granuloma, foreign body) is
  sometimes challenging.
- The *lung* parenchyma is best visualized in the
  lateral view. It is visible in the dorsal part of the
  coelomic cavity as a honeycombed structure.
  This pattern is caused by the parabronchi being
  viewed end-on. Infection of lung tissue can be
  seen as focal (e.g. aspergillosis) or diffuse–
  homogenous (e.g. bacterial infection)
  radiodensities. These alterations often involve the
  caudal part of the lung tissue. Sometimes
  abscesses or granulomas can form well defined
  radiodense areas within the lung.
- The size of the *air sacs* varies significantly
  depending on the respiratory cycle and the size
  of other inner organs. In healthy birds, delineation
  of the different air sacs is often difficult.

Radiographic alterations of the air sacs include focal or diffuse radiodense areas (e.g. aspergillosis) and thickened air sac walls (e.g. aspergillosis, obesity). 'Air trapping' occurs in cases of severe aspergillosis, with increased pressure within the air sac leading to massive air sac extension.

Digestive system, liver and spleen

- The *liver* can be assessed in both views. Assessment of the size is best in the ventrodorsal view. However, the 'hourglass' shape as described for psittacine birds (formed by the heart, liver and intestines) is not as typical in pigeons and raptors. In pigeons the size of the intestines is larger, whereas in raptors the size of the intestinal shadow depends on the time of feeding. A filled intestinal tract can spread the liver shadow, leading to a larger appearance of this organ. In cases of liver enlargement, the proventriculus (gizzard) can be displaced dorsally (caudally) and the air sacs can be distended. Contrast studies might be necessary to outline the shape of the liver.
- The *proventriculus*, *gizzard* and *intestines* can be assessed in both views. In pigeons, the gizzard normally contains certain amounts of grit, but grit overload is always a sign of intestinal disease. Even though the normal intestinal shadow in pigeons is larger, in cases of intestinal infections a swelling of the intestinal loops can sometimes be diagnosed. In raptors, the size of the proventriculus, gizzard and intestines is strongly dependent on the food content, and interpretation is difficult. Foreign bodies can be seen only if they are radiodense.
- The *spleen* is usually only visible in the lateral view, depending on its size. An enlarged spleen is always an indication of infectious disease, especially chlamydophilosis.

Urogenital tract

- The *kidneys* are located in the caudodorsal part of the coelomic cavity, embedded in the pelvic bones and around the vertebral column. They can be assessed mainly in the lateral view. They appear smaller in pigeons than in raptors and passerine birds. Kidney enlargement is often visible in the cranial part of the kidneys. Sometimes it can be difficult to differentiate kidney enlargement from active gonads.
- The *gonads* are situated cranioventrally to the kidneys, with their size strongly dependent on the sexual activity of the bird. Sex differentiation is only possible radiologically if eggs are present, or, in some cases, if both testes can be seen. Depending on the reproductive status, the size of the female reproductive organs can increase enormously and fill a large part of the coelomic cavity. In this case a displacement of the other organs and the air sacs occurs physiologically.

Radiologically detectable alterations in the urogenital system include neoplasia, calcinosis of the kidneys, and egg binding with egg shell alterations (see Chapter 21). Gout (urate deposition) is barely visible radiographically unless secondary calcinosis occurs. An increased density of the kidneys can be associated with gout but can also be caused by dehydration.

Cardiovascular system

- The *heart* is situated in the cranioventral part of the coelomic cavity, with the pericardium connected to the inner surface of the sternum. It can be assessed in both views. Measurements of the cardiac silhouette have been published for geese and psittacine birds, both indicating that, in the ventrodorsal view, approximately 50–60% of the width of the thorax can be considered as a normal heart size. However, radiological assessment of cardiac alterations is of limited value, and ultrasonography should be performed in every case of suspected heart disease. In falcons during the flying session, the cardiac silhouette tends to appear slightly larger in comparison to birds during resting periods.
- The *vessels* can best be assessed in the lateral view. An increased radiodensity of the great vessels indicates possible atherosclerosis. Diagnosis of atherosclerosis is challenging and should always include blood chemistry.

Contrast radiography

Contrast studies (Figure 11.8) are useful procedures for obtaining additional information.

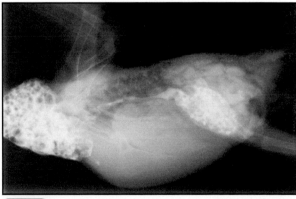

11.8 Lateral view of a racing pigeon 2 hours after oral administration of barium sulphate (20 ml/kg). The gastrointestinal tract is demonstrated, with a crop containing food, a small proventriculus and a gizzard containing grit.

Indications include:

- Examination of an organ's size, shape, content or position
- Determination of an organ's function
- Assessment of the size of neighbouring organs
- Examination of the thickness and condition of hollow structures.

Typical indications therefore include the demonstration of alimentary tract lesions (e.g. constipation, obstruction) and organ displacements. Contraindications are severely debilitated or dehydrated birds and suspected perforations in the gastrointestinal tract (barium sulphate). Starving the bird for some hours is advantageous to prevent regurgitation (emptied crop).

Barium sulphate

Barium sulphate is the main contrast medium for gastrointestinal use in birds, in a suspension with concentration between 25 and 40%. The suspension should be warmed to body temperature and can be diluted with water. The contrast medium is given via crop gavage in a dosage of 20 ml/kg body mass.

- It is important to hold the bird upright for approximately one minute after the application, in order to prevent regurgitation and aspiration, as massive lung damage can occur.
- An additional fluid substitution is recommended, especially in birds with diarrhoea or fluid loss.
- Anaesthesia should be avoided after the administration of contrast medium.

Passage times vary greatly between different species and between individuals (Figure 11.9). First radiographs should be taken 5 minutes after administration, with further radiographs depending on the passage time. In the UK, if horizontal beam radiography is to be used the RPA should be consulted.

	Pigeons	Canaries	Raptors
Crop	0	0	0
Ventriculus	5–15	5–10	10–15
Intestines	30–60	10–20	30–120
Cloaca	60–120	30–45	90–120

11.9 Approximate time (minutes after administration) of organ demonstration after application of barium sulphate (20 ml/kg body mass) via crop gavage.

Alternatively, barium may be placed directly into the proventriculus by means of a tube from the mouth. Where imaging of the crop is not required, this technique saves time and number of exposures. The first plates should be taken immediately after placing the barium.

Air

The use of air as a negative contrast medium is described but rarely administered. Nevertheless it is used wherever present for the interpretation of radiographs (air sacs; air within crop/proventriculus/intestines).

Iodinated contrast media

Iodinated contrast media can be given for gastrography, sinography, urography, angiocardiography and myelography. Use for gastrography is indicated in cases of suspected perforations. It is administered in a dosage of 10 ml/kg body mass (solution containing 250 mg iodine/ml). In comparison with barium sulphate, the opacity is less and the passage time is much faster. Sinography can be indicated in cases of chronic sinusitis, suspected foreign bodies and obstructions. Dosages of 0.1–1.0 ml (solution containing 150–250 mg iodine/ml) are instilled directly into the nares or the sinus. After the examination, the contrast medium should be flushed out with sterile saline solution.

Angiocardiography, urography and myelography have been described in birds but to date these techniques are not standard procedures and further studies are necessary to evaluate their role in avian medicine.

References and further reading

Krautwald-Junghanns ME, Tellhelm B, Hummel G *et al.* (1992) *Atlas of Radiographic Anatomy and Diagnosis of Cage Birds.* Paul Parey, Berlin

McMillan M (1994) Imaging techniques. In: *Avian Medicine: Principles and Application*, ed. BW Ritchie, GJ Harrison and LR Harrison, pp. 246–261. Wingers, Lake Worth, FL

Nemetz LP (2006) Principles of high-definition digital radiology for the avian patient. In: *Proceedings 27th Annual Meeting Association of Avian Veterinarians, San Antonio*, pp. 39–49

12

Advanced non-invasive imaging techniques

Michael Pees and Michael Lierz

Ultrasonography

Examination of the heart, liver, spleen, gastrointestinal system and urogenital system has been described. There are still limitations because of the anatomical peculiarities of birds (particularly the air sac system), but ultrasonography provides unique information for some indications, especially the examination of the cardiovascular and the urogenital systems. Although sonographic presentation of the inner organs in healthy birds may sometimes be difficult, organ enlargements and fluid accumulations in diseased birds improve the image quality significantly.

Equipment
Due to the relatively small size of many birds and their high heart rates, there are some special demands.

- Probes with small coupling surfaces (micro-curved or phased-array probes) are the most suitable for coupling.
- An ultrasound frequency of at least 7.5 MHz (the author's recommendation is 10 MHz) should be used to obtain images of sufficient resolution.
- The ultrasound examination should be recorded (digital motion loops or video sequences) to reduce the time of the examination, so that the assessment can be done afterwards without further stress for the bird.
- For echocardiographic examinations, the device used should provide a frame rate of 100 or more frames/second to get images from defined cardiac stages (systole and diastole). This is important due to the high heart rates in birds. A Doppler function (colour and spectral Doppler) and an electrocardiography (ECG) trigger option are useful for the examination.

> **For small birds, a stand-off might be necessary for the examination (the easiest way is to fill the finger of a latex examination glove with some water-soluble acoustic gel and use it as a stand-off).**

Patient preparation and approaches
In order to reduce artefacts from the filled gastro-intestinal tract, the bird should be fasted before examination.

- In passerine birds the fasting time should be not more than 2 hours (though fasting is not normally necessary in softbills).
- Pigeons should be fasted for 12 hours and raptors up to 48 hours.

Except for Doppler echocardiography, anaesthesia is not necessary. However, in birds that are not used to handling and if the procedure takes more than a few minutes, sedation can help to reduce stress and facilitate the examination. The patient may be held by an assistant in either dorsal or lateral (using the flank area) recumbency or in a standing position. In patients with clinical signs of cardiac disease or dyspnoea, the examination should be performed with the bird in an upright position.

There are two possible approaches for ultrasound examination in birds: the ventral approach behind the sternum and the parasternal approach behind the last rib.

- For the ventral approach the transducer is coupled in the median line directly behind the caudal end of the sternum (Figure 12.1).

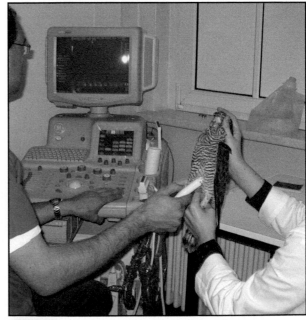

12.1 Ultrasonographic examination of a Sparrowhawk. The transducer is placed in the median line behind the sternum. Feathers should be either parted or plucked in the area of contact.

- The parasternal approach can be used in pigeons and some raptor species. For this approach, the scanner is placed between the last rib and the pelvic bones on the right side of the bird.

Since feathers impede the contact between scanner and skin they have to be plucked or parted. This is easier after the application of some commercial water-soluble acoustic gel.

Examination procedure

In comparison with other techniques, ultrasound assessment is much more subjective and more dependent on personal experience. It is advisable to use an examination protocol. The authors normally start the examination of the body cavity with the evaluation of the liver, followed by the heart, the gastrointestinal system and finally the urogenital system.

Liver

The transducer is first directed cranially to visualize the liver tissue (Figure 12.2). The liver parenchyma appears coarsely granular, with a uniform texture throughout. Intrahepatic vessels are visible as anechoic channels. In species with a gall bladder (e.g. falcons) this structure is generally visible as a round to oval anechoic structure. In fasted birds the gall bladder is generally enlarged.

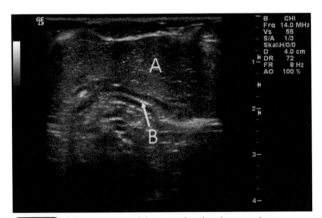

12.2 Ultrasonographic examination in a racing pigeon, ventral approach. The healthy liver tissue (A) is of average echogenicity and homogenous structure. The intestines (B) can be demonstrated with hypoechoic walls and hyperechoic content.

The transducer is swept until the whole liver has been examined. Typical findings are an enlarged (or reduced) size, irregular swollen edges, an increased echogenicity of the parenchyma or focal parenchymal lesions and dilated liver vessels. If necessary, ultrasound-guided biopsies may be taken according to the procedure in mammals.

Heart

The heart is visualized behind the liver with the probe directed craniodorsally. After identification of the heart, the transducer is swept laterally to visualize the organ section by section. First the sagittal view

(perpendicular to the sternum) is examined, then the transducer is rotated 90 degrees to obtain a second plane of view. Before measurements are taken, the probe has to be adjusted to the maximum extent of the ventricles.

The heart can be examined using B-Mode (2-D echocardiography). The size of both ventricles, the wall thickness of the interventricular septum and the contractility of the ventricles can be measured (Figures 12.3 and 12.4). Reference values have been reported for pigeons and raptors (Figure 12.5). The use of Doppler echocardiography is documented for some raptor species, and blood flow velocities have been measured (Figure 12.6).

Common findings in birds with cardiovascular disease include arrhythmias, hypertrophies and dilatations/wall thinning of the ventricles and alterations of the pericardium, including pericardial effusion, often combined with ascites and liver congestion.

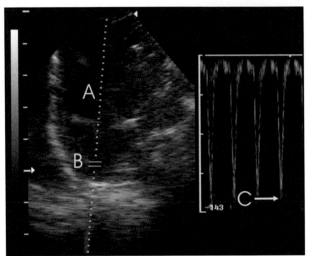

12.3 Ultrasonographic examination in a Common Buzzard, spectral Doppler examination, ventral approach. The velocity of the aortic outflow is demonstrated (C). A = left ventricle; B = left atrium.

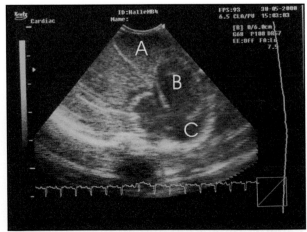

12.4 Ultrasonographic examination in a Common Buzzard, ventral approach. The liver (A) is used as an acoustic window. The heart is demonstrated with left ventricle (B) and the left atrium (C).

Parameter		Diurnal raptors[a] (Boskovic *et al.*, 1999)	Pigeons (Schulz, 1995)
		Ventromedial approach	Parasternal approach
Body mass (g)		720 ± 197	434 ± 52
Left ventricle	Length systole (mm)	14.7 ± 2.8	17.9 ± 1.0
	Length diastole (mm)	16.4 ± 2.7	20.1 ± 1.4
	Width systole (mm)	6.3 ± 1.1	5.2 ± 0.4
	Width diastole (mm)	7.7 ± 1.2	7.4 ± 0.6
	Width fractional shortening (%)	not given	27.2 ± 4.5
Right ventricle	Length systole (mm)	12.7 ± 2.7	not given
	Length diastole (mm)	13.9 ± 2.5	9.9 ± 0.8
	Width systole (mm)	2.1 ± 0.6	not given
	Width diastole (mm)	2.5 ± 0.8	4.0 ± 0.5
IVS	Thickness systole (mm)	1.9 ± 0.6	3.8 ± 0.1
	Thickness diastole (mm)	1.9 ± 0.5	3.3 ± 0.2

12.5 2-D echocardiography: important measured and calculated parameters in raptors and pigeons (mean value ± standard deviation), IVS = interventricular septum. [a] Including Common Buzzard, Sparrowhawk, Goshawk, Red Kite.

Parameter	*Falco* spp.	Common Buzzard
Diastolic inflow left ventricle (m/s)	0.21 ± 0.03	0.14 ± 0.01
Diastolic inflow right ventricle (m/s)	0.21 ± 0.04	0.14 ± 0.02
Systolic outflow aortic root (m/s)	0.95 ± 0.07	1.18 ± 0.05

12.6 Velocities of intracardiac blood flow, values obtained under anaesthesia. (Data from Straub *et al.*, 2001).

Gastrointestinal system

For the examination of the gastrointestinal system, the transducer is swept to the left side of the body cavity. The gizzard is easy to identify due to its large muscles and possible content of grit or food (Figure 12.7). The proventriculus can be seen occasionally on the right side. The small intestines can only be demonstrated clearly with high examination frequencies (at least 10 MHz). The peristalsis, wall thickness and wall layers can be assessed.

Common findings in birds with gastrointestinal disease are increased or decreased peristalsis as well as an enlargement of the intestines and the intestinal wall.

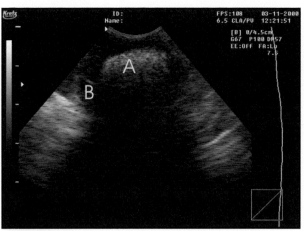

12.7 Ultrasonographic examination in a racing pigeon, ventral approach. The gizzard is always easy to identify due to the hyperechoic content (A, grit) and the hypoechoic wall (B). Beyond the gizzard, no structure can be demonstrated (acoustic shadowing).

Urogenital system

The urogenital system, lying behind the intestines, is examined starting with the presentation of the kidneys. The kidneys should be scanned in a cross-section to identify the tissue. In healthy birds, they are not recognizable in most cases. With pathological situations, such as an increased kidney size (swelling), tumours or ascites the demonstration of kidney tissue is usually possible. If identified, the whole extent of the organ can be demonstrated in a longitudinal section.

The visibility of the testes and ovary depends on the status of sexual activity: immature and inactive gonads are normally not visible in the ultrasound image. Therefore sex determination with transcutaneous ultrasonography is only possible in female birds with large follicles or eggs present. The use of intracloacal ultrasonography in birds has been described, but is limited to larger species and special equipment (Hildebrandt *et al.*, 1995).

In birds with urogenital tract disease, common alterations found in the ultrasonographic examination include organ enlargements, cystic alterations of the ovary and the kidneys, eggs without calcified shells and thickening of the oviduct (inflammatory processes and laminated eggs) and tumours.

Computed tomography

CT is an advanced radiographic technique that provides unique information about the inner structures of the body (Figures 12.8 to 12.11). It is a three-dimensional non-invasive technique with cross-sectional scans. These scans provide information without disturbing superimpositions of the organs. The bird is examined in either an axial or longitudinal direction, with 0.5–2 mm slice thickness. The X-ray absorption is calculated for small volume elements and displayed as individual grey shades. Densitometric measurements, given in Hounsfield Units (HU), can be used to identify and assess the tissues and organs.

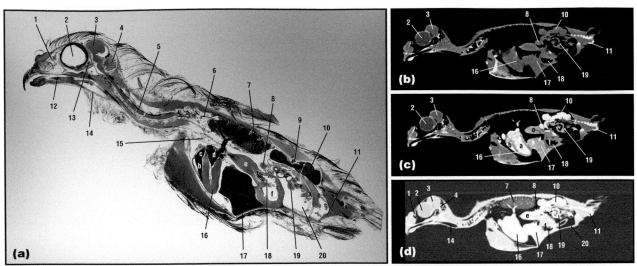

12.8 **(a)** Plastination of a falcon in sagittal view. (courtesy of HC Biovision). **(b–d)** CT scans: **(b)** plain scan; **(c)** 50 seconds after contrast medium; **(d)** with lung filter applied. 1 = conchae; 2 = orbit; 3 = cerebrum; 4 = cerebellum; 5 = spinal cord; 6 = paravertebral ganglia; 7 = lung; 8 = spleen; 9 = external iliac artery; 10 = kidney; 11 = cloaca; 12 = tongue; 13 = optic nerve; 14 = trachea; 15 = oesophagus; 16 = heart (a = left ventricle; b = right ventricle; c = right atrium; d = left atrium); 17 = liver; 18 = ventriculi (e = proventriculus; f = ventriculus); 19 = intestinal loops; 20 = air sac.

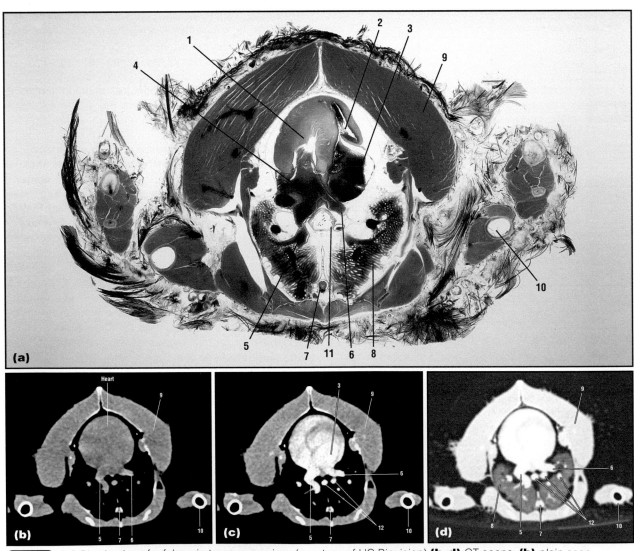

12.9 **(a)** Plastination of a falcon in transverse view. (courtesy of HC Biovision) **(b–d)** CT scans: **(b)** plain scan; **(c)** 50 seconds after intravenous iodine contrast medium; **(d)** with lung filter applied. 1 = left ventricle; 2 = right ventricle; 3 = right atrium; 4 = left atrium; 5 = left pulmonary artery; 6 = right pulmonary artery; 7 = spinal cord; 8 = lung; 9 = breast muscle; 10 = humerus; 11 = oesophagus; 12 = vessels.

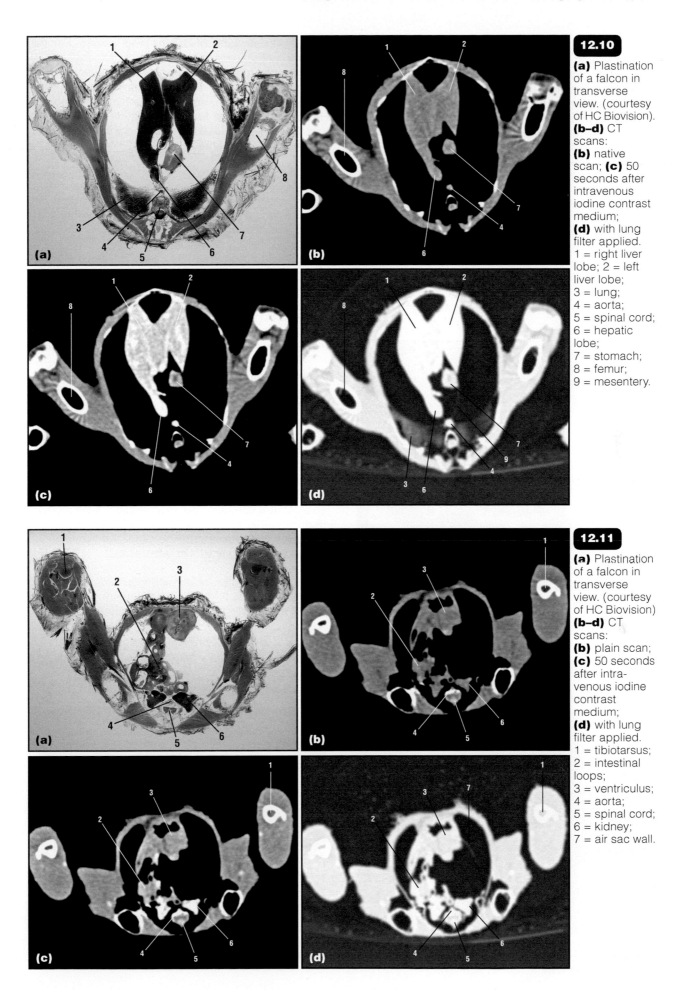

12.10
(a) Plastination of a falcon in transverse view. (courtesy of HC Biovision). **(b–d)** CT scans: **(b)** native scan; **(c)** 50 seconds after intravenous iodine contrast medium; **(d)** with lung filter applied.
1 = right liver lobe; 2 = left liver lobe;
3 = lung;
4 = aorta;
5 = spinal cord;
6 = hepatic lobe;
7 = stomach;
8 = femur;
9 = mesentery.

12.11
(a) Plastination of a falcon in transverse view. (courtesy of HC Biovision) **(b–d)** CT scans: **(b)** plain scan; **(c)** 50 seconds after intra-venous iodine contrast medium; **(d)** with lung filter applied.
1 = tibiotarsus;
2 = intestinal loops;
3 = ventriculus;
4 = aorta;
5 = spinal cord;
6 = kidney;
7 = air sac wall.

In order to reduce movement artefacts and stress, the bird should be anaesthetized for the examination. The use of fixation plates (as described in Chapter 11) is also possible.

For the examination the bird is placed in dorsal or ventral recumbency. Small birds can be positioned with the longitudinal axis crosswise to the gantry table and examined with longitudinal (sagittal) scans. Larger birds (raptors) should be scanned in axial (transversal) scans, with the longitudinal axis parallel to the table.

In the authors' experience, common indications for the use of CT are respiratory diseases (especially sinusitis, pneumonia (Figure 12.12) and air sacculitis), skeletal abnormalities (Figure 12.13), liver and kidney alterations and space-occupying processes. In these cases, CT is a valuable technique that provides more sensitive information in comparison with conventional radiography. The technique allows accurate localization of organs and lesions. For the diagnosis of respiratory disease (e.g. aspergillosis) it is very useful to assess the trachea and syrinx as well as the structure of the pulmonary tissue, giving detailed information on the extent of the disease. However, references for CT examination are still rare and systematic studies are necessary to evaluate the potential of this technique.

Magnetic resonance imaging

MRI is a recent technique based on measurements of the tissue response to a magnetic field stimulus. Since this response is different depending on the biochemical properties of the tissues, a two-dimensional section through the body can be produced. Since the signal intensity depends mainly on the proton response in the tissue, MRI is of special value for the assessment of soft tissue and fluids.

Depending on the type of signal measurement, two major weightings can be used to assess tissue:

- T1 images (fat as bright signal; fluid as dark (low) signal)
- T2 images (fluid bright; fat as grey (medium) signal).

Bone tissue is of low signal intensity (dark).

The main indication for MRI examinations in birds is soft tissue enlargement (e.g. suspected neoplasia or inflammatory processes). In the authors' experience, MRI is useful for the examination of the kidneys (Figure 12.14), liver, eye, central nervous system and all cases of space-occupying processes (neoplasia, granulomas (Figure 12.15), abscesses).

MRI examinations are much more time-consuming than CT and this is the limiting problem for its use in avian medicine. A standard examination normally takes 20–45 minutes. Since anaesthesia is required, and the bird has to be held in a fixed position, there is an increased risk of circulatory collapse, especially in weakened patients.

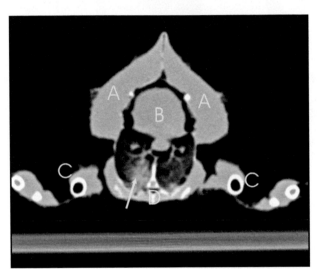

12.12 CT of a Eurasian Kestrel, axial view. A radiodense area within the left lung tissue can be seen (arrowed). A = pectoral muscle; B = heart; C = humerus; D = spinal column.

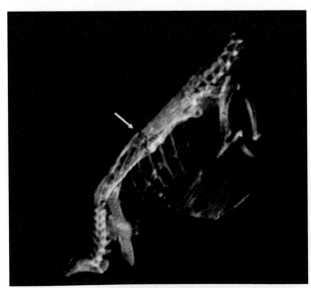

12.13 CT of a Eurasian Kestrel, three-dimensional reformation. A fracture of the spinal column is demonstrated (arrow).

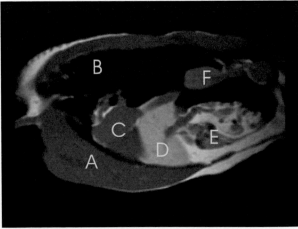

12.14 MRI of a Goshawk, T1-weighted. A = pectoral muscle; B = lung; C = heart; D = liver; E = intestines (with fat); F = kidneys.

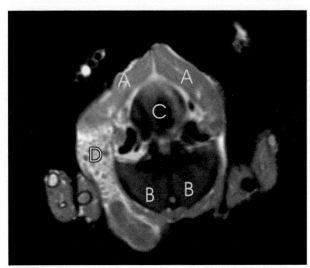

12.15 MRI of a Peregrine Falcon, T1-weighted. A granulomatous mass could be identified on the pectoral wall (diagnosis: mycobacteriosis). A = pectoral muscle; B = lungs; C = heart; D = granulomas.

Another problem is the detail resolution, which is low in comparison with CT and radiography, making it difficult to assess organs, especially in small birds.

However, since the MRI technique is unique and provides information different from all other imaging techniques, it should be taken into account at least in special cases, after the failure of other diagnostic means. With ongoing technical progress, this technique will probably become more important for birds in the future.

References and further reading

Boskovic M, Krautwald-Junghanns ME, Failing K *et al.* (1999) Möglichkeiten und Grenzen echokardiographischer Untersuchungen bei Tag- und Nachtgreifvögeln (Accipitriformes, Falconiformes, Strigiformes). *Tierärztliche Praxis* **27**, 334–341

Gumpenberger M (2001) The use of computed tomography in avian and reptile medicine. *Seminars in Avian and Exotic Pet Medicine* **10**(4), 174–180

Hildebrandt T, Görlitz F, Thielebein J, Pitra C and Talsness CE (1995) Transintestinal ultrasonographical sexing. In: *Proceedings of the European Committee of the Association of Avian Veterinarians*, pp. 37–41

Krautwald-Junghanns ME, Schulz M, Hagner D *et al.* (1995) Transcoelomic two-dimensional echocardiography in the avian patient. *Journal of Avian Medicine and Surgery* **9**, 19–31

Krautwald-Junghanns ME, Stahl A, Pees M, Enders F and Bartels T (2002) Sonographic investigations of the gastrointestinal tract of granivorous birds. *Veterinary Radiology and Ultrasound* **43**(6), 576–578

Pees M and Krautwald-Junghanns ME (2005) Avian echocardiography. *Seminars in Avian and Exotic Pet Medicine* **14**(1), 14–21

Pees M, Kiefer I, Ludewig E *et al.* (2006) Comparative ultrasonographic investigations of the gastrointestinal tract and the liver in healthy and diseased pigeons. *Veterinary Radiology and Ultrasound* **47**(4), 370–375

Schulz M (1995) Morphologische und funktionelle Messungen am Herzen von Brieftauben (*Columba livia* forma domestica) mit Hilfe der Schnittbildechokardiographie. Doctoral thesis, Giessen

Straub J, Pees M, Schumacher J *et al.* (2001) Doppler-echocardiography in birds. In: *Proceedings of the European Association of Avian Veterinarians*, pp. 92–94

13

Endoscopy, biopsy and endosurgery

Michael Lierz

Introduction

The first routine use of endoscopy in birds occurred in the late 1970s for sexing monomorphic species. In the past few years it has become important for diagnostic purposes (including biopsy) and more recently for endoscopy-guided surgery. The direct visualization of organs allows a direct assessment of the organs (size, shape, colour, surface, early alterations) and is therefore superior to radiography as a diagnostic tool for a certain organ. However, endoscopy does not replace radiography: the latter allows an overview of the whole body of the bird, while visible alterations can be differentiated by endoscopy. In addition, radiography gives valuable information about the risk of endoscopy (e.g. in ascites) and gives guidance as to the site of entry, depending on where a pathological alteration has been detected.

As endoscopy is an invasive technique and sudden movements of the bird must be avoided to prevent tissue trauma from the tip of the endoscope, the patient needs to be anaesthetized.

Using endoscopy as a diagnostic tool is a simple procedure; the difficulties lie more in interpretation of the images, especially with the many different bird species and their anatomical perculiarities. The veterinary surgeon should take every opportunity to practise the technique, beginning with dead or euthanased birds, followed by a necropsy to understand the results of endoscopic evaluation.

Technical requirements

The existence of air sacs in birds provides a unique opportunity to employ endoscopy as a diagnostic tool without the need for insufflation. Therefore the technical requirements are low. It is advisable to acquire a complete endoscopy set-up from one company, so that all parts are compatible.

Basic equipment should include:

- Curved small forceps
- Scalpel blade or small scissors
- Resorbable suture (1–1.5 metric (4/0–5/0))
- Haemostatic agents and vascular clips and suture
- Light source (xenon or halogen light)
- Light cable
- Endoscope
- Working channel
- Biopsy and grasping forceps.

Endoscope selection

In avian endoscopy, rigid endoscopes are the first choice as they are of use for most indications. Flexible endoscopes might be used in gastroscopy (crop, proventriculus, ventriculus) but these procedures can often also be done with larger (25–30 cm) rigid endoscopes. Endoscopes with several single lenses are cheaper but the image is of lower quality (especially contrast). Endoscopes with rod lenses (HOPKINS) are more expensive but of better quality and are recommended. Equipment from different manufacturers should be compared so that the best quality (border sharpness, depth of focus) can be selected.

Specifications

- Diameter and length:
  - Diameter 1.9 mm: smallest with acceptable image
  - Diameter 2.7 mm: best compromise between excellent image and small diameter for small patients, useful for most indications in avian practice (recommended)
  - Diameter 4 mm: excellent image, especially for photo-documentation; superior for larger patients (Figure 13.1).
- Length: variable, not less than 13 cm; 19 cm is standard and recommended.
- For passerine birds: 1.2 mm semi-rigid endoscopes.
- Viewing angle:
  - 0 degrees: straightforward, similar view if turning around its optical axes, superior for photo-documentation

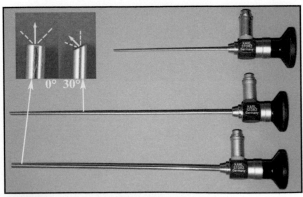

13.1 Different endoscopes, top to bottom: 1.9 mm, 2.7 mm, 4 mm diameter. The inset shows 0 and 30 degrees viewing angles. (© Michael Lierz)

– 30 degrees forward oblique telescope, allows visualization of a larger area by rotating the endoscope around its own optical axes (recommended as first choice).

Biopsy forceps:

- Flexible forceps matching selected working channel.
- 1.8 mm diameter.
- Elliptical mouth: grasps deeper into tissue.
- Round mouth: not as deep as elliptical mouth (recommended).
- Flexible grasping forceps for granuloma and foreign body removal.

Accessories:

- 22 gauge flexible infusion–aspiration needle, with Teflon cover for puncturing of cysts or direct application of medication (Figure 13.2).
- Photo-documentation including videos:
  - Essential for forensic cases
  - Useful to show results to bird owner.
- Equipment for endoscopy-guided surgery (Figure 13.3a).
- Mobile endoscopy unit including light source, camera, monitor and digital storage system in one unit, very useful for home visits.
- Diode laser for endoscopy-guided procedures.
- HF-electosurgery unit for endoscopic use.
- Fixation plate for birds, for correct positioning of the patient (Figure 13.3b).

Cameras: Generally the use of a camera and monitor system is vital for endoscopy-guided surgeries. The direct view through the endoscope is adequate for routine use in small animal practice to evaluate pathological alterations in the patient. However, images of alterations of the gonads when sexing a bird are regularly requested by clients (especially if the bird is for sale) and for such purposes a commercial digital camera can be used, though professional systems are of great advantage.

Trolleys: The motivation to organize equipment for a short endoscope is often low. Having all the equipment ready for use on a trolley is invaluable: the equipment can be removed easily from the surgical theatre (which helps to protect the equipment) and all the components can be managed with a single electrical switch. However, these trolleys are expensive and are not essential for the practice.

Care of equipment
Endoscopes are very sensitive to bending and torsion. They should only be used within a working channel.

Cleaning and disinfection
The manufacturer's recommendations should be followed.

- Heat sterilization is not advisable, even if recommended by the manufacturer; it may lower the lifetime of the endoscope (heat expansion and retraction of lenses may loosen them).

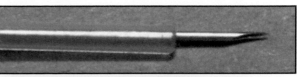

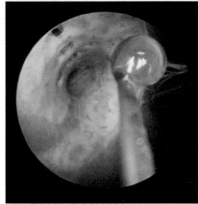

13.2

A Teflon tube with a flexible 22 gauge needle makes the precise endoscopic application of medicines and the performance of aspiration biopsy (e.g. cysts) easily possible.
(© Michael Lierz)

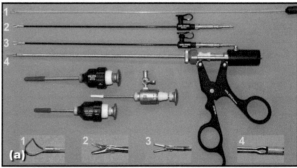

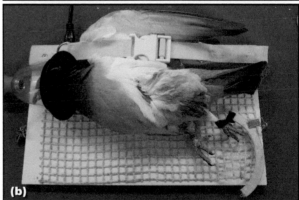

13.3 **(a)** Basic set of equipment for endoscopy-guided surgery in birds, connectable to a radiosurgery unit. 1 = monopolar sling; 2 = monopolar scissors; 3 = monopolar grasping forceps; 4 = bipolar coagulation forceps. **(b)** Fixation plate for birds, specially designed for endoscopic procedures. (© Michael Lierz)

- Gas sterilization is uncommon, as it is large scale.
- Disinfection bath:
  - Disinfectant and duration of bath according to manufacturer's recommendations
  - Clean before (e.g. blood, tissue material)
  - No permanent storage of endoscopes within the bath: will lead to precipitate on the lens (milky picture) and may decrease flexibility of forceps and scissors.
- Rinse equipment with sterile water after disinfection bath (to avoid irritation in next use).
- Dry with sterile towel or alcohol.

Preparation and contraindications

Pre-endoscopic fasting is required as the bird is anaesthetized and because the gut should be emptied to allow a better visualization of the abdominal cavity. Preoperative preparation, especially if dealing with sick or traumatized birds, is similar to that required for other surgical techniques.

Obesity may reduce the view in the body cavity, which can increase the risk of organ damage by the endoscope or other inserted equipment. In moulting birds removal of growing feathers can lead to bleeding, which can also reduce the view. The most important contraindication to laparoscopy is ascites. Insertion of the endoscope may allow the abdominal fluid to enter the respiratory tract, thus drowning the bird.

Laparoscopy

The choice of endoscopic approach to the body cavity depends on the diagnostic goal. For sexing and in routine diagnostic cases the approach is from the left side, as in most birds females have only a left ovary. A right-sided approach is chosen if alterations on that side are suspected from radiography. However, it is highly recommended that all organs within the body cavity should be assessed, as unsuspected lesions can be present. The approach can be between the last two ribs or, preferably (as more flexible for exploration of the whole cavity), caudal to the last rib.

1. The bird is placed in lateral recumbency on its right side, with the wings extended dorsocranially. The left leg may be pulled either cranially or caudally.

2. To allow surgical preparation and disinfection, a few feathers over the intended incision area are plucked.

3. For orientation, an area with the last rib as cranial border, the iliotibialis muscle as caudal border and the spine as dorsal border is visible (Figure 13.4a). The incision is made in the middle of this area, starting 0.5 cm ventral to the acetabulum. The iliotibialis muscle, which can mask the correct approach, is pushed caudally with the forceps or a trocar (Figure 13.7b) to visualize the fascia. By increasing the pressure with the forceps or trocar the abdominal wall and the underlying air sac are penetrated, accompanied by a 'pop' when penetration is complete. The procedure is similar if the approach between the last two ribs has been chosen. Instead of the fascia, the intercostal muscle is penetrated.

4. In either method, the preferred caudal thoracic air sac is reached (Figure 13.4c). In some cases this air sac is missed and the abdominal (Figure 13.4d) or cranial thoracic air sac is penetrated. Penetration of fascia and air sac must be performed vertical to the body wall, with a cranioventral orientation of the forceps, as a dorsal orientation might damage the kidney and lead to fatal bleeding. The necessity for a blunt instrument cannot be overemphasized, since it is difficult to control the exact level of penetration during this 'popping through' step, and serious damage with accompanying haemorrhage can occur if a sharp trocar or other pointed instrument is used.

5. After insertion, the endoscope is held at its tip by thumb and forefinger, with the ball of the thumb on the bird or the table (Figure 13.5). This

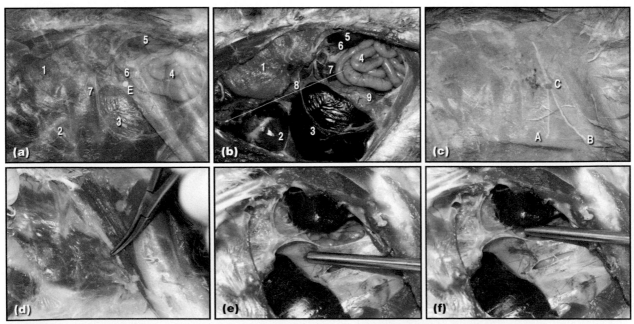

13.4 Laparoscopy. **(a)** Internal organs to be evaluated through the entrance (E). 1= lung, 2 = heart, 3 = liver, 4 = intestine, 5 = kidney, 6 = spleen, 7 = proventriculus. **(b)** The arrow shows the direction of the endoscope for full exploration of the body cavity. 1 = lung, 2 = heart: 3 = liver, 4 = intestine, 5 = kidney, 6 = gonads and adrenal gland, 7 = spleen, 8 = proventriculus, 9 = ventriculus. **(c)** Triangulation from behind the last rib (A) with the cranial border of the iliotibialis muscle (B), identifies the site of entry into the body cavity (C). **(d)** The iliotibialis muscle is pushed caudally using curved forceps. Increasing the pressure punctures the body wall and either **(e)** the caudal thoracic air sac or **(f)** the abdominal air sac is entered. (© Michael Lierz)

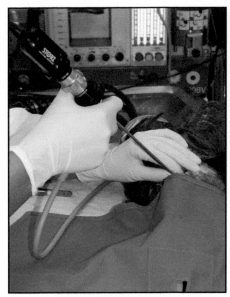

13.5

Correct handling of the endoscope. The hand should be in contact with the bird. (© Michael Lierz)

In larger birds, or those with opaque air sacs, the abdominal air sac may need to be punctured in order to obtain a clear view of the triangle involving the adrenal gland, the gonad and the cranial division of the kidney.

7. Cranial to this triangle, the caudal aspect of the left lung will be visible. Necessary further punctures of air sacs do not harm the bird as they quickly self-close. Ventrally, the kidney, the ureter, and uterus or ductus deferens are visible. Further ventrally, intestinal loops can be seen. Turning the view cranioventrally, the proventriculus/ventriculus, liver and in some cases spleen are visible (Figure 13.6b). Pulling the endoscope back into the caudal thoracic air sac, the air sac, liver, proventriculus and the lung opening to the air sac can be detected (Figure 13.7a). Depending on the bird's size, this lung entrance allows a retrograde scoping of the lung, including smaller bronchi (Figure 13.7b,c).

8. Slowly pushing the endoscope cranially, the cranial thoracic air sac is entered and further parts of the lung and liver, along with the beating heart, are visible (Figure 13.8a). With practice, the endoscope can be slowly guided further cranially towards the heart base (Figure 13.8b). As well as the main vessels, the brachial plexus can be investigated (Figure 13.8c).

allows permanent contact with the bird and prevents an uncontrolled deeper insertion of the endoscope or instruments (causing potentially severe tissue damage) in case of bird movement.

6. First, the caudal thoracic and abdominal air sacs are visible. In small birds with clear air sacs, the gonads may be visualized without further advancement of the endoscope (Figure 13.6a).

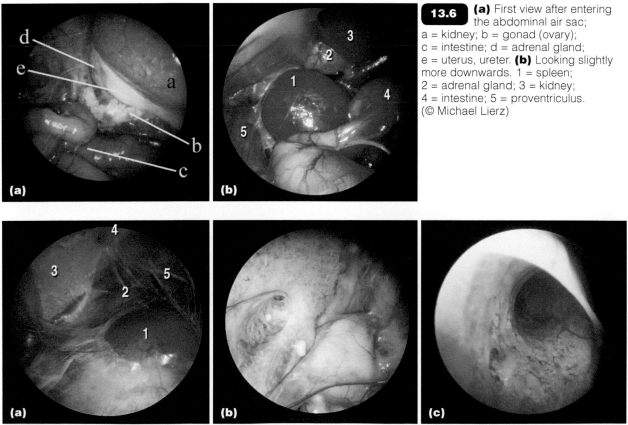

13.6 **(a)** First view after entering the abdominal air sac; a = kidney; b = gonad (ovary); c = intestine; d = adrenal gland; e = uterus, ureter. **(b)** Looking slightly more downwards. 1 = spleen; 2 = adrenal gland; 3 = kidney; 4 = intestine; 5 = proventriculus. (© Michael Lierz)

13.7 **(a)** First view after entering the caudal thoracic air sac. 1 = liver; 2 = proventriculus; 3 = lung; 4 = retrograde entrance to the lung; 5 = hole in air sac, made by surgeon to enter the abdominal air sac. **(b,c)** The connection between the caudal thoracic air sac and lung allows a retrograde internal exploration of the lung, evaluating the honeycomb structure. Such a view is not possible performing a tracheobronchoscopy. (© Michael Lierz)

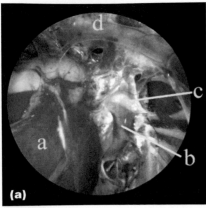 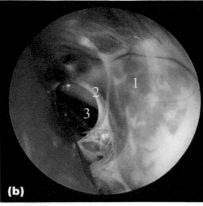 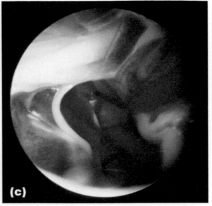

13.8 **(a)** Overview after turning the endoscope cranially. a = liver; b = heart; c = heart fat; d = lung. **(b)** Pushing the endoscope further cranially. 1 = heart; 2 = left brachiocephalic trunk; 3 = space for pushing the scope further cranial to the thyroid gland. **(c)** Passing the heart to evaluate the bird further cranially, the brachial plexus can be seen. (© Michael Lierz)

9. Guiding the endoscope over the heart base even more cranially, the trachea can be seen. Following the trachea, the thyroid glands are visible (Figure 13.9).
10. After endoscopy, the skin is closed using one or two single knots or tissue glue.

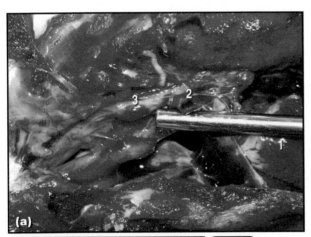

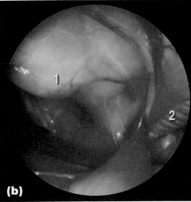

13.9

(a) Direction of the endoscope to evaluate the thyroid gland; 1 = heart, 2 = left brachiocephalic artery, 3 = thyroid gland. **(b)** The same view; 1 = thyroid gland, 2 = trachea. (© Michael Lierz)

Direct liver approach
The bird is positioned in dorsal recumbency. The abdominal wall is entered through the ventral midline. A layer of fat may be present just under the skin in the area directly caudal to the caudal aspect of the sternum. A loop of duodenum with the lobe of pancreas (Figure 13.10) is located above (ventral to) the liver.

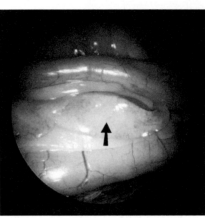

13.10

Within the duodenal loop, the pancreas (arrowed) is visible. (© Michael Lierz)

Gonads and sexing
DNA methods allow non-invasive sexing of many monomorphic avian species but, other than the determination of gender, no additional information is achieved using this technique. Using endoscopy it is possible to investigate all organs, which is of importance especially during pre-purchase examinations. In addition it is possible to assess gonad activity and functionality (physiological breeding performance). When dealing with rare avian species the result is usually more reliable than using DNA methods, since accidental or deliberate manipulation by dealers or owners (e.g. sending a feather from a different bird, contamination by feather dust of a different bird) are possible using DNA methods.

Gonads are visible ventrally at the cranial pole of the kidney (see Figure 13.6). In most avian species only the left ovary is present, but in some juvenile females the rudimentary right ovary can still be seen. In close contact to the ureter, the ductus deferens or the uterus is visible. Gonad size varies according the bird's breeding status and allows judgement about previous breeding (laying) activities. The size of the testes can increase by several times during the breeding season in some species (especially pigeons and passerine birds). The physiological appearance of the gonads varies enormously between species and it is important to know the particular species prior to performing the procedure. In questionable cases of the sex or presumed abnormalities, the right body side can be viewed for clarification.

Females

From the ovary a suspensory ligament crosses the cranial pole of the kidney towards the dorsal body wall. This ligament is the main evidence for sexing, as in juvenile birds (chicks) the ovaries are difficult to detect (Figure 13.11a). This ligament must be carefully assessed when examining breeding birds, as in case of damage or absence the breeding performance of the bird is questionable. Removal of this ligament is a procedure for sterilization in female birds. The left ovary may be flat with a cobblestone appearance in birds with inactive ovaries, or may appear as a cluster of grapes with follicular development. The ovary is generally of yellowish-white colour. Sometimes pigmentation occurs (Figure 13.11b). Inflammation of follicles may be present, reducing the bird's reproductive performance (Figure 13.11c).

Males

In males the above-described ligament is absent (Figure 13.12a). The paired white (in some species pigmented) testes are usually oval (Figure 13.12b) with two or three vessels crossing the surface. In birds with clear air sacs, both testes may be visualized from the left lateral approach. In rare cases (hermaphrodites) both ovary and testis are visible (Figure 13.12c). Testicular biopsy is a very valuable tool for the investigation of infertility in breeding birds.

Tracheobronchoscopy

The anaesthetized bird is placed in a standing position with the neck extended (which is most important). For a very short procedure the time between the 'cut-off' of the anaesthesia and waking of the bird is long enough for evaluation. For longer procedures, air-sac perfusion anaesthesia should be chosen (see Chapter 10). The diameter of the endoscope should be a maximum of two-thirds of the tracheal diameter, allowing the bird to breathe or air to pass in case of perfusion anaesthesia.

After placement of a beak speculum (to prevent damage to the endoscope) the tongue is pulled cranially and the endoscope enters the larynx (Figure 13.13). The endoscope can then be advanced gently from the larynx into the trachea up to the bifurcation.

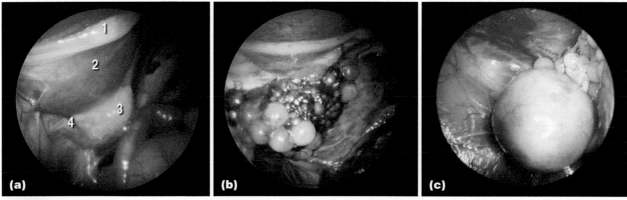

13.11 Sex determination in females. **(a)** In juvenile females the suspensory ligament (1) of the ovary is already visible (2 = kidney; 3 = ovary; 4 = adrenal gland). The gonads are sometimes very difficult to distinguish as they are very small in juvenile birds. **(b)** In some species the ovary may be pigmented. **(c)** A swollen discoloured follicle is a sign of folliculitis. (© Michael Lierz)

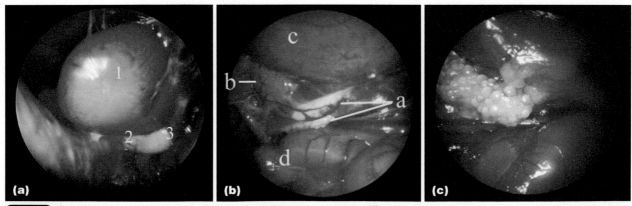

13.12 Sex determination in males. **(a)** Although the gonad is very difficult to assess in juveniles, the missing suspensory ligament indicates a male bird (unless it has been removed for sterilization). 1 = kidney; 2 = adrenal gland; 3 = juvenile testis. **(b)** Sometimes both testes (a) are visible (b = adrenal gland; c = kidney; d = intestine). **(c)** In very rare cases of hermaphroditism, both testis and ovary are visible. (© Michael Lierz)

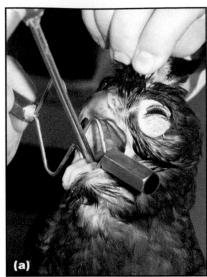

13.13

Tracheoscopy.
(a) Correct positioning, extending the neck and using a beak speculum.
(b) The opening of the trachea is located at the base of the tongue.
(© Michael Lierz)

Gastroscopy

Gastroscopy allows evaluation of the oesophagus, crop and proventriculus. Prior to gastroscopy, a fasting period is important to prevent a reduced view due to food. As the oesophagus, crop and proventriculus are hollow organs, expansion is necessary for a detailed investigation.

The bird is positioned in ventral recumbency, with the head lower than the body (Figure 13.14). In addition it is recommended that breathing and

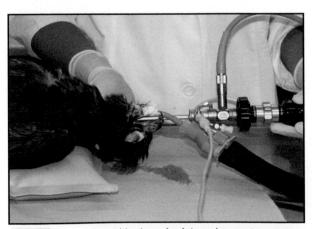

13.14 Correct positioning of a falcon for gastroscopy. Intubation and a head position lower than the body avoids aspiration of fluid. (© Michael Lierz)

Expansion

Expansion can be performed using insufflation with air or fluids (water, saline). As an air-insufflation pump is expensive, water pressure due to a gradient, or cheaper aquarium pumps can be used. Mucosal structures float when fluids are used, which makes them better assessable; water also allows removal of food or mucus.

A working channel with two taps, one as a water inlet and the other as an outlet, is needed. In addition a third channel for biopsy or grasping forceps is recommended.

The water inlet tap is attached to a normal infusion tube, which is connected to an infusion bottle at a higher level. A second infusion tube is connected to the water outlet, ending in a collecting bin. The two taps are used to regulate the amount of water within the digestive system, expanding the organ for examination. To avoid aspiration, the water should not be rinsed out of the oral cavity. It is vital that the water is warmed, as cold water leads quickly to hypothermia.

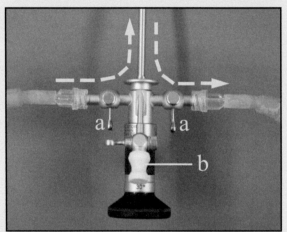

Endoscope within a working channel for fluid expansion of hollow organs. a = taps; b = working channel for additional instrument; arrows = fluid direction.

Air insufflation has some safety advantages but has disadvantages (no washing, etc.). In addition some anatomical structures (e.g. papillae) are only visible using water expansion.

anaesthesia should be controlled via an endotracheal tube. The endoscope is inserted into the oesophagus and gently advanced under visual control.

Gastroscopy can also be performed using a flexible gastroscope but requires additional equipment, which is usually not necessary for most avian patients. In larger birds a long gastroscope might be of advantage, but it is also possible to introduce the rigid endoscope via an ingluviotomy.

As gastroscopy is perfomed using a working channel, mucosal biopsy can easily be performed and is of great diagnostic value. Using grasping forceps or sling cages, removal of foreign bodies is also possible.

Cloacoscopy

The bird is placed in dorsal recumbency. Expansion is similar to gastroscopy (see above). In addition to the cloaca, the ureter, rectum and (in sexually active females) uterus can be examined. Faeces and urine are always present and need to be removed for a more detailed examination. The presence of urine leads to ostia of the ureter (Figure 13.15). Fresh blood within the faeces can be investigated, as it may originate from the cloaca, intestine, ureters or uterus.

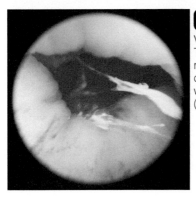

13.15 View into the cloaca. The white stripes represent the passing of urine within the washing fluid. (© Michael Lierz)

Endoscopy-guided biopsy

Endoscopy-guided biopsy allows sampling of organs under direct visualization. Samples can be taken from altered areas; and complications, such as bleeding, are directly visible. During a routine endoscopic procedure, preparations should always be made for biopsy as unexpected abnormalities are common (Lierz *et al.*, 1998). Biopsy is very important in the early diagnosis of disease and the decision is often made too late.

In general, biopsy of the lung, liver, kidney, spleen, gonads, proventriculus, ventriculus, thyroid gland and mucosal membranes of oesophagus, crop and cloaca is possible using biopsy forceps within a working channel. Indications for biopsy are given in Figure 13.16.

With biopsy of hollow organs with a thin wall (oesophagus, crop, proventriculus, cloaca), there is increased risk of perforating the organ; therefore the procedure should be reserved for the advanced endoscopist.

Aspiration biopsy is possible using a long flexible needle with a Teflon cover (see Figure 13.2). Cyst puncture and lavage sampling are best done using this needle.

Where there is a general alteration of an organ the biopsy sample should be taken from its border (e.g. liver, Figure 13.17a), as there are fewer vessels. For an air sac biopsy, the entrance hole of the endoscope is the preferred area (Fig. 13.17b). Where there are focal alterations these should be sampled.

Finally it must be considered that endoscopic procedures, in particular tissue biopsy, lead to changes in certain blood values. Increases in urea, uric acid, GLDH, AST and ALT have been measured after liver biopsy (Lierz *et al.*, 1998). Therefore blood sampling must be performed before endoscopy and biopsy.

Organ	Indications
Kidney	Polyuria, polydipsia. Increased blood levels of uric acid, potassium. Kidney swellings and increased density on radiograph. Visible alterations in colour, shape, surface during endoscopy
Liver	Increased blood levels of bile acids, cholinesterase, and combination of AST, ALT, GLDH (without CK increase). Enlargement of liver shadow on radiograph. Liver swelling, colour changes, alterations during endoscopy
Air sac	Milky appearance or coatings during endoscopy
Lung	Pathological appearance during endoscopy. Increased density in lung shadow on radiograph
Spleen	Suspected systemic infections, especially *Chlamydophila*. Spleen enlargement on radiography. Spleen enlargement or colour changes during endoscopy
Gonads (especially testes)	Infertile clutches. Assessment of a breeding bird for sale. Enlargement of testes in 'off breeding' seasons. Changes in colour or shape during endoscopy
Oesophagus, crop, proventriculus	PDD diagnosis. Coatings or pathological changes on mucosa during endoscopy
Thyroid gland	Suspected hypothyroidism

13.16 A selection of indications for tissue biopsy.

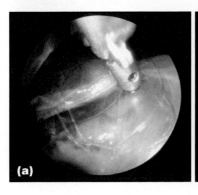
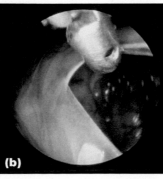

(a)   (b)

13.17 Biopsy sites. **(a)** In the case of a diffuse alteration of the liver, the sample is taken from its border. **(b)** In the case of a diffuse alteration of the air sac, the sample is taken from the entrance hole for the endoscope. (© Michael Lierz)

Endoscopic findings

Basically, all body entrances can be used for endoscopic evaluation and sampling using flexible forceps and a working channel.

Figure 13.18 summarizes normal appearance and common abnormalities of body organs viewed by endoscopy.

Organ and physiological appearance	Alteration	Common causes
Air sac Clear and transparent, just a few vessels and sometimes little fatty infiltrates (Figure 13.19a) Pathognomonic images are rare: alterations should be investigated by biopsy	Increased vascularity (Figure 13.19b), thickening of air sac wall	Mild inflammation, early infection or environmental (smoke, spray)
	Granulomas (Figure 13.19c), foreign material (e.g. pus) (Figure 13.19d)	Aspergillosis, foreign bodies, bacterial infection
Lung Pink-reddish colour, prominent structure Bronchi can be entered through caudal thoracic air sac	Blur of structures, colour changes (yellow), sometimes foreign material (Figure 13.20)	Pneumonia, gout
	Haemorrhages	Trauma
	Focal black spots	Anthracosis (birds from cities, smoking owners)
Trachea, bronchi, thyroid glands Whites tubes with complete tracheal rings. Thyroid glands: lens-shaped, light red, attached to trachea near the syrinx (see Figure 13.9)	Glassy colour of thyroid glands	Hypothyrodism (biopsy)
Kidney and sacral plexus Three parts, brown-red-orange colour, star-shaped structure on surface; adrenal gland and gonad at cranial pole, ventrally attached ureter and uterus (deferent duct). With a 30 degree endoscope the sacral plexus (ischiadic nerve) is detectable dorsal to the kidney (lameness diagnostics) (Figure 13.21a). Kidney biopsy often rewarding	Star-shaped structure not visible (kidney swelling) (Figure 13.21b)	General disease or kidney problem (biopsy)
	Yellow to white foci on surface	Uric acid: gout or dehydration
	Yellow colour (Figure 13.21c)	Obesity
	Pale colour	Anaemia
	Single yellow–white spots	Abscesses, neoplasia, cysts
Gonads and sexing See text and Figures 13.11 and 13.12		
Adrenal gland Slightly cranial to gonads, usually yellow and small (Figure 13.12b). May vary in size, colour and shape; might be confused with gonads or obscured by active gonads	Increase in size and/or vascularization	Stress or associated with disease
Proventriculus Elongated usually white organ, dorsal to liver with smooth surface (see Figures 13.6 and 13.7)	Focal haemorrhages	Ulceration, foreign bodies
Ventriculus Not visible in all routine examinations, massive muscular structure. In raptors, much thinner compared with passerines and pigeons	Focal haemorrhages	Ulceration, foreign bodies
Intestine Tube-like structure, smooth surface with many vessels, colour depends on ingesta, usually grey	White foci, foreign material (pus) (Figure 13.22)	Endoparasites, bacterial granulomas (*E. coli*), peritonitis
	Visible particles of ingesta (thin wall)	Ulcerative enteritis (*Clostridium perfringens*)
Pancreas Within the duodenal loop, white-yellow colour, homogenous structure (see Figure 13.10)	Colour changes, glassy appearance, uneven surface (biopsy), petechiae	Pancreatitis, neoplasia, PMV, avian influenza
Liver Uniform brown-red colour. Liver border sharp (Figure 13.23a) Liver is central organ of metabolism, liver biopsies very rewarding, even without visible alterations (changes in liver blood values as indication)	Rounded liver border (Figure 13.23b)	Generalized disease, infections, fatty liver
	Uniform yellow colour	Fatty liver
	Swollen, yellow-grey, mealy appearance	Amyloidosis
	Red areas (Figure 13.23c)	Haemorrhages (trauma), siderosis
	Multiple white foci (Figure 13.23d)	Necrosis (hollow) (herpesvirus, salmonellosis), abscesses (prominent) (tuberculosis, other bacteria), neoplasia
	Coating of liver capsule	Often in conjunction with air sac coatings (bacterial, fungal, parasitic infections)

13.18 Organ evaluation: normal appearance, common alterations and possible reasons. (continues) ▶

Organ and physiological appearance	Alteration	Common causes
Spleen Reddish-purple-brown (see Figure 13.6), sometimes speckled. Dorsal to proventriculus, ventral to kidney, often in between intestinal loops. Always consider spleen biopsy	Increased size (Figure 13.24)	Immune response (disease, check for *Chlamydophila*)
	Yellow colour	Obesity, fatty spleen
	White foci	Necrosis (e.g. herpesvirus) Granulomas (tuberculosis)
Heart and pericardium Pericardium transparent, fat at heart base and tip. Main heart vessels as thick white tubes. Next to heart: brachial plexus (fine yellow-white cross-stripe net shape) (see Figure 13.8)	Milky pericardium	Pericarditis, pericardial effusion (drain with 22 gauge flexible needle)
	Missing heart fat	Starvation, chronic disease, guarded prognosis
Tracheobronchoscopy – trachea Mucus light red (pink), shiny, visible closed tracheal rings, no exudates (Figure 13.25a)	Swollen red mucosa, hidden tracheal rings	Tracheitis (viral, bacterial, fungal, parasitic)
	Exudates, worms	Bacterial or parasitic infection
	Granulomas (especially at syrinx), foreign bodies (Figure 13.25b)	Fungal or bacterial infection, foreign bodies
	Strictures, tumours	
Gastroscopy – oesophagus, crop, proventriculus Surface varies with species. Usually oesophagus smooth (Figure 13.26), crop with furrows and proventriculus with papillae. Mucosa homogenous light red-pink.	Plaques, haemorrhages, focal dark red areas	Trauma, ulcerations, irritations due to foreign bodies, infections
	Yellow coating	Trichomoniasis, wet pox, candidiasis, hypovitaminosis A
	Yellow-white spots	Trichomoniasis, capillariosis
Cloacoscopy – cloaca Divided into three parts, mucous membrane light red (pink), in some species with papillae (see Figure 13.15)	Reddening of mucosa	Irritation, inflammation, infection
	Cauliflower appearance	Papillomatosis, neoplasia

13.18 (continued) Organ evaluation: normal appearance, common alterations and possible reasons.

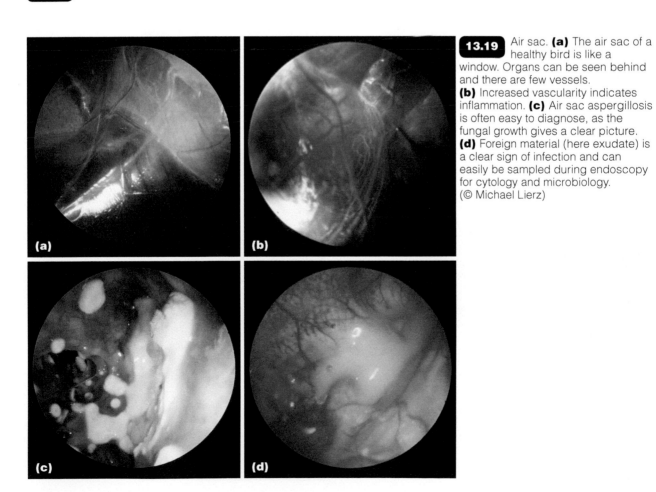

13.19 Air sac. **(a)** The air sac of a healthy bird is like a window. Organs can be seen behind and there are few vessels. **(b)** Increased vascularity indicates inflammation. **(c)** Air sac aspergillosis is often easy to diagnose, as the fungal growth gives a clear picture. **(d)** Foreign material (here exudate) is a clear sign of infection and can easily be sampled during endoscopy for cytology and microbiology. (© Michael Lierz)

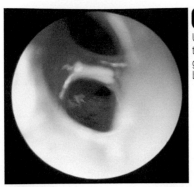

13.20
Urate crystals within the lung indicate gout. (© Michael Lierz)

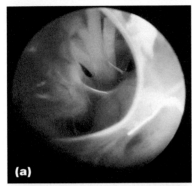
(a)

13.21
Kidney and sacral plexus. **(a)** Above the kidney the sacral plexus is visible. A 30 degree endoscope makes this evaluation much easier. **(b)** Loss of structure of the kidney indicates severe swelling. **(c)** Yellow-white foci within the kidney may be gout but may also be a sign of exsicosis (reversible deposits of urate within the tubuli). If the cause is gout, the foci persist following fluid therapy. (© Michael Lierz)

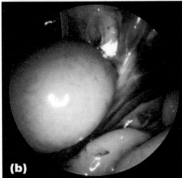
(b)

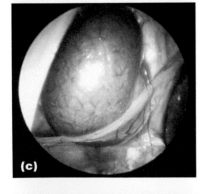
(c)

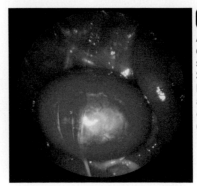

13.22
Exudate between the intestinal loops is often a sign of peritonitis or may be egg material (egg peritonitis). (© Michael Lierz)

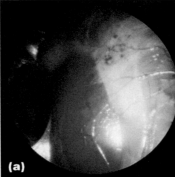
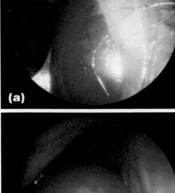
(a)

13.23
Liver. **(a)** Normal appearance, with homogenous brown-red colour and a sharp liver border. **(b)** A rounded liver border represents swelling and is a strong indication for biopsy. **(c)** Colour change is always pathological. Here, haemosiderosis is seen. **(d)** Multiple white foci are necrosis or granulomas/ tubercles. Differentials are *E. coli*, salmonellosis, tuberculosis or herpesvirus infection. (© Michael Lierz)

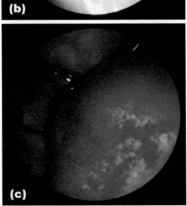
(b)

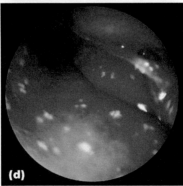
(c)

(d)

13.24
A swollen spleen is often seen with systemic infections. Spleen biopsy may be of value if the agent cannot be detected elsewhere. (© Michael Lierz)

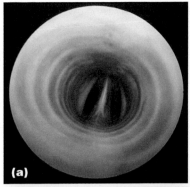

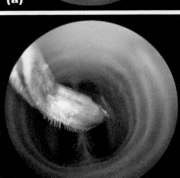

13.25

Trachea. **(a)** Normal appearance of the trachea and bifurcation. The complete tracheal rings are clearly visible. **(b)** A foreign body (awn) in the trachea of a falcon after transportation on straw. As it had just happened, the tracheal mucosa shows only a slight reaction. (© Michael Lierz)

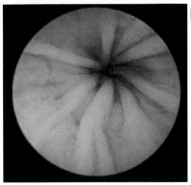

13.26

The oesophagus of a healthy falcon. (© Michael Lierz)

Complications during and after endoscopy

Haemorrhage is the main complication during endoscopy. In particular the kidney can be damaged during penetration of the air sac at the beginning of a laparoscopy. Perforations of the proventriculus and lethal peritonitis might occur. If there is major haemorrhage, attempts should be made to halt the bleeding using electrocoagulation, diode laser (endoscopy-guided) or sterile sticks of cotton wool. In addition the bird should be placed at an angle of 45 degrees with the head lifted to prevent blood entering the lungs and to allow the blood to drain into the caudal air sacs.

After endoscopy, subcutaneous emphysema might occur rarely in cases of excessive air sac damage. Closure of these defects is pointless. The emphysema is drained regularly until the defect closes itself.

In cases of insufficient cleaning or sterilization of equipment, internal granulomas or abscesses can occur, and the risk of transmitting disease increases. Birds from different sources should therefore not be examined one after another on the same day, as sufficient sterilization of equipment cannot be guaranteed. For this reason, regular surgical 'sexing' sessions organized by breeder clubs are not recommended.

Surgical endoscopic procedures

Endoscopy-guided surgery is a very recent innovation in avian medicine (Hernandez-Divers, 2005; Lierz and Hafez, 2004, 2005). The results are promising, as it represents a lower impact on the bird compared with a laparotomy.

There are several different techniques.

- Using a single-entry technique, a single instrument is directed through a working channel into the visual field of the endoscope. The instrument cannot be manipulated independently of the endoscope.
- Using a double-entry technique, an additional cannula with trocar (as a channel for an instrument) is placed, enabling the surgeon to work with two different instruments.
- Using triple-entry techniques, two cannulae are placed in addition to the centrally placed endoscope. The approaches to the avian coelom are chosen according to the procedure performed.

To start with, endoscopy-guided surgery requires a profound knowledge of the internal anatomy of the bird and advanced skills in performing laparotomic and laparoscopic procedures. Once familiar with endoscopy in birds, the next step of performing such surgeries is very near.

Indications
Endoscopy-guided obliteration of air sac granulomas or papillomas using electrocauterization or laser can be performed. In particular, endoscopy-guided diode lasers have been used successfully to obliterate granulomas within the trachea or air sac in emergencies to restore respiratory function. Additional procedures include tumour resection as well as sterilization and castration (Lierz and Hafez, 2005).

Instrumentation
The development of 2 mm and 3 mm human paediatric laparoscopy equipment has accelerated the development of endosurgery in birds. A variety of instruments are available and necessary:

- 2–3 mm dissection forceps, scissors, grasping forceps (in which parts should be monopolar and therefore connectable to the radiosurgery unit)
- Bipolar forceps and monopolar sling (essential)
- Cannulae (2.5 mm or 3.5 mm, according to instrument size) with trocars, for introducing instruments into the surgical field. After insertion the trocar is removed, leaving the cannula in place. The material of such a unit is stainless steel, plastic or graphite
- (For advanced surgeons) palpation probes, needle holders and knot tiers.

The main problem with endosurgery is the maintenance of haemostasis. Therefore a radiosurgery unit for connection to the endosurgical instruments is vital. Laser units can be used but they are not routinely available in veterinary practice.

Surgical procedure

Preparation for endosurgery (single- or double-entry technique) is similar to a routine endoscopic examination, pulling the left pelvic limb caudally. For sterilization the approach is from the left side (female birds) or from both sides (male birds). The additional cannula using the double-entry technique is placed cranioventral to the endoscope between the last two ribs (Figure 13.27). Using the triple-entry technique the same approaches can be used, placing the second trocar ventrocaudal to the endoscope (Figure 13.28). Because of the advantageous angle to the gonad and the larger surgical field, the following approach (which can also be used for the other techniques described above) may be of advantage.

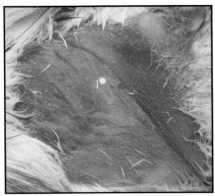

13.27
Double-entry technique for minimal invasive surgery in birds: sites for (1) additional working channel for instruments and (2) entrance of the endoscope. (© Michael Lierz)

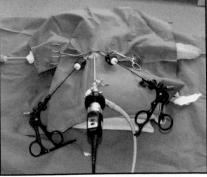

13.28
Triple-entry technique for minimal invasive surgery in birds: sites for (1) entrance of the endoscope and (2) two additional working channels for instruments. (© Michael Lierz)

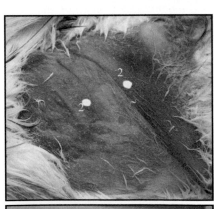

1. Placing the bird as described above, the pelvic limb is pulled cranially.
2. Ventral to the medial flexor cruris muscle, the endoscope is introduced caudal to the last rib.
3. One cannula is inserted caudal to the endoscope through the external oblique abdominal muscle just caudal to the mid-point of the pubis.
4. This double-entry technique can be extended by introducing a second cannula cranial to the endoscope into the last or second-last intercostal space (Figure 13.29).

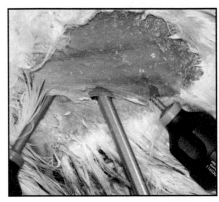

13.29
Triple-entry technique for minimal invasive surgery by pushing the leg cranially and entering the body cavity ventral to the leg muscles. (© Michael Lierz)

When using a multiple-entry technique it is very important to keep the approaches of the instrument ports and the endoscope as far apart from each other as possible to ensure the correct triangulation of the endoscope and instruments within the bird (Figure 13.30). Therefore the triple-entry technique is only possible in birds weighing more than 400 g. For sterilization and in most cases of castration the single- or double-entry technique is sufficient.

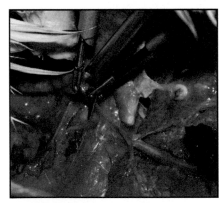

13.30
Correct triangulation of endoscope (middle) and instruments is vital for successful surgery. (© Michael Lierz)

The endoscopist controls the endoscope and the instrument when using the single- or double-entry technique. With a triple-entry technique the endoscope is placed on a sandbag or is handled by an assistant while the endoscopist controls both instruments. The radiosurgery or diode laser unit is activated by a foot-pedal.

Sterilization of female birds

The ovary is a very fragile organ and its endoscopic removal presents a high risk of lethal haemorrhage. In addition the total removal of all hormone-producing tissue is very difficult. Therefore female birds are sterilized rather than ovariectomized.

In very young females or in young raptors, the juvenile ovary can be vaporized using a diode laser (Figure 13.31). This procedure is not possible with larger ovaries as full tissue removal is not reliable.

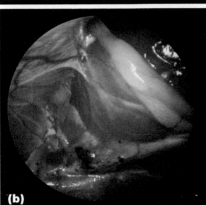

13.31

Female sterilization. **(a)** A diode laser can be used to vaporize the gonads (here ovary) in juvenile birds. **(b)** Cranial pole of the kidney of a female falcon 6 months after sterilization using a diode laser. Ovarian tissue is absent. (© Michael Lierz)

In juvenile birds, grasping forceps can be introduced through the endoscope's working channel (single-entry technique). The infundibulum is grasped and the oviduct removed from underlying tissue by gently pulling. In this way it is possible to remove almost the entire oviduct without much bleeding. Such females develop normally (including the ovary) and are hormonally active, as has been shown in cockatiels (Pye *et al.*, 2001). As an alternative the oviduct can be obliterated by monopolar or bipolar grasping forceps. In some cases it has been noticed that the oviduct fills with egg albumen during sexual activity and this might lead to problems. Therefore the complete removal of the oviduct is recommended.

In adult birds, the oviduct should be removed using a double- or triple-entry technique. The oviduct is fixed with grasping forceps and obliterated as far cranial as possible using mono- or bipolar grasping forceps through a second entry port. A second obliteration is performed slightly behind the first one. The oviduct is then cut between both obliterations using monopolar scissors. The same is performed at the most caudal part of the oviduct that can be reached.

Vasectomy

In juvenile birds, the deferent duct can be grasped and removed by pulling with grasping forceps through the endoscope's working channel. Using this method in Japanese quail (Jones and Redig, 2003), it was

demonstrated that the testes would develop normally and that the testosterone blood levels would increase with sexual maturity in the same way as in unsterilized males. In addition, the sexual behaviour of such males was unchanged.

As an alternative, the deferent duct can be obliterated by electrosurgery. In adult birds, endoscopy-guided sterilization is only possible using a double- or triple-entry technique. Grasping forceps are used to elevate the testis from the underlying tissue, which also elevates the deferent duct. Using a second entry port, scissors are introduced to cut the deferent duct (Figure 13.32). It is also recommended that at least 1 cm of the duct is removed, to reduce the chances of functionality being re-established if the two ends reunite (Figure 13.33).

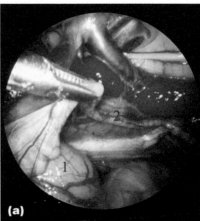

13.32

Sterilization of an adult male bird. **(a,b)** The deferent duct is lifted and cut with scissors. The procedure must be performed at two places to remove at least 1 cm of the duct to prevent reunion. **(c)** Remnants of the deferent duct 5 months after sterilization. (© Michael Lierz)

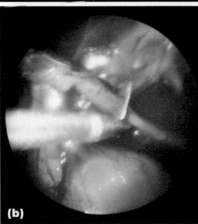

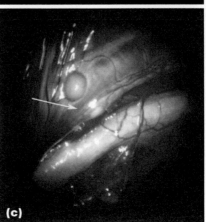

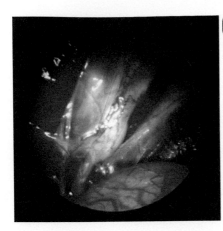

13.33
Reunion of the two ends of a deferent duct after it was cut, without having a section removed. (© Michael Lierz)

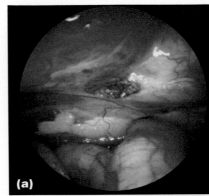

(a)

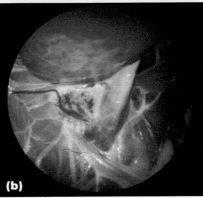

(b)

13.34
Castration of a juvenile male bird. **(a)** Immediately after vaporization of the testis using a diode laser. **(b)** 6 months later. Testicular tissue is no longer visible. (© Michael Lierz)

Castration

The double- or triple-entry technique is used for castration. Especially in adult birds, the triple-entry technique is of advantage as it allows a better view into the surgical field. Grasping forceps are used to elevate the testis from the kidney. The mesorchium can be cut using monopolar coagulation scissors. Then the testis can be removed.

In adult birds, the blood supply to the testis is increased, necessitating additional obliteration of the blood vessels by monopolar or bipolar coagulation forceps. The risk of lethal haemorrhage is very high in male birds during sexual activity and therefore castration must be avoided during that time.

In juvenile birds, the testis can be grasped and removed with a radiosurgical sling, obliterating the vessels when closing the sling. In juvenile raptors, the testis is very small and closely attached to the adrenal gland and kidney vessel (see Figure 13.12a). In such cases removal of the testis is impossible. Using a diode laser, both testes can be vaporized successfully with only a low risk (Figure 13.34).

Risks

As with diagnostic endoscopy, there is a much greater risk of lethal haemorrhage during endosurgery. Therefore sterilization and castration of juvenile birds is always preferable to surgery in mature birds, as the blood supply to the genital tract is much less. On the other hand, the structures of the genital tract are sometimes difficult to distinguish from other tissues (adrenal gland, kidney, ureter, blood vessels) or are attached to other organs (depending on the species), leading to further difficulties. The procedure requires more experience and training. When using coagulation or laser techniques it is vital to avoid any damage to underlying tissue, especially to the kidney and ureter.

References and further reading

Baileys RE (1953) Surgery for sexing and observing gonad condition in birds. *Auk* **70**, 497–500

Birkhead TR and Pellatt JE (1989) Vasectomy in small passerine birds. *Veterinary Record* **125**, 646

Hernandez-Divers SJ (2005) Minimally invasive endoscopic surgery of birds. *Journal of Avian Medicine and Surgery* **19**, 107–120

Hochleithner M (1997) Endoscopy. In: *Avian Medicine and Surgery*, ed. RB Altman *et al.*, pp. 800–805. WB Saunders, Philadelphia

Jones R and Redig PT (2003) Endoscopy guided vasectomy in the immature Japanese quail (*Coturnix coturnix japonica*). In: *Proceedings of the 7th Conference of the European Association of Avian Veterinarians and the 5th Scientific Meeting of the European College of Avian Medicine and Surgery*, pp. 117–123

Lierz M (2004) Endoskopie. In: *Leitsymptome bei Papageien und Sittichen*, ed. M Pees, pp. 185–194. Enke Verlag, Stuttgart

Lierz M (2006) Diagnostic value of endoscopy and biopsy. In: *Clinical Avian Medicine, Vol. II*, ed. G Harrison and T Lightfoot, pp. 631–652. Spix, Palm Beach, FL

Lierz M, Ewringmann A and Goebel T (1998) Blood chemistry values in wild raptors and their changes after liver biopsy. *Berlin Muenchen Tierärztliche Wochenschrift* **111**, 295–301

Lierz M and Hafez HM (2004) Endoscopic guided surgery in birds – sterilisation and castration. In: *Proceedings of XIV DVG-Conference about avian diseases, Munich*, pp. 26–31

Lierz M and Hafez HM (2005) Endoscopy guided multiple entry surgery in birds. In: *Proceedings of the 8th Conference of the European Association of Avian Veterinarians and the 6th Scientific ECAMS Meeting, Arles, France, April 2005*, pp. 184–189

McDonald SE (1987) Endoscopic examination. In: *Companion Bird Medicine*, ed. EW Burr, pp. 166–174. Iowa State University Press, Ames, IA

Pye GW, Bennett RA, Plunske R and Davidson J (2001) Endoscopic salpingohysterectomy of juvenile cockatiels (*Nymphicus hollandicus*). *Journal of Avian Medicine and Surgery* **15**, 90–94

Taylor M (1994) Endoscopic examination and biopsy techniques. In: *Avian Principles and Application*, ed. BW Ritchie *et al.*, pp. 327–354. Wingers Publishing, Lake Worth, FL

14

Soft tissue surgery

Neil A. Forbes

Introduction

To be a successful avian surgeon the sympathetic handling of soft tissues is mandatory. Avian surgery requires exactness in view of small body size and increased metabolic rate, as any errors are magnified. Surgery on birds <2 kg requires microsurgical techniques and equipment as well as a significant degree of manual dexterity. For avian surgery to be safe and effective, haemorrhage, tissue trauma, anaesthetic time and anaesthetic and metabolic complications must all be minimized and good postoperative care (including analgesia) must be provided.

Equipment

Microsurgical instruments

Only the tips of the instruments should be miniaturized; the handles should be of normal length. Counterweights minimize digital fatigue, though this is not relevant until one has a considerable surgical caseload, which may take some years. Care of such instruments is important: they are expensive and fragile, and will not last long if abused.

Relatively few instruments are required in an avian surgical kit. The essentials include fine-pointed scissors, needle holders, 2 pairs of artery forceps, atraumatic grasping forceps (e.g. Harris ring-tip forceps) and a retractor (e.g. Alm) (Figure 14.1).

Where possible, handles should be round in outline, so that instrument-tip movement can be accomplished by a finger-rolling action rather than the traditional wrist movement. Spring-loaded locking instruments will also greatly assist in preventing finger fatigue.

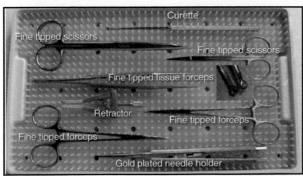

14.1 Typical surgical kit for avian surgery (note inset of Harris ring-tip forceps).

Magnification

Some form of magnification is essential for all patients <1 kg. A bifocal surgical lens, attached to a rechargeable halogen light source (hence no trailing light cables or attachments to immobile light sources), with a variable focal distance is ideal but the cost is significant. If that cost is prohibitive, various much improved loupes are available, with long-life but rapidly rechargeable batteries and very bright LED bulbs. Their quality is highly variable and so different models should be tested. Their disadvantage is that they have a fixed focal distance: movement of the head away from the optimum distance can lead to a sensation of 'motion sickness', but this is easily overcome with practice.

It is essential that good magnification and, in particular, bright powerful illumination are available in order to see within the body cavities. The greater the magnification, the shorter the focal distance, and hence the closer the clinician will be to the surgical tissues. This should be considered in relation to table height and standing or sitting height.

Other equipment

Surgical drapes

Before surgery, only a minimal area of plumage should be plucked (to minimize body heat loss and hypothermia). Excessive wetting of the skin should be avoided, in particular with labile fluids such as alcohol (in view of heat loss due to latent heat of evaporation and intoxication through skin absorption). The accurate visualization of respiration is essential for monitoring depth of anaesthesia. For all these reasons the use of sterile clear plastic surgical drapes maintained on the skin with an aerosol surgical spray adhesive is advantageous.

Haemoclips

Haemoclips (and applicators) are essential for clamping intra-abdominal vessels for which, in view of their position, ligation is precluded. Care and practice are required in the safe and effective application of clips.

Sterile cotton buds

These are invaluable for applying 'point pressure' to control haemorrhage, as well as moving tissues in an atraumatic manner.

Material	Reaction	Duration	Advantages	Disadvantages	Indications
Catgut	Intense	Still present at 120 days, i.e. much slower disintegration than in mammals	None	Intense irritation. Poor strength and knot holding	None
Polyglactin 910	Greatest (greater than in mammals)	Short – completely gone by 60 days, i.e. quicker than in mammals	Rapidly absorbed	Causes intense inflammatory reaction and facilitates tracking and adherence of bacteria	Only use where the benefit of speed outweighs the effect of inflammatory response
Polydioxanone	Minimal	Hydrolysis is still ongoing at 120 days, i.e. slower than in mammals	Minimal reaction, long duration. Monofilament, hence less tissue damage. Minimal risk of bacterial tracking and adherence	Long duration	Majority of surgical avian situations, in particular body wall and tendon repairs
Nylon, steel	Minimal	Non-absorbable	Minimal tissue reaction and long duration	Stiffness can cause local irritation and then self-trauma. More commonly associated with postoperative haematoma, seroma and caseogranuloma	Few indications, as polydioxanone is adequate for most situations that require long-term strength

14.2 Common suture materials and their applications in avian surgery.

Suture materials

The finest material, with the least number of sutures, should be used. A suture material that does not permit capillary action (i.e. no multifilament) and that causes minimal tissue reaction (i.e. monofilament nylon or polydioxanone, but not polyglactin) should be used. Common suture materials are considered in Figure 14.2.

The duration of maintenance of suture strength must be appropriate to the speed of tissue healing. Tendons, ligaments and fascia heal slowly (50% strength in 50 days) and should be repaired using polydioxanone or nylon.

Suture sizes in birds vary, but generally range from 0.7 to 2 metric (3/0–6/0). Taper-point needles are preferable to cutting needles, as reduced iatrogenic cutting by the needle is likely to occur.

Dressings

Birds tolerate bandages or dressings poorly. In areas where some additional support is required over a suture line, hydrocolloid dressings (Figure 14.3) may be sutured in place. Such dressings will promote healing whilst also providing protection to the area (Figure 14.4).

Planning for microsurgery

An ergonomic operating position is important. A seated position is recommended in order to achieve greater forearm control and hence hand stability (Figure 14.5). Control of hand tremor is unimportant until the surgeon is using magnification, at which point it is essential. Slight instrument movements are exaggerated when magnified and the surgeon's natural ability to control such movements is reduced by magnification.

When planning avian surgery, other distractions and stresses such as time constraints should be eliminated.

Trade name	Manufacturer
Tegasorb Tegasorb THIN	3M
Hydrocol	Bertek (Dow Hickam)
BGC Matrix	Brennen
Comfeel (multiple presentations)	Coloplast
DuoDERM CGF DuoDERM (multiple presentations) SignaDRESS Sterile	ConvaTec
DermaFilm HD DermaFilm Thin	DermaRite
Granuflex	Convatec
Restore (multiple presentations)	Hollister
NU-DERM	Johnson & Johnson
Ultec	Kendall
ExuDERM (multiple presentations)	Medline
RepliCare (multiple presentations) Cutinova Hydro Cutinova Thin	

14.3 Examples of hydrocolloid dressings.

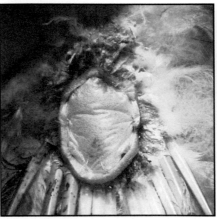

14.4
Peregrine Falcon after preen gland removal, oversewn with hydrocolloid dressing.

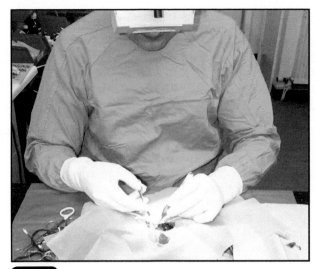

14.5 Surgeon in sitting position with forearm support.

- The veterinary surgeon's fine muscle control may be impaired if excessively strenuous exercise has been taken in the previous 24 hours.
- Caffeine intake should be neither increased nor reduced.
- All risks and possible complications should be assessed prior to surgery so that they can be confidently dealt with should they occur.
- Small infrequently used instruments are those most likely to have been misplaced. Steps should be taken to ensure that all the necessary equipment for a procedure is available and sterile prior to anaesthetic induction.
- The operating table must be stable against movement of people or machinery in the vicinity. Staff should be advised not to touch or knock the table during surgery, as even slight patient movements result in significant surgical risks.

No surgeon should commence surgery unless wholly familiar with avian anatomy. 'Fresh' cadaver surgery can be used for anatomical familiarization and in order to become experienced at tissue handling and at evaluating what traction and trauma can be placed on delicate structures without causing lasting damage in a living bird. Cadavers that are not fresh will have undergone severe tissue changes, which might give an unrealistic impression of the minimal trauma that living tissues would tolerate.

Radiosurgery

Radiosurgery is invaluable, but training and care are required. Correct utilization of radiosurgery will not cause excessive tissue damage or delayed wound healing (Turner *et al.*, 1992) but will facilitate incision in the absence of significant haemorrhage, as well as giving accurate control of any bleeding points (using the bipolar forceps).

Radiosurgery employs high-frequency alternating current to generate energy. There are two electrodes: active and indifferent. The active electrode should remain cool. Radiosurgical units use radiofrequency current (as opposed to electrical current used in diathermy) and this is received at the indifferent plate. Direct contact between the patient and the plate is not required, thus removing any risk of contact-point heat generation that otherwise could lead to tissue necrosis in the patient.

Haemorrhage control

The control of haemorrhage is essential to prevent significant blood loss and to facilitate uninterrupted visualization of the surgical field, thus reducing surgical time and increasing the precision of surgery. Bipolar forceps are invaluable for controlling point haemorrhage, even in the presence of a liquid blood-filled field. The two points of the bipolar forceps constitute the two separate electrodes (active and indifferent), so there is no need for a ground plate. Intraoperative sterile switching from monopolar to bipolar is essential to facilitate effective mono- and bipolar use. Cautery with the monopolar head is ineffective in a wet (e.g. bloody) field.

Incisions

The optimum frequency for incisions is 3.8–4.0 MHz. This frequency provides a precision focus of the energy in a minimal area.

To minimize lateral heat (and hence collateral tissue damage), the smallest possible electrode size is always used. For the same reason the electrode should be in contact with the tissue for the minimum time possible. Once a tissue has been cut, the operator should not return to the same tissue with a single wire within 7 seconds, or 15 seconds if using a loop electrode.

Excessive sparking or lateral heat should not occur as long as the power setting is not too high. If the power is too low, the electrode drags; this in turn increases the lateral heat and tissue damage (this can also occur when trying to cut through fat). Any excessive tissue damage will delay postoperative tissue healing.

Waveforms

A fully filtered waveform is ideal, as this minimizes lateral heat.

- Fully filtered, fully rectified (90% cutting, 10% coagulation) current should be used for cutting skin and for biopsy.
- Fully rectified (50% cutting, 50% coagulation) current should be used for dissection with haemostasis.
- Partially rectified (10% cutting, 90% coagulation) current should be used for coagulation.

Surgical lasers

Laser surgery is now more readily available and affordable. Electrical energy excites a 'lasing medium' (carbon dioxide, diode or argon) contained in an optical laser chamber. As the medium returns to a more organized state it loses energy, generating photons as electromagnetic radiation or light. These photons are focused via lenses and fibres into a focused and controlled beam. Lasers provide non-contact but accurate tissue penetration with minimal lateral damage.

The type of lasing compound affects the wavelength and frequency of radiation. Carbon dioxide lasers can operate with a focused beam for cutting, or a defocused beam for vaporizing tissues. Tissue penetration and collateral thermal injury with carbon dioxide lasers are very limited (0.05–0.2 mm) as compared with diode lasers, which create 0.3–0.6 mm thermal injury from the incision site (Bowles *et al.*, 2006). However, carbon dioxide lasers can only seal vessels up to 0.6 mm, whilst diode lasers can seal vessels up to 2 mm and can also operate in a fluid environment. Diode lasers have the ability to operate via endoscopes, facilitating minimally invasive endoscopic surgeries (see Chapter 13). Argon lasers are not generally used in avian surgery.

There is no doubt that the application of surgical lasers will have a growing place in avian surgery during the next few years (Bartels, 2002). The main advantages are reductions in oedema, postoperative swelling, lateral damage, healing times and postoperative pain, enabling more extensive surgeries (e.g. orchidectomy) to be performed.

Patient preparation

The patient must be assessed in relation to energy and nutritional status, as well as circulatory fluid or blood deficit, and any abnormalities should be corrected. Intraoperative and postoperative hypothermia, analgesia, sepsis and shock must be controlled. Presurgical patient preparation is important (see Chapter 10).

Skin preparation

Sufficient feathers are removed (ideally, not flight feathers) to enable adequate sterile access to the operative site. Adjacent feathers may then be retracted from the surgical field and held in place with adhesive tape. The minimization of the area of feather removal, whilst still enabling intraoperative control of sepsis, is beneficial in the control of intra- or postoperative hypothermia.

In the author's practice, skin preparation is performed using iodine-based alcoholic tincture disinfectant. An aerosol surgical adhesive is applied to the skin and a sterile transparent drape is applied.

Surgery of the skin and adnexa

Soft tissue wounds and injuries

Birds typically have very thin skin, with minimal soft tissue structures (in particular on the extremities). Desiccation and devitalization of subcuticular tissues following loss of skin integrity is common.

A decision must initially be taken as to whether a skin deficit will heal by first or second intention. Closing the skin, or covering it with hydrocolloid or vapour membrane dressings to prevent desiccation, is essential in all cases. Tissue damage, necrosis, organic contamination or significant bacterial or fungal infection will preclude first-intention healing (Redig, 1996). In the majority of cases, debridement and irrigation will facilitate first-intention closure.

The commonest site for skin deficit is the cranium (subsequent to trauma whilst in flight). In these cases a bipedicle cervical or advancement graft may be used to move loose skin from the lower neck up over the deficit. Because avian skin is typically very thin, free skin grafting tends not to be successful.

Skin closure may be achieved with vertical or horizontal mattress sutures (as opposed to single interrupted sutures) where the potential for wound site tension is a risk. Raptor wounds are generally best protected or covered to prevent self-trauma. Hydrocolloid dressings (see Figure 14.3) may be sewn in place over a wound to stimulate healing as well as simultaneously providing protection to the wound.

On occasions neck restraint collars may need to be used in order to prevent self-trauma whilst wounds heal.

Surgery of the propatagium

The propatagium is essential in order to enable normal flight. It is a delicate structure with limited vascular supply. Direct blunt or electrical trauma, or avascular necrosis consequent to bandaging, can lead to significant soft tissue loss (Figure 14.6).

The propatagium comprises two layers of skin (reinforced by an elastic web), one dorsally and one ventrally, with a propatagial ligament enclosed within the leading edge. The ligament has collagen sections at either end, with an elasticated section in the middle (pars elastica). The propatagium receives its blood

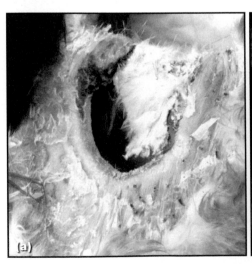
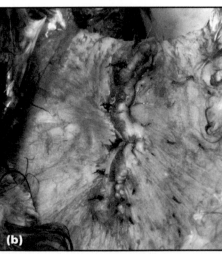

14.6 **(a)** Harris' Hawk with significant propatagial loss following electrocution. **(b)** The same patient following surgery. This bird regained normal flight 4 weeks later.

supply from the radial artery and branches of the subscapular artery, which runs just caudal to the propatagial ligament.

In the event of injury, the two sides of the dorsal aspect of the ligament should be rejoined, as should the two sides of the ventral aspect. Any defect or deficit of the propatagial ligament should be removed and the fresh ends joined. A moderate shortening of the propatagial ligament can be tolerated by most raptors, as the structure will stretch postoperatively to accommodate the shortening. Following surgery, a single piece of hydrocolloid dressing, cardboard or radiology film should be cut to cover the dorsal and ventral propatagium, proximal and distal to the wound (akin to two pieces of bread making a sandwich around the propatagium). This material is sewn dorsal to ventral and is kept in place for at least 2½ weeks. The material prevents stretching of the healing tissue until significant strength has been generated.

Feather cysts

These are rare in raptors but common in passerines, in particular Norwich and Gloster Canaries, which have been genetically selected to produce soft fluffy feathers, predisposing them to abnormal follicular development making cysts more likely to occur. Certain individual breed lines within a Canary flight can be more susceptible to the problem.

Each feather cyst should be accessed individually. If there is a chance that the next follicular development will be normal as long as a particular cyst is resolved, that cyst should be surgically opened (under general anaesthesia), cleaned out and managed by second-intention healing, whilst watching carefully for recurrence of the cyst. The surgeon should be aware that feather follicles have a rich blood supply and so these patients are prone to significant blood loss, which is a significant concern for a small bird.

A more serious cyst, or one managed conservatively that recurs, should be surgically removed together with the dermal papilla from which it develops. Care must be taken in dissecting down around the feather cyst, towards its base, so that all the cyst or feather shaft is removed together with the dermal papilla, but without affecting the blood supply to adjacent feather follicles. If this can be achieved without the use of radiosurgery, so much the better, as the latter might increase the risk of collateral follicle damage. The cyst or follicle is approached from the dorsal aspect, but on following it down to the papilla, access to remove the cranial aspects may require a ventral approach. A tourniquet and topical haemostasis are likely to be required.

Uropygial (preen) gland

The uropygial gland may suffer from ductal blockage, gland abscessation or neoplasia. Blockage is often overcome by application of digital pressure, resulting in a jet of thick waxy and oily secretion. Infection and neoplasia can be difficult to differentiate as both result in a significant inflammatory response. Adenoma, adenocarcinoma and squamous cell carcinoma may occur. Biopsy should always be performed in cases of doubt. Preen gland adenocarcinoma is the only avian adenocarcinoma likely to be cured by surgery; in part this is because it is diagnosed at an earlier stage than those affecting internal organs.

Abscesses are treated by curettage and topical and systemic antibiosis. Preen gland neoplasia requires careful surgical excision. The gland itself has a significant blood supply and radiosurgery or laser surgery is invaluable. The gland is bordered ventrally by fibrinous connective tissue that attaches firmly to the dorsal surface of the pygostyle and caudal vertebrae. Surgical removal must extend to the connective tissue layer, which is relatively avascular in comparison with the gland itself. In many species the two sides of the gland are separated by a central septum; in early cases in these species it is possible to perform a unilateral gland removal. The skin overlying the gland should be preserved so as to facilitate postoperative closure.

Neoplasms

Birds suffer from a range of cutaneous, subcutaneous and internal neoplasms. These should be approached in a similar manner to those in other species. Masses may be aspirated for cytological examination, biopsy samples may be harvested, or masses removed and submitted for histopathology.

Lipoma

This benign tumour of fat tissue is represented in raptors, pigeons and passerine birds infrequently, compared with psittacine birds. Total surgical removal is generally curative.

Xanthoma

This non-neoplastic mass typically occurs on extremities, especially anatomical regions where there has been trauma or haemorrhage. Xanthomas are defined as intradermal deposits of cholesterol clefts with an associated inflammatory reaction. This author has also removed a confirmed xanthoma from an infraorbital sinus (Lanner Falcon) and two from the lumen of the trachea (Harris' Hawk). The exact appearance varies but they are often seen as yellowish plaques under the skin, diffuse thickening or lobulated masses, which will sometimes ulcerate.

Xanthomas tend to be highly vascularized and invasive by nature. Reduction of the dietary fat may assist, but surgical removal at any early stage is usually recommended. Following removal, if the skin cannot be closed the deficit may be covered with a hydrocolloid dressing (e.g. Granuflex or tissue glue) on the extremity of the wing (which is the commonest site), and the distal limb amputated. Histology is always indicated, as this is also a common site for fibrosarcoma.

Squamous cell carcinoma

This is the commonest neoplasm in raptors (Forbes et al., 2000) and is found most often in the Peregrine Falcon and Harris' Hawk . The predilection sites are pre-femoral or the ventral aspect of the wing. Typically there is overlying skin ulceration with secondary bacterial or yeast infection.

Surgical removal with a 1 cm margin is typically curative. Metastasis to lung and bone has been reported. If there is recurrence, topical 5-fluorouracil has been reported by Paterson (1997) and has also proven efficacious for the author when used in this situation in birds.

Papillomas

Papillomas are relatively common and have been found on the digits, cloaca, glottis and crop. Those that can be removed surgically should be (choice of technique will be dictated by the nature and position of the mass); those that do not lend themselves to surgery are typically self-limiting. In terms of visual appearance the main differential is that of pox (dry form), though the latter tends to be erythematous, ulcerated initially and self-curing in 6–8 weeks.

Fibrosarcoma

This has been reported in a number of sites, in particular the metacarpus. These neoplasms tend to be locally malignant, but do not tend to metastasize. Complete surgical removal is typically curative.

Gastrointestinal and reproductive tract techniques

Tongue damage

Due to growth of the lower beak, where the lateral aspects of the rhamphotheca roll dorsally and medially, tongue damage is frequently seen when the aperture in the tip of the rhamphotheca is no longer sufficiently large for the tongue tip to fit through. In this situation, the excessive beak material interfering with the tongue is removed with a dremel. Discoloration of the tongue may occur with microbacterial abscessation as well as *Capillaria* spp. infestation (see Chapter 18).

Oropharynx

Abscessation can occur above the hard palate or within the sinus structures. Obstruction of drainage from the infraorbital sinus results in a swollen fluid-filled infraorbital sinus. Culture and sensitivity testing together with cytology should be undertaken and appropriate therapeutics administered. In the case of *Pseudomonas* spp. infections in particular, an area of palate may become necrotic and require surgical removal.

The palatine area is served by a copious blood supply. Surgery to remove the necrotic mass should not be undertaken until there is a clear demarcation between viable and non-viable tissue; in this way haemostasis should not be a significant problem.

Oesophagus and crop

Oesophageal stricture formation may occur after infections (trichomoniasis, capillariasis, candidiasis), tube-feeding trauma, thermal or caustic trauma, foreign body ingestion or iatrogenic surgical trauma. Where strictures occur, the eliciting cause must be determined and addressed. If necessary, a pharyngostomy tube (see later) may be placed during supportive and medical care. If a stricture remains it may be relieved by serial mechanical dilation, achieved by passing tubes or cannulae of increasing size periodically over a period of several weeks.

Ingluviotomy

This technique is commonly indicated for the relief of 'sour crop'. The crop's function is to accommodate ingested food until such time as it is passed into the stomach. In a raptor, food will normally pass from the crop into the stomach within 6–10 hours of feeding. Any food remaining in the crop will be held at close to 41°C, and such food will rapidly putrefy in the absence of acid or digestive enzymes, leading to life-threatening toxaemia. Impactions are less life-threatening in non-meat-eating birds, but the cause of the impaction will still need to addressed. In normal breeding pigeons, a milky substance is produced by both male and female pigeons, which is a nutritional and immunological solution for feeding to youngsters (see Chapter 27).

'Sour crop' in a meat-eating bird will be evident from the foetid oral odour. Such patients are more critical than they appear and these are genuine emergency cases. The crop should be emptied as soon as possible and any toxins flushed out. Surgery should not be delayed for medical stabilization, but as soon as the bird is anaesthetized intravenous fluid therapy, antibiosis, NSAIDs and anti-emetics should be administered. In the author's opinion, this is best achieved by opening the crop wall, dropping any food out and flushing the internal lumen, with immediate or next-day closure. If extension of the anaesthesia to facilitate same-day closure is felt to be life-threatening, closure should be delayed for 12–24 hours. There are many different approaches to this common problem (see Chapter 23).

An ingluviotomy may also be indicated for the retrieval of any outsize ingested foreign object, the placement of an ingluviostomy tube or, on occasions, to enable proventriculoscopy.

1. The bird is placed in dorsal or lateral recumbency, entubated, with the head elevated above the level of the crop.
2. A probe is placed per os into the crop, to delineate the position of the organ.
3. The skin is incised over the left lateral crop wall, close to the thoracic inlet.
4. The crop wall is localized and isolated.
5. An incision site is selected to avoid large blood vessels and so as not to interfere with postoperative feeding or tube placement.
6. Stay sutures are placed in the crop and an incision one-third to one-half the length of the skin incision is made (as it will stretch to equal that of the skin).
7. Crop closure is achieved with 0.7–1.5 metric (4/0–6/0) synthetic monofilament absorbable material using a single or double continuous inversion pattern, followed by separate skin closure.

Crop or oesophageal lacerations

These may occur following traumatic tube feeding or external trauma (e.g. talon punctures from another raptor). In pigeons, wire-strike injuries often result in extensive lacerations involving the skin of the ventral neck. Crop punctures are often not recognized at the time of trauma but rather later, when a significant build-up of foetid toxin-producing decaying food material has developed subcutaneously. A significant active inflammatory reaction will be present. Surgical exploration, closure of the crop wound, drainage (pharyngostomy tube placement if required), fluid therapy, analgesia, anti-inflammatory and antibiotic therapy may be required, prior to surgical skin closure some days later.

Oesophagostomy or ingluviostomy tube placement

Tube placement is required in situations where the mouth, proximal or distal oesophagus, or crop needs to be bypassed. Such situations may include orthopaedic conditions of the beak and head, or trauma, infection, neoplasia, severe parasitic infestations, or strictures affecting any part of the gastrointestinal tract between the mouth and the proventriculus, or simply in a bird so weak that it is unable to feed itself.

1. The bird is anaesthetized, intubated and placed in lateral recumbency.
2. A metal feeding tube is placed by mouth and tented up in an appropriate position in the cervical oesophagus (cranial to the crop).
3. The skin is prepared and a small incision is made over the end of the feeding tube.
4. A rubber or plastic feeding tube (which can be connected to a feeding syringe) of appropriate size is passed via the incision into the oesophagus, and advanced caudally. The tube is passed via the crop and distal (thoracic) oesophagus into the proventriculus.
5. A skin suture is placed around the tube. Tape is placed either side of the feeding tube as it exits the skin incision and is sutured to the skin.
6. The capped feeding end is then enclosed in a bandage wrap around the neck or attached to the bird's back.

Regular small meals (smaller than if feeding into the crop) are administered and care is taken to flush the tube clean after each use. Such a tube may be left in place for several weeks if necessary. The tube is best fixed in place using a 'Chinese finger-trap' pattern around the tube, which is then secured to the skin. Alternatively tape may be placed either side of the tube, and the tape in turn is sewn to the skin.

Laparotomy

The caudal thoracic and abdominal air sacs receive fresh air from the trachea. It is important to appreciate that laparotomy is impossible without opening the posterior air sacs and that this has a profound effect on both the effectiveness of inhalant anaesthesia and on intraoperative heat loss. Once a laparotomy incision is made, openings around the surgical site may be packed off, or plugged with abdominal organs. Alternatively, parenteral anaesthetic agents may be used (see Chapter 10). During any laparotomy procedure, the bird's head should be raised at 30–40 degrees to prevent any surgical irrigation fluid from entering the lung field.

Left lateral laparotomy

This is the most useful approach and is used for access to the gonads, left kidney, oviduct, ureter, proventriculus and ventriculus. The bird is placed in right lateral recumbency. The wings are reflected dorsally, whilst the left leg is restrained in a dorsolateral direction (Figure 14.7).

1. Pluck the operative site.
2. Locate the anatomical landmarks: ribs 7 and 8 (last two ribs) at the level of the uncinate process, and the caudal point of the pubis.
3. Prepare the surgical site.
4. Incise the skin between the left leg and the abdominal wall (to allow further abduction).
5. Extend the skin incision caudally to the caudal extent of the pubis and cranially to over the cranial edge of the 7th rib at the level of the uncinate process.
6. Locate the superficial medial femoral artery and vein as they traverse dorsal to ventral across the lateral abdominal wall medial to the coxofemoral joint (Figure 14.8).
7. Use bipolar cautery to seal these vessels, dorsal and ventral to the intended site of muscle incision (level of the uncinate process).
8. Taking great care not to incise any underlying viscera, create a muscle incision from the caudal extent of the pubis to the caudal aspect of the 8th rib.
9. Approach the 8th rib with bipolar forceps from the caudal direction, closing the forceps around either side of the cranial aspect of the 8th rib and apply cautery to seal the intercostal vessels (Figure 14.9). Then cut the rib, just below the uncinate process, with strong scissors. Repeat the process with rib 7.

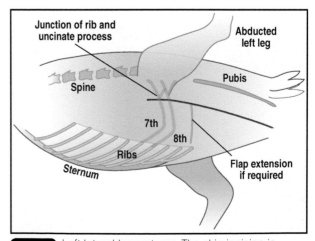

14.7 Left lateral laparotomy. The skin incision is shown as a red line.

10. Insert a small retractor (e.g. Heiss or Alm) between the cut rib ends to enable full visualization of the abdominal cavity. The Lone Star retractor system (Figure 14.10) is invaluable for such surgeries.
11. The air sac wall is broken down with blunt dissection. The oviduct is located dorsal to the intestine and ventral to the kidney. It is white in comparison with the intestine and has longitudinal rather than circumferential muscle striations.

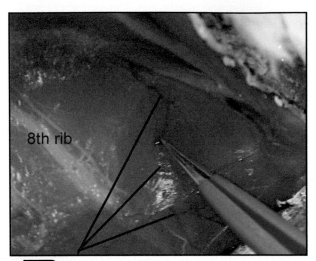

4.8 Superficial medial femoral artery and vein.

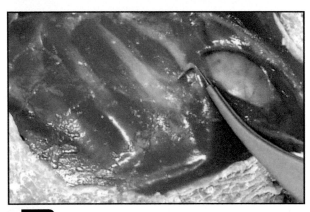

4.9 Bipolar cauterization of intercostal artery.

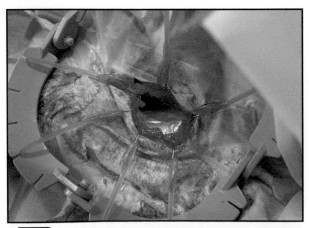

4.10 Lone Star retractor.

12. On completion of the surgery the incision is closed using 0.7–1.5 metric (4/0–6/0) absorbable monofilament synthetic material in a continuous or interrupted pattern in two layers. The intercostal muscles are apposed and no attempt is made to rejoin the transected ribs.

Salpingohysterectomy

This procedure is rarely indicated for medical reasons in raptors (compared with parrots). However, in certain countries it is now illegal to fly a fertile hybrid falcon; therefore salpingohysterectomy and vasectomy of falcons is likely to become a more widely requested procedure (Lierz and Hafez, 2005).

In a similar vein, the control of pigeon populations in built-up areas is becoming an increasingly important issue and there is no doubt that population control is the most effective method of dealing with the problem. Until such time as an effective, safe and reliable method of immunological neutering for birds is achieved, surgical neutering may be called on. Surgical neutering of both male and female birds is best achieved outside the breeding season, using minimally invasive endoscopic techniques (see Chapter 13).

As the avian ovary is firmly attached to the dorsal abdominal wall, its removal is challenging and often dangerous. In order to prevent further egg laying, all of the oviduct and uterus may be removed instead. A review of ovariectomy techniques is given by Echols (2002).

Surgical salpingohysterectomy is indicated consequent to egg peritonitis in cases where future breeding is contraindicated, or where there is unresolved egg binding (dystocia) with egg or remnants left in the oviduct in cases where future breeding potential is of lesser concern than the long-term health of the bird.

1. The ventral suspensory ligament of the oviduct is located and broken down by blunt dissection, from a caudal to a cranial direction (Figure 14.11).
2. As the opening of the infundibulum is approached, it should be gently lifted laterally, in order to visualize the significant blood vessel coursing between the ovary and the infundibulum. This vessel should be clamped off with one or two haemoclips.
3. The dorsal suspensory ligament of the oviduct has regular significant blood vessels. These are best coagulated with bipolar forceps using the 'Harrison technique'. Holding the oviduct in a ventral position, the bipolar forceps are advanced from the infundibulum in a dorsal direction, maintaining a line parallel with the ventral border of the kidneys. The forceps are closed, current is applied and the forceps are pulled cranially through the ligament to the infundibulum, cauterizing all vessels in the process. The process is repeated as the ligament is followed caudally, care being taken not to stray far from the dorsal wall of the oviduct lest the ureters are accidentally cauterized.

4. A cotton bud is placed per vent into the cloaca, to delineate the cranial extent of the cloaca. The base of the oviduct is then clamped off using haemoclips, just cranial to the cloaca (Figure 14.12).

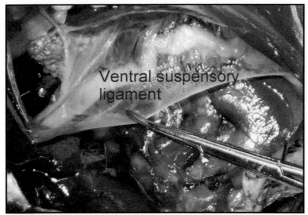

14.11 Blunt dissection of the ventral suspensory ligament of the oviduct.

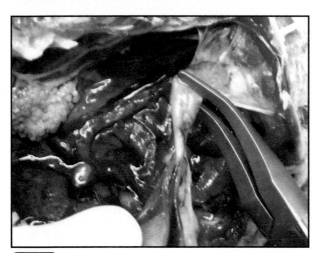

14.12 Clamping of uterine stump.

Caesarean section

Where a hen is suffering from egg binding and either the egg and hen are of high financial or conservational value, or she is suffering from egg binding that is not responsive to medical support or per cloacal egg content suction and implosion, caesarean section may be considered as an alternative.

1. Depending on the position of the egg, a midline incision (usually) or a caudal left lateral incision is made. If the egg is in the distal oviduct, a ventral midline approach will give optimum access (see below).
2. The initial incision is made in the midline a third of the distance from pubis to sternum and then extended in either direction as is necessary to achieve access to the oviduct. The midline musculature is incised with great care to avoid damage to any internal viscera or organs. The oviduct is incised directly over the bound egg, avoiding any prominent blood vessels.

3. After egg removal, the oviduct is inspected and the cause of binding determined and rectified. If correction is not possible, salpingohysterectomy may be indicated at a later date but would be inappropriate at this time, due to the excessive combined surgical stress where the egg binding will have already have caused a significant degree of stress. Moreover salpingohysterectomy is most safely conducted when the organ is not active, i.e. small in size and relatively avascular.
4. The oviduct is closed with a single interrupted or continuous inversion suture pattern, using 1.5 metric (4/0) or finer absorbable material.

Ventral midline laparotomy

This approach gives poor visibility of the majority of the body cavity, but it does facilitate surgery of the small intestine, pancreatic biopsy, liver biopsy or cloacopexy and is used in diffuse abdominal disease such as peritonitis, egg binding and cloacal prolapse.

The bird is placed in dorsal recumbency, the midline prepared and the legs abducted caudally. The skin of the abdominal wall is tented and an initial incision is made using scissors or the single wire radiosurgical electrode or laser. Care is required to prevent iatrogenic visceral damage and the risk is minimized by creating the incision caudally over the cloaca, rather than over the small intestine. The incision is extended with fine scissors. This approach can be extended along the costal border cranially and to the pubis caudally to create a flap on one or both sides of the midline to increase access. This approach is particularly useful for access to the caudal uterus and cloaca.

Uterine torsion

Egg binding may arise subject to a range of causes. If the condition does not respond to medical support, and particularly if there is a markedly swollen abdomen, torsion of the oviduct should be considered (Harcourt-Brown, 1996). In such cases the oviduct may have suffered a torsion through which no egg can pass. A number of eggs in a varying state of decay may be present in the proximal oviduct.

For torsion to occur, typically a traumatic breach will have occurred in the dorsal oviductal suspensory ligament through which the oviduct will have passed. Many such patients are in poor condition and represent a high surgical risk. Once the bird has been stabilized, a ventral midline surgical approach is used to access the oviduct. On occasions the torsion may be reduced (often surgical drainage of the oviduct is required first) and the breach of the suspensory ligament repaired. Alternatively a salpingohysterectomy may be performed.

Orchidectomy

This may also be performed via the left lateral approach. The testicles (like the ovaries) are attached to the dorsal abdominal wall, adjacent to the aorta, and connected only by a short testicular artery. The left testicle is identified, the caudal pole is elevated and a haemoclip is placed under the testicle (Figure 14.13). The testicle is then incised over the clip. Once achieved, a further clip is applied in a more

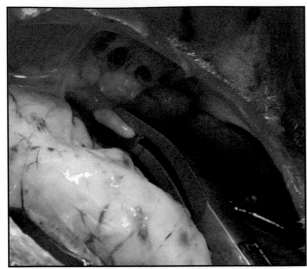

14.13 Haemoclip application to left testis on caudomedial aspect.

craniad position and so on. If any testicular tissue is left, there is a possibility of regeneration. Access to the right testicle will be more difficult and requires blunt dissection through the air sac wall, or via a fresh incision on the contralateral abdominal wall. A similar removal process may then be performed on this testicle.

Proventriculotomy/ventriculotomy

Proventriculotomy for access to the proventriculus is most commonly indicated for the removal of foreign objects that are not retrievable per os or ingluvies with rigid or flexible endoscopes. In raptors, the majority of objects that are ingested are either digested or returned as a pellet (including most foreign bodies), but this is not the case in other birds under discussion here. Access to the ventriculus is achieved by one of three routes.

Raptors: In birds with a less muscular or well defined ventriculus (e.g. raptors), access is general and the exact incision site is less critical. Access is gained via the left lateral laparotomy approach; sufficient exposure is necessary to visualize the suspensory membranes and to avoid the proventricular vessels along its greater curvature. In raptors the proventriculus and ventriculus are found as two discrete but confluent areas. Depending on the size of the patient, it is advantageous to pack off the abdomen, behind the ventriculus, with saline-soaked gauze swabs to minimize the potential effect of any leakage. In view of the lack of mesentery for overlying the ventricular or proventricular incision after closure, it is advantageous if the incision can be made at a point where the suture line can be covered over with the liver. Suction should be available to remove enteric contents in a controlled manner. An endoscope may be passed into the gut via the incision in both cranial and caudal directions to verify that all foreign objects have been removed. The incision is closed in two continuous layers (opposed then inverted) using 0.4–1.5 metric (4/0–8/0) synthetic absorbable monofilament material.

Suture placement in normal gut surgery includes the submucosa in view of its greater collagen content. However, the avian proventriculus has minimal collagen and so greater care is required. As birds have no mesentery, enterotomy carries a higher risk of post-operative peritonitis. The liver may take the role of the mesentery in overlying the closed isthmal incision. Care should be taken to minimize collateral damage during incision and repair of the isthmus. It has been demonstrated (in turkeys) that the entire neural network situated within the isthmus must remain intact for normal gastroduodenal motility to occur. The ventricular suspensory ligaments are not repaired.

Pigeons and passerine birds: In herbivorous, insectivorous and granivorous birds (many passerine species), a more muscular ventriculus is present. The ventriculus (grinding stomach) has four muscular bands, which attach to each other with extensive aponeurosis. These bands of muscle are arranged asymmetrically to facilitate a grinding and rotary crushing action.

1. A transabdominal (i.e. from side to side, just caudal to the caudal edge of the sternum) incision is made to approach the ventriculus.
2. The abdominal air sac is broken down to gain access to the ventriculus.
3. A small fatty ligament found on the surface of the ventriculus is carefully removed, whilst making every attempt to maintain the integrity of the gastric blood vessels.
4. The thin-walled muscle area on the caudal aspect of the ventriculus is located. This muscle is generally a paler colour and is palpably thinner, being located on the caudal edge of the ventriculus and often appearing as a slight 'out-pouching' from the contour of the ventriculus. The muscle fibres in this area are positioned in a different direction to the main fibres of the central muscular section of the organ.
5. A stab incision is created in this thin area of muscle, parallel in direction to the muscle fibres.
6. Once any foreign material has been removed, the muscle is closed with a series of fine single interrupted appositional (rather than inverted) sutures in one layer. Inversion of the suture line is generally impossible in this area.

Some authors recommend entry into the ventriculus via the thick muscular wall, but in this author's hands the access achieved via this approach is less satisfactory.

Yolk sacculectomy

In neonatal chicks, the presence of an infected or unretracted yolk sac necessitates surgical removal. Following induction of anaesthesia, the bird is placed in dorsal recumbency. If the yolk sac is external, a purse-string suture is placed around its base and the yolk sac is removed. If the yolk sac is internal, the chick is prepared for surgery, with fluid therapy, antibiosis and analgesia. At what is judged to be the optimal time, surgery is undertaken.

Under isofluorane anaesthesia, a small incision is delicately created cranial to the umbilicus. This incision is extended around the umbilicus and the umbilical stump is excised. The yolk sac is exteriorized and the duct (joining the yolk sac to the small intestine) is ligated. Care is taken to avoid rupture or spillage of the yolk sac contents. The abdominal incision is closed in two layers. Survival rates for such surgery in sick chicks is not good, hence the care taken to optimize their condition prior to surgery.

Organs prolapsed through the cloaca

Apart from partial cloacal prolapses, or prolapsed cloacal masses (papilloma, neoplasia or mycobacterial granuloma), total prolapses can occur where the entire cloaca is prolapsed to reveal the colonic, urethral and oviductal junctions (Figure 14.14). Alternatively, the oviduct or colon may be prolapsed. Differentiation of the tissues involved is important and is achieved by assessing the size and appearance of the structures present.

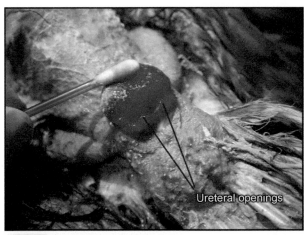
Ureteral openings

14.14 Cloaca prolapsed in a Harris' Hawk, with the ureteral openings indicated.

Birds presented with such prolapses are typically suffering severe shock. Fluid therapy, analgesia and anti-inflammatory therapy are all mandatory. If a colonic or uterine prolapse is present, there must inevitably be an intussusception. Pushing the offending organ back through the cloacal opening and placing a purse-string suture will not lead to a satisfactory outcome (though this a recommended and acceptable action if immediate referral for extensive surgery is an option). Such cases require an immediate midline (with or without flap) laparotomy and reduction or removal of the intussusception, which may contain a length of devitalized gut; an enterectomy will be required to remove this. Intussusception has also been seen secondary to linear foreign bodies or following enteric infections.

If tissues have remained vital, a pexy should be performed to a suitable internal structure to maintain the reduction. If the bird is particularly shocked or weakened, then rather than resecting and rejoining the gut at one surgery it may be prudent to create a stoma or a loop jejunostomy or colostomy, with reattachment several days later (VanDerHeyden, 1993). Midline flap incisions provide optimal access.

Microsurgical instrumentation and techniques are mandatory. Blood vessel appositional clamps (e.g. Acland clamps) are invaluable in order to maintain occlusion of the cut gut ends and appositional positioning whilst suture placement and gut closure are achieved (Figure 14.15). These vascular clamps are designed to avoid tissue slippage, whilst maintaining low pressure to avoid tissue damage. Clamps may be used individually, or conjoined (attached to a bar or clamped together), so that both ends of the tissue are adjacent to each other.

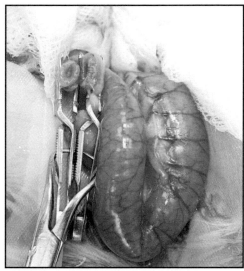

14.15 Appositional blood vessel clamps used to facilitate gastrointestinal tract anastomosis.

Intestinal anastomosis

Intestinal anastomosis is performed with an end-to-end technique using 0.2–0.7 metric (6/0–10/0) material with a simple appositional method. If the gut is <2 mm in diameter, six to eight simple interrupted sutures are used (similar to a blood vessel anastomosis). If the gut is >2 mm in diameter a continuous pattern should be used. The advantages of a continuous pattern are that it reduces surgery time, yields improved apposition and so reduces risk of leakage, reduces tissue irritation and achieves improved endothelialization. Care should be taken not to overtighten a continuous pattern, as this would cause a purse-string and compromise food passage across the repair site. Sutures are initially placed at 12 o'clock and 6 o'clock; then sutures are placed in the caudal section of gut (Figure 14.16a).

Further sutures are placed in the caudal section. The right clamp is rotated anticlockwise, and the left clamp clockwise, to bring the two (previously lateral) edges into apposition (Figure 14.16b) in readiness for inversional suture application.

If the sections of gut being joined are of unequal size, or where end-to-end anastomosis is technically difficult for other reasons, a side-to-side or side-to-end technique may be used. If using a side-to-side method, the end sections may be closed with sutures or haemoclips. One section of gut is offered up to the side of the other and the back of the anastomosis is sutured (Figure 14.17a). An aperture is then created in both proximal and distal segments (Figure 14.17b).

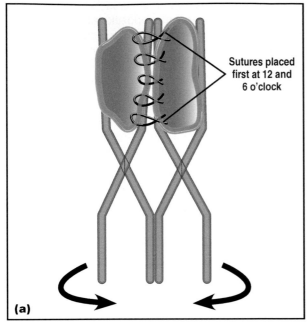

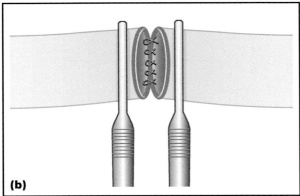

14.16 End-to-end intestinal anastomosis. Rotating the clamps in opposite directions brings the edges into apposition.

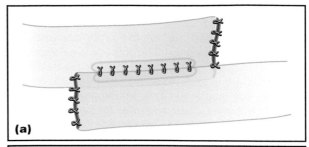

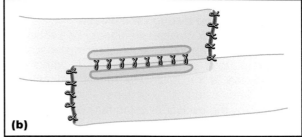

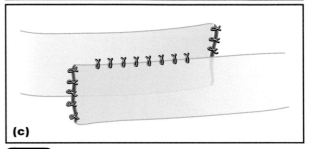

14.17 Side-to-side intestinal anastomosis.

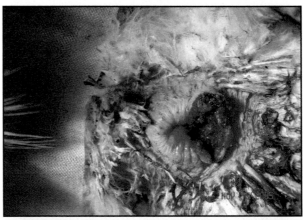

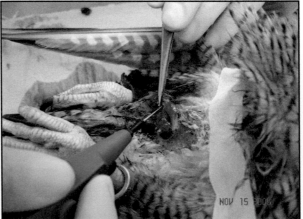

14.18 Electrosurgical removal of cloacal tumours. (Courtesy of Michael Lierz)

The two apertures are then apposed, prior to the lateral edges of each aperture being closed with a series of inversional sutures (Figure 14.17c). If necessary, the front repair sutures may be pre-placed.

When passing needles through fine tissue, it is important that the needle is encouraged to follow its natural curvature, otherwise an excessive needle hole is created. The arcing instrument action achieved by finger rolling of round-bodied instruments minimizes this problem.

Cloacoliths and cloacal tumours

Cloacoliths are firm rough-surfaced aggregations of urates. They are uncommon and the pathogenesis is unclear. This author has experienced them most frequently in birds that have recently undergone extended nesting or brooding behaviour, such that they may not have voided faeces as frequently as normal. Birds present with repeated straining, often passing scant traces of blood. The condition is readily diagnosed on digital exploration of the cloaca. The bird is anaesthetized; the cloacolith may be fragmented with artery forceps, and removed piecemeal. Analgesics and antibiosis should be administered.

Cloacal tumour removal is shown in Figure 14.18.

Respiratory tract surgery

Damage to the glottis can occur subsequent to hunting injuries. Surgical management is challenging and should be considered on a case-by-case basis.

Tracheotomy

This procedure is most commonly indicated in the treatment of syringeal aspergilloma or retrieval of a tracheal foreign body, which are not amenable to endoscopic or laser surgical techniques. The bird is placed in dorsal recumbency, with the head directed towards the surgeon. The head of the bird should be elevated at 45 degrees to the tail, so as to facilitate interoperative visualization into the thorax.

A skin incision is made adjacent to the thoracic inlet. The crop is identified, bluntly dissected and displaced to the right. The interclavicular air sac is entered and the trachea is elevated.

The sternotrachealis (attached bilaterally to the ventral aspect of the trachea) is separated from the trachea and transected. Stay sutures may be placed into the trachea in order to draw it into an anterior direction. In most species it is impossible to completely exteriorize the syrinx. A tracheotomy may now be performed, cutting one half of the tracheal circumference, through the ligament between adjacent tracheal cartilages (using a no. 11 scalpel blade) (Figure 14.19). Any tracheal foreign body or aspergilloma may then be removed by suction or traction with fine forceps.

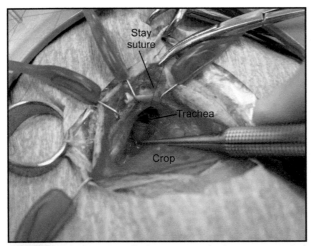

14.19 Tracheotomy: lesion exposed prior to removal of aspergilloma.

The incision is repaired with single interrupted sutures (0.7 metric (6/0) polydiaxonone, two or three sutures only) placed to include two rings either side of the incision.

If additional access is required, the superficial pectoral muscles may be elevated and an osteotomy of the clavicle performed. On closure the two ends of the clavicle are apposed but not rejoined.

The muscle is replaced and sutured into position. The crop is sutured back into place, to create an airtight repair over the interclavicular air sac, using a continuous suture pattern and absorbable suture material. The skin is closed in a routine manner.

Trachectomy

In cases where a severe tracheal stenosis occurs following trauma (including recent intubation) or severe fungal infection of cartilage where tracheal rings have become involved, tracheal resection and removal of the affected tissue are indicated. Depending on the site of the lesion, most species can cope with removal of up to five tracheal rings. In such cases close apposition of cartilages following surgery, using a suture material that elicits minimal tissue reaction (e.g. polydiaxonone), is used in order to minimize the risk of intraluminal granuloma formation. Trauma to tracheal tissues during surgery must be minimized. It is preferable to place sutures in the trachea at the time of resection, to facilitate apposition and anastomosis. Two to four sutures are used (depending on patient size) and are all pre-placed before any are tied.

Sinus surgery

Sinusitis can be difficult to resolve medically. Even daily sinus flushing with appropriate antibiosis and hyaluronidase may fail to resolve an infected sinus, or parasitic infestation of the sinus (e.g. *Cyathostoma* spp.). In such cases the initial task is to locate which sinus is infected and to determine its exact anatomical position. This is best achieved by magnetic resonance imaging (MRI), computed tomography (CT) or iodine contrast radiography. Surgical access is gained to the offending sinus and the sinus is opened or trephined. The infected sinus should be cleaned out and drainage maintained for at least a week.

Biopsy

Liver

Liver biopsy should be performed in cases of hepatomegaly, hepatopathy, endoscopic confirmation of abnormal appearance or where two consecutive bile acid levels are elevated in excess of 25% above the normal upper limit. The commonest findings are haemochromatosis, amyloidosis, chronic active hepatitis, hepatic lipidosis, toxic insult and cirrhosis.

With the patient in dorsal recumbency a 2–3 cm incision through skin and then abdominal musculature is created parallel to, and 0.5 cm caudal to, the caudal edge of the sternum (marked B on Figure 14.20), just lateral to the midline (A on Figure 14.20). The liver will

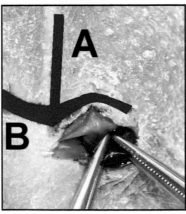

14.20

Liver biopsy, 1 cm left lateral of midline, 0.5 cm caudal to sternum.

be identified beneath the sternum. Two fine artery forceps are triangulated to isolate a wedge of liver tissue (1 cm wide and 0.75 cm deep). The segment of liver is removed and the forceps are removed a minute later. Alternatively, a monopolar loupe electrode may be used to harvest a biopsy sample. In such cases, the power is activated prior to making contact with the tissues, ensuring a sufficient margin between the incision and the tissue to be examined. Cauterized tissue yields poor histopathological results.

Liver biopsy can be performed endoscopically (see Chapter 13), but the author prefers the open approach, as it renders improved access, greater ability to achieve haemostasis (should this be a problem) and an improved sample size.

Pancreas

A number of pancreatic diseases have been reported in a range of avian species (Graham and Heyer, 1992; Speer, 1998; Ritzman, 2000); little research into the clinical significance of amylase and lipase levels has been reported, though a fourfold increase in amylase level may be suggestive of pancreatic pathology. Histopathology is currently the diagnostic tool of choice. Clinical signs associated with avian pancreatitis include anorexia, abdominal discomfort (colic), weight loss, polyuria, polydipsia, abdominal distension, polyphagia, or foetid pale bulky faeces, but many cases are asymptomatic.

To obtain a biopsy sample the bird is anaesthetized, intubated and placed in dorsal recumbency. A small (1–2 cm) craniocaudal incision is made in the mid-abdominal region. Care is taken not to damage underlying viscera. The ascending and descending loops of the small intestine (in which are found the dorsal and ventral lobes of the pancreas) are readily located and exteriorized. If no lesions are readily apparent in other areas of the pancreas, the most distal aspect of the organ is harvested. The distal pancreatic lobe should be gently elevated prior to biopsy sample collection to ensure that the arterial supply to the distal portion is not damaged during collection. The incision is closed in a routine manner.

Kidney

This is indicated where clinical signs or elevated levels of creatinine and uric acid suggest that there is renal pathology. Renal biopsy is best achieved endoscopically (see Chapter 13).

Other procedures

For abdominal air sac placement see Chapter 10. For digital tendon repair see Chapter 16.

Devoicing

Devoicing birds is a high-risk procedure with an uncertain outcome in both the short and long term and is ethically questionable. Legislation varies between nations: it is illegal in the UK and a number of other countries.

Postsurgical care

Postsurgical care greatly affects the outcome of any procedure. Prevention of self-trauma, a rapid recovery, sufficient analgesia and fluid, thermal and nutritional support as well as the minimization of stress are vital.

References and further reading

Antinoff N (2001) It isn't always PDD: three cases with proventricular enlargement. In: *Proceedings of the Annual Conference Association of Avian Vets, Denver*, pp. 35–37

Bartels KE (ed.) (2002) Lasers in medicine and surgery. *Veterinary Clinics of North America* **32**(3)

Bowles HL, Odberg E, Harrison GJ and Kottwitz JJ (2006) Soft tissue diosorders. In: *Clinical Avian Medicine Vol II*, ed. GJ Harrison and TL Lightfoot, pp. 775–829. Spix, Palm Beach, FL

Doolen M (1994) Crop biopsy – a low risk diagnosis for neuropathic gastric dilation. In: *Proceedings of the Annual Conference Association of Avian Vets, Denver*, pp. 193–196

Echols SM (2002) Surgery of the avian reproductive tract. *Seminars in Avian and Exotic Pet Medicine* **11**(4), 177–195

Forbes NA, Cooper JE and Higgins RJ (2000) Neoplasms of birds of prey. In: *Raptor Biomedicine III*, ed. JT Lumeij *et al.*, pp. 127–146. Zoological Education Network, Lake Worth, FL

Graham DL and Heyer GW (1992) Diseases of the exocrine pancreas in pet, exotic and wild birds: a pathologist's perspective. In: *Proceedings of the Annual Conference Association of Avian Vets, Denver*, pp. 190–193

Harcourt-Brown NH (1996) Torsion and displacement of the oviduct as a cause of egg-binding in four psittacine birds. *Journal of Avian Medicine and Surgery* **10**(4), 262–267

Hernandez-Divers SJ (2002) Diode laser surgery: principles and applications in exotic animals. *Seminars in Avian and Exotic Pet Medicine* **11**(4), 208–220

Hernandez Divers SJ (2005) Minimally invasive endoscopic surgery of birds. *Journal of Avian Medicine and Surgery* **19**, 107–120

Krautwald-Junghans ME, Tellhelm B, Kostka VM and Tacke S (1999) Surgical removal of ventricular foreign bodies from an adult ostrich (*Struthio camelus*). *Veterinary Record* **145**, 640–642

Krautwald-Junghans ME, Kaleta EF, Marshang RE and Pieper K (2000) Untersuchungen zur Diagnostik und Therapie der papillomatose des avwaren gastrointestinaltraktes. *Tierärztliche Praxis* **28**(K), 272–278

Lierz M and Hafez HM (2005) Endoscopy guided multiple entry surgery in birds. In: *Proceedings of the 8th Conference of the European Association of Avian Veterinarians and the 6th Scientific ECAMS Meeting, Arles, France, April 2005*, pp. 184–189

Lumeij JT (1994) Gastroenterology. In: *Avian Medicine: Principles and Application*, ed. BW Ritchie *et al.*, pp. 482–521. Wingers, Lake Worth, FL

McCluggage D (1992) Proventriculotomy: a study of selected cases. In: *Proceedings of the Annual Conference Association of Avian Vets, Denver*, pp. 195–200

Paterson S (1997) Treatment of superficial ulcerative squamous cell carcinoma in three horses with topical 5-fluorouracil. *Veterinary Record* **141**, 626–628

Redig PT (1996) Avian emergencies. In: *Manual of Raptors, Pigeons and Waterfowl*, ed. PH Beynon *et al.*, pp. 30–41. BSAVA, Cheltenham

Ritzman TK (2000) Pancreatic hypoplasia in Eclectus Parrot (*Eclectus roratus polychloros*). In: *Proceedings of the Annual Conference Association of Avian Vets, Denver*, pp. 83–87

Stewart JS (1991) A simple proventriculotomy technique for the ostrich. *Journal of Avian Medicine and Surgery* **5**(3), 139–140

Taylor M and Murray M (1999) A diagnostic approach to the avian cloaca. In: *Proceedings of the Annual Conference Association of Avian Vets, Denver*, pp. 301–304

Tomaszewski E, Phalen DN and Wilson VG (1999) Synchronicity, papillomas, and herpes disease. In: *Proceedings of the Annual Conference Association of Avian Vets, Denver*, pp. 219–221

Turner RJ, Cohen RA, Voet RL, Stephens SR and Weinstein SA (1992) Analysis of tissue margins of core biopsy specimens obtained with 'cold knife', CO_2 and Nd:YAG lasers and a radiofrequency surgical unit. *Journal of Reproductive Medicine* **37**(7), 607–10

VanDerHeyden N (1993) Jejunostomy and jejuno-cloacal anastomosis in Macaws. In: *Proceedings of the Annual Conference Association of Avian Vets, Denver*, pp. 35–37

Van Sant F (2001) The hazards of non food item ingestion, In: *Proceedings of the Annual Conference Association of Avian Vets, Denver*, pp. 72–77

Wishnow KI, Johnson DE, Grignon DJ, Cromeens DM and Ayala AG (1989) Regeneration of the urinary bladder mucosa after complete surgical denudation. *De Voe Journal of Urology* **141**, 1476–1479

15

Hard tissue surgery

Jean-Michel Hatt

Introduction

Raptors, pigeons and passerine birds cover a wide range of body weights from just a few grams in the Canary to >10 kg in the Andean Condor. Birds may originate from the wild and from different captive management systems, such as cagebirds and also birds kept for special purposes such as falconry. These aspects have a significant impact on the type of trauma that is likely to occur, the therapy that needs to be applied and the degree of return to normal function that will have to be achieved for an outcome to be considered successful. Causes of injuries include flying into hard objects (windows, cars), collision with wires or projectiles, biting (especially beak trauma) and entrapment. Predisposing factors for fractures need to be considered, such as metabolic bone disease, bone infections (e.g. mycobacteriosis) and neoplasia.

In general, wild birds, especially raptors, will require the highest degree of restitution of function if the bird is to be released and survive and reproduce in the wild. Racing pigeons, which have to be able to fly long distances, and falconry birds, which are expected to hunt at extremely high speeds, also pose a significant challenge to hard tissue surgery. On the other hand, birds kept all year round in a cage (including many passerine species) may live well even though a limb is no longer fully functional.

The choice of technique used will reflect the type of bird, the damage, the surgical skills of the veterinary surgeon and financial constraints. Radiography is of great importance for diagnosis. Exact positioning and use of good quality fine-definition screens are prerequisites for the correct diagnostic work-up.

This chapter gives an overview of the current techniques that are of most interest for the practitioner. Methods that require a high degree of surgical skills and expensive equipment have not been included; also older techniques that are not of use frequently, such as certain complex types of splint, have been omitted. The fact that most avian patients requiring orthopaedic surgery will generally weigh <1 kg implies that both special surgical equipment and miniaturized implants will be used. Recent developments in human osteosynthesis have produced a large variety of such miniaturized and lightweight materials, which are excellent for avian surgery.

Although the author has taken great care to collect scientific data from as many sources as possible, large parts of this chapter still reflect personal observations. It is to be hoped that in the future the information given here will be subjected to scientific analysis to allow a transition from experience-based to evidence-based hard tissue surgery in birds in general and especially in birds of prey.

Anatomy and physiology

Some anatomical aspects that are of great importance for hard tissue surgery should be emphasized. Birds have a lightweight fused skeleton. The cortex is in general 50% of that of a mammal of comparable body weight. Trabeculae act as struts and stabilize the large medulla. An important aspect for avian orthopaedics is that birds tend to have a higher degree of comminuted fractures compared with mammals (Schuster, 1996). This is due to the fact that the amount of inorganic substances, such as hydroxyapatite, is 84% in the avian bone whereas in the mammalian bone it averages 65%. Comminution results in sharp fractures that carry a higher risk of skin penetration, resulting in open fractures (Figure 15.1). This risk is further increased by the fact that avian bones are covered by less soft tissue than those in mammals.

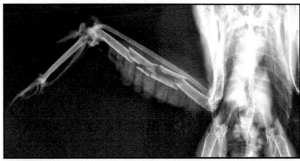

15.1 Red Kite with a highly comminuted diaphyseal ulnar fracture. The sharp edges of the bone may damage the skin and cause an open fracture. Note the soft tissue swelling around the fracture. The radius is intact and such types of fracture may heal with coaptive bandages, as long as there is no major dislocation of fragments.

A unique characteristic of certain avian bones is that they are pneumatized. Such bones (i.e. humerus, coracoid, pelvis, and in some birds also femur and sternum) have a direct connection to air sacs. Therefore, contamination of the fracture site may rapidly develop into a respiratory tract disease. Another noteworthy characteristic of avian bone is the development of medullary bone. This occurs in females during egg production periods under the influence of oestrogen. Bone trabeculae grow from the endosteum; they act as calcium stores for egg shell formation.

Examination

Upon presentation, orthopaedic problems may manifest as lameness, wing droop, paresis, swelling or open wounds. A thorough examination should not only localize the orthopaedic disorder but also recognize other damage, such as haemorrhage of internal organs. Special attention has to be given to the eye, especially the posterior chamber, where haemorrhages frequently occur around the pecten oculi as a result of trauma (see Chapter 25).

A more detailed examination is best carried out under general anaesthesia. Usually this will also include radiographic examination, or other methods of diagnostic imaging. It must be remembered that two radiographs need to be taken with orthogonal views and that it may be advisable to take radiographs of the unaffected contralateral limb for comparative purposes and to aid reconstruction of a physiological form of the injured bone.

Bone healing

Few data are available regarding bone healing in birds (Bush *et al.*, 1976; West *et al.*, 1996; Clark *et al.*, 2005). From studies in the humerus of pigeons it appears that the endosteal surface is at least as active histologically as the periosteal surface. Woven bone is present along the endosteal surface 4 days after osteotomy and it is subsequently replaced by lamellar bone. The majority of callus tissue during healing is derived from the periosteal surface, and the blood supply from the surrounding tissue is very important. The intramedullary circulation appears to be less important in avian bone healing than in mammals. It has even been observed that the reformation of intramedullary circulation is not imperative for osseous union.

Bone healing may occur as primary or secondary healing. Primary bone healing occurs if excellent stabilization is provided and results in only minimal callus formation. In avian medicine primary healing is rarely possible and secondary healing is frequent, which is characterized by stages of inflammation, soft callus formation and subsequent hard callus formation, and finally remodelling. In chickens it has been shown that maximum callus formation in the radius was achieved in 2–3 weeks (Hulse and Hyman, 2003). This coincides with personal observations that in many cases implants such as external fixators can safely be removed after 3 weeks. In the chicken study, complete bone healing occurred at day 42.

Complications in bone healing are non-unions and delayed unions. They are usually the result of prolonged instability and/or infection at the site of the fracture. A non-union is defined as the absence of a bridging ossification with persistent interfragmentary tissue consisting of non-mineralized fibrocartilage (Kaderly, 1993). This fibrocartilage is avascular. The treatment of this condition must therefore include the removal of fibrocartilage and opening of the medullary cavity to allow revascularization and development of resorptive channels for remodelling. A form of non-union is pseudoarthrosis and it has been described in the fractured tibiotarsus of a wild White-tailed Sea Eagle (Lierz *et al.*, 2001). In this case it was noteworthy that, although there were no external signs of an open fracture, the fracture site was contaminated with soil.

Equipment

Equipment for hard tissue surgery is likely to reflect the skills of the surgeon and also the techniques most frequently used in a particular setting. Basic avian orthopaedics may be performed with very limited surgical equipment. Avian bones not only heal faster than mammalian bones, but also the risk of complications, such as non-union and osteomyelitis, appears subjectively to be less frequent in birds than in mammals, though scientific evidence for this observation is lacking.

The small size of avian patients requires the use of surgical equipment that is adapted to the anatomical conditions. A selection of appropriate instruments is shown in Figures 15.2 and 15.3.

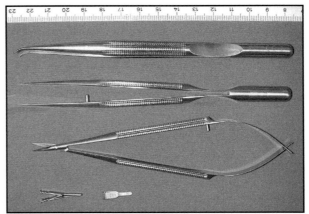

15.2 Atraumatic surgery necessitates the use of special surgical equipment such as microsurgical forceps and scissors. Note the large size and curvature of the handles and the counterweight. The blood vessel clamps are very useful in case of haemorrhage.

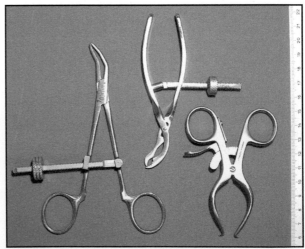

15.3 Useful instruments for avian orthopaedics (from left): angled Doolen bone-holding clamp (5½ inches); Verbrugge-Rogalski bone forceps (1.5 mm × 4 inches); a Guelpi-Neroma retractor (3½ inches).

The recent development of implants in human orthopaedics has also brought about a large choice for the avian surgeon. In particular, miniaturized implants have found several applications.

Pins

There is a large variety of pins used in avian medicine (Figure 15.4). The simplest and cheapest are hypodermic needles used as intramedullary pins in small birds. Such pins have especially been used successfully in diaphyseal tibiotarsal fractures in birds with a body weight <500 g. In large birds, Steinmann intramedullary pins are preferred. These are smooth pins usually with a trocar point on both ends. They are typically available in diameters from 1.6 to 6.3 mm. For smaller species, Kirschner (K-) wires and very small threaded pins may be preferred; they are available with a diameter of 0.8 mm. For external skeletal fixation (ESF), half-pins (which pass through one side of the limb and both bone cortices) or full pins (which pass through both sides of the limb and the bone) may be used.

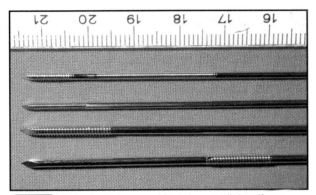

15.4 Selected pins used in avian medicine (from top): negative profile miniature half-pin with roughened surface; negative profile half-pin with a very small thread width; positive profile (rolled-on) half-pin; positive profile full-pin. Positive profile pins are less likely to break than negative profile pins, which is of importance especially in birds >1 kg.

Threading

There are threaded and non-threaded pins and the thread may be partially threaded or centrally threaded. Partially threaded half-pins have a thread that starts directly behind the trocar point and expands over a variable length. In centrally threaded pins the central area of the pin has a thread that starts at a variable distance behind the trocar point.

Non-threaded pins should only be used as full pins in ESF in birds. The avian cortex is too thin to allow stable half-pin positioning that will not carry a significant risk of becoming loose. This is also true when pins are positioned at an angle of 30–40 degrees.

Negative profile pins: The thread is cut into the shaft, which results in a decreased core diameter. These pins were typically used in the early days of veterinary ESF. Negative profile pins tend to break at the thread/non-thread junction and are not considered to have adequate strength for veterinary patients; nevertheless, such pins may still be used, especially in birds <1 kg. In the author's experience, pin fracture

is rare if pins with a very short negative thread are used. This results in the thread/non-thread junction being placed in the medullary cavity, which protects it from cyclic loading and failure from metal fatigue. Negative profile pins are cheaper than positive profile pins and can be placed without pre-drilling, which reduces surgery time. The thread width should be adapted to the cortex so that two threads are placed in the cortex for satisfactory stability.

Positive profile pins: These have a uniform core diameter and are therefore much less susceptible to breaking or bending. Drilling of a pilot hole is highly beneficial for pin placement.

The Miniature INTERFACE™ fixation half-pins (IMEX™ Veterinary Inc., Longview, Texas) are an excellent choice for external fixation in birds. They are available with a shank diameter as small as 0.9 mm and they are typically 75 mm long. The central area of the pin shank is factory-roughened to enhance the interface between the acrylic frame and the pin. These pins are successfully placed without pre-drilling.

Drills and chucks

Pins may be placed with a hand chuck of suitable size; for small patients a miniature hand chuck is available. Hand placement is more prone to oversized pin holes due to wobbling and, as a consequence, pins may become loose. Low-speed power-drill pin placement does not result in significantly increased temperature and thermal necrosis is not an issue; it is therefore preferable and has the additional advantage of reducing surgery time. Unless it is causing significant trauma, a pin that has been drilled too far through the opposite cortex should not be moved backward, as this increases the size of the pin hole.

Plates

Plates are not commonly used in birds. Exceptions are fractures of the pelvic limb in long-legged birds and fractures of the coracoid, especially in large raptors. Figure 15.5 summarizes the advantages and disadvantages of plating *versus* ESF. The reasons for not using plating are the lack of miniaturized plates and the brittleness of avian bone which, with its thin cortices, will not hold implants well. Recent research

	Advantages	Disadvantages
Plating	First intention healing possible. Well suited to bones with important soft tissue covering. Potentially causes less discomfort	Open reduction increases risk of infection. Removal of plates is invasive. Increased costs
External skeletal fixation	Closed fracture reduction sometimes possible. Dynamization of fracture possible by earlier removal of selected pins. Application needs less time	First intention healing rarely achieved. Use may be limited in certain fractures due to space limitations. Fixator may be mauled by bird, or bird may get caught

15.5 Advantages and disadvantages of plating *versus* external skeletal fixation in avian orthopaedics.

into human maxillofacial surgery has resulted in the development of very small plates such as the titanium maxillofacial miniplate Compact 1.0 (Stratec Medical, Oberdorf, Switzerland) (Figure 15.6). These plates have been used successfully in cats and toy-breed dogs (von Werthern and Bernasconi, 2000). In birds they have been used successfully in psittacids and in pigeons up to 500 g to treat fractures of the tibiotarsus and the ulna. Using self-tapping screws reduces surgery time (Levitt, 1989).

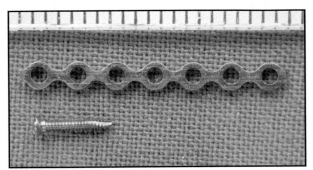

15.6 The titanium maxillofacial miniplate, Compact 1.0 (Stratec Medical, Oberdorf, Switzerland) is cuttable and mouldable. The screws are self-tapping.

An advantage of miniaturized plates is that they can be modelled for best fit along the bone surface. However, this softness also makes them more prone to bending and fracture. Miniplates are not intended for the repair of bones loaded under torsion. In birds, leverage exerted on an ulnar fracture is significantly higher than in companion animals, due to a different relationship of muscle insertions to joints. The use of longer plates in birds compared with similar fractures in small animals has been recommended (Howard, 1990). A longer plate distributes bending forces in a more uniform manner.

Plates should be placed on the tension side of a bone but, to the author's knowledge, the tension side of avian bones have not yet been determined. Double plating is strongly recommended.

External fixators

ESF is the method of choice in most situations requiring hard tissue surgery. The system may be of limited use in very complicated fractures and in fractures that are in close proximity to a joint. The advantages of ESF are its minimal damage to vascularity and excellent stability. In some cases closed fracture reduction is possible, which additionally minimizes vascular damage and the risk of fracture infection.

The most frequently used ESF types are the uniplanar type 1 splint, the uniplanar type 2 splint and the so-called tie-in external fixation type (a combination of intramedullary pin and external fixation) (Figure 15.7). The configuration of the type 2 splint uses more space and its use is usually possible only distal to the elbow or the stifle. Biplanar configuration ESF is very rarely used in birds.

When choosing an ESF system, weight is an important consideration. Figure 15.8 compares the weights of three different systems.

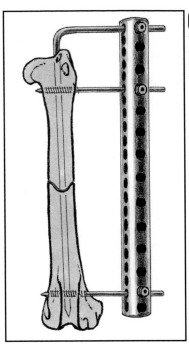

15.7 Tie-in external skeletal fixator in a femur. This type of fixator is often the method of choice in femur and humerus fractures. (Drawing by Matthias Haab.)

System	Weight (g)	Source
Polymethylmethacrylate 6 × 67 mm	2	Hatt *et al.* (2007)
FESSA system 6 × 67 mm with 6 screws	6	Hatt *et al.* (2007)
Kirschner System with 6 clamps	44	Reichler *et al.* (1997)
Menard System with 6 clamps	47	Reichler *et al.* (1997)

15.8 Weight of different systems of connecting bars for external skeletal fixation. (Data from Hatt *et al.*, 2007)

Clamps and connecting bars

Traditionally, Kirschner–Ehmer or Meynard clamps have been used. Steinmann pins are used as fixation pins and connecting bars. Connecting rods are also available in titanium, carbon fibre and aluminium. Compared with stainless steel, titanium is twice as strong and carbon fibre five times as strong, which may allow the use of smaller rods and thus reduce the weight of the system. The connecting bar should always be positioned far enough (typically 1 cm) from the body to allow for swelling and callus formation without entrapment of the skin in the connecting bar.

The most proximal and distal fixation pins are driven through small skin incisions into the two fragments perpendicular to the bone. A connecting bar with clamps is slid on to the end pins with the anticipated number of 'open' clamps in the middle. The fact that adding a clamp at a later stage is somewhat complicated and that the surgeon therefore has to anticipate exactly the number of pins is a disadvantage of the Kirschner–Ehmer and Meynard systems. More recently the IMEX-SK™ external skeletal fixation system has been developed, which, according to the manufacturer, supports the use of positive profile pins directly through the primary clamp bolt, allows the surgeon to add a fixation clamp easily as needed, and provides the freedom to utilize a great variety of pin diameters and styles. The small apparatus may be used in raptors and pigeons.

Tubular fixators

A disadvantage of the clamps is that they add significant weight. Additionally, the width of the clamp limits the distance between pins to approximately 5 mm. This disadvantage does not occur if a tubular fixator is used, which combines the function of both connecting rod and clamps. In the author's experience the FESSA (Fixateur Externe du Service de Santé des Armées) tubular external fixator has proved to be very useful for a wide range of fracture types. The FESSA tubular external fixator is lightweight and was specifically developed for use in complex fractures of the hands and feet in humans (Meyrueis *et al.*, 1993).

The FESSA (Figure 15.9) is made of stainless steel and different models are available with diameters of 6, 8 and 12 mm, for which pins of up to 2 mm and 2.5 mm, respectively, may be used. The length of the fixators varies from 30 to 118 mm. To elongate the system further, a linear or angular combination of two fixators is possible. A system of screws and holes used to attach the pins in the tube replaces the connecting rod and clamps in other ESF systems. Minimum distance between pins is 2 mm. The pins may be placed perpendicular or, by exiting through the neighbouring hole, at an angle of approximately 30 degrees (as shown in Figure 15.9). The fixator may be used in different ways, such as a type 1, type 2, or type 3 external fixator or as a tie-in fixator.

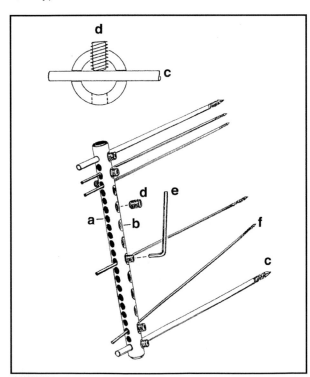

15.9 Schematic view of the components of the FESSA external fixator. Tube with (a) gliding and (b) threaded holes, (c) Kirschner pins, (d) screws and (e) allen key. Fixation of pin (c) perpendicular or (f) at 30 degree angle. (Reproduced from Hatt *et al.*, 2007, with permission)

Polymethylmethacrylate

An alternative to using rods or tubes as connecting bars is polymethylmethacrylate. PMMA can be modelled according to the bone form and allows free-form bars. This is especially useful in bones that are curved and also allows placement of pins at a very small distance. Instead of inserting first the most proximal and distal pin and connecting them to a rod, the surgeon inserts all necessary pins. The free ends of the pins may be bent at 90 degrees; PMMA is mixed until it is of doughy consistency and applied around the pins. PMMA can also be injected into a latex tube (Penrose drain) which has been placed over the free ends of the pins at a distance of 1–2 cm from the bone (Figure 15.10). It is recommended that the pin holes should be marked on the latex tube with a pen to avoid distortion due to the elasticity of the latex. The latex will slide more easily over the pins if these are covered with a drop of alcohol.

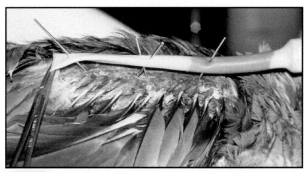

15.10 PMMA being injected into a latex tube (Penrose drain). When hardened this will be the connection bar of a type-1 external skeletal fixator.

With free-form bars the small area of contact between the cement and the smooth pin surface may result in instability. It is therefore strongly recommended that the miniature INTERFACE™ fixation half-pins discussed above are used.

When using PMMA the alignment of the pins can be difficult and displacement of the fracture may occur until the connecting bar is in place and the PMMA has hardened. Once it has hardened, changes are not possible. These disadvantages have been solved by first applying a connection bar with clamps, which is replaced by a PMMA bar once the fracture reduction is considered satisfactory. Partial dismantling for dynamization is more complicated with the PMMA bar than with the FESSA system or clamps.

Complications

The most common complication in ESF is drainage around a fixation pin. Restriction of activity and cleansing of the pin site with 2% hydrogen peroxide has been advocated in mammals and is also recommended for birds (Egger, 1998).

Perioperative management

Stabilization

Since fractures and luxations are usually the result of trauma, the patient may need to be stabilized prior to surgery, with treatment of shock, haemorrhage and sepsis. Treatment may include fluid therapy and re-feeding (see Chapter 7).

Whereas fractures and torn tendons may still be treated successfully after several days, luxations should be restored within 3 days. Fractures may be stabilized temporarily with external coaptation with a bandage or a splint. In certain situations temporary internal fracture fixation such as a reduced tie-in external fixator may be applied.

In open fractures, wound management is important. When necrotic or foreign material is in a wound, surgical debridement needs to be carried out to reduce the risk of infection and sepsis and improve wound healing. In addition to removing tissue with the scalpel, the wound should be flushed with a 2% polyhexanide solution (Lavasept) or iodophores such as undiluted Betadine solution. Special care must be taken with pneumatized bones (e.g. humerus) that foreign material is not further introduced into the respiratory system by flushing, thus resulting in respiratory tract disease.

Analgesia

Pre- and postoperative management must also include analgesia (see Chapter 10). Not using analgesia because it results in the bird not using a damaged limb and hence results in less stress on the implant is not acceptable. Fractures have to be treated in such a way that the animal can use the limb as needed.

Antibiotics

It is advisable to treat any bird with antibiotics before surgery. Uncomplicated cases can be maintained on cephalosporins, enrofloxacin or amoxicillin/clavulanate. It should be kept in mind that certain antibiotics, such as enrofloxacin, cause irritation at the site of injection and therefore should preferably be given subcutaneously or orally, and never into the pectoral muscles.

In a bird that presents with an open wound, special attention needs to be given to antibiotic treatment (e.g. clindamycin) that will be effective against the development of osteomyelitis. Antibiotic-impregnated PMMA beads have been implanted with success. The author has also had good results with gentamicin sponges: the antibiotic is released for approximately 3 days; the collagen carrier is resorbed after 3 months.

There are different opinions about concurrently using antimycotics in these situations. In birds that are especially prone to respiratory mycosis (e.g. Goshawk, Snowy Owl), it may be advisable to combine antibiotic treatment with an antimycotic, such as itraconazole or voriconazole.

Antibiotic treatment is generally continued for one week after surgery, but if osteomyelitis is considered a risk the treatment will have to be prolonged to 2 or more weeks. Antimycotic treatment will be given for at least 3 weeks.

Postoperative management

Postoperative wound management should start 24 hours after surgery. If a bandage has been applied, it needs to be removed and the surgical site inspected. Pin tracts of external fixators are inspected for signs of infection and treated with an iodinated ointment such as Betadine. Fistulae are explored and sequestra are removed if necessary. Sutures and pin tracts with signs of infection should be treated with an antibiotic ophthalmic ointment such as a combination of bacitracin, neomycin and polymyxin (Vetropolycin®, Pharmaderm). Where there are complications, especially infection, performing culture and sensitivity testing is highly recommended. In addition the husbandry of patients needs to be continuously monitored, and improved if necessary.

In uncomplicated cases bandages should be removed within 3 days of surgery. If the bandage has to be left in place for a prolonged time, physical therapy should be initiated within a week postoperatively. Without physical therapy there is a significant risk of permanent loss of flexibility of joints. Physical therapy is also of great importance to inhibit contraction of tendinous structures such as the propatagium. Contraction of the propatagium may result in an altered conformation of the leading edge of the wing, or a wing that is incapable of full extension. Physical therapy will be applied once or twice a week and in most cases will be carried out with the patient under general anaesthesia. Extension followed by flexion should be carried out carefully as far as the joint allows. The exercises should take 5–10 minutes.

Radiographs are taken immediately postoperatively and after approximately 2 weeks. Uncomplicated fractures in birds will be stable after 2–3 weeks and implants can be removed. Dynamization by removing only some pins of an external skeletal fixator may promote healing. The callus can usually be palpated but radiographically it may not yet be evident. For an arthrodesis, implants have to remain for a longer period, typically 6 weeks or more.

Accommodation

For the best possible fracture healing, it is important that the bird is kept in a quiet place after surgery. Birds may have to get used to an implant and may become agitated for some time. The author recommends keeping the bird in a box with smooth walls in order to prevent feather damage and climbing. The size of such a box is usually smaller than that of a cage, but should in any case allow the bird to stand or perch close to the ground in a physiological position. Additional protection of feathers is recommended with a tail guard and padding of carpal joints.

If complete darkness is considered necessary, phases of light should be given at regular intervals (every 2–4 hours) to allow the bird to feed. In large birds of prey, one feeding a day is acceptable. Only when the bird is calm and has resumed feeding should it be transferred to a more spacious cage or an aviary.

Common techniques

Cage rest

In very small birds up to 200 g and with fractures of non-weight-bearing bones, cage rest for 3 weeks may be an acceptable method of therapy, especially in young growing birds. Fracture healing will occur within

3–4 weeks. For birds that will be flown outside their cage this method may not be suitable, since a complete return to function is less likely than with surgical fixation. Exceptions are fractures of the ulna or the radius. As long as the dislocation is only of minor concern, cage rest might be acceptable since the healthy bone will act as a splint (see Figure 15.1).

External coaptation

This method is rarely appropriate as the sole method of fracture repair in birds. The prolonged immobilization of joints and frequently poor alignment of the fracture typically prohibit a full return to function. The most likely condition for external coaptation is in very small birds (<200 g) and in cases with metabolic bone disease, when bones are too soft to hold implants. An important exception for the use of bandages and splints in larger birds is as a method of initial immobilization, such as for the stabilization of a critically ill patient or for referral to a specialized clinic where surgery can be performed. Figure 15.11 summarizes different methods of external coaptation in relation to the affected bone.

Any method of external coaptation will only be successful if the joints proximal and distal to the fracture are adequately immobilized. The most commonly used external coaptation is the figure-of-eight bandage around the wing (Figure 15.12). If the fracture involves the elbow or the humerus the bandage is also applied around the body. The unaffected wing should not be bandaged. Care must be taken to allow the bird normal respiration.

A frequently used type of splint is the Altman splint (Figure 15.13). These splints have often been used with success, especially in small passerine birds, to immobilize fractures of the tibiotarsus and the tarsometatarsus. Splints have been created from different materials such as veterinary thermoplastic, wood or metal, and special tapes. The appropriate material is mainly influenced by the body weight of the patient and the location of the fracture. Tibiotarsal fractures can easily be treated with tapes in small passerine birds, but thermoplastic splints are more suitable in fractures of the digits or metacarpal bones, especially in larger birds.

Fracture	Figure-of-eight bandage	Altman tape splint	Other type of fixation	Comments
Coracoid/clavicle/scapula	✓			Figure-of-eight bandage also around the thorax. Cage rest alone 5–6 weeks, possible if no wing droop. Surgery recommended in coracoid fractures, especially when fracture ends are dislocated
Humerus	✓			Figure-of-eight bandage also around the thorax. Bandage only for short-term stabilization, prior to surgery
Radius/ulna	✓			Bandaging alone may be satisfactory in simple fractures if only ulna or radius affected. Beware of synostosis between radius and ulna, as well as propatagial contraction
Carpometacarpus	✓		Cranial U-shaped splint	Splint made of thermoplastic, moulded around metacarpus
Pelvis				Cage rest for 5–6 weeks. Prognosis good as long as no neurological deficits
Femur			Whole-body wrap with affected leg	Recommended only in birds below 200g body weight. Femur should not be immobilized in extended but in a perching position, since this will automatically bring the fracture ends into physiological apposition
Tibiotarsus		✓		
Tarsometatarsus		✓		In small birds especially, coaptation recommended, due to risk of damaging tendons or vascularization with surgical implants
Phalanges			Tape splint with a shoe	See Figure 15.24

15.11 External coaptation for the immobilization of different fracture types in birds of prey, pigeons and passerine birds. (Note: in birds with a body weight above 200 g, bandages are usually not recommended as the sole method of treatment of long bone fractures).

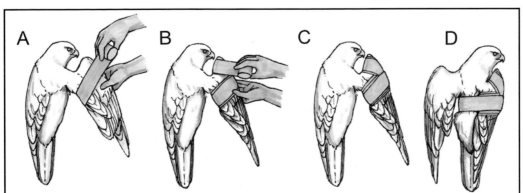

15.12 Figure-of-eight bandage for the immobilization of the wing (A–C). If the fracture involves the elbow or humerus, the bandage is also applied around the body (D). (Drawing by Matthias Haab)

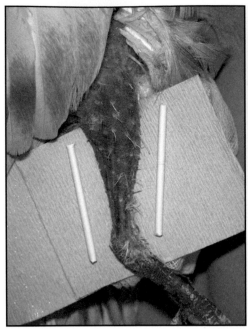 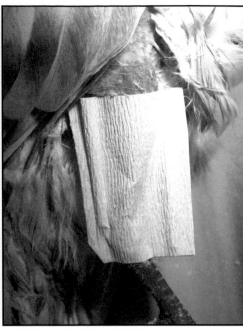

15.13
Altman splint for the immobilization of a tibiotarsal fracture. Ear-cleaner tips have been integrated into the splint to give additional stability.

A special type of bandaging in birds of prey, especially during rehabilitation, includes tail sheets (see Chapter 6) and carpal protection splints. These are intended to protect retrices and joints, respectively, against damage, the ultimate goal being that captivity does not lead to further damage in a bird intended for release.

All bandages and splints must be monitored closely for soiling, slippage, vascular compromise and other signs that replacement is required.

The major disadvantage of external coaptation is the instability and immobilization of the joints adjacent to the fracture, which may result in joint pathology if no adequate physiotherapy is used. With external coaptation, bone healing will take approximately twice as long as following osteosynthesis.

Internal fixation

The methods applied are intramedullary pinning, plating and ESF. Figure 15.14 includes suggested methods of internal fixation in relation to the affected bone. A prerequisite for internal fixation is physiological bone quality and a patient that is stable enough to undergo surgery. Cerclages, hemicerclages and interfragmentary wires are rarely used, because they have a negative effect on vascularization.

Fracture	External fixation	Internal fixation	Other type of fixation	Comments
Coracoid/clavicle/scapula		Intramedullary pin or plating		Clavicula and scapula usually 5–6 weeks' cage rest. In captive birds and little dislocation of fragments of coracoid, cage rest for 5–6 weeks is good therapeutic option. If wing droop present, figure-of-eight bandage put around thorax is advisable
Humerus	Intramedullary pin/external skeletal fixation tie-in		In very distal fractures where fragment does not allow insertion of external pins, cross-pinning with K-wires is option	See Figures 15.17–15.19. Use of sole intramedullary pin without external fixation only if full return to flight not prerequisite
Radius/ulna	External fixation and intramedullary pinning of diaphyseal fracture of ulna with dorsal type-1 external skeletal fixator recommended if both bones fractured or where complete restitution to be achieved (e.g. falconry birds)	For stabilization of radius		Conservative therapy with figure-of-eight bandage may be satisfactory if only one of two bones fractured and no significant displacement of fragment. Plating of ulna (see Figure 15.20) has been successfully performed in pigeons using miniplates
Carpometacarpus	Type-1 or tie-in external fixator			In smaller birds splints may be best treatment option

15.14 Suggested methods for surgical fracture management in birds of prey, pigeons and passerine birds. (continues) ▶

Fracture	External fixation	Internal fixation	Other type of fixation	Comments
Pelvis				Cage rest for 5–6 weeks. Prognosis good as long as no neurological deficits
Femur	Intramedullary pin/external skeletal fixation tie-in		Fractures of trochanter and proximal femur may be repaired using tension-band wiring system with K-wires and cerclage wire (Figure 15.21). Distal fractures may be treated with Rush pins or cross-pinning (Harcourt-Brown, 2002) (Figure 15.22)	In small birds splints or intramedullary pinning alone are acceptable therapeutic methods
Tibiotarsus	Type-2 or a tie-in external fixator	Especially in small and medium-sized birds		Postoperatively transitory neuroparalysis may result in non-weight-bearing for 3–5 days. Both affected and unaffected foot should be bandaged during that time to protect from bruising and pododermatitis, respectively
Tarsometatarsus	Type-2 external fixator			In smaller birds splints may be best treatment option
Phalanges			Tape splint	See Figure 15.24

15.14 (continued) Suggested methods for surgical fracture management in birds of prey, pigeons and passerine birds.

External skeletal fixation

ESF is often the method of choice in avian orthopaedics. In particular, comminuted fractures (which frequently occur in birds) are well suited. In contrast to mammals, sequestra formation is unlikely and the fragments will be incorporated into the fracture and add stability. Fragments should be left in place, as long as they are not necrotic. Fixators are applied to most bones of thoracic and pelvic limbs.

An important advantage of ESF is the minimal trauma to osseous vascularity and surrounding soft tissue. Furthermore, as no implants are applied to the fracture site itself, vascularization of the fracture site is not impaired, which is of major importance for the healing process.

Uniplanar type 1 fixators are mainly used in fractures of the ulna or metacarpus. It is important to use threaded pins of approximately one-third of the bone width and they must be well inserted in the contralateral cortex. Uniplanar type 2 fixators may be applied to the tibiotarsus and the tarsometatarsus, as there is enough space for the medial connecting rod. In most cases non-threaded pins will result in satisfactory stability. Unless centrally threaded pins are used, care must be taken to insert at least one pin at an angle of 30 degrees to the bone. If all pins are inserted perpendicular to the bone, the entire fixator system may become unstable. Centrally positive profile pins may be used for additional stability.

Tie-in fixators are usually used in the humerus and femur, but may also be suitable for ulnar or tibiotarsal fractures. The tie-in method combines intramedullary pinning with a uniplanar type 1 external skeletal fixator. The intramedullary pin must fill 50–60% of the medullary cavity and should not exit within the joint. In bones that taper, such as the tibiotarsus, pin diameter should be adjusted accordingly. The free end is bent at a 90 degree angle to be parallel to the other pins (see Figure 15.7). When bending the pin it is very important that no force is transferred to the bone. The use of locking pliers is highly recommended.

As a general rule for type 1 or type 2 external fixators, at least two pins are inserted in each fragment. Tension forces on long bones may be significant in birds. To reduce the risk of occurrence of refracturing proximal or distal to the fixator, the external fixator should cover at least 70% of the bone's length.

Postoperatively, gauze is wedged between the connecting bars and the skin to provide mild compression and to absorb fluids. Together with the connecting bar it is wrapped with adhesive bandage. The gauze is removed after 2–3 days. A coaptive bandage may be applied for the first 2–3 days after surgery.

Plating

The use of plates needs special expertise and usually results in high costs, both for the implants and the equipment. Application is more traumatic than intramedullary pinning or ESF and in most cases needs additional exposure of the fracture. However, plating is more likely to result in first intention healing with very little callus formation.

Currently the results obtained with intramedullary pinning and ESF are still satisfactory in most circumstances. From reports it appears that the coracoid is well suited for plating, especially in larger birds (>1 kg). Plating can be an option in long bone fractures where one of the fragments is too small for the placement of two or three pins. The development of small cuttable and mouldable plates offers new options, and the 1.0 mm and 2.0 mm miniplates from Synthes have significant potential. They may be used with self-tapping screws, with a very narrow thread width, which allows application in bones with very thin cortex, and both makes application easier and requires less time. Most problems in plates are related to bending and breaking rather than screw pullout (Howard, 1990; Christen *et al.*, 2005). It is recommended that all holes of a plate are filled, to reduce the risk of plate breaking. Double plating is preferable where possible and is similar to ESF. In long bones the author recommends that 70% of the bone length should be plated, to counteract the leverage.

Whenever possible plates should be removed when the fracture has healed. In birds kept outside, removing plates may be necessary because of possible pain from cold conduction, especially where only a little soft tissue covers the plate, as on the ulna and the tibiotarsus. Cold conduction is less of a problem with indoor cagebirds and personal experience with leaving plates in place has not revealed any problems; in particular, bone lysis below the plate has not been observed.

Bone grafts

Avian bone is characterized by a thin and very brittle cortex and fractures are frequently comminuted. In general the risk of sequestration in birds is minimal compared with mammals. Therefore, whenever possible, fragments should remain at the fracture site.

When cortex is lost, bone grafts provide a stable absorbable matrix for the ingrowth of host bone. Autogenous grafts are not readily available, especially in smaller birds, without causing a risk of fracture at another site. Storage of allografts is often limited due to the large number of avian species that are presented in the veterinary practice. Therefore the main research interest has focused on xenografts. Cortical allo- and xenografts in pigeons did not contribute to callus formation and there was an increase in foreign body reaction, sequestrum formation and wound infection (MacCoy and Haschek, 1988). The use of xenogenic canine and ratite intramedullary cortical bone pins gave more promising results in pigeons and resulted in uncomplicated healing. Ratite cancellous grafts resulted in increased new bone production when applied in artificial non-union ulnar fractures in pigeons (Mathews *et al.*, 2003). Cancellous autografts may be collected from the sternum. However, further work is needed on bone grafts to develop an adequate method that will be useful under situations other than experimental.

Fractures of the thoracic limb

Fractures of the thoracic limb usually occur following a hard frontal or lateral impact, which is more likely in birds that can reach considerable speed, e.g. for falconry or in aviaries.

Coracoid

In most birds the coracoid is a large bone, which together with the clavicle and the scapula forms the thoracic girdle. Its main action is to support the wing and counteract compression of the thorax by the main flight muscles. The coracoid lies just lateral to the brachiocephalic trunks and the subclavian and common carotid arteries.

The coracoid typically fractures when the bird hits an object with high speed. Cagebirds rarely reach such high speeds and this fracture therefore is more common in birds flown outside. With the exception of wing droop, a coracoid fracture may result in very few or no clinical signs as long as the bird is perching. When the bird is flying the instability in the girdle will result in inability to obtain lift. Captive pigeons, raptors and passerine birds will be observed hopping around instead of flying from one perch to another.

Palpation of the coracoid in small birds is challenging. Typically there are two types of injury: transverse diaphyseal fractures and a tear of the tendinous articulation with the sternum. The former typically results in a significant transverse displacement of the proximal part of the coracoid, which is easily diagnosed by radiography. The fragment may impact on the crop or trachea. A tear of the articulation may be more difficult to diagnose and may only result in the formation of an asymmetry between the two distal ends of the coracoids (Figure 15.15). A prerequisite for diagnosis is perfect ventrodorsal positioning for radiography.

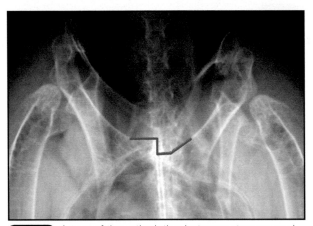

15.15 A tear of the articulation between sternum and right coracoid in a Common Buzzard results in the formation of an asymmetry (line).

Therapeutic options range from simple cage rest to intramedullary pinning and plating of the coracoid. In captive birds with little dislocation of fragments, cage rest for 5–6 weeks is a good option. If wing droop is present, a figure-of-eight bandage around the thorax is advisable. In these cases physical therapy twice weekly should be applied, otherwise ankylosis of the elbow and shortening of the tendon of the propatagium may occur. Malunion and shortening will occur and may interfere with flying. Therefore, if return to full function is necessary, internal fixation appears to be the method of choice. In a study by Holz (2003) it was found that more birds treated surgically could be released to the wild than conservatively treated birds. This reflects a superior overall degree of restitution with surgery.

Surgery may include intramedullary pinning (Figure 15.16) or plating. Access to the coracoid is via a ventral approach by a combination of blunt and sharp dissection and reflection of the pectoral muscles: the superficial muscles are reflected caudally and the deep pectoral muscles are reflected cranially.

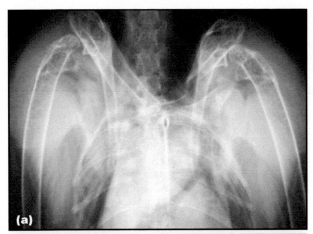

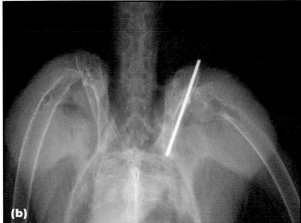

15.16 Tawny Owl with a diaphyseal fracture of the left coracoid with rotation of the proximal fragment, **(a)** before and **(b)** after intramedullary pin placement.

Special care must be taken not to damage pectoral vessels and nerves. Retrograde intramedullary pin placement is chosen from the fragment closest to the shoulder. When advancing the pin, care must be taken not to enter the sternum or the thoracic cavity. Bandaging (figure-of-eight bandage) may or may not be required, but cage rest for 3 weeks is recommended.

A diaphyseal fracture can also be stabilized with one or two miniplates. Physiotherapy twice a week is recommended. Plates on the coracoid may be left in place.

Scapula
Fractures of the scapula are rare and are usually diaphyseal transverse or oblique. They result from a trauma to the back. There usually are no clinical signs; diagnosis is made by radiography. Treatment usually is 5 weeks of cage rest.

Clavicle
Collision injury may in rare cases lead to fractures of the clavicle. Diaphyseal transverse fractures are present. There usually are no clinical signs, though occasionally wing droop may be observed. Diagnosis is made by radiography. This bone is well supported by pectoral muscle and there is only minor dislocation. Treatment is usually 5 weeks of cage rest.

Humerus
Wrong handling, impact or fighting can result in humeral fractures. These are typically diaphyseal transverse or oblique fractures, with one or more fragments. Proximal fractures are well supported by muscles. Wing rotation is frequently observed and luxation, possibly with rupture of the tendon of the supracoracoideus muscle, may also be present. Due to contraction of the biceps and the pectoral muscles, the distal fragment overlaps the proximal fragment. In oblique fractures perforation of the skin is frequent. It should be kept in mind that the humerus is connected to the clavicular air sac and open fractures may result in respiratory tract disease.

Clinical signs, besides inability to fly, are frequently minimal. In distal fractures the rotation of the wing is observed. Upon palpation of the humerus, instability and crepitation are obvious. The diagnosis is corroborated by radiography.

Treatment options should whenever possible include internal fixation. External coaptation such as figure-of-eight bandaging is contraindicated because it causes displacement, which has a negative influence on healing.

For internal fixation the intramedullary pin/external skeletal fixation tie-in is generally the method of choice, because it results in excellent longitudinal and rotational stability (Figure 15.17).

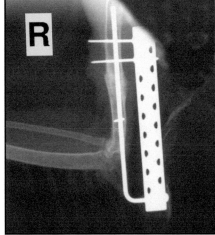

15.17 Tie-in fixator in the humerus of a Kestrel. The fracture has healed without exuberant callus formation.

The bird is positioned in ventral recumbency and the affected wing is stretched out laterally. A lateral approach is chosen and the intramedullary pin is inserted in a normograde fashion from a site just proximal to the distal humeral condyles (Figure 15.18). When choosing the point of entry it must be taken into consideration that there must be enough space for a second pin more distally but still proximal to the epicondyle. The normograde pin insertion is usually chosen in closed diaphyseal fractures, where the distal fragment is smaller. The pin is introduced through a skin insertion proximal to the dorsal epicondylus of the humerus. The fracture is reduced and the pin is driven proximally until it enters the cortex of the proximal humerus. The free part of the pin which exits is then bent at a 90 degree angle approximately 2 cm away from the skin. Special attention has to be given to the radial nerve, which crosses over the distal part of the humerus.

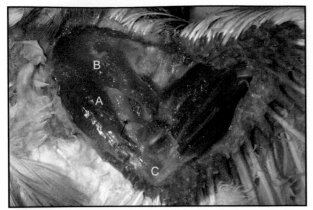

15.18 Dorsal view of the humerus in a pigeon after removal of skin for better visualization of anatomical structures, deltoideus major (A), pars propatagialis of the deltoideus muscle (B), dorsal condylus of the humerus (C), radial nerve crossing the humerus (arrow).

Fracture reduction is possible without opening of the fracture. If the fracture has to be accessed at the proximal humerus, this is done dorsally between the major deltoid muscle and the pars propatagialis. Subsequently the distal pin is inserted just distal to the point of exit of the intramedullary pin. Care should be taken not to insert the pin over the epicondyle, due to potential damage to ligaments and tendons. The third pin is inserted into the proximal humerus in the free edge of the crista deltopectoralis of the dorsal tubercle parallel to the other pins (Figure 15.19). Before insertion of the proximal pin, the wing is folded against the body to bring the bone into physiological alignment. The three pins are then connected to each other with an appropriate connection bar. If the FESSA system is used, the tubular fixator will be applied when the intramedullary and the first pin are in place and the third pin will be set through one of the holes of the fixator.

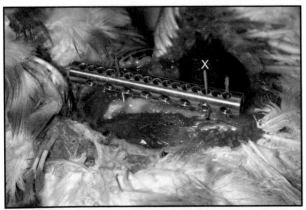

15.19 Dorsal view of the humerus with a tubular external fixator. The distal ends of the pins have not been shortened. The skin has been removed for better visualization. The intramedullary tie-in pin has been marked (X).

As an alternative, the retrograde method is chosen if the distal fragment is larger, starting at the proximal fragment. The pin is driven from the fracture site towards the shoulder to exit the proximal humerus at the dorsal tubercle. The fracture is reduced and the pin is driven into the distal fragment. The free part of the pin is then bent at a 90 degree angle approximately 1–2 cm away from the skin. A second pin is then inserted just distally in the crista deltopectoralis parallel to the intramedullary pin. The wing is folded against the body for physiological alignment and the third pin inserted just proximal to the dorsal epicondyle of the humerus. A fourth pin between the third pin and the fracture is rarely necessary.

In very distal fractures, where the fragment does not allow insertion of external pins, cross-pinning with K-wires may be used, as described for the femur.

The choice of a sole intramedullary pin without ESF should only be taken if full return to flight is not a prerequisite. A normograde insertion of the pin from the distal fragment as described above may also be used. The diameter of the pin should be at least 50% of the bone cavity. Following surgery the wing has to be kept in a figure-of-eight bandage for 3 weeks, with physiotherapy twice a week to avoid ankylosis. Callus formation will take more time (approximately 5 weeks) than with the tie-in method. In comminuted fractures this method is not recommended.

Ulna and radius

In wild birds fractures of the ulna and radius are frequent, especially when a collision with a wire occurs. It is important to differentiate between fractures of one or both bones. If only one of the bones is fractured, no clinical signs will be obvious. In birds where the ulna, which is larger than the radius, is intact, birds may even be able to fly a short distance. If both bones are fractured wing droop will be noted, with the wing tip touching the perch. In nervous birds, torsion of the wing may occur.

Fractures may be diagnosed upon palpation. For a definitive diagnosis and exact evaluation of the fracture, radiography is necessary.

Conservative therapy with a figure-of-eight bandage may be satisfactory if only one bone is fractured and when there is no significant displacement of the fragment. The bandage is applied to the wing, without attaching the wing to the body. The unaffected bone will act as a splint. A possible complication is contraction of the propatagium as a result of prolonged immobilization. This will prevent physiological extension of the wing. In addition there is a risk of synostosis between the ulna and radius, which will prevent the normal action of the two bones sliding longitudinally in relation to each other, when the wing is flexing and extending during flight. Therefore regular physical therapy is important.

ESF and intramedullary pinning of a diaphyseal fracture of the ulna with a dorsal type 1 external skeletal fixator is recommended if both bones are fractured or in cases where complete restitution is to be achieved (e.g. falconry birds). The ulna is approached by bluntly separating the common digital extensor and supinator muscles. An alternative is the application of a tie-in fixator. The intramedullary pin is introduced in a normograde fashion entering at the caudolateral aspect of the ulna distal to the olecranon. Enough space must be left for a second pin, which will be introduced in this fragment between the olecranon and intramedullary pin. The pin is first introduced at almost 90 degrees to the bone and the angle is gradually reduced to achieve alignment with the long axis of the ulna. The fracture is then reduced and the pin advanced until it engages in the cortex. Care should be taken not to enter the carpometacarpal joint. The additional pins are then applied as in the humerus, with the first pin entering between the intramedullary pin and the olecranon. In the distal fragment one or two pins are introduced in the distal extremity of the ulna, without damaging the carpometacarpal joint. To reduce the risk of synostosis between radius and ulna, the radius may be reduced with an intramedullary pin in a retrograde fashion starting at the distal fragment.

Plating of the ulna has been successfully performed in pigeons using miniplates (Figure 15.20). Plates should be removed when the fracture has healed, as the little soft tissue that covers the ulna does not give adequate protection from cold conduction.

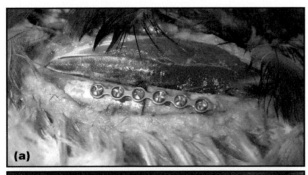

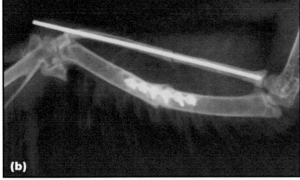

15.20 Plating of the ulna in a pigeon, **(a)** intraoperative view and **(b)** radiography after 4 weeks. There is a bridging callus on the ulna; the radius has been fixed with an intramedullary pin for additional stability.

Carpometacarpus

Projectile impact or squeezing may cause fractures; in most cases these are comminuted. The major challenge is to keep the blood supply unaffected. The wingtip is supplied by only one artery; if this artery is damaged, wingtip necrosis is likely to occur.

Clinical signs are usually restricted to drooping or rotation of the wingtip. Crepitation may be palpated. The extent of the fracture is assessed by radiography.

In simple and closed fractures the application of a cranial U-shaped splint and a figure-of-eight bandage for 3 weeks has been successful. Thermoplastic material can easily been moulded around the carpometacarpus.

In highly comminuted or open fractures the application of a type 1 or a tie-in external fixator is recommended. The approach is from the dorsal side. For the tie-in method the intramedullary pin is introduced retrograde into the major carpometacarpal bone to exit at the dorsal side of the proximal end without entering the joint or damaging the radius. The fracture is reduced and the pin is advanced into the distal fragment until it engages in the cortex. It is advisable to use a pin of only one-third of the width of the major carpometacarpal bone, because a pin needs to be inserted into the proximal and distal fragments. The intramedullary pin is then bent at 90 degrees and the three pins are stabilized with an external fixator bar.

In small birds such as pigeons and passerine species ESF may not be practical. In these birds intramedullary pinning with a Kirschner wire or a hypodermic needle and bandaging will be the method of choice. Another option is to use the calamus of the primary feathers as 'external pins' and join them with thermoplastic such as Hexcelite, Veraform or polypropylene. Fixation will be left in place for 3–4 weeks.

Fractures of the vertebral column

Fractures of the vertebral column typically occur just cranial or caudal to the synsacrum. Depending on the amount of damage to the lumbosacral plexus, there may be neurological deficits. If the lumbar and sacral parts of the plexus are damaged, the withdrawal reflex of the limbs will be absent. A space-occupying mass in the kidney or the pelvic canal may impinge on the lumbosacral plexus and its nerve, causing paresis or reduced withdrawal reflex in the limb. A hanging tail, flaccid vent and over-distended cloaca that is easily expressed indicate lower motor neuron damage to the pudendal nerve or its spinal roots. If the innervation of the cloaca is damaged uncontrolled voiding of excreta will result, with soiling of pericloacal feathers.

Radiography may not always be helpful for diagnosis, especially when there is very little or no dislocation. Myelography or computed tomography may be more suitable for diagnostic work-up.

If there is paralysis of the pelvic limbs and cloaca the prognosis is grave and euthanasia must be discussed. If there is only minor damage to the nerves, 5–6 weeks of cage rest may result in recovery.

Fractures of the pelvic limb

Pelvis

Pelvic fractures are rare and usually no clinical signs are obvious. Lameness or hyperaesthesia may be present if the lumbosacral plexus is affected. If there is severe dislocation of one or several fragments, possible problems with defecation or oviposition should be considered. Pelvic fractures are often accompanied by other fractures. Possible disconnection between the synsacrum and pelvis might occur. Radiographic interpretation of the pelvic anatomy might be difficult, especially if the gastrointestinal tract is full. Prognosis is good as long as there are no neurological deficits. Cage rest for 5–6 weeks is the treatment of choice.

Femur

Open fractures are rare in the femur. The bone is well protected by the iliotobialis and medial femorotibialis muscles, the body wall and the flexor cruris and medial part of the puboischiofemoralis muscles. These strong muscles result in dislocation and contraction of the fracture. The femur typically shows transverse diaphyseal fractures, with little or no comminution. Clinical signs include lameness, with inability to grasp an object. Upon palpation, crepitation may be obvious. However, due to the large muscles, palpation can be challenging. Radiography will be indispensable for diagnosis and for making the therapeutic choice.

Different types of splints, e.g. Spica or Thomas splints, have been described for conservative therapy. These splints are less effective than internal fixation. If conservative therapy is nevertheless chosen, the leg should be immobilized not in an extended but in a perching position, since this will automatically bring the fracture ends into physiological opposition.

In small birds (<300 g), sole intramedullary pinning is an acceptable surgical method. If the curve of the bone is lost this does not seem to have a significant adverse effect on functional use of the leg. The pin is inserted in a retrograde fashion from the fracture in the proximal fragment. The pin exits at the major trochanter and is subsequently pushed into the distal fragment until it engages in the cortex beneath the knee. There is little rotational stability, and healing will take 4–6 weeks. The approach to the femur is lateral. The iliofibularis muscle must be moved caudally and the cranial iliotibialis and external femorotibialis muscles are moved cranially. Care must be taken not to damage the ischiadic artery and nerve, which lie beneath the iliofibularis muscle caudal to the femur.

In larger birds a tie-in fixation is the method of choice. The intramedullary pin is introduced as described before. The free end exiting at the hip is bent laterally at 90 degrees. A distal pin is introduced from lateral to medial in the condyles. A proximal pin is introduced a short distance distal to the head of the femur. This pin must be smaller as it shares the marrow cavity with the intramedullary pin. The free ends are attached to a connecting bar.

Fractures of the trochanter and the proximal femur may be repaired using a tension-band wiring system with K-wires and cerclage wire (Figure 15.21). Distal fractures may be treated with Rush pins or cross-pinning as described by Harcourt-Brown (2002) (Figure 15.22).

Tibiotarsus

In captive birds the tibiotarsus, especially the proximal one third, is the most frequently affected bone. In birds of prey a major cause is when the leash used to tether the birds is too long, allowing the bird to get up speed when bating. The tibiotarsus is also the bone most frequently affected when metabolic bone disease is present.

> **Clinical signs are lameness, with the leg usually kept hanging behind the perch (in contrast to paralysis of nerves, where the leg is kept in a 'hand for a kiss' position on the perch).**

Fractures are usually diaphyseal with or without comminution, depending on whether it was a high- or low-energy impact. The tibiotarsus is surrounded by little soft tissue and both palpation and surgical access to the fracture are easy.

In very small birds (<200 g) an Altman tape splint will be the method of choice for diaphyseal fractures. It is important to include the femorotibial and the intertarsal joints in the bandage (see Figure 15.13).

Intramedullary pinning of the tibiotarsus is probably the orthopaedic intervention in birds with the longest tradition. Surgical approach to the tibia is from craniomedial between the cranial tibial and the gastrocnemius muscles, to avoid the lateral veins,

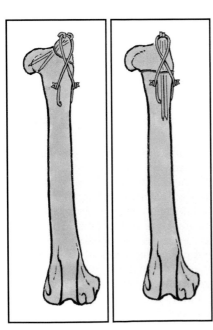

15.21 Fractures of the trochanter are usually stabilized with two pins and tension-band fixation. Twist knots are formed on both sides of the figure-of-eight tension band to allow symmetrical tightening. (Drawing by Matthias Haab)

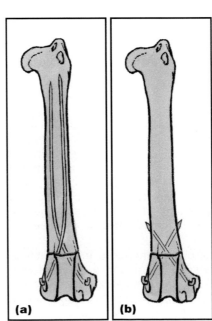

15.22 Fixation of fractures of the distal metaphysis of the femur may be treated with **(a)** Rush pins or **(b)** cross-pins. (Drawing by Matthias Haab)

(a) (b)

arteries and nerves. The pin is then advanced retrograde into the proximal fragment to exit on the cranial aspect of the proximal tibia, thus avoiding the patellar tendon and cruciate ligaments. The pin is then pushed towards the intertarsal joint. This method offers excellent alignment but poor rotational stability. Fracture healing will take approximately 5–6 weeks.

A modification of this method is to use nickel–titanium alloy pins, which have a 'memory' and can be bent at 180 degrees and will spring back to the normal position. The pins can be inserted into both fragments from the site of fracture, without needing to exit near a joint. These pins are not removed following fracture healing.

The repair of fractures of the distal tibiotarsus is complicated by two tendons. The tendon of insertion of the cranial tibial muscle runs over the cranial surface of the intertarsal joint through a fibrous retinaculum. The tendon of insertion of the long digital extensor muscle runs under the fibrous supratendinal bridge, on the cranial aspect of the bone deep to the cranial tibial muscle. The free running of these tendons should not be compromised.

In comminuted fractures the method of choice is a uniplanar type-2 external skeletal fixator (Figure 15.23). Two pins are inserted into the proximal and distal fragment each. Positive profile full pins may be used for the highest degree of stability. In the author's experience Steinmann pins work well in birds up to 1 kg. Approach to the bone is from the craniomedial aspect. The most proximal and distal pins are inserted first and connected with the connection bar, at a distance to restore the physiological length of the tibiotarsus. The distal pin should be placed 2–3 mm proximal to the condyles. Care must be taken not to damage the long digital extensor tendon and the medial metatarsal vein. The proximal pin is introduced just cranial to the fibula. Subsequently a second pin is inserted into each fragment. One of these pins needs to be inserted at an oblique 30 degree angle to the

bone, to avoid instability of the bone fragments. A type-2 external fixator will result in the fastest healing and can usually be removed after 2 weeks.

For tibiotarsal fractures with little or no comminution, Redig (2002) recommended lateral tie-in ESF. The intramedullary pin is either introduced at the tibial table on the lateral aspect of the femorotibial joint and passed normograde into the proximal and distal fragments, or introduced at the fracture site and retrograded at the stifle. In either case the patellar tendon has to be displaced to protect it against pin penetration.

Postoperatively, transitory neuroparalysis may result in non-weight-bearing for 3–5 days. Both the affected and unaffected foot should be bandaged during that time to protect from bruising and pododermatitis, respectively.

Tarsometatarsus

In most birds of prey this bone is long, flat and C-shaped. Fractures are commonly caused when birds get caught in the leg band and they tend to be comminuted. Clinical signs are similar to a tibiotarsal fracture. The foot is frequently rotated laterally.

Surgical access is difficult due to the large number of ligaments and tendons. In particular the flexor tendon in the flexor groove has to be avoided. It runs in the groove on the caudal aspect of the tarsometatarsus. A uniplanar type-2 external fixator is the method of choice in comminuted fractures. When applying an external fixator it should be noted that the artery and nerve lie dorsally, and the veins laterally and medially.

In birds <200 g an Altman tape splint can be recommended. As with all splints, the joint proximal and distal to the fracture must be included.

Other alternatives include the use of external coaptation, though this is an area where it is very easy to damage a tendon, especially in birds where the bone is slightly curved around the tendon sheath.

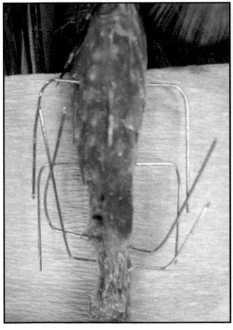 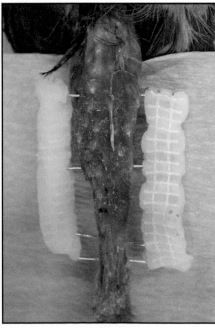

15.23 Uniplanar type-2 external skeletal fixator in the tibiotarsus of a pigeon. In this small bird Kirschner wires have been used and the connecting bar is made of veterinary thermoplastic.

Phalanges

Squeezing, tearing or biting wounds often result in fracture and significant soft tissue trauma. The fracture is usually closed. Malposition and/or deviation of the affected digit and even lameness may be clinical signs. Automutilation may be a result, especially if innervation of the digit is impaired. Cage rest or tape splints are usually the method of choice. Splints may be manufactured as a shoe on to which the digits will be taped (Figure 15.24). Cardboard may be used in small birds, such as passerines; in larger birds Hexcelite, Veraform or polypropylene is preferable. When splints are used a stiff toe may result, and physical therapy is recommended as a preventive measure.

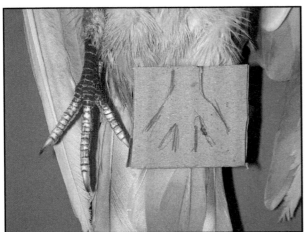
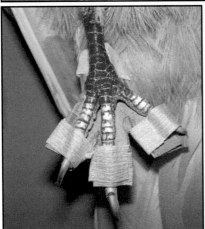

15.24 Phalangeal fractures in small birds (generally below 200 g body weight) can be treated with splints. Regular physical therapy is important to minimize the risk of a stiff toe due to adhesions.

Digit amputation

With open or comminuted fractures, amputation of the affected digit has to be contemplated. However, the consequences for a bird of prey will have to be taken into consideration. The first and second digits are of great importance and amputation may preclude the patient's future use as a falconry bird.

Amputation of a digit can be performed either by disarticulation or by mid-diaphyseal cut. It is essential to clean the feet carefully before surgery, since they are commonly soiled with faeces and urine. To reduce haemorrhage a tourniquet is applied proximally. The skin is incised distally to the joint or diaphysis in the dorsal two thirds of the digit. Radiosurgery or a scalpel blade may be used. The joint is disarticulated proximal the affected bone, with the help of rongeurs. The diaphyseal cut is made with a saw; in small passerine

birds a scalpel could be appropriate. The remaining plantar skin is cut distally enough at a point to allow a flap to be pulled dorsally. Skin closure in a simple interrupted pattern is made with 1–1.5 metric (4/0–5/0) non-absorbable monofilament suture material. The tourniquet must be removed, and a bandage is applied for 3 days postoperatively.

Beak repair techniques

Diseases of the beak are rarer in raptors, pigeons and passerine birds than in psittacines and there is less force acting on the beak. The major problems that affect birds of prey in particular are overgrowth and trauma.

Trauma

The major reason for beak trauma is collision or entrapment. Part of the beak may be lost or the beak may be fractured. Such problems are usually presented as an emergency, especially when there is significant bleeding. Treatment should aim at preventing a worsening of the condition and at guaranteeing that the bird can feed normally. In passerine birds, which have a high metabolic rate, anorexia can quickly result in a life-threatening condition.

Clinical signs of beak trauma are usually obvious and the history may indicate what happened. If fractures are suspected, radiography is an important diagnostic aid. It is necessary to use high-quality films with high detail such as dental or mammography films (see Chapter 11). Figure 15.25 shows a fracture of the mandible in a Tawny Owl. Subluxation of the upper beak might also occur.

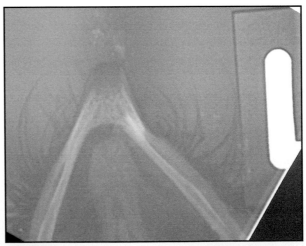

15.25 Radiograph of a fracture of the left mandible of a Tawny Owl. Dental film was used for high resolution.

Therapy is aimed at allowing the bird to feed normally as soon as possible. If an open wound is present it should be carefully cleaned with, for example, a diluted chlorhexidine solution or a 2% polyhexanide solution, to avoid development of an infectious process. Minor damage to the beak may be treated by applying cerclage wires (Figure 15.26), PMMA or bioactive glass.

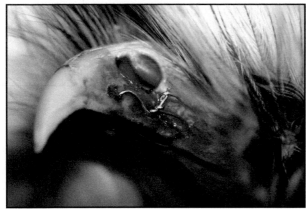

15.26 Fracture of the upper beak in a Great Grey Owl immobilized with a cerclage wire.

If a large part of the beak is missing, the prognosis should be evaluated carefully. A beak prosthesis will only be of temporary help, but may allow an initial period of inability to ingest food to be overcome. If the prosthesis is not supported with implants in the bone, it is likely to fall off within a few days. If an open wound is present, there is a significant risk of a prosthesis hiding the development of an infectious process. Thus the use of a prosthesis is not warranted as long as the bird is feeding.

It might be necessary to feed the bird artificially at first. Analgesics and antibiotics are used as for the perioperative management of an osteosynthesis. The healing process is likely to take several months. If there is malformation, regular beak trimming may become necessary.

Overgrown beak
This condition is rare in pigeons and passerine birds but frequent in raptors, especially falcons. Captive management often does not allow adequate use and wear of the beak, and the rich diet in captivity also promotes beak growth. Trauma may result in malformation and irregular wear, which also leads to overgrowth. The clinical signs are an obviously malformed beak and possibly anorexia. Chapter 8 gives details of beak trimming.

If malformation is present, such as a scissor beak, this can be corrected with a prosthesis. The prosthesis is applied to the tip of the beak and increases its length. The length and direction of the prosthesis will be such as to form a scissor in the opposite direction, which will result in a temporary overcorrection. The prosthesis is left in place for 8 weeks and the patient needs to be monitored carefully to avoid permanent overcorrection. In chicks, the direction of the beak may be corrected by physical therapy: the beak is pushed into the physiological position 6–8 times a day.

Joint luxation

Disease of joints may be traumatic (luxation, fractures that involve the joint), infectious (septic arthritis, e.g. *Salmonella*, *Escherichia coli*, *Mycoplasma*) or metabolic (e.g. articular gout). In birds of prey the most frequent joint disease is traumatic, whereas in pigeons infection, especially salmonellosis, frequently manifests in the elbow. This condition is discussed in more detail in Chapter 29.

Traumatic injuries are emergencies not so much because of survival, but because of prognosis. By 3 days after luxation the joint will show fibrosis and therapy will be unsuccessful. Especially in wild birds, which are frequently only caught several days after the injury occurred, joint disease is often a reason for euthanasia because full restitution of function is unlikely. In captive birds the impairment may be of lesser importance and surgical arthrodesis will be an option in certain cases.

Particularly with luxations, tendons may be damaged, but they can be repaired and this does not need to be done immediately. After 4–6 weeks the sheath will have reacted with granulation tissue. This highly vascularized tissue can be used to cover the suture. It is important to suture both the tendon and the sheet. A bandage is applied for 4–6 weeks.

Shoulder girdle
Clinical signs of a luxation in the shoulder girdle are subtle and may involve a minor lateral rotation of the wing. Palpation of an instability or crepitation may be difficult for the inexperienced veterinary surgeon. The shoulder is well surrounded by muscles. Radiography is important for diagnosis and additional fractures should be looked for. Treatment will involve repositioning and bandaging for 2–3 weeks. Prognosis is good for cagebirds, but full restitution is rare in birds that are flown.

Elbow
Luxation of the elbow is frequent in raptors and typically occurs when the bird gets caught, e.g. in a wire. The bird will show wing droop and inability to extend the wing fully, and swelling will be noted on palpation. There is little soft tissue around the elbow, which makes diagnosis easier than in the shoulder.

Diagnosis is made by radiography with lateral and anteroposterior views. In most cases there is a caudodorsal luxation involving both the radiohumeral and the ulnohumeral joints (Figure 15.27). In cases of doubt radiography is performed with maximal bending and stretching. With ruptured ligaments the joint space will be abnormally wide.

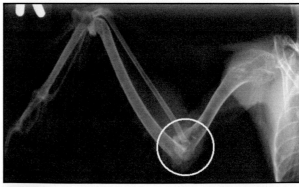

15.27 Elbow luxation in a Hobby. In most cases a caudodorsal luxation involving both the radiohumeral and the ulnohumeral joints is present, as in this case (circled).

Both closed and surgical reduction have been described. Success rates vary from 25% to 50%, depending on the author. Reduction is attempted under general anaesthesia. The distal humerus is grasped with one hand, whilst the other hand holds the radius and ulna. The joint is flexed and the radius and ulna are rotated, applying pressure so that the radius is forced into alignment with the dorsal humeral condylus. When repositioning has occurred (which can be felt as a 'pop'), the elbow is slowly extended. The joint is subsequently immobilized with a transarticular type-1 external skeletal fixator involving the humerus and ulna for 7–10 days.

A surgical treatment has been described by Helmer and Redig (2006) whereby the elbow joint is approached dorsally and the tendon of origin of the supinator muscle transected. Subsequently the ulna is leveraged into alignment with the humerus, using a periostal elevator. The supinator tendon has to be resutured and a pseudocollateral ligament is created by suturing the triceps tendon to the common digital extensor tendon. The joint will also need to be immobilized with a transarticular type-1 external skeletal fixator. A figure-of-eight bandage is recommended during the first 5–7 days after surgery. After removing the bandage, physical therapy under general anaesthesia is performed two or three times a week. If reluxation occurs following removal of the fixator, the joint should be reassessed for ruptured tendons which need to be sutured. Surgical arthrodesis might be the last resort.

Carpus

Clinical signs of luxation in the carpus are similar to the condition termed 'angel wing' in growing waterfowl, i.e. an outward rotation of the wingtip. The carpal bone is usually luxated in a ventral direction. Diagnosis may be difficult for the inexperienced veterinary surgeon and it is advisable to perform radiography on both wings for comparative purposes. Fractures may also be present. Under general anaesthesia the carpus is extended and the wingtip is abducted laterally. At the same time the metacarpal bone is pushed dorsally with the thumb. After repositioning, the wing is wrapped in a figure-of-eight bandage for 7–10 days.

Hip joint

The hip joint in birds involves the head of the femur, which articulates with the acetabulum, and the trochanter of the femur, which articulates with the antitrochanter of the pelvis, allowing some birds to perch on one leg. The femoral head is connected to the acetabulum by the femoral ligament and supported by thickenings of the joint capsule. The ventral collateral and the round ligament have major roles in maintaining the proper position of the femoral head. Dislocation can only occur by rupturing the ligament and often avulsion fracture of the femoral head will be present. The caudodorsal joint capsule is frequently torn. The femur is in most cases dislocated in a dorsal or craniodorsal direction and the leg is held in a non-weight-bearing extended position.

Diagnosis is made by radiology. It is recommended that radiographs are taken of both joints for comparative purposes. Exact lateral positioning is a prerequisite for the determination of the direction of the dislocation. In cases where the luxation is not older than 3 days, repositioning followed by 3 weeks of cage rest is a treatment option. If a surgical approach to the joint is necessary, this should be made from the caudolateral approach between the iliotibialis and the iliofibularis muscles. Harcourt-Brown (2002) described a method by which the iliotiobial and iliofibular muscles are used to stabilize the hip joint. MacCoy (1989) successfully used a femoral head ostectomy with a muscle sling made from the iliofibularis muscle in two psittacine birds. An alternative to this method has been described where, after removing the head of the femur, the sutures are placed from the femoral trochanter to the cranial rim of the acetabulum and to the ala prae-acetabularis. Surgery is followed by 3 weeks of cage rest. It is important to prevent flying during recovery, due to the negative impact on the joint when landing. Surgical methods appear to be superior to slings or splints, which result in pseudoarthrosis or muscle contraction without significant clinical improvement.

The use of pins and transfixation is not recommended because of the proximity of the kidney, blood vessels and nerves to the acetabulum.

Femorotibial joint (stifle)

The femorotibial joint is similar to that of mammals and contains two menisci, cranial and caudal cruciate ligaments and collateral ligaments. The fibula does not engage in the joint. Clinical signs of luxation are paresis, with rupture of the cranial and caudal cruciate ligaments as well as collateral ligaments. The tibiotarsus is frequently dislocated caudally. In luxations that have just happened and where only minor disruption of ligaments is suspected, repositioning and cage rest for 3 weeks have been successful.

In more severe cases, with complete disruption, surgical intervention is necessary. In an attempt to save the joint, repair of ligaments and use of replacement ligaments with Teflon suture material may be tried. Hypodermic needles are used to drill holes in the bone and the suture material is then threaded through the needle. Often transarticular external fixation will be the method of choice, resulting in arthrodesis. Different methods have been described, such as transarticular type-1 external skeletal fixators or intramedullary pins in the proximal tibiotarsus and the distal femur which exit at the knee and are joined with acrylics in a partially flexed perching position. For the initiation of the process it is important to remove joint cartilage with rongeurs or a drill.

A frequent complication of stifle disease is bumblefoot on the contralateral foot. Even with successful arthrodesis, unequal weight-bearing may be present and this predisposes birds to pododermatitis. During cage rest after surgery, the feet should therefore be bandaged (see Chapter 16).

Intertarsal joint

Most frequently, dislocation in the intertarsal joint involves the tendon of the flexor hallucis longus muscle. The tendon bursts out of its position and lies to the lateral aspect of the tibial cartilage, usually as a sequel to trauma. The bird is unable to use its leg. If seen within a day or two of the event, the tendon is easily repositioned surgically. The tunnel that the tendon occupied is readily identified and the tendon can be repositioned. The tear is repaired with polydioxanone. Postsurgically the bird should be kept in a deep narrow container to avoid the tendency for the leg to splay and therefore repeat damage. In chronic cases of tendon displacement it is better to leave the tendon rather than attempt repositioning surgically.

Phalangeal joints

Phalangeal joints may be dislocated without permanent ligament damage. Replacement is done under general anaesthesia, without external support. If a collateral ligament is broken and there is no additional trauma, the ligament should be repaired with polyglactin suture material.

Acknowledgements

Matthias Haab from the Department of Horses, Vetsuisse Faculty, University of Zurich, is very much thanked for his drawings (Figures 15.7, 15.12, 15.21 and 15.22).

References and further reading

Ackermann J and Redig P (1997) Surgical repair of elbow luxations in raptors. *Journal of Avian Medicine and Surgery* **11**, 247–254

Bush M, Montali RJ, Novak GR and James AE (1976) The healing of avian fractures: a histological xeroradiographic study. *Journal of the American Animal Hospital Association* **12**, 768–773

Christen C, Fischer I, von Rechenberg B, Flückiger M and Hatt J-M (2005) Evaluation of a maxillofacial miniplate compact 1.0 for the fracture repair in pigeons (*Columba livia*). *Journal of Avian Medicine and Surgery* **19**, 185–190

Clark WD, Smith EL, Linn KA, Paul-Murphy JR and Cook ME (2005) Use of peripheral quantitative computed tomography to monitor bone healing after radial osteotomy in three-week-old chickens (*Gallus domesticus*). *Journal of Avian Medicine and Surgery* **19**, 198–207

Clippinger TL, Bennett RA and Platt SR (1996) The avian neurological examination and ancillary neurodiagnostic techniques. *Journal of Avian Medicine and Surgery* **10**, 221–247

Egger EL (1998) External skeletal fixation. In: *Current Techniques in Small Animal Surgery, 4th edn*, ed. MJ Bojrab, pp. 941–950. Williams & Wilkins, Baltimore

Harcourt-Brown NH (1996) Foot and leg problems. In: *BSAVA Manual of Raptors, Pigeons and Waterfowl*, ed. PE Beynon *et al.*, pp. 147–168. BSAVA, Cheltenham

Harcourt-Brown NH (1999) *Birds of Prey: Anatomy, Radiography & Clinical conditions of the Pelvic Limb*. Zoological Education Network, Greenacres, Florida

Harcourt-Brown NH (2000) Tendon repair in the pelvic limb of birds of prey: part II surgical considerations. In: *Raptor Biomedicine, III edn*, ed. JT Lumeij *et al.*, pp. 217–237. Zoological Education Network, Lake Worth, FL

Harcourt-Brown NH (2002) Orthopedic conditions that affect the avian pelvic limb. *Veterinary Clinics of North America: Exotic Animal Practice* **5**, 49–81

Hatt J-M (2007) Affektionen des Schnabels. In: *Kompendium der Ziervogelkrankheiten. 3. Auflage*, ed. E-H Kaleta and M-E Krautwald-Junghanns, pp. 152–156. Schlütersche, Stuttgart

Hatt J-M, Christen C and Sandmeier P (2007) The tubular external skeletal fixator (F.E.S.S.A.): clinical application in fracture repair in 28 birds. *Veterinary Record* **160**, 188–194

Helmer PJ and Redig PT (2006) Surgical resolution of orthopedic disorders. In: *Clinical Avian Medicine*, ed. GJ Harrison and TL Lightfoot, pp. 761–773. Spix, Palm Beach, FL

Holz PH (2003) Coracoid fractures in wild birds: repair and outcomes. *Australian Veterinary Journal* **81**, 469–471

Howard PE (1990) The use of bone plates in the repair of avian fractures. *Journal of the American Animal Hospital Association* **26**, 613–622

Hulse D and Hyman B (2003) Fracture biology and biomechanics. In: *Textbook of Small Animal Surgery, 3rd edn*, ed DH Slatter, pp. 1785–1792. WB Saunders, Philadelphia

Kaderly RE (1993) Delayed union, nonunion and malunion. In: *Textbook of Small Animal Surgery, 2nd edn*, ed. D Slatter, pp. 1676–1685. WB Saunders, Philadelphia

King AS (1991) *A Color Atlas of Avian Anatomy*. WB Saunders, Philadelphia

King AS and McLelland J (1984) *Form and Function in Birds*. Academic Press, New York

König HE and Liebich H-G (2001) *Anatomie und Propädeutik des Geflügels*. Schattauer, Stuttgart

Levitt L (1989) Avian orthopedics. *Compendium on Continuing Education for the Practicing Veterinarian* **11**, 899–929

Lierz M, Lierz U and Brunnberg L (2001) Surgical management of a pseudoarthrosis in a white-tailed sea eagle (*Haliaeetus albicilla*). *Proceedings of the 40th International Symposium on Diseases of Zoo Animals and Wildlife, Rotterdam, Institute of Zoo and Wildlife Research* **40**, 295–297

MacCoy DM (1989) Excision arthroplasty for management of coxofemoral luxation in pet birds. *Journal of the American Veterinary Medical Association* **194**, 95–97

MacCoy DM and Haschek WM (1988) Healing of transverse humeral fractures in pigeons treated with ethylene oxide-sterilized, dry stored, only cortical xenografts and allografts. *American Journal of Veterinary Research* **49**, 106–111

Mathews KG, Danova A, Newman H, Barnes HJ and Philips L (2003) Ratite cancellous xenograft: effects on avian fracture healing. *Veterinary Comparative Orthopaedics and Traumatology* **16**, 50–58

Meyrueis JP, Masselot A and Meyrueis J (1993) Etude mécanique comparative tridimensionnelle de fixateurs externes. *Revue de Chirurgie Orthopédique* **79**, 402–406

Orosz SE, Ensley PK and Haynes CJ (1992) *Avian Surgical Anatomy: Thoracic and Pelvic Limbs*. WB Saunders, Philadelphia

Redig PT (2002) Orthopedic fixation for long bone fractures of raptors and other large birds: pelvic limb. In: *Proceedings of the Annual Conference of the Association of Avian Veterinarians, Monterey*, pp. 323–335

Reichler IM, von Werthern CJ and Montavon PM (1997) Der tubuläre fixateur externe (F.E.S.S.A.): klinische Anwendung zur Frakturversorgung bei 6 Zwerghunden und 20 Katzen. *Kleintierpraxis* **42**, 407–419

Schuster S (1996) *Untersuchungen zur Häufigkeit, Lokalisation und Art von Frakturen beim Vogel*. Doctoral Thesis, University of Giessen

von Werthern C and Bernasconi C (2000) Application of the maxillofacial miniplate compact 1.0 in the fracture repair of 12 cats and two dogs. *Veterinary Comparative Orthopaedics and Traumatology* **13**, 92

West PG, Rowland GR, Budsberg SC and Aron DN (1996) Histomorphometric and angiographic analysis of bone healing in the humerus of pigeons. *American Journal of Veterinary Research* **57**, 1010–1015

16

Raptors: disorders of the feet

Tom Bailey and Chris Lloyd

Anatomy

Figure 16.1 illustrates the normal foot (see also Chapter 5). The functions of the feet and limbs of raptors are:

- To support the weight of the body
- To act as a rudder during some flight manoeuvres
- To cushion the impact of landing
- To catch, hold and kill prey
- To help to regulate body temperature
- To help to preen those parts of the body inaccessible to the beak
- To act as courtship signals in some species.

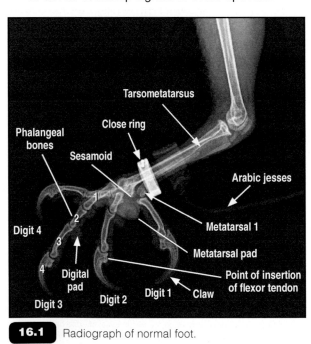

16.1 Radiograph of normal foot.

Disorders of the foot

Disorders are presented here in alphabetical order.

Abscesses

Injuries to the skin often result in large hard subcutaneous abscesses on the dorsal aspect of the foot in raptors (Figure 16.2). *Staphylococcus* spp. are the bacteria most commonly isolated from these lesions. Avian pus is very thick or solid; consequently surgical removal of abscess and capsule is recommended.

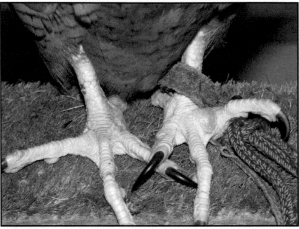

16.2 Abscess on the dorsal aspect of the foot of a falcon.

Flushing the defect with a diluted disinfectant such as F10SC or povidone–iodine, and the use of antibiotic-impregnated beads may be useful in some cases.

Avipox virus

Avipox virus is a large DNA virus discussed in more detail in Chapter 19. Four forms of disease are recognized in birds, but this chapter is only concerned with the cutaneous form that affects the feet of raptors (see also Chapter 24).

The dry form is the most common in raptors. It is characterized by papular lesions mainly on the skin around the beak, eyes and non-feathered parts of the legs distal to the tarsometatarsus. Typically the cutaneous form appears as small papules that develop into vesicles that progress to crusty lesions 5–15 mm in diameter, but the lesions can become very large in young birds, Gyrfalcons or immuno-suppressed adults. Secondary infections with bacterial and fungal pathogens are common. Following severe infections pigmented skin can become discoloured and there may be extensive scar tissue formation or talon loss that requires corrective surgery. The differential diagnosis list for the cutaneous form includes abscess, dermatitis, insect bites and neoplasia. A definitive diagnosis of avian pox can be made through histopathological examination, PCR testing or viral culture of biopsy samples.

While there is no specific treatment for infection with avipox virus, secondary bacterial, fungal or *Chlamydophila* infections that contribute to morbidity can be treated. Shoemaker *et al.* (1998) described the successful surgical excision of pox lesions from the foot of a Goshawk. Laser, electrocautery and chemical cautery using silver nitrate pencils can also be used to treat cutaneous vesicles in the early stages (Lierz, 2000). Non-specific treatment includes antibiotics to control any secondary infections, multivitamin supplementation and application of topical ointments and/or antiseptic foot baths. Mosquito proofing and possibly vaccination can provide some protection. Birds with pox lesions of the feet will often mutilate the toes and a modified hood may be required in this instance (see Figure 16.18).

Bumblefoot

Bumblefoot is a common condition of captive raptors and has been recognized since medieval times, when it was referred to as '*podagre*'. It is a frustrating disease to treat and it is important to consider each case of foot disease as a separate entity. Bumblefoot has been described as a pododermatitis although the authors feel that this is an inadequate description. The disease is characterized by superficial abrasions, ulceration, and cellulitis or abscessation of the plantar epithelium. Left untreated, the condition becomes debilitating with common sequelae including necrosis, tendonitis, septic arthritis and osteomyelitis. Secondary problems also arise, including infection of other joints, valvular endocarditis and (particularly in Gyrfalcons and Gyr-hybrids in the Middle East) amyloidosis. Captive falcons have the highest incidence of bumblefoot within the bird of prey group (Riddle, 1980). Accipiters, Red-tailed Hawks and Harris' Hawks that develop bumblefoot often respond much better to treatment than falcons and some clinicians consider that this is because these 'broadwings' bear less weight on the centre of their feet compared with falcons (Sullivan, 2006).

Causative factors

Numerous authors have suggested aetiologies for bumblefoot, which is a multifactorial condition that results from a combination of factors that damage the integrity of the foot. Husbandry factors such as dietary deficiencies, levels of inactivity, obesity, talon overgrowth and poor perching surfaces all contribute to the degradation of the integrity of the skin and tissues of the base of the foot. The factors that are considered by most authors to contribute to the aetiology of bumblefoot are:

- Overgrown talons, causing weight to be redistributed to the metatarsal pad, making it more susceptible to trauma and bruising
- Self-puncturing of the bottom of the foot by overgrown talons or foreign bodies
- Poor perch design – hard abrasive surface texture, poor anatomical shape
- Bruising to the plantar surface of the foot (this can have multiple aetiologies, such as persistent bating from a perch by a tethered raptor, hitting a lure too hard, or being housed in a small aviary with fixed perches)

- Poor nutrition
- Damage to the contralateral foot resulting in an asymmetrical weight distribution
- Lack of exercise and weight gain.

Remple and Al-Ashbal (1993) considered that repeated trauma of the foot leads to devitalization of the skin and subsequent colonization by pathogenic staphylococci. Harcourt-Brown (1996) postulated that the formation of bumblefoot depends on a decrease in blood supply to the skin and subcutaneous tissues and is analogous to a bed sore in humans.

With inappropriate pressure on the plantar areas often being one of the initiating factors, the plantar scab over the lesion leads to even more pressure on underlying tissues, resulting in local ischaemia and disrupting wound healing. *Staphylococcus* spp. are responsible for a variety of superficial and invasive infections and are usually associated with a breakdown of host defence systems. In bumblefoot, there appears to be an inadequate heterophil response during the acute phase of the inflammatory reaction, eventually leading to a chronic granulomatous inflammatory reaction and insulating the pathogens from the humoral and cellular immune response (Remple and Al-Ashbal, 1993).

Heidenreich (1995) considered that the sudden cessation of flying in falconry birds at the end of the falconry season leads to circulatory problems and metabolic imbalances resulting from a surplus of protein and insufficient utilization of energy. This leads to oedema in the lower parts of the body and swelling of the metatarsal pads and toes. Lierz (2003) demonstrated a regular increase in blood circulation in the feet of falcons after training and considered that if the training of a falcon stops suddenly (also comparable to sudden captivity in wild birds) this interferes with the blood circulation of the feet, contributing to the development of bumblefoot. This may explain the beneficial effects of continuing to fly a falcon on the healing of early bumblefoot lesions. Lierz was able to show that the incidence of bumblefoot could be reduced by changing the training methods after the hunting season and 'detraining' the bird.

Presentation and classification

The principal presenting sign of bumblefoot is swelling and inflammation of the plantar surface of the foot. The most common locations for lesions are the metatarsal pad in the centre of the foot, the pads under the middle phalangeal joint of digits II, III and IV or the distal digital pad of digits I and II. Swellings and scabs represent the final stages of a condition that starts with the erosion of the papillated epithelium. Consequently, in the battle to prevent this disease, the early recognition by falconers and veterinary surgeons of the loss of papillation and erythema of the bottom of the foot is vital.

Many classification schemes have been proposed to grade bumblefoot lesions and these different classifications can be confusing, even for clinicians familiar with the disease. The type of bumblefoot lesions seen vary between geographical regions, probably because of the different species, diets, environmental conditions (humidity) and most importantly the different types of falconry furniture and aviary perching materials that are used. Remple (1993) suggested a five-stage classification of the disease, which provides a useful and practical guide (Figures 16.3 and 16.4). It is important to remember that no two cases are identical, that the progression of the condition often surprises even experienced clinicians and that it is not always easy to pigeonhole a case into a category. Clinical challenges in treating bumblefoot include the poor tissue regeneration and healing caused by pressure necrosis and the reduction of vascular perfusion, and the poor delivery of systemic antibiotics to the infected areas. Consequently, treatment failure is not unusual.

Class	Description	Prognosis
I	Early insult or lesion characterized by thin flattened epithelium or proliferative lesions causing hypertrophy of the epithelium to form a corn. May be hyperaemia of the skin but no infection of underlying tissues in Class I lesions. Wild-caught Gyrfalcons susceptible to particular form of bumblefoot presenting as pale ischaemic spot in centre of foot, probably caused by combination of pressure and bruising, and rapidly progressing to grade III unless immediate corrective steps taken to change management	Excellent
II	Characterized by infection[a] of subcutaneous tissues but with no gross swelling of affected feet. Can be caused by puncture with localized infection or develop from local ischaemic necrosis caused by penetrating corn or scab	Good
III	Characterized by infected hot swollen and painful feet without apparent damage to deep vital structures. Swelling can be serous (usually following puncture followed by acute inflammation), fibrotic (chronic encapsulating reaction) or caseous (chronic necrotic inflammatory reaction)	Good to guarded
IV	Characterized by infection of deep vital structures producing tenosynovitis, arthritis and/or osteomyelitis but retaining pedal function. Can be fibrotic or caseous	Guarded to poor
V	End-stage disease with loss of pedal function	Grave

16.3 Classification scheme for bumblefoot in falcons (Remple, 1993). [a] Secondary microbial infection includes: *Staphylococcus aureus*, *S. epidermidis*, *Corynebacterium*, *Escherichia coli*, *Streptococcus faecalis*, *Pseudomonas*, *Bacteroides*, *Clostridium*, *Candida albicans* and *Aspergillus*.

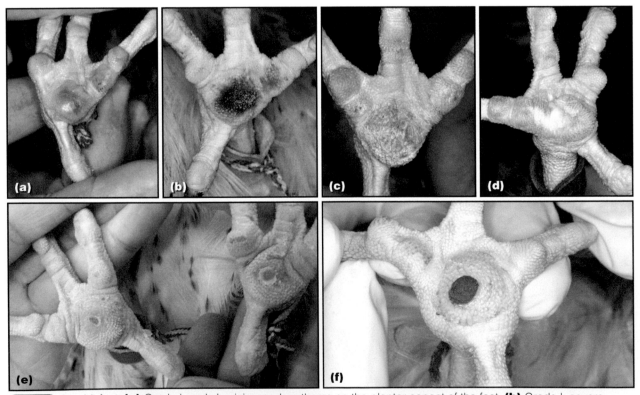

16.4 Bumblefoot. **(a)** Grade I: early bruising and erythema on the plantar aspect of the foot. **(b)** Grade I: severe bruising on the plantar aspect of the foot. **(c)** Grade I: dry proliferative lesions causing hypertrophy of the epithelium to form a corn. **(d)** Grade I: a fracture on the contralateral foot resulted in pressure necrosis of the skin of the plantar aspect of this foot, which had not been bandaged. **(e)** Grade II: small superficial scabs. **(f)** Grade III: an infected small (5 mm) but deeply penetrating scab; the foot is swollen. (continues) ▶

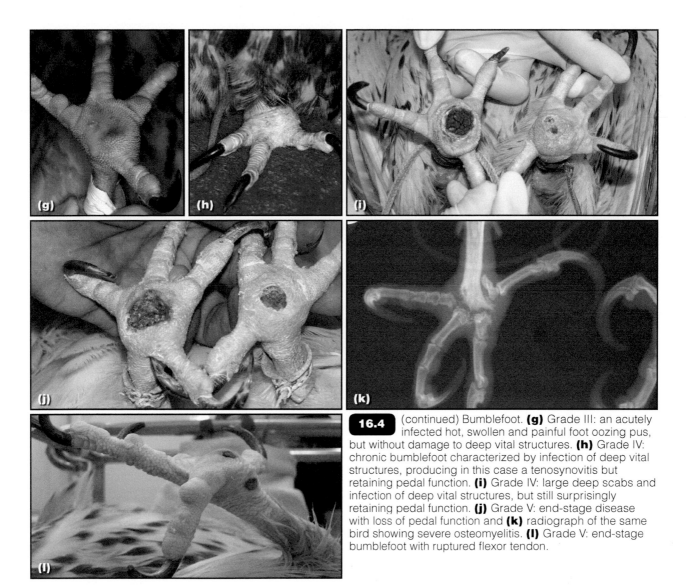

16.4 (continued) Bumblefoot. **(g)** Grade III: an acutely infected hot, swollen and painful foot oozing pus, but without damage to deep vital structures. **(h)** Grade IV: chronic bumblefoot characterized by infection of deep vital structures, producing in this case a tenosynovitis but retaining pedal function. **(i)** Grade IV: large deep scabs and infection of deep vital structures, but still surprisingly retaining pedal function. **(j)** Grade V: end-stage disease with loss of pedal function and **(k)** radiograph of the same bird showing severe osteomyelitis. **(l)** Grade V: end-stage bumblefoot with ruptured flexor tendon.

Diagnosis

Diagnosis is based on the appearance of the foot as assessed during clinical examination. It is always easier to examine raptor feet under anaesthesia. In order to classify the lesions, radiographs should be taken to determine whether foot bones are involved. It is important to wear gloves during examination of the feet as *Staphylococcus* spp. are an important pathogen in bumblefoot. The feet should be palpated and compared for heat and swelling. Microbiology and cytology samples should be collected from exudates. Sensitivity testing should be conducted on all isolates. If there is a loss of pedal function caused by osteomyelitis of several digits and the metatarsus and damage to the flexor tendons, the prognosis is hopeless and euthanasia should be recommended.

It is important always to assess both feet. Even in rare cases of unilateral bumblefoot the apparently healthy foot must be re-checked regularly, as weight-bearing on one leg leads to alterations.

Management changes for all bumblefoot cases

The following management changes should made in all classes of bumblefoot, regardless of the stage of development:

- Give a balanced diet with multivitamin and mineral supplementation (see Chapter 17)
- Use artificial turf (e.g. Astroturf) to cover all perching surfaces. Astroturf perches can also be wrapped in soft leather or towels (which can be more easily cleaned) to provide a springy surface for raptors recovering from painful foot lesions
- Reduce the weight of the bird to its flying weight
- Increase exercise; trained birds should continue to be flown.

Class I lesions will often respond to these management changes complemented with daily massaging of the feet while applying topical creams, such as aloe vera preparations or yeast extract and shark liver oil (Preparation H). Povidone–iodine painted on the bottom of the foot hardens the skin in early cases where the epithelium is thinner and has not lost its integrity. Sports gels containing heparin, sodium, dimethylsulfoxide and dexpanthenol are useful for cases of bruised feet. In order to maximize the chances of a positive clinical outcome and to minimize the chances of recurrence, it is important to discuss management changes with the owner before embarking on treatment or surgery.

Therapy and surgery

The therapeutic goals for treating cases of bumblefoot include:

- Reducing swelling and inflammation
- Debriding necrotic tissue
- Establishing drainage in infected cases
- Eliminating pathogens and protecting the wound from further infection
- Promoting granulation and healing by appropriate dressings and bandaging.

Birds with infected and swollen feet but no scab formation: These birds often respond to antibiotics and analgesics. Oral lincomycin, marbofloxacin or amoxicillin/clavulanate should be given for 7–10 days. Topical application of a mixture of dimethylsulfoxide (DMSO) gel and sodium fusidate ointment (equal parts) or DMSO gel and piperacillin to the swollen parts of the feet are helpful in reducing swelling. In these cases either the owner can apply the topical creams or the feet can be bandaged after applying the creams and rechecked every 24–48 hours. DMSO-based ointments should not be used for more than a week before surgery or healing may be inhibited.

Birds with epithelial changes (scabs): These birds will require surgical investigation to varying degrees, bandaging, antibacterial therapy and analgesics as well as the management changes previously discussed. There are two treatment options:

- Surgery, debridement of infected and necrotic material and primary closure
- Removal of the scab, debridement of the defect and treatment as an open wound to heal by granulation and secondary intention with regular bandage changes. These cases can be closed at a later stage depending on the progress of the healing.

Although primary closure should be the desired goal, not all cases of bumblefoot can be treated this way. Some defects are too large, there may be too much infection to allow closure and in many birds the epithelium is so poorly vascularized that defects will not close by primary intention. Surgical cases do fail and when this happens the original defect will have

become larger, delaying resolution. Before embarking on surgery and primary closure it is important to be confident that the skin surrounding the defect is healthy, well vascularized and viable. If it is, then the chances of breakdown of the surgical site are considerably reduced. The closure of large plantar defects resulting from severe bumblefoot, using axial pattern, composite transposition flaps (arterial pedicle grafts), is discussed in detail by Remple (2001). VetBioSIST (Cook, Australia), a naturally occurring extracellular matrix derived from pig small intestine submucosa, has been used by Chitty (2000) in successfully repairing bumblefoot lesions in a Harris' Hawk and a Himalayan Griffon Vulture, but the authors would be cautious over its use in large falcons.

Bandages and 'bumblefoot shoes': Remple (1993) and Riddle and Hoolihan (1993) developed a new protocol for bumblefoot: surgery followed by foot casting that involves precise anatomical fit to the shape of the falcon's foot. These casting methods have been adapted over the years and bumblefoot shoes (Figure 16.5) have been made from neoprene, orthopaedic thermoplastic material, memory foam used to make horse saddles, foam exercise mats or from children's foam swimming noodles. The principles for all these 'shoes' and 'foot casts' are similar: they are constructed so that pressure is removed from the plantar surface of the foot. The soft shoes compress considerably over time and should be changed regularly to ensure that pressure is kept from the healing plantar surface. Complications of rigid casts include post-casting constrictive toe oedema and pressure sores on the digital pads; pressure sores are rarely seen with foam shoes.

In the Middle East it is common for falconers who present bumblefoot cases during the hunting season to request that surgery is *not* performed on their birds; instead they prefer to have bandage changes until the hunting season is finished. Although contrary to the veterinary 'gut feeling' of wanting to intervene heroically with scalpel and suture, many cases will resolve with topical creams to encourage granulation and once- or twice-weekly bandage changes (Figure 16.6). The exercise of flying and the fact that the bird is kept at its flying weight are probably factors that contribute to the success of less invasive procedures. Products that the authors use to encourage granulation in open bumblefoot lesions include:

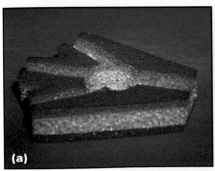
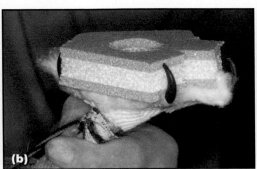
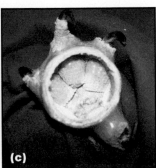

16.5 **(a)** Foam bumblefoot shoe. **(b)** Shoe in position on the foot. The central hole allows topical treatment. **(c)** Foot cast. (c, © Michael Lierz)

- Collagen dressing (e.g. Collamend, Genitrix Animal Health and Nutrition, UK; Promogran, Johnson and Johnson, UK)
- Medical hydrosylate Type I Collagen ointment (e.g. Collasate postoperative dressing, PRN Pharmacal, USA)
- Hydrogel with alginate (e.g. Nu-gel, Johnson and Johnson, UK)
- Intra-site gel (Smith and Nephew, UK)
- Honey (unpasteurized), adopted from old falconry traditions (Figure 16.7).

The authors are cautious of using hydroactive dressings on bumblefoot wounds, because in some cases the moist environment created by these dressings retards healing, encourages tissue necrosis and can be associated with secondary *Candida* infections. The timescale for recovery and healing of the feet using bandages depends on class and size of deficit, and can take 2–6 months.

Bumblefoot surgery: A mixture of fucidin and DMSO gel, or Preparation H, combined with bandages and bumblefoot shoes along with parenteral antibiosis can be given for 5–7 days to loosen up the scab and provide a sensible period of preoperative antibiotics. Where open infected lesions are present, daily wet-to-dry debriding bandages or povidone–iodine-soaked swabs may be useful in cleaning the surgical site. In the case of an encapsulated abscess within the foot, the use of extensive presurgical antibiosis should be reconsidered, as most antibiotics are unable to penetrate the capsule. This might lead to antibiotic concentrations below

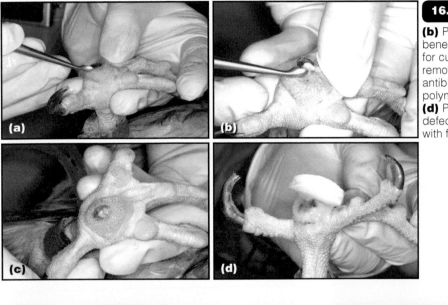

16.6 **(a)** Removal of scab on a Grade III bumblefoot. **(b)** Plug of infected caseous material beneath the scab. Swabs may be taken for culture. Necrotic material should be removed by curettage. **(c)** Implanting antibiotic-impregnated polymethylmethacrylate beads. **(d)** Placing Melolin dressing over the defect, which has also been covered with fucidin cream.

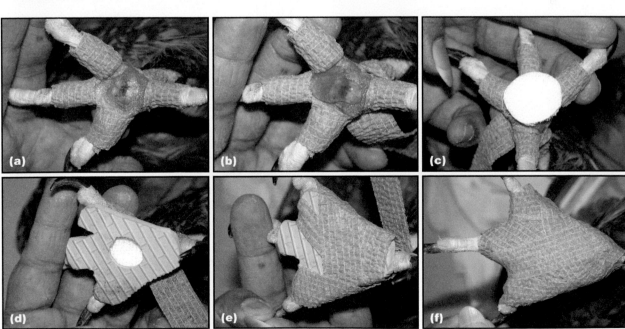

16.7 Treatment of a Grade II bumblefoot defect using honey and bumblefoot shoes: **(a)** defect after cleaning and the application of conforming bandage to the digits to prevent pressure ulcers caused by the shoes; **(b)** honey applied to the defect; **(c)** Melolin pad applied to the defect; **(d)** bumblefoot shoe positioned over the dressing; and **(e,f)** shoe positioned in place using conforming bandage.

inhibitory concentrations and therefore might induce resistance. In such cases antibiotic application is recommended shortly before surgery.

When bumblefoot surgery is undertaken the bird should be anaesthetized. Surgery is facilitated by the use of a padded device that supports the foot while the raptor is in dorsal recumbency (Figure 16.8), so that the digits can be held in hyperextension with towel clamps or tape (Remple, 1993). During surgery bleeding can either be controlled by an assistant placing digital pressure around the mid-tarsometatarsal region or by using a tourniquet placed in the same position.

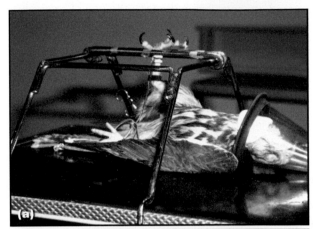

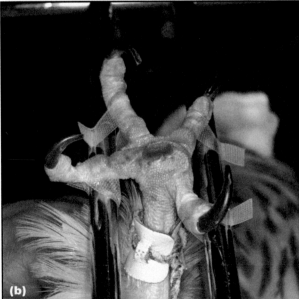

16.8 **(a)** Surgery is facilitated by the use of a padded device that supports the foot while the raptor is in dorsal recumbency. **(b)** A foot positioned in the device for surgery.

Before any incision is made, the integument should be evaluated carefully to determine the direction and extent of the elliptical incision. After the foot has been scrubbed and prepared for surgery the scab should be removed and swabs of the deep internal tissues cultured for bacteriology and mycology. Fibrotic and exudative material can be removed by curettage using a small Volkmann's scoop. This allows curettage without damage to vital structures. Irrigation with a solution of disinfectant such as F10 accompanies curettage. Once the wound has been cleaned to healthy vascular tissue the wound is sutured. Incision edges should be cut back until they are actively bleeding and near-perfect apposition of skin edges with little pressure on the suture line enhances the chances of successful first intention healing (Figure 16.9). Simple interrupted sutures using 1.5 metric (4/0) nylon are generally used, but tension relieving 'near–far/far–near' suture patterns have been used in some cases.

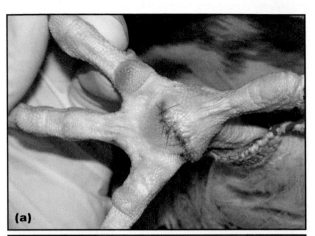

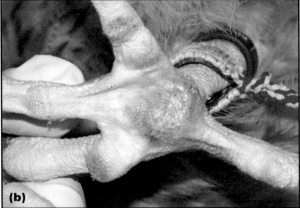

16.9 **(a)** Bumblefoot surgery showing placement of sutures; and **(b)** healed foot in the same bird one month after removal of sutures.

Bandaging and aftercare are an important part of the surgical procedure. Sodium fucidate cream or Dermisol cream is applied to the surgical site with a non-adhesive dressing (e.g. Melolin, Smith and Nephew, UK) and the foot is bandaged with non-adhesive elastic wrap (e.g. Vetrap, 3M Animal Care Products, USA). Hydroactive wound dressings (e.g. Duoderm, Convatec, USA) have been used by many authors. The use of shoes to protect the incision from pressure is also recommended.

Postoperatively the bird should be kept in a perch-free room on thick foam pads covered with artificial grass to further reduce pressure on the feet (Figure 16.10). As the bird has bandaged feet, food must be cut into bite-sized pieces. Antibiotic therapy based on the results of sensitivity testing should be continued for a minimum of 14 days, or until first intention healing has taken place. The feet should be checked daily and bandages changed two or three times a week, depending on the progress of healing. If healing is satisfactory, sutures can be removed in

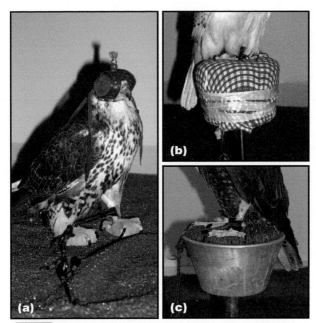

16.10 **(a)** Hospital ward for patients after bumblefoot surgery. Birds are housed on artificial grass on top of foam to minimize pressure on the healing feet. **(b)** Padded perch to manage a Gyrfalcon that has thin skin on the plantar foot following bumblefoot surgery. **(c)** Maintaining captive raptors on textured substrates such as Astroturf is one of the more important ways of minimizing the possibility of birds developing bumblefoot.

stages after 21 days. It is wise not to remove all the sutures in one go because of potential weakening of the freshly healed scar. Once all the sutures are removed the feet should be wrapped for a further 7–10 days. Most authors consider that the time to full recovery of the integrity of the foot is about 4–6 months after surgery, and it is important to discuss this timescale and costs with the owner of the bird before embarking on treatment.

Recurrence and treatment of unresponsive bumblefoot cases: It is not uncommon to have cases of bumblefoot where the surgical site fails to heal by primary intention, or where large defects fail to granulate (Figure 16.11). It is important when embarking on the

treatment of bumblefoot cases, especially given the length of time successful cases take to heal, to have conducted a comprehensive investigation of the health of the bird before embarking on lengthy treatment. Chronic renal disease, amyloidosis, aspergillosis, and fatty liver and kidney syndrome are conditions that will reduce the chances of successful foot healing. The sesamoid of the metatarsophalangeal joint is occasionally found to be infected in unresponsive bumblefoot cases in falcons; surgical removal of the sesamoid removed the chronic source of infection and allowed the bumblefoot to be cured.

Antibiotic-impregnated polymethylmethacrylate beads and antibiotic-impregnated gels: The more chronic forms of the disease affecting tendons and joints tend to respond poorly to systemic antibiotics. The use of antibiotic-impregnated polymethylmethacrylate beads (AIPMMA) in conjunction with aggressive surgical debridement is an effective method for delivering antibiotics into infected ischaemic sites and their use improves the response rate to therapy (see Figure 16.6). The beads allow a higher local concentration of antibiotics than can be achieved with systemic therapy. The methods for using and making these beads are reviewed by Remple and Forbes (2000). The authors regularly use piperacillin, ceftazidime and amikacin AIPMMA and have recently used amphotericin-impregnated beads to treat stubborn cases of bumblefoot with *Candida* infections. The beads should be removed after 7–10 days, although it has been shown that they are histologically non-reactive and consequently they can be left in place indefinitely.

Recently a doxycycline gel (Doxirobe™ gel, Pfizer Animal Health) has been used as part of the intralesional treatment of bumblefoot (Kummrow *et al.*, 2007). Once solidified, Doxirobe™ remains in the lesion for several weeks, serving both to protect the tissue and to provide local antibiotic delivery. This approach utilizes not only the initial antimicrobial affects of doxycycline but also its beneficial actions in modulating the host's immune response over the longer term, through the local release of sub-antimicrobial doses (Thomas *et al.*, 2000).

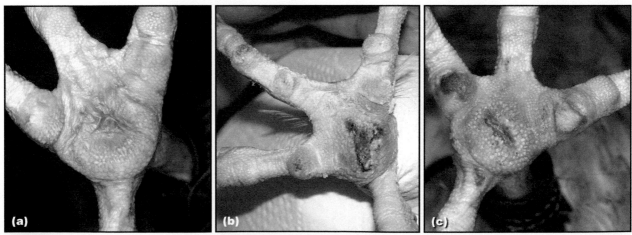

16.11 **(a)** Although the surgery to repair the bumblefoot defect has been successful in this case, the skin is very thin and bumblefoot can easily recur if the bird is not managed well. **(b)** Breakdown of a surgical site after unsuccessful surgery. **(c)** Pressure ulcers caused by poorly fitting bumblefoot shoes.

Prevention

Bumblefoot can be prevented by good husbandry (see Management changes, above), including the provision of psychological security with appropriately designed and constructed perches. Frequent examination of the raptor's feet will enable detection of early changes such as erythema and smoothing of the dermal papillae, which often precede the formation of bumblefoot lesions.

Bumblefoot complications: amyloidosis

Amyloidosis is an emerging and significant disease in falcons in the Middle East (McKinney, 2002) and is associated with chronic inflammatory or infectious stimuli such as bumblefoot in falcons. Gyrfalcons and Gyr-hybrids appear to be very susceptible to this disease, which commonly occurs in birds that are being treated for or have had a history of treatment for bumblefoot. This condition is fully discussed in Chapter 20. The stress of long-term care in birds suffering from bumblefoot can often leave them susceptible to diseases such as aspergillosis and clostridial enterotoxaemia

Constriction injuries of limbs and toes

Constriction injuries to the legs or toes of falcons are often seen. Metatarsal or more commonly digital constrictions occur when thin jesses become twisted or entangled about the feet (Figure 16.12). Digital constrictions can also occur secondary to circumferential constriction caused by pox scabs as well as by entanglement of toes in bandage material. The constrictions initially cause oedema and, if untreated, necrosis of the digit distal to the constriction. The cause of the constriction should be removed (scabs should be debrided or incised to prevent further vascular compromise) and hydroactive dressings applied to the affected digit. Damage to

flexor tendons is common. Complete healing can take many months and if unsuccessful may result in amputation of the toe.

Infectious swellings, insect bites, pox, neoplasia and trauma to the leg can cause constriction injuries to the metatarsus where there is a closed ring. The resulting tissue swelling can cause the ring to become too tight, leading to pressure necrosis. Rings should be removed from such birds and wounds treated as previously discussed (but see Chapter 37).

Corns

Corns have been discussed above in the section on Bumblefoot.

Cutaneous mycobacteriosis

Mycobacteriosis is found in raptors worldwide. Primary cutaneous lesions can appear as subcutaneous granulomas. The skin appears thickened because of the accumulation of macrophages in the dermis and subcutis. Diagnosis is confirmed by biopsy and a combination of histopathology, DNA probes or culture (see Chapter 19).

Distraction of the first metatarsal bone

This condition is almost exclusively seen in hawks, particularly goshawks and Harris' Hawk. It is considered to be caused by frequent repetitive concussion to the plantar surface of the foot. Affected birds are presented with an inflamed soft swelling on the medial aspect of the distal tarsometatarsus. Radiography reveals the first metatarsal bone to be slightly rotated and displaced in a proximoplantar direction (Figure 16.13). Sometimes a plug of purulent material develops in the metatarsal fossa which will need to be removed surgically. Treatment consists of antibiotics, analgesics and sodium fusidate ointment over the swelling.

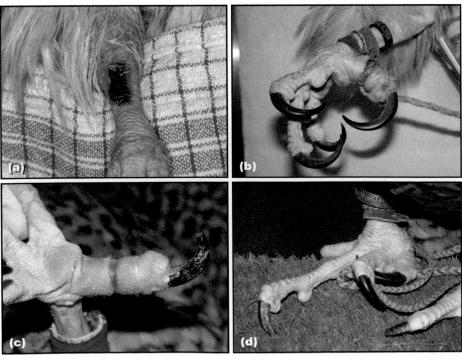

16.12 **(a)** An abrasion to the dorsal aspect of the metatarsus caused by constriction of the jesses. **(b)** A constriction of the first phalanx can occur with some jesses (in this case Arabian style). **(c)** A similar case after using hydroactive dressings and bandaging. **(d)** In this case the tendon has been damaged.

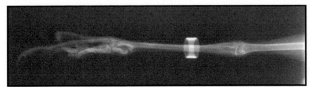

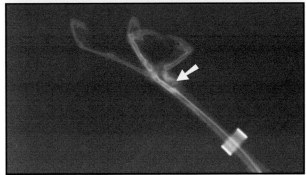

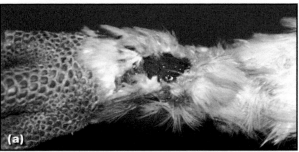

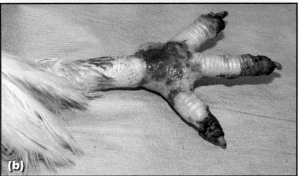

16.13 Radiographs of distracted talon in a Sparrowhawk. This is an old lesion that has become infected. Note area of lucency (arrowed) at base of P1. (© John Chitty)

Dry feet

Raptors kept in dry environments or on poor planes of nutrition are often presented with dry and cracking skin on their feet (Figure 16.14). Improving the diet and daily applications of aloe vera and vitamin E cream will usually resolve the problem.

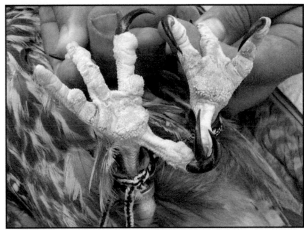

16.14 Poorly keratinized and dry feet in a malnourished falcon.

Dry gangrene of the skin

Sometimes after surgery to the foot, the skin around the surgical site will lose its blood supply and die (Figure 16.15a). Many factors are likely to implicated in this problem, including pre-existing poor skin or previous bruising to the area, often because of the initial traumatic injury for which the bird was presented. The use of some topical medications (DMSO jelly) can occasionally be associated with skin necrosis (Figure 16.15b). Severe cases where deeper structures such as muscles and ligaments are affected may require euthanasia. Less severe cases can be treated with debridement and hydroactive dressings. Dry gangrene also occurs after electrocution injuries.

16.15 **(a)** Gangrene caused by a *Salmonella* infection. **(b)** Necrosis of the skin caused by overuse of DMSO cream in a badly bruised foot.

Erysipelothrix infection

Erysipelothrix rhusiopathiae is an occasional cause of disease in eagles and hawks. Rats, mice and birds (including poultry) are considered to be reservoirs for the bacterium, and disease usually follows injury to the skin. Only the acute form is seen in raptors and clinical signs comprise pronounced swelling and red discoloration of skin. Early treatment is necessary as the disease follows a rapid course and death will ensue within 2–3 days. Tetracycline, doxycycline and penicillin are effective first-choice antibiotics to treat this infection, backed up by sensitivity testing.

Frostbite

Frostbite of the toes has been observed in tropical species housed in extremely cold conditions. The condition has been reported in Harris' Hawks in Canada (Hudelson and Hudelson, 1995) and King Vultures, Indian Black Vultures and the Bateleur in Germany (Heidenreich, 1995). The toes are especially vulnerable to frostbite and the condition presents initially as swelling, followed by devitalized and discoloured skin caused by epidermal and dermal necrosis. In the early stages, slow warming of the affected feet can help to minimize tissue damage. This is done by gently massaging the feet in cold and then gradually warmer and warmer water baths to stimulate blood flow. If necrosis is not complete, the appropriate treatment is debridement of the lesions followed by the application of hydrocolloid dressings. Amputation of the toes may be necessary where there is complete necrosis.

Haematomas

Subcutaneous haemorrhages and bruising are often found on the feet, usually following fighting with quarry. If there are no external injuries, antibiotics are generally not necessary but analgesics and anti-inflammatory drugs may be indicated. Where two raptors fight, injuries are often undetected and an antibiotic course of 5 days is recommended to prevent septicaemia. Larger bruises can be treated with topical products for sporting injuries containing heparin and DMSO. Temporary bandaging of the feet with pressure-relieving shoes whilst still allowing daily application of creams may be required for a short period to prevent the skin from becoming devitalized.

Pelvic limb oedema in accipiters

Heidenreich (1995) described a condition called pelvic limb oedema in wild-caught Goshawks. This condition occurs a few days after the bird is withdrawn from hunting and is given an excess of food. Initially the condition presents as soft swellings of the legs followed by localized bump-like lesions. Heidenreich recommended the use of topical products that encourage blood flow to the area, but stated that the condition can take many weeks to resolve. The condition can be avoided by ensuring that birds that are ending their hunting season are gradually brought down to an inactive phase and have food levels increased slowly.

Phalangeal fractures and dislocations

The phalangeal bones are often fractured in hunting accidents or during training when a falcon strikes a lure too hard (Figure 16.16a). Each digit has a large flexor tendon surrounded by a tendon sheath on the plantar aspect. These structures form an effective splint. Harcourt-Brown (1996) considered that splinting the digit can result in trapping of the flexor tendon and joint in the developing callus, resulting in a non-functional toe. In his opinion digital fractures rarely need support and heal best if left unsplinted. Riddle and Hoolihan (1993) used casts in the treatment of toe fractures in falcons and reported that they were well tolerated and resulted in healing in all cases. The authors routinely use splints made of Vet-Lite (Kruuse, Belgium) to support fractures of the first phalanx of falcons and see few problems (Figure 16.16b). Large phalangeal bones such as those in vultures can be repaired with laterally placed full-pin fixation (Harcourt-Brown, 1996).

Dislocations are common in falcons and can occur without any serious ligament damage. The joint can be returned to its normal position with manual manipulation under general anaesthesia. If collateral ligament damage does occur, it should be repaired with fine-gauge PDS. Ball bandages for 5 days are also helpful.

Ball bandages

Ball bandages are a useful method for immobilizing the toes and feet, especially after surgery of the flexor or extensor tendons or after phalangeal fractures (Figure 16.17). Harcourt-Brown (1996) recommended taping the toes to half a flexible ball and covering the foot with a bandage for 3–4 weeks after tendon surgery. Assisted feeding will be needed during this period as the bird will be unable to hold its food to feed.

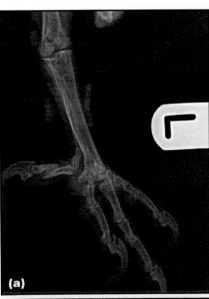
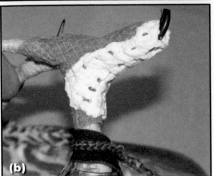

16.16
(a) Radiograph of a phalangeal fracture of the first digit.
(b) Splints made of Vet-Lite to support a fracture of the first phalanx in a falcon.

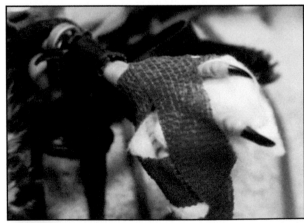

16.17 Ball bandage. A simple bandage with a large wad of cotton wool (some prefer to use half a squash ball) held in place with elasticated cohesive dressing. The bandage must be kept dry and the talons must protrude such that the toes are able to flex and extend slightly, thus preventing adhesions between healing bone and tendon. The bandage should be removed after 3–5 days. (© John Chitty)

Self-mutilation

Self-mutilation to the foot and digits is an occasional problem in falcons, particularly birds that have been recently trapped from the wild. Sometimes raptors will pick at and pull off foot bandages following surgery (Figure 16.18a); in other cases, birds that have lost talons will mutilate their feet. In severe cases the

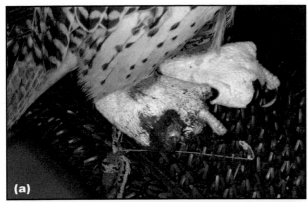

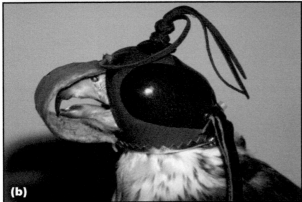

16.18 **(a)** Self-mutilation in a bird with bandaged feet following bumblefoot surgery. **(b)** This hood has been adapted to prevent auto-mutilation.

birds can cause such severe mutilation that one or more toes will need to be amputated. Analgesics should always be given to birds that have had surgery or injuries to the feet. Birds that start to self-mutilate should be fitted with specially adapted hoods (Figure 16.18b).

Septic arthritis
The most common joints to be affected with septic arthritis are the interphalangeal joints (Harcourt-Brown, 2002). The infection may enter from a scab under the talon, a penetrating injury such as a bite, or secondary to injuries caused by avipox infection, fractures or extensive bruising. Antibiotic therapy should be based on sensitivity results, while cytology will also help to guide initial therapy. Radiography of the foot is an important part of determining prognosis. Any lytic changes to the phalangeal bones make the prognosis poor and amputation of the digit may be necessary. In cases with no radiographic evidence of bony change, treatment involves daily irrigation of the joint with saline and 0.25–0.5 ml of intra-articular lincomycin or tobramycin. Systemic antibiotics are also recommended.

Talon disorders
Talons grow continuously from their base and injuries to this zone of proliferation can cause abnormalities in the development of the horny tissue of the claws. If the nail bed is injured, the talon will either be unable to regrow or will develop abnormally, with serious implications for any hunting bird.

Broken (Figure 16.19) and shed claws are a common cause of presentation and can also be a complication of some diseases such as avipox. Minor damage to claws can result in a surprising amount of bleeding for the size of injury. Cautery with silver nitrate sticks or potassium permanganate crystals will usually stop the bleeding. If the claw is torn off, exposing the underlying phalangeal bone and germinal epithelium (Figure 16.20a), the area must be cleaned with dilute disinfectant and covered with a hydrocolloid dressing to prevent the germinal epithelium drying out. These dressings should be changed first after 48 hours and subsequently every 5–7 days. Removing the fibrin clot will allow regrowth of the claw.

A technique utilizing cyanoacrylate glue is widely used in falcon hospitals in the Middle East (Figure 16.20b). Once the exposed bone has been cleaned and is dry it is covered with layers of 5-minute epoxy glue or 'super glue' mixed with talcum powder and antibiotic powder (e.g. clindamycin or piperacillin). Four or five layers are applied, shaping the material in the form of an artificial claw. This will also protect the germinal epithelium from further damage and the artificial nail is shed after a few weeks. Antibiotics

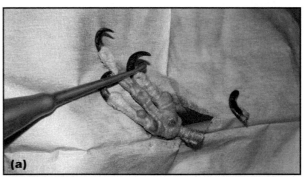

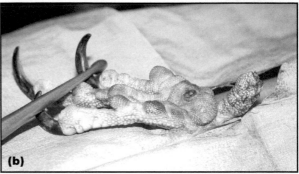

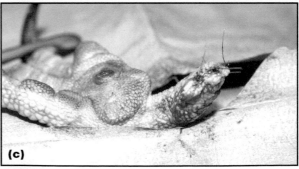

16.19 Removal of a damaged nail on the hallux.

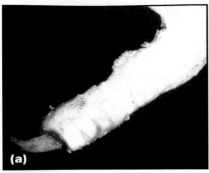
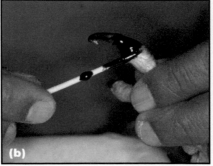
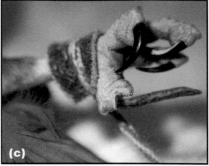

16.20 **(a)** A falcon's nail has been torn off, exposing the underlying phalangeal bone. **(b)** Repairing a lost claw using cyanoacrylate glue. **(c)** Severely overgrown nails resulting in 'corkscrew claws'.

should be given to all cases of claw loss along with analgesics, because some birds will be irritated by the loss of a claw and will self-mutilate. It will take 4–8 months for the new claw to regrow fully.

In nature, raptors keep their talons in shape through a combination of diet and contact with a diverse range of rough perching surfaces. Insufficient wear of the talons occurs when captive birds are fed on soft food and kept on unsuitable perches. In such cases talons sheaths are retained (thickening and dulling the talon) or overgrowth occurs causing deformities such as a corkscrew talon (Figure 16.20c). Trimming or coping is necessary to return the claws to normal.

Tendon injuries

Severed flexor or extensor tendons may occur following bites from prey such as squirrels, infection of the claw and distal phalangeal bone, constriction injuries or as a sequel to bumblefoot. The tendons are poorly vascularized and are nourished via the tendon sheath fluid. Joining tendons by an end-to-end anastomosis fails because there is no healing response at the joined ends. Harcourt-Brown (2000b) comprehensively reviewed tendon repair in raptors. To summarize his findings: a blood supply to the severed ends must be obtained from the tendon sheath, either by allowing the tendon ends to adhere to the tendon sheath and vascularize, or by suturing the tendon to the tendon sheath soon after the injury. After 3–4 weeks the tendon ends are vascularized and they can be joined. After surgery a ball bandage (see Figure 16.17) should be applied to the feet to prevent the muscular activity of the bird from breaking down the repair.

Tendon sheath infections

The flexor and extensor tendon sheaths are contiguous from the distal phalanx to just proximal to the intertarsal joint. Tendon sheath infections often progress from infections of the distal interphalangeal joint or bumblefoot lesions (Figure 16.21). Antibiotic therapy should be based on sensitivity results of aspirates from the tendon sheath, and cytology should also be performed to guide initial therapy. The usual isolate is *Staphylococcus*. Infections of tendon sheaths are often stubborn to treat and almost always require irrigation of the sheath to drain purulent material as well as systemic antibiotics.

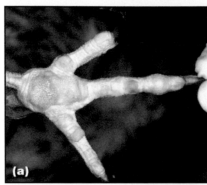
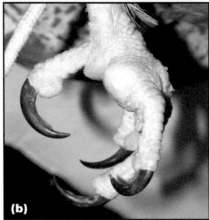

16.21
(a) Tendinitis caused by *Staphylococcus* spp. in a Saker Falcon.
(b) Infected interphalangeal joint.

Toe injuries

The tendon of insertion of the extensor digitorum longus muscle is more complex in the falcon than in the hawk. This tendon is more frequently severed in toe injuries in trained hawks than in falcons, resulting in loss of function of the digit. Harcourt-Brown (2000b) considered that this is partly due to the single branch of the tendon to digits II and IV in the hawk, compared with the double branch of the tendon to each toe in the falcon, as well as the different prey species hunted by these two groups of birds.

Squirrel bites are a common cause of loss of function of the digit. The typical squirrel bite is on the foot or leg, a couple of millimetres long, and appears innocuous. It is therefore often left untreated other than staunching blood flow and initial cleaning. Unfortunately, these bites often introduce bacteria and erosive infections commence. These may not be apparent for a few weeks, by which time there may be osteomyelitis and/or tenosynovitis. Post-infection tendon rupture can result. It is therefore recommended that squirrel bites should be seen as a matter of urgency, the wound thoroughly irrigated, and antibiosis instigated. Typically a 14-day course of amoxicillin/clavulanate is used in the first instance.

Wounds

Wounds are common in falconry birds that are being used for hunting. Wounds to the feet often heal more slowly than on other parts of the body, possibly due to poorer vasculature. Injury to the scaly skin of the tarsometatarsal region occurs more commonly in hawks than in falcons. Harcourt-Brown (2000) considered that this difference is because hawks bate more frequently than falcons and if jesses are not kept supple abrasions of the skin result. These injuries can result in a bacterial dermatitis. Eagles are susceptible to digital infections that occur secondary to cracks caused by dry skin.

Treatment of skin lacerations requires prompt surgical debridement and freshening of the skin edges before closure. Temporary immobilization of the wounded area may be necessary. Talon punctures caused by crabbing injuries (fighting between two hawks) are susceptible to clostridial infections. Such injuries should be flushed with hydrogen peroxide and the bird given antibiotics.

Amputation of the digit

Amputation of the digit in raptors is considered when tendon damage, skin loss or septic arthritis has caused loss of function. If the functionless toe does not interfere with the use of the foot, it may be kept and stabilized by performing an arthrodesis. The skin, subcutaneous tissues, tendons and tendon sheaths are incised and retracted proximally from the damaged phalangeal bone. The phalangeal bone should be cut so that none of the joint remains. The flexor and extensor tendons and their associated sheaths should be sutured over the end of the bone and the skin sutured over the top of this. The suture material used is 1.5–2 metric (3/0–4/0) PDS and the toe should be lightly bandaged with either a hydroactive dressing or Dermisol and a non-absorbent dressing such as Melolin. It is important to consider the function of the digit to be amputated. A raptor would be greatly affected by the loss of the hallux or digit II and less so by the amputation of digit IV.

References and further reading

Berners J (1486) *The Boke of St Albans*. Printed at St Albans by the Schoolmaster Printer. Reprinted (1881) Elliott Stock, London
Blome R (1683) *Hawking or Faulconry*. Facsimile edition (1929). Cresset Press, London

Brown L (1997) *Birds of Prey*. Chancellor Press, London
Chitty J (2000) The use of Vet Bio SIST in bumblefoot management. In: *Proceedings of the European Association of Avian Veterinarians*, pp. 489–491
Cooper JE (2002) *Birds of Prey: Health and Disease*. Blackwell Science, Oxford
Forbes NA, Cooper JE and Allchurch AF (2000) Neoplasms of birds of prey. In: *Raptor Biomedicine III*, ed. JT Lumeij *et al.*, pp. 127–146. Zoological Education Network, Lake Worth, FL
Fox NC (1995) *Understanding the Bird of Prey*. Hancock House Publishers, Surrey, British Columbia
Harcourt-Brown N (1996) Foot and leg problems. In: *BSAVA Manual of Raptors, Pigeons and Waterfowl*, ed. NA Forbes and N Harcourt-Brown, pp. 147–168. BSAVA Publications, Cheltenham
Harcourt-Brown N (2000a) *Birds of Prey: Anatomy, Radiology and Clinical Conditions of the Pelvic Limb*. [CD ROM]. Zoological Education Network, Lake Worth, FL
Harcourt-Brown N (2000b) Tendon repair in the pelvic limb of birds of prey. In: *Raptor Biomedicine III*, ed. JT Lumeij *et al.*, pp. 201–239. Zoological Education Network, Lake Worth, FL
Harcourt-Brown N (2002) Orthopedic conditions that affect the avian pelvic limb. *Veterinary Clinics of North America: Exotic Animal Practice* **5**, 49–81
Heidenreich M (1995) *Birds of Prey: Medicine and Management*. Blackwell Science, Oxford
Hudelson S and Hudelson P (1995) Dermatology of raptors: a review. *Seminars in Avian and Exotic Pet Medicine* **4**, 184–194
Kummrow M, Murray M and Bailey TA (2007) Successful treatment of bumblefoot lesions in a peregrine falcon (*Falco peregrinus*) with Doxirobe. In: *Proceedings of the European Association of Avian Veterinarians, Zurich*, pp. 101–104
Lierz M (2000) Possible therapy for early pox lesions. *Exotic DVM* **2.3**, 88–90
Lierz M (2003) Aspects of the pathogenesis of bumblefoot in falcons. In: *Proceedings of the 7th Conference of the European Association of Avian Veterinarians and 5th Scientific Meeting of the European College of Avian Medicine and Surgery, Tenerife*, pp. 178–184
McKinney PA (2002) Amyloidosis in falconiformes. In: *Proceedings of the Australian Chapter: American Association of Avian Veterinarians, Surfers Paradise Conference*, pp. 257–264
Mueller M, Wernery U and Koesters J (2000) Bumblefoot and lack of exercise among wild and captive bred falcons tested in the United Arab Emirates. *Avian Diseases* **44**, 676–680
Redig P (1993) Bumblefoot treatment in raptors. In: *Zoo and Wild Animal Medicine Current Therapy 3*, ed. ME Fowler, pp. 181–188. WB Saunders, Philadelphia
Remple JD (1993) Raptor bumblefoot: a new treatment technique. In: *Raptor Biomedicine II*, ed. PT Redig *et al.*, pp. 154–160. University of Minnesota Press, Minneapolis
Remple JD (2001) The use of axial pattern, composite transposition flaps (arterial pedicle grafts) to close large plantar defects resulting from severe bumblefoot in raptors. In: *Proceedings of the European Association of Avian Veterinarians, Munich*, pp. 55–61
Remple JD and Al-Ashbal AA (1993) Raptor bumblefoot: another look at histopathology and pathogenesis. In: *Raptor Biomedicine II*, ed. P Redig *et al.*, pp. 92–98. University of Minnesota Press, Minneapolis
Remple JD and Forbes NA (2000) Antibiotic impregnated polymethylacrylate beads in the treatment of bumblefoot in falcons. In: *Raptor Biomedicine III*, ed. JT Lumeij *et al.*, pp. 255–266. Zoological Education Network, Lake Worth, FL
Riddle KE (1980) Surgical treatment of bumblefoot in raptors. In: *Recent Advances in the Study of Raptor Diseases*, ed. JE Cooper and AG Greenwood, pp. 67–73. Chiron, Keighley, Yorkshire
Riddle KE and Hoolihan J (1993) A form-fitting, composite-casting method for avian appendages. In: *Raptor Biomedicine II*, ed. PT Redig *et al.*, pp. 161–164. University of Minnesota Press, Minneapolis
Shoemaker NJ, Dorrestein GM and Lumeij JT (1998) An avipoxvirus infection in a goshawk. *Avian Pathology* **27**, 103–106
Sullivan T (2006) Bumblefoot revisited. *American Falconry* **43**, 58–60
Thomas J, Walker C and Bradshaw M (2000) Long-term use of subantimicrobial dose doxycycline does not lead to changes in antimicrobial susceptibility. *Journal of Periodontology* **71**, 1472–1483
Wilson H, Roberts R, Northrup N, Hernandez-Divers S and Latimer K (2005) Radiation tolerances doses to Cobalt-60 teletherapy in psittacine birds. In: *Proceedings of 26th AAV Conference and Expo, August 9–11, Monterey, California*, pp. 57–58

17

Raptors: nutrition

John Chitty

Introduction

Properly balanced nutrition is fundamental to the correct husbandry and performance of the captive raptor. They require a diet balanced in terms of quality, quantity and affordability that should reflect their requirements for water, carbohydrate, protein, fat and micronutrients (vitamins and minerals).

In simplistic form, raptors eat meat. However, simple provision of meat is not sufficient. Raptors are *whole-carcass feeders*. Failure to provide whole carcasses of prey of an appropriate size for the raptor will result in selective feeding and nutritional imbalance.

Ideally raptors should be fed as close to their natural diet as possible. They can be broadly considered in the groups shown in Figure 17.1 but these generalizations should only be used as a guide. Most raptors will take any source of meat when their preferred source is unavailable. Detailed information is available in Ferguson-Lees and Christie (2001).

In captivity, full choice of natural prey is rarely available and so some compromise is necessary. Formulated rations have been proposed and marketed but have gained little popularity, the vast majority of falconers preferring fresh or frozen carcasses as food sources.

Feeding a good quality whole carcass
This implies the feeding of a complete prey item that is appropriate to the size of the raptor, such that the raptor can ingest the entire carcass, including all body organs. The prey should have been reared on a good quality complete diet (appropriate to its species) and have been kept in an appropriate hygienic husbandry system. That is to say, only healthy prey should be fed to the raptor. Prey should be killed in a humane manner and the carcass stored and defrosted in such a way that degradation of tissues and contamination by toxins or microorganisms is minimal.

Nutritional requirements vary according to life stage, with extra or specific needs during breeding, rearing, growth and performance. These needs will be discussed and compared with 'baseline' diet later in the chapter.

The raptor gut and digestive physiology are discussed in Chapter 5. It is a fairly simple system with a poorly developed ventriculus, as little grinding of food is necessary, and relatively undeveloped large bowel/caecum, as they do not need to ferment food. It is important to note that raptors can be divided into two groups: those with crops (diurnal birds of prey – the Falconiformes) and those without (owls). This has an impact on volumes that can be fed at each meal.

Castings

All birds of prey produce castings. These are the regurgitated 'indigestible' parts of the carcass (feathers and fur; also bones in owls). The volume, appearance and timing of casting varies according to diet fed and, to a lesser extent, the individual bird. Experienced falconers monitor castings very closely, as variance from the normal often indicates a digestive upset. In particular, failure to produce a casting (containing material from which the bird would normally produce a casting) within 12–16 hours of a feed should be treated as an urgent medical problem.

Type of diet	Species	Comments
Mammals	Large eagles (*Aquila* spp.); Kestrels; smaller owls (e.g. Barn Owl)	Many eagles will also take carrion
Birds	Northern Sparrowhawk; larger falcons (e.g. Peregrine, Saker, Gyrfalcon)	
Mixed mammals/ birds	Northern Goshawk and other large accipiters; larger owls	
Fish	Osprey; fish eagles (*Haliaetus* spp., e.g. Bald Eagle, African Fish Eagle)	Most fish feeders (with exception of Osprey) will also take land-based prey or carrion as necessary
Insects	Hobby; Merlin; Little Owl	Many insect feeders will also feed on birds (e.g. Hobby, Merlin) or small mammals (e.g. Little Owl)
Carrion	Vultures; condors	
Fully mixed	Kites; Common Buzzard	

17.1 Natural diets of selected raptor species.

Nutrients

Energy

Energy is the fundament of diet. These birds eat, primarily, to fulfil their daily calorie requirements.

Energy is derived from fat, carbohydrate and protein. Of these, fat represents the major source in terms of *gross energy* (GE), being approximately twice as 'energy-dense' (measured in kJ/g) as protein or carbohydrate.

Carbohydrates are not an important component of the raptor diet. While the raptor brain is dependent on glucose (as in other species) and glycogen stores are built up in muscle and liver to act as a store of readily available energy, the natural diet is not carbohydrate-rich. Therefore carbohydrate stores are built up by conversion of other dietary components.

GE is only the energy that enters the digestive system. Digestion is not 100% efficient, nor is all the energy actually available for digestion. *Indigestible energy* is removed in the form of castings, faeces and urine. *Metabolizable energy* (ME) is the remaining energy available from the diet, i.e. GE minus the energy lost in castings, faeces and urine.

A general case can be made for a basic dietary calculation that, for birds fed vertebrate prey, ME from the diet is 75% (±7%) of GE (Kirkwood, 1981; Robbins, 1993), though there is some variation between food sources and species. For example, ME from day-old cockerels (DOCs) has been estimated at 85% (but only 71% when fed to Kestrels) and from mice 75% (Forbes and Flint, 2000).

The *basal metabolic rate* (BMR) is the amount of energy needed to 'stay alive' and can be calculated in raptors as follows:

$$BMR = 78 \times \text{body weight (kg)}^{0.75}$$

On top of BMR, further dietary energy is needed to meet extra physiological stress, such as growth, performance, breeding and thermoregulation. Any shortfall in energy intake will be made up from body stores. In general this will come from fat stores laid down in times of dietary energy excess. However, inactive birds will utilize protein stores (muscle) in cold weather, which means that falconers need to increase not only dietary fat but also dietary protein in winter.

As stated, birds eat to fulfil their daily energy requirements. In raptors, this means they hunt when hungry. This is the basis of falconry training: birds are kept hungry to encourage hunting behaviour (see Chapter 2). To achieve this, falconers monitor weight and body condition very closely during the flying season. An experienced falconer will have an excellent knowledge of the individual bird's hunting performance in relation to its body weight and feeding regime. Any variance from this may represent disease and should be taken seriously, meriting in-depth investigation in spite of a bird that often overtly seems well. Such variances include:

- Failure to gain or lose weight in expected proportion to changes in feeding
- Failure to hold expected body condition in relation to body weight

- Failure to hunt in an expected manner ('lazy' or easily tired) given weight and/or body condition
- Excessive or reduced appetite in relation to body weight or condition.

Thus the bird is judged on a combination of its *weight*, *body condition* and *performance*.

At the start of each flying season the weight of the bird is usually reduced to an expected (based on previous seasons) or estimated (based on other birds of similar size) body weight before training. This is a part of the manning procedure (see Chapter 2).

Kirkwood (1981) studied rates of weight loss in starved raptors. Rates of energy loss did not vary significantly between species, which indicated that the same type of tissue was being broken down in each case. The rate of loss (g/day) was shown to be 28.27 × body weight $(kg)^{0.723}$; the time to achieve 25% body weight loss was 9.7 × body weight $(kg)^{0.276}$ days.

The presence of body weight in these equations indicates that larger birds are much more capable of withstanding fasting than smaller birds.

Energy excess

Energy excess is very unlikely in the trained bird during the flying season, but this tightly regulated feeding contrasts with the feeding of aviary birds, which are often fed to excess in spite of doing little or no exercise.

Hepatic lipidosis (Figure 17.2) is common in aviary birds, especially those in permanent breeding aviaries and zoological collections. While prolonged calorie excess is a major factor, other factors may also play a part. In particular, fatty liver–kidney syndrome of Merlins is well described (Forbes and Cooper, 1993) and it is proposed that the feeding of DOCs to birds that feed predominantly in the wild on insects may result in a higher proportion of fat to protein in the diet and a high proportion of avidin, resulting in binding of dietary biotin and reduced hepatic gluconeogenesis.

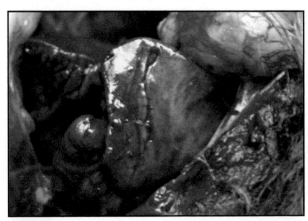

17.2 Hepatic lipidosis in an owl. The bird had been kept in an aviary all its life. (© John Chitty)

Atherosclerosis in older birds may be a consequence of long-term excessive dietary energy and reduced activity, though genetic factors may also be involved.

In both conditions, signs may be minimal or absent, with birds dying spontaneously when stressed.

Aviary birds should be handled on several occasions through the year to allow assessment of body weight and condition and, therefore, modification of diet if necessary. Serum cholesterol measurements may also be of assistance in screening for potential hepatic lipidosis or atherosclerosis cases. Values >8 mmol/l are of concern, as is a finding of low-density lipoprotein greater than high-density lipoprotein.

Energy deficiency

Energy deficiency is seen regularly in trained birds. The most frequent presentation is a thin bird that collapses during or immediately after flight.

Diagnosis is from the typical history; blood samples will reveal a profound hypoglycaemia. Blood glucose levels are very variable in raptors, but it is more common to see a hyperglycaemia as a consequence of stress. Blood glucose should always be measured patient-side both for immediate results and to avoid an artefactual hypoglycaemia due to poor blood storage or inappropriate anticoagulant.

Response to intravenous glucose should be rapid. Many falconers carry glucose or gluconeogenic compounds for immediate oral use should this happen in the field.

In most cases, the history reveals a 'starved' bird and clearly there is a fundamental problem with the management technique for that particular bird that needs addressing by the falconer. In essence it is a problem normally seen with inexperienced falconers and much less commonly with the more experienced. Increased feeding and a short break from training will enable weight gain. The bird should then be flown at a higher weight, given suitable breaks during hunting, or fed during hunting trips.

In some cases, however, hypoglycaemia may be the result of an underlying disease process, such as parasitism, malabsorption or hepatic disease. A thorough history and clinical investigation are recommended for any case of hypoglycaemia (even those that seem 'simple'), particularly for those that fail to gain weight with increased feeding.

As described earlier, smaller birds are less able to withstand periods of starvation and so it is of little surprise that this is most common in smaller species used for falconry, especially the Sparrowhawk. This is one of the reasons that those new to falconry should begin with larger birds.

In this author's experience hypoglycaemia is also often seen in second-season Harris' Hawks. The falconer will have worked out an 'ideal flying weight' during the first season and put the bird to moult in an aviary in the close season. They then bring the bird out, man it and reduce the weight to the previous 'ideal', failing to take into account any growth that will have occurred during this time. Typically, these birds will be thin (even emaciated) in spite of being at the stated weight. It should always be emphasized that body weight *and* condition should be assessed together.

Essential fatty acids (EFAs)

It is likely that raptors do have certain requirements for these. However, good quality carcasses should contain adequate levels and so supplementation is unlikely to be necessary unless specific clinical syndromes suggest otherwise (e.g. dry scaly skin or brittle feathers, or signs consistent with allergy).

Protein

Protein is the staple of the raptor's diet. It may be utilized for energy, but is mainly used for tissue growth and repair. Protein should comprise 15–20% of the diet (Cooper, 2002). The limiting factors are the quality and type of protein available in the diet.

Proteins are made up of chains of amino acids. There are 20 of these, of which nine are deemed essential: arginine, isoleucine, leucine, lysine, methionine, phenylalanine, threonine, tryptophan and valine. Tyrosine and cysteine are termed semi-essential; they can be synthesized from phenylalanine and methinonine, respectively, provided that these essential amino acids are available in sufficient quantity. The remaining amino acids are non-essential and can be synthesized by the raptor from other dietary components.

If the bird is eating a good quality whole-carcass diet, sufficient essential amino acids should be present and deficiencies are rarely seen. Failure to absorb and process protein due to gastrointestinal disease, parasites or metabolic disease may result in temporary 'deficiencies' that are evidenced by stress- or fret-marks in growing feathers.

This author has also seen some birds with poor quality beak and talon growth that have apparently responded fully or partly to methionine supplementation. It is most likely that this is due to specific metabolic inability to process this amino acid rather than absolute dietary deficiency.

Water

All raptors require daily access to fresh clean drinking water. Ideally it should be provided in open dishes so that the bird can bathe as well as drink. Failure to provide access to water will deprive the bird of choice and it may be unable to drink when it most needs to. This will exacerbate or even cause disease.

It may be necessary to remove water dishes for part of a day, perhaps before flight (to avoid clogged feathers) or after noon in winter (to reduce incidence of wingtip oedema and necrosis syndrome). Nonetheless, water should be available for at least part of each day.

It has often been opined that raptors should obtain all dietary water from prey items, but wild raptors do drink. In captivity most are fed thawed frozen food, a process that loses some of the 'natural' water from the carcass. Birds also need additional water in hot weather, after exercise or when sick.

As with all aspects of feeding, observation of the bird's regular drinking habits is essential. In this way polydipsia may be readily detected and clinical investigation undertaken.

Micronutrients

Calcium, phosphorus and vitamin D

It is impossible to discuss one of these micronutrients without addressing the others.

- Vitamin D is required as D3 and is ingested in both active and inactive forms from prey items. Activation of Vitamin D3 in the raptor requires access to unfiltered sunlight each day. Inactive vitamin is excreted from the preen gland; it is spread over the plumage and re-ingested during preening.
- Calcium and phosphorus are readily available from whole carcasses, provided that bones can also be ingested, i.e. the prey is small enough to avoid selective 'picking' by the bird.

The ratio between these minerals is vital. Ideally it should be between 1:1 and 2:1. Deficiency of calcium or vitamin D3 (or relative excess of phosphorus) will result in:

- Reproductive failure (soft-shelled eggs, egg binding, egg-related peritonitis)
- Nutritional secondary hyperparathyroidism (generally referred to as 'rickets' in young birds) (Figure 17.3). This will most commonly be seen in second or third clutches during a breeding season. Females lay down stores of calcium before the first clutch in the form of increased bone density and intramedullary hyperostosis. These stores may become depleted with successive clutches and bone deformities may develop in chicks. Renal disease in the female bird may produce a similar syndrome (Forbes and Rees Davies, 2000). Otherwise disease is seen in birds reared in the total absence of unfiltered sunlight (or artificial UV-B light) and those fed on deficient diets during rearing.
- Neurological signs (usually in growing birds or breeding females). Signs include tremors, weakness or fits. Typical signalment should arouse clinical suspicion and assessment of plasma ionized calcium levels is diagnostic. Total calcium measurement may be misleading as this value includes protein-bound 'inactive' calcium.

Excess calcium in the diet is unlikely to cause a clinical problem, as the excess will not be absorbed from the diet. However, overdosage of activated vitamin D3 supplements should be avoided, as it will result in hypercalcaemia and mineralization of soft tissues, especially the kidneys.

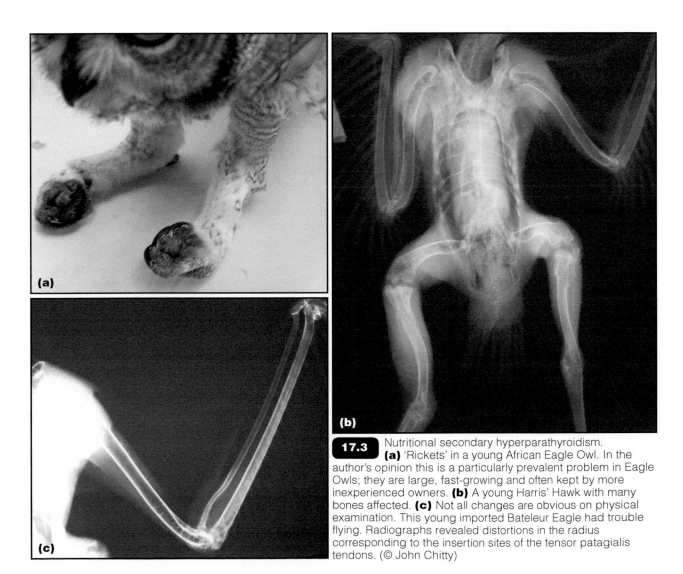

17.3 Nutritional secondary hyperparathyroidism. **(a)** 'Rickets' in a young African Eagle Owl. In the author's opinion this is a particularly prevalent problem in Eagle Owls; they are large, fast-growing and often kept by more inexperienced owners. **(b)** A young Harris' Hawk with many bones affected. **(c)** Not all changes are obvious on physical examination. This young imported Bateleur Eagle had trouble flying. Radiographs revealed distortions in the radius corresponding to the insertion sites of the tensor patagialis tendons. (© John Chitty)

Other minerals and electrolytes

Given a good quality whole-carcass diet, deficiency or excess of these components is extremely unlikely and clinical syndromes are correspondingly rare. Iron supplementation may be required after blood loss or haemolytic episodes.

Other fat-soluble vitamins

Vitamin A: Vitamin A is stored in the liver (and to a lesser extent in fat) and so should be available in required amounts from almost all whole-carcass items. Deficiency is seen occasionally, especially if only eviscerated carcasses or muscle meat are given or poor quality food is provided. Signs include:

- Weight loss and failure to grow properly
- Poor hatch rates
- Xerophthalmia
- Opacification of the third eyelids and enlargement of the lachrymal glands (this may result in infection or keratoconjunctivitis sicca)
- Hyperkeratosis of the eyelids
- Squamous metaplasia resulting in lesions/infections of the mucous membranes, especially the mouth and conjunctivae
- Squamous metaplasia of the ureters resulting in renal disease
- Vitamin A deficiency has also been implicated in bumblefoot pathogenesis (Heidenreich, 1997; Cooper, 2002).

Diagnosis is by suggestive signs (see above), biopsy (showing squamous metaplasia) and nutritional analysis (a diet of eviscerated DOCs may be suggestive).

Therapy involves diversification of the diet and oral supplementation of vitamin A. Injectable vitamin A is rarely indicated in the author's opinion; the pathogenesis of the disease is slow and recovery will be accordingly slow. There is also the risk of overdosage with both oral and injectable preparations, though it is less common when given by mouth. Signs of excess vitamin A are very similar to those of deficiency.

Vitamin E: Vitamin E is an antioxidant. It is stored in body fat and so, while deficiency should be rare, any spoilage of the carcass will deplete vitamin E stores.

Opinions vary on the likelihood of deficiency. Klasing (1998) stated that vitamin E concentrations in the tissues of chicks, mice, rats and quail are low and so deficiency is likely in raptors fed these. However, Forbes and Flint (2000) stated that levels in rats and chicks should be adequate. Both sources agree that levels in quail are low unless these birds are fed vitamin E-supplemented diets.

Requirements vary between species, with piscivorous birds having a higher requirement (Klasing, 1998).

Vitamin E is essential for fertility, red blood cell formation and stabilization of cell membranes. Deficiency will result in:

- White muscle disease (a muscular dystrophy in young birds)
- Reduced libido in males
- Reduced fertility
- Reduced hatchability and chick survival and thrift
- Splayed legs
- Encephalomalacia
- Oedema around neck, wings and ventrum (possibly linked to cardiac lesions or white muscle disease).

Serum vitamin E has been assessed in raptors. While tissue analysis is generally recommended for absolute diagnosis of deficiency, this is simply not practical in the clinical situation. The finding of low plasma α-tocopherol levels appears to indicate the current feeding of a diet deficient in vitamin E and therefore implies deficiency (M Lierz, 2007, personal communication).

Vitamin E excess is unlikely to cause clinical signs. However, all fat-soluble vitamins compete for absorption from the gut; therefore excess vitamin E may result in deficiency of vitamins A, D or K.

Vitamin K: Deficiency is highly unlikely, but clinical signs of haemorrhage and failure of coagulation will occur in coumarol toxicity.

Water-soluble vitamins

Vitamin C: Adequate levels are synthesized in the liver and so dietary deficiency is not a clinical entity in these species.

B-vitamins: There are many B-vitamins and good quality whole-carcass feeding should provide them. Dietary deficiency is rare, but the following may be seen.

- **Thiamine (B1)** deficiency may occur, especially in fish eaters fed thawed frozen fish, where activation of thiaminase will destroy the available vitamin. To avoid this, frozen fish should be thawed in boiling water or (preferably) only fresh fish should be used. In both cases, a B1 supplement should be given.
  - The author has also seen this deficiency in a young Red Kite and juvenile Saker hybrid (Figure 17.4) and in both cases it was more

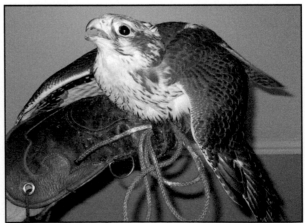

17.4 Thiamine deficiency in a juvenile Saker hybrid. The bird is unable to stand and is throwing its head upwards ('stargazing'). (© John Chitty)

likely that deficiency was the result of a metabolic disorder or inability to absorb or process thiamine, rather than absolute deficiency. This opinion was also voiced by Forbes and Rees Davies (2000) in describing thiamine-responsive fits in certain lines of Harris' Hawk.

- – Signs are dramatic, with incoordination progressing to seizure. Classically, affected birds will 'stargaze'.
- – In one study (Carnarius *et al.*, 2005) plasma thiamine levels in healthy Northern Goshawks ranged from 44 to 162 μg/l (fed and starved). A young bird with clinical signs of thiamine deficiency had a plasma level of 2.2 μg/l. However, while plasma levels will confirm diagnosis, this will not be particularly useful in the immediate clinical setting as the time delay in getting results will be a problem. Therefore suspicious cases should be given therapeutic doses of thiamine to assess effect.
- – Response to injectable thiamine is rapid and 4 mg thiamine/kg injected intramuscularly should produce clinical improvement. Thereafter oral supplementation and dietary modifications should maintain response.
- **Riboflavin (B2)** deficiency has been reported (Forbes and Rees Davies, 2000) in very young chicks, which had curled toes.
- **Pyridoxine (B6)** deficiency has been associated in other species with poor appetite and growth, poor feathering and neurological signs. Malformation of collagen fibres may also lead to abnormalities in bone and cartilage development. Pyridoxine toxicity has been reported in pigeons after administration of 90–100 mg/bird (Peeters *et al.*, 1977; Brown and Julian, 2003) and some falconers have reported sudden death in their falcons after administration of a multivitamin tablet containing 50 mg pyridoxinium chloride (in addition to 50 mg thiamine hydrochloride, 5 mg folic acid and 0.05 mg cyanocobalamin) (M Lierz, 2007, personal communication).

Available foods

Wild-caught prey

This seems the obvious alternative to free hunting by the bird. There are a number of problems associated with this type of feeding, whether the prey is shot, caught by the bird itself, or picked up as roadkill.

Toxins

Wild-caught prey may contain various potential toxins, including alphachloralose, coumarol rodenticides and, especially, lead. Certainly any shot quarry should be regarded as a possible source of lead, as shot will be scattered through the carcass (see Figure 26.2). Some falconers will only use quarry that has been 'head shot' with a rifle; they will then discard the head. However, most bullets will fragment on impact so this is still a large risk.

Infectious agents

Various infectious agents can be contracted from wild-caught quarry. Of particular importance are trichomoniasis ('frounce') (see Chapter 18), salmonellosis, *Escherichia coli*, mycobacteriosis, campylobacteriosis, chlamydophilosis, paramyxovirus, orthomyxovirus (influenza) and herpesvirus, as well as various enteric parasites. Many of these may be contracted from wild pigeon or doves, many of which are carriers of trichomoniasis, salmonellosis, chlamydophilosis, paramyxovirus and herpesvirus. Some advocate feeding pigeon meat after it has been frozen for several weeks and then defrosted. While this will remove trichomonads it will not prevent viral infection or transmission of most bacteria. Therefore feeding wild pigeon is not recommended.

Most birds are allowed to feed briefly on any quarry they have caught. Ideally, the bird should be allowed to deplume feathers and then be removed from the quarry at the earliest opportunity, only being allowed to continue feeding after a thorough inspection of the carcass (Figure 17.5). While the quarry may have appeared fit and well in flight, it could be that the hunting raptor 'selected' a weaker individual in hunting, or the quarry may be carrying lead shot.

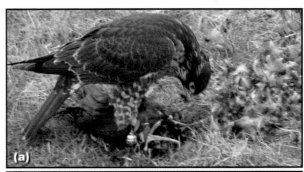
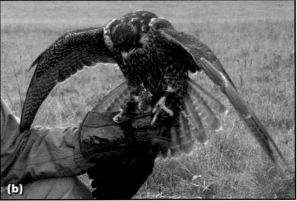

17.5 **(a)** Falcon feeding on its captured quarry. Many birds 'deplume' quarry and discard most of the feathers. **(b)** After a brief feed the bird is removed, the quarry is opened and inspected, and a small portion of breast meat is fed on the fist. (© John Chitty)

Commercial foodstuffs

Because of the potential problems associated with wild-caught prey, feeding tends to be based on commercially available foodstuffs. The nutritional content of some of these is summarized in Figure 17.6 and their advantages and disadvantages are considered below.

NUTRIENT TYPE														
FOOD TYPE	Chicken egg	DOC Strain 1	DOC Strain 2	DOC	DOC	DOC	DOC	Quail (male)	Quail (female)	Quail	Quail Vit E+	Rat Weaner	Rat	Rat	Rat
CATEGORY / AGE		1 day	1 day	1 day	1 day	1 day	1 day	6 weeks	6 weeks	6 weeks	7 weeks	5 weeks	11 weeks		11 weeks
SEX		Male	Male	Male	Male	Male	Male	Male	Female	Mixed	Mixed	Mixed	Male		Mixed
SAMPLE SIZE					200		200	3	3	18	100	200	3		75
PREPARATION METHOD	No shell				whole	skinned	de-yolked	plucked	plucked		plucked				eviscerated
Moisture (%)	75.3	72.4	73.6	75	76.1	77.8	78.5	65.1	65.6	67	66.6	72.5	64.3	65.6	68.3
Gross Energy (kcal/kg DM)	14700	6020	6000	6100	6162	6000	6042				5565	5756		5780	6305
Crude fibre (%DM)	trace	0.8	1.1		0.4		2.8				3.3	2.9		2.4	1.3
Protein (%DM)		62.2	62.5	60	72.4	59.2	69.3	64.9	71.6	47.4	58.7	59.6	63.4	62.8	62.1
Lipid (%DM)		24.2	23.4	28.1	22.6	26.9	20	33.2	26.3	25.8	27.8	25.5	34.9	22.1	31.5
Ash (%DM)		7.4	7.1	7.1	7.5	8.1	8.8	9.6	12	10.3	13.5	10.5	7.5	10	6.6
Calcium (%DM)	0.9	1.36	1.24	1.2		1.4								2.06	
Phosphorus (%DM)		1.0	0.94	0.9		0.9				3.8				1.48	
Protein (g/100g)	12.5				17.3		14.9				19.6	16.4			19.7
Nitrogen (g/100g)	10.02														
Lipid (g/100g)					5.4		4.3				9.3	7			11.3
Ash (g/100g)					1.8		1.9				4.5	2.9			2.1
Vitamin A – Retinol (IU/100g)	634				496.7		363.3	3299	6644	9010	3633.3	816.7	6824		4000
Vitamin B1 – Thiamine (mg/100g)	0.06	1.6	1.06		0.06		0.07				0.18	0.31		1.33	0.21
Vitamin E – α-tocopherol (IU/100g)	14				40.7		21.4	4.16	7.93	4.5	10.1	9.6	21.05		15.6
Ca:P ratio	0.28:1	1.36:1	1.32:1	1.3:1	1.49:1	1.5:1	1.17:1				1.54:1	1.21:1		1.39:1	1.33:1
Calcium (mg/100g)	50				775		680	3268	4361		2140	1010	2286		5930
Phosphorus (mg/100g)	178				521		581				1390	838			4470
Copper (mg/100g)	0.014	0.33	0.34		0.264		0.268	0.266	0.302	0.29	0.48	0.847	0.13	0.45	0.18
Iron (mg/100g)	1.44	3.4	3.19		5.23		5.57	8.5	11.24	7.14	11.1	6.74	4.3	5.89	4.79
Magnesium (mg/100g)	10				36		33.1	57.9	75.3	66	74.8	59.5	24.7		30.2
Manganese (mg/100g)	0.024	0.08	0.06		<0.1		<0.01	0.66	0.85		0.417	0.92	0.29	0.25	<0.1
Zinc (mg/100g)	1.1	2.99	3.63		2.96		2.89	5.5	5.43	5.7	3.88	3.73	3.5	4.33	2.14
Sodium (mg/100g)	126				370		371				204	254			114

17.6 Nutritional content of various raptor foodstuffs. DOC = day-old cockerel. (Forbes and Flint, 2000; reprinted with kind permission of Honeybrook Farm Animal Feeds) (continues)

FOOD TYPE CATEGORY	Mouse	Mouse	Mouse	Mouse	Mouse	Chicken	Chicken	Guinea pig	Sparrow	Pigeon	Pheasant	Crow	Rabbit	Hare	Beef	Beef
AGE	12 weeks		12 weeks				6 weeks	10 weeks								
SEX	Male		Mixed				Male	Male								
SAMPLE SIZE	3		200				3	3	11							
PREPARATION METHOD					skinned		plucked	decapitated	plucked	lean	lean	lean	lean	lean	lean	washed
NUTRIENT TYPE																
Moisture (%)	66.9	64.9	66.9	64.4	67.7	66.5	67.7	69.3	68.38	72.2	72.4	69.6	74.2	74.8		
Gross Energy (kcal/kg DM)	5840		5923	6500	6900	5930			5393	6100	5520	5780	5890	5990	1149	819
Crude fibre (%DM)	1.7		1.5	1.7		2			0.43							
Protein (%DM)	56.1		58.9	42.7	44.8	56.7	64	58.9	64.58							
Lipid (%DM)	24.9		29.9	46.5	41	26.9	47.2	45.4	15.93	20.7	0	8.6	5	11.7		
Ash (%DM)	10.4		9.7	7.6	10.3	9.5	10.4	8.9	10.62							
Calcium (%DM)	2.38			1.7	2.3	1.94			2.94							
Phosphorus (%DM)	1.72			1.2	1.5	1.4			2.35							
Protein (g/100g)			19.5							13	14.8	11.3	14.4	13.8	20.7	14.4
Nitrogen (g/100g)																
Lipid (g/100g)			9.9												5.7	4.2
Ash (g/100g)			3.2													
Vitamin A – Retinol (IU/100g)	65734		13533				3559	1999								
Vitamin B1 – Thiamine (mg/100g)			0.02			0.85										
Vitamin E – Alpha-tocopherol (IU/100g)	7.44		5.9				6.14	2.98								
Ca:P ratio	1.38:1		1.51:1	1.2:1	1.5:1	1.39:1			1.25:1						0.05:1	0.08:1
Calcium (mg/100g)	3208		2110				2455	2946							30	40
Phosphorus (mg/100g)			1400												660	490
Copper (mg/100g)	0.38		0.549			0.45	0.27	0.6	1.26							
Iron (mg/100g)	7.64		13.3			4.91	9.76	5.19	59.2							
Magnesium (mg/100g)	43.2		72.2				53.6	63.7	30							
Manganese (mg/100g)	0.53		0.709			0.3	1.1	0.66	1.14							
Zinc (mg/100g)	4.4		4.87			5.28	7.41	6.44								
Sodium (mg/100g)			273													

17.6 (continued) Nutritional content of various raptor foodstuffs. (Forbes and Flint, 2000; reprinted with kind permission of Honeybrook Farm Animal Feeds)

Day-old cockerels (DOCs)

Cheap and easily available, these are the staple of most raptor diets. They have had a bad press in recent years as it is felt that they are capable of transmitting disease (especially salmonellosis and *E. coli*) and are too high in fat and low in calcium. However, good quality DOCs have a good protein level, are less fat than commercially available rodents, contain good levels of fat-soluble vitamins, and an excellent calcium to phosphorus ratio – provided they are fed with the yolk sac left in. Many falconers remove the yolk sac to 'reduce levels of infection', but this reasoning is false. Removal of the yolk sac will also remove the main source of calcium and fat-soluble vitamins, resulting in a carcass that is no longer nutritionally balanced. If the yolk sac appears unsuitable for feeding, the whole chick should be condemned (Figure 17.7). It is also worth checking that chicks have not been defrosted and re-frozen; this would be apparent as red legs on the chicks and the entire batch of chicks should be discarded (Figure 17.8).

One potential problem with feeding whole chick is that it is messy. Some raptors will accumulate material under the talons, leading to an erosive dermatitis. This will track in, resulting in osteomyelitis and, often, loss or damage to the flexor tendon and its attachment (Figure 17.9). Attention must be paid to cleanliness if feeding raptors on chicks.

A particular worry is the feeding of DOCs to Mauritius Kestrels. This species has a particular sensitivity to the adenoviruses that may be found in the chicks.

3–4-week-old chickens: Some raptor breeders buy DOCs alive and raise them under controlled conditions: vitamins and other supplements can be added to their drinking water and also their fat content can be regulated. At the age of 3–4 weeks they are large enough to be a meal and can be fed freshly slaughtered as a whole-carcass meal. This food is particularly valuable during the breeding season, especially for falcons, but the work load and space requirements for rearing the chicks may be limiting.

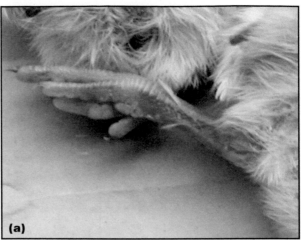
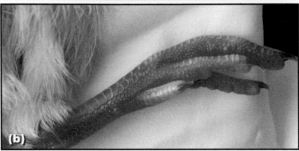

17.8 **(a)** Normal leg colour of a defrosted day-old cockerel. **(b)** Reddened leg of a DOC that has been defrosted, refrozen and then thawed again. This should not be fed to a raptor. Given the potential problems of feeding avian prey (possibly carrying avian pathogens) to raptors, it is vital that storage and handling of DOCs is optimal. (© John Chitty)

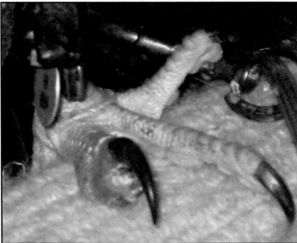

17.9 Infected digit 2 of a Harris' Hawk resulting from a dermatitis caused by an accumulation of food debris under the talon. Note how the toe appears 'knocked up', indicating rupture of the flexor tendon or destruction of its attachment. (© John Chitty)

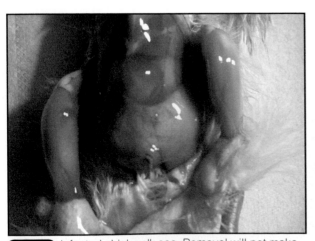

17.7 Infected chick yolk sac. Removal will not make this chick an acceptable food item; note how wet the carcass is. The whole chick must be discarded. (© John Chitty)

Quail

These have gained popularity as an alternative to DOCs, but care must be taken as to which sort of quail are fed (Figure 17.10). Only quail that have been specifically bred and reared for feeding to raptors should be used.

Type	Description	Advantages	Disadvantages
5-week culls	Males	Small and low fat, lacking yolk-sac	Low in fat-soluble vitamins
6–8-week prime birds	Produced specifically as a feedstuff	Good quality well balanced feedstuff with adequate calcium levels and good Ca:P ratio	May be low in vitamin E
8-month ex-layers	Females with large active ovaries	Cheap and good levels of fat-soluble vitamins	Very fat. Potential source of pathogens after being in intensive production systems. Care should be taken with vaccinated birds (live vaccine may adversely affect raptors). Not recommended
Vitamin E-enhanced prime birds	As prime birds but enhanced vitamin E	Good vitamin E levels	Expensive. May not carry any great advantage over DOCs

17.10 Types of quail fed to raptors.

Rodents

When feeding rodents, the size of the animal must be chosen with regard to the size of raptor to ensure that the raptor can take as much of the carcass as possible.

Rats: Rats are a very good source of calcium and fat-soluble vitamins as well as being high in protein. They are often high in fat and some raptors find them unappetizing; they are also hard to prepare and reasonably expensive.

The fat content can be controlled if rats are bought live and maintained by the falconer to control their feeding. Where rats are slaughtered and are to be stored frozen, it is important to eviscerate the carcass partially (intestine and gut, but not liver, kidney and heart) before freezing, as rats take some time to defrost completely – and during that time bacteria may leave the gut and contaminate the meat.

Mice: Mice are an excellent source of protein and calcium, but expensive even if produced in a home-run 'mouse farm'. They can be very high in fat (see rats, above).

Other rodents: Rodents such as hamsters and guinea pigs are often available for feeding. Hamsters probably offer little advantage over mice, but guinea pigs are relatively cheap and offer a good quality alternative to rats and mice. However, the fur is loose and many believe that this will result in excessive amounts of casting and possible gut impaction. The carcass should therefore be skinned and eviscerated (as the very large gut is unlikely to be eaten by the raptor) before feeding.

Rabbit and hare

Both are excellent sources of protein and calcium for larger birds. They are also relatively low in fat. However, they need careful preparation: the gut should be removed (as with guinea pigs) and, if fed to hawks, the long bones and spine need to be broken into pieces, otherwise gut impaction may result (Figure 17.11).

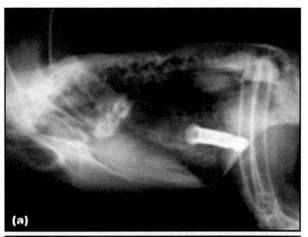

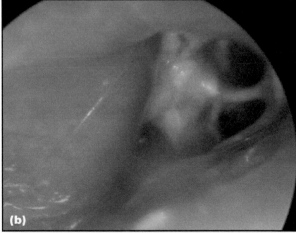

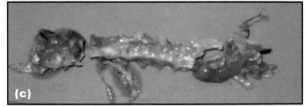

17.11 Rabbit vertebrae obstructing the distal oesophagus. **(a)** Harris' Hawk. Note the placement of an air sac tube. On initial presentation the bird was dyspnoeic due to penetration of the oesophageal wall and a purulent pneumonia. **(b)** Northern Goshawk: endoscopic view. **(c)** Post-endoscopic removal. The spine has been fed as too large a piece. (© John Chitty)

Beef

Many falconers like to feed beef, especially to sick birds or to their favourite, which is generally anthropomorphic feeding. While the protein content is excellent, the calcium:phosphorus ratio is poor and no practical amount of supplementation will improve it. Beef feeding may be of use when flying birds in public demonstration as feeding carcasses (even chick legs) may be aesthetically unacceptable. It is vital in such cases to use only minimal amounts of beef as a reward, to avoid unbalancing the diet.

Large joints of meat (beef, lamb or horse) may be supplied to larger eagles or vultures. In these cases the joints should be pounded first so that the bones are shattered, enabling some improvement in the Ca:P balance. There have been suggestions that feeding horse meat (Heidenreich, 1997) or pork (Schöneberg, 2004) may lead to gout; therefore the use of both these meat sources should be avoided.

Feeding prepared meats intended for humans, such as mince, sausages and bacon, is not recommended even for short periods when desperate. Bacon, in particular, has been associated with toxicity.

Fish

Although fish-eaters (Osprey, Fish Eagle) can be fed on mammal-based diets, they do enjoy fish and this should form some part of the diet. Fresh whole trout is ideal, but farmed fish is much more fatty than wild-caught. If frozen fish is to be used, it should be defrosted in boiling water and B-vitamin supplements should be added.

Food preparation

It is of no use obtaining good quality food if preparation methods are unhygienic. Standard precautions should be taken with frozen food:

- It should be defrosted in a clean fridge used only for the raptor food
- It should never be defrosted in open areas where vermin may contaminate it
- Only enough for the next day's feed should be taken out and defrosted each time, to avoid spoilage.

All tools and equipment (knives, boards, etc.) should be maintained in a hygienic manner as if being used in preparing food for human consumption. A major problem area is the falconer's bag, which should be thoroughly cleaned and disinfected after each hunting trip.

Supplements

In general, supplementation of vitamins and minerals should not be required in the adult non-breeding bird. These areas should be addressed in the basic diet. If the diet is fundamentally poor, the addition of various micronutrients is unlikely to address the main problem and definitely will not improve the state of the macronutrients.

Specific need for supplements

If supplements are to be used, they should only be those recommended and developed for raptors. These should be balanced and heavy doses of single fat-soluble vitamins should be avoided. All supplements should be used precisely according to the manufacturer's instructions.

The use of any supplements should be directed towards specific requirements at specific times, e.g. growth and rearing, breeding, moulting. *During all these periods, basic feeding should be increased with particular attention to protein content and quality.*

Growth and rearing

Addition of a calcium/vitamin D3/fat-soluble vitamin mix is beneficial.

Breeding

Female birds lay down calcium stores approximately a month before breeding. The addition of a calcium/vitamin D3 supplement and a vitamin E supplement is recommended for males and females during this period. However, it is vital to use these supplements only in the quantities recommended by the manufacturer in order to avoid overdosage

Moulting

Use of an essential amino acid/fat-soluble (especially vitamin A) vitamin mix during the moulting period may assist in feather growth and in speeding up moult.

Probiotics

Probiotics are often used in raptors. As the birds do not have a fermenting gut it is unclear what role the gut flora (and therefore the probiotics) may play. It has been proposed that probiotics 'block' more pathogenic bacteria, in which case they may be used during times of stress (e.g. manning, transport), when they will certainly do no harm and the electrolytes that are included in most mixtures will certainly help.

Rangle

This is the deliberate feeding of stones to captive hawks or falcons so that they then cast up the stones. The aim is to 'cleanse' the stomach, removing apparent fat deposits and thus making the bird hungrier and a better hunter. Some falconers recommend doing this up to once a month during the hunting season.

There is little evidence to show that it works and, given the risk of damage to the gut and obstruction, this is a practice that may be better avoided.

In the Middle East this procedure is traditionally performed using ammonium chloride (*schnather*). Many cases of toxicity have resulted and this practice is certainly not recommended.

Hand-rearing

Attention must be paid to the normal adult diet and to any changes that adult raptors would normally make when rearing young in the wild. The basic rules are as follows:

- Maintain a good (2:1) calcium:phosphorus ratio. Calcium and vitamin D3 supplements should be used
- Avoid excessive protein loads. This may result in rapid soft tissue and feather growth, which may overload soft bones, predisposing to deformities (e.g. 'angel wing')
- Chicks should be restricted in small pots to prevent excessive movement and splay leg
- In the first few days of life the chick's gut is sterile. Absolute cleanliness must be observed in the rearing room
- Probiotics may be useful
- Food should be slightly wetted with clean fresh water immediately before being offered to the chick
- Young vultures require food to be part-digested. This is best achieved by soaking food in a commercial pancreatic supplement (for dogs with exocrine pancreatic insufficiency) for half an hour before feeding
- Only small pieces of food should be fed at a time. Crop filling should be assessed and attention quickly sought if the crop is slow to clear.

Feeding in special circumstances

Pre-transport

In general, birds should travel with an empty crop; ideally they should have cast before travel. The exception is experienced hunting birds that may be used to being fed immediately after hunting and before the trip home. Nonetheless even these birds should not undertake long journeys with a full crop. The danger is that they regurgitate while hooded or confined, resulting in choking.

Sick or recovering birds

It is not essential to feed casting matter. Thin birds that need building up during or after illness can be 'half-crop' fed. Essentially, the bird is fed little and often. Only a half-crop of food (without skin or bone) is given. The bird is fed again as soon as the crop is empty and this continues through the day. This technique is also useful for birds that have problems holding weight and can be utilized while awaiting results from the clinical investigation and during therapy.

Fluid feeds may be used in very sick inappetent birds. In the short term the foods marketed for other species (e.g. Critical Care Formula, Vetark) are excellent as they provide electrolytes and simple carbohydrates.

Over the longer period, protein and fat need to be provided. The critical care diets marketed for cats and ferrets are appropriate in these cases. The quantity that can be tube fed at each time will depend on the size of the bird and whether or not it has a crop (see Chapter 8).

Vomiting birds should be fed smaller volumes more frequently (after the vomition has been controlled).

In all cases, normal carcass food should be introduced little by little as the bird starts to respond to the sight of it. Meat should not be left in with the patient (it may be tempted to eat after the food has begun to deteriorate) but should be shown to the bird and then left for 30–60 minutes only. If the bird has not fed after this time, tube feeding should be continued and the exercise repeated later that day or the next day.

References

Brown TP and Julian RJ (2003) Other toxins and poisons. In *Diseases of Poultry, 11th edn*, ed. YM Saif, p. 1143. Iowa State Press, Ames, IA

Carnarius M, Hafez HM, Henning A, Henning HJ and Lierz M (2005) Central nervous symptoms caused by thiamine deficiency in juvenile Goshawks (*Accipiter gentilis*). In: *Proceedings of the 8th Conference of the European Association of Avian Veterinarians. Arles, France; April 24–30th*, pp. 151–158

Cooper JE (2002) *Birds of Prey: Health and Disease*. Blackwell Science, Oxford

Ferguson-Lees J and Christie DA (2001) *Raptors of the World*. Christopher Helm, London

Forbes NA and Cooper JE (1993) Fatty liver-kidney syndrome of Merlins. In: *Raptor Biomedicine*, ed. PT Redig *et al.*, pp. 45–48. Chiron Publications, Keighley

Forbes NA and Flint CG (2000) *Raptor Nutrition*. Honeybrook Farm Animal Feeds, Evesham

Forbes NA and Rees Davies R (2000) Practical raptor nutrition. In: *Proceedings of the 21st Annual Conference & Expo of the Association of Avian Veterinarians, Portland, Oregon. Aug 30th–Sept 1st*, pp. 165–171

Heidenreich M (1997) *Birds of Prey Medicine and Management*. Blackwell Science, Oxford

Kirkwood JK (1981) Maintenance energy requirements and rate of weight loss during starvation in birds of prey. In: *Recent Advances in the Study of Raptor Diseases*, ed. J Cooper and M Greenwood, pp. 153–158. Chiron Publications, Keighley

Klasing KC (1998) *Comparative Avian Nutrition*. CAB International, Wallingford

Peeters N, Viaene N and Devriese L (1977) Poisoning in pigeons after administration of vitamin B6 (pyridoxine). *Poultry Abstracts*, **4**, 108

Robbins CT (1993) *Wildlife Feeding and Nutrition, 2nd edn*. Academic Press, San Diego

Schöneberg H (2004) *Falknerei – Der leitfaden für Prüfung und Praxis*. Verlag Peter N Klüh, Germany

18

Raptors: parasitic disease

Neil A. Forbes

Introduction

Free-living birds tolerate their parasites but are not confined to a limited physical space, which means that their immediate environment is not subjected to an escalating level of contamination. In contrast, captive raptors are often maintained in a confined space, such that any infected raptor host will constantly contaminate their immediate environment. When the infestation involves parasites with direct life cycles, or where intermediate hosts (e.g. snails, arthropods or earthworms) are present within the bird's environment, life cycles can be completed and endemic levels of parasitism and clinical disease are common. Raptor keepers must therefore test for, treat, control and prevent an environmental build up of such parasites.

Ectoparasites

Lierz et al. (2002) demonstrated a 97% prevalence of ectoparasites in wild injured raptors in Germany. The parasites include arachnids of the order Acarina (ticks and mites) and insects of the orders Mallophaga (biting lice) and Diptera (flies).

Ticks

Both soft (Argasidae) and hard (Ixodidae) ticks cause disease in raptors, the former predominantly in tropical areas and the latter in temperate areas. The main significance of ticks is as vectors for blood-borne protozoal infections such as *Haemoproteus* and *Babesia*, though they can also transmit viruses, bacteria and rickettsiae.

Clinical disease

Monks et al. (2006) demonstrated that a seasonal and regional tick-related syndrome causes significant mortality and morbidity in cage and aviary birds (50% being raptors) in the UK: 60% of cases reported occurred in August or September, but all months except January and February were represented. Disease-carrying ticks universally attached around the head, eyelids (Figure 18.1) or neck. Birds were presented with localized oedema and subcutaneous haemorrhage, often spreading to the choana and oropharynx. In this survey 60% of affected raptors survived. During the period of the survey, in each year over 95% of cases occurred within a tight time window of some 14 days. All ticks were identified as *Ixodes frontalis*, a specific bird tick.

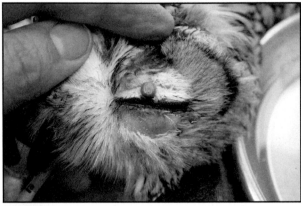

18.1 *Ixodes frontalis* on a European Eagle Owl.

Samples from ticks and affected birds were submitted for PCR testing for *Borrelia burgdorferi sensu lato*, *Babesia* spp., *Bartonella* spp. and *Ehrlichia* spp., but all tests yielded negative results.

Monks et al. (2006) considered it likely that ticks found close to aviaries had fallen off infected birds (which might have been roosting in overhanging trees) during the tick season in the previous year. The ticks were subsequently triggered by meteorological changes, then located the nearest bird and attached themselves to it. At the time of attachment, the ticks would be very small, but would swell as they engorged with blood. On occasions birds were found dead, sometimes with the tick still attached but sometimes with just a tell-tale area of subcutaneous haemorrhage on the head or neck. In other cases the bird was recognized as being unwell and was presented to a veterinary surgeon.

Sick birds were treated with fluid and nutritional support, antibiosis and anti-inflammatory therapy, and 75% of the treated birds recovered.

The findings of this survey indicate that tick-infected birds should be presented for therapy to a veterinary surgeon. When one bird is affected, seasonal and geographical indicators indicate that other birds in the vicinity are at risk of infection.

Treatment

All birds were given fluid therapy, NSAIDs and antibiotics and it was demonstrated that survival rates were significantly improved in cases where a therapeutic course of oxytetracycline was administered (Monks et al., 2006).

Control: Any affected birds and all in-contacts should be treated with a single dose of fipronil spray at 7.5 mg/kg (3 ml/kg), applied directly to the skin. An effective and bird-safe environmental parasiticide should be applied to all aviary floors in the vicinity (e.g. permethrin or cypermethrin plus pyriproxyfen or (s)-methoprene). Where sites have suffered losses in one year, the ground should be treated prophylactically with an appropriate bird-safe pesticide in at least August and September in subsequent years. The use of suspended flights and free-range poultry (to scavenge for ticks) is an environmentally sympathetic alternative.

Mites

Dermanyssus gallinae
The red poultry mite (Figure 18.2a) tends to feed on its host only at night, hiding away in crevices and cracks in adjacent woodwork during the day. Mites are most easily seen on the host with a light after dark. They will be recognized as small (circa 0.5 mm) round brown, red or black mites, at times accumulating around feather shafts. Heavily infested nestlings may suffer weight loss, lethargy, weakness and even collapse due to anaemia. The host should be treated with permethrin or fipronil at 7.5 mg/kg (3 ml/kg) and the environment should be treated with permethrin or cypermethrin plus pyriproxyfen or (s)-methoprene.

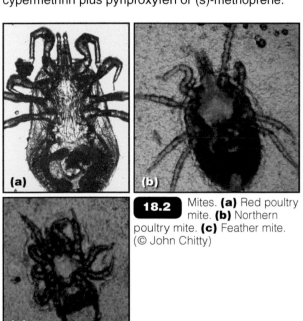

18.2 Mites. **(a)** Red poultry mite. **(b)** Northern poultry mite. **(c)** Feather mite. (© John Chitty)

Ornithonyssus
The northern poultry mite (Figure 18.2b) spends all of its life on the host. The mite is easily controlled by treating the host with permethrin or fipronil at 7.5 mg/kg.

Quill mites
Quill mites (*Harpyrhynchus* spp.; Figure 18.2c) are rare in raptors. Mites enter a developing blood feather. As the feather matures, a circumferential constriction forms around the shaft of the feather, which then breaks off at that point, releasing the mites to enter a fresh blood feather. Mites feeding in developing blood feathers are susceptible to avermectins at a dose of 0.2 mg/kg is diluted 1:11 with propylene glycol and applied to the skin at a dose of 0.2 ml/kg body weight, weekly on four occasions.

Cnemidocoptes
Cnemidocoptes, more commonly responsible for scaly leg or face in canaries and budgerigars, can cause cere and leg lesions in raptors (see Chapter 24). Treatment is with avermectins, as above. All in-contact birds should be treated.

Feather lice (Mallophaga)
Feather lice (Figure 18.3) that feed exclusively on dead feather material are most prevalent on captive raptors. They cause considerable irritation and in an otherwise healthy bird would be removed by the host during normal preening. The lice are readily visible on inspection of the underside of feathers. They may also be noted scurrying in a sideways crab-like fashion between feathers, particularly when the host is anaesthetized (in response to the concurrent reduction in body temperature). Eggs may be visible on feathers (Figure 18.4), typically attached to the feather vein adjacent to the shaft.

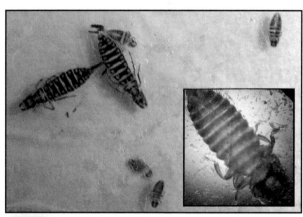

18.3 Lice from Oriental White-backed Vulture. The longer thinner parasites are adapted to the remiges, while the shorter ones are from the body feathers. The close-up view identifies the short species as typical chewing lice (Mallophaga). (© John Chitty)

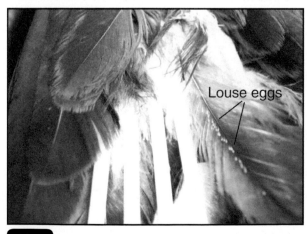

Louse eggs

18.4 Louse eggs on a Harris' Hawk.

The presence of significant numbers of feather lice is typically an indication that the bird is unwell or has some physical impediment to normal preening (e.g. a spinal injury or arthritis).

Treatment

Treatment is with a single application of fipronil spray at a dose of 7.5 mg/kg (3 ml/kg), applied directly to the skin rather than the plumage.

True flies (Diptera)

Hippoboscidae

Louse or flat flies (Figure 18.5) are regularly found on birds of prey as well as on certain of their prey species (corvids in particular). The flies resemble household flies but are flattened dorsoventrally and are difficult to squash. They act as vectors for a variety of pathogens (including some blood parasites, e.g. *Leucocytozoon* and *Haemoproteus*) and should be eliminated when found. The flies are effectively controlled with a single application of fipronil at 7.5 mg/kg (3 ml/kg).

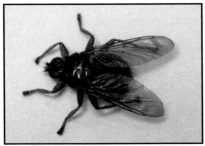

18.5

Flat-fly (Hippoboscidae). (© John Chitty)

Blowflies

Blowflies are the cause of myiasis, or fly strike, in sheep. They are unusual in raptors in the UK but, in the author's experience, infestation occurs most commonly in wild injured raptors during the summer months, when they are severely debilitated and are suffering an open wound. The bird should be treated with antibiosis, fluid therapy, anti-inflammatory agents and an insecticide (e.g. F10 Insecticidal Spray).

Endoparasites

Endoparasites are common in free-living adult raptors (54–80% prevalence) (Smith, 1993; Ferrer *et al.*, 2004), in which they cause minimal clinical disease unless the bird is suffering concurrent illness, nutritional shortage (commonest in inclement weather and during dispersal at the end of rearing) or trauma. Endoparasites seen in raptors include the following groups.

- Nematodes (roundworms) are common in captive and free-living raptors. Clinical disease is common in young birds (as they have yet to develop an immunity) as well as in free-living birds that have suffered concurrent disease or injury. These parasites may be gut-active or act on the respiratory system.
- Cestodes (tapeworms) rarely cause clinical disease, even in wild birds.

- Trematodes (flukes) are found as several species in raptors, but are not commonly of clinical significance.
- Protozoa (unicellular organisms) include *Trichomonas gallinae*, several coccidian species and tissue cryptosporidians. They also include haemoparasites that may be transmitted by mosquitoes, flies or ticks, according to the species of parasite, which means that vector control is relevant.

Gut-active nematodes

Ascarids

These roundworms are one of the commonest endoparasites of wild and captive raptors. Disease prevalence is compounded by the fact that they generally have direct life cycles, such that ingestion of defecated eggs (Figure 18.6) will cause immediate reinfection of the host. The problem is compounded as the ova are generally resistant and will survive for up to a year in the environment, though they are not infective for 2 weeks after shedding. Once ingested, the prepatent period (from infection to faecal shedding of ova) is generally 5–6 weeks; thus a reinfected bird can test negative for a considerable period.

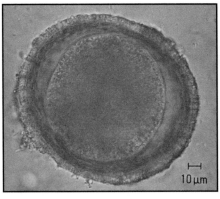

18.6

Ascarid egg. (© Michael Lierz)

- *Clinical disease* is most commonly found in young birds, who may suffer from weight loss, lethargy or on rare occasions where heavy infestation occurs, gut blockage.
- *Treatment:* fenbendazole or avermectins.
- *Control:*
  - Regular screening (twice a year, i.e. after the flying season and again after the moult, prior to retraining for a new season)
  - Environmental parasite control (see later).

Capillaria spp.

These are common and problematical parasites of free-living and captive raptors. The thread-like worms, 1–5 cm long, are located in the oropharynx or intestine. Infection may on occasions be recognized by white lesions on a bird's tongue or oropharynx (Figure 18.7a). They usually have a direct life cycle but use earthworms as a paratenic host. The prepatent period is 3–4 weeks. The parasite is particularly common in species that naturally feed on earthworms (e.g. Common Buzzard, Red-tailed Hawk, Red Kite).

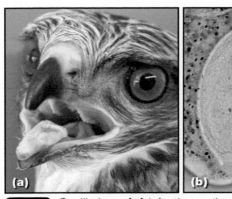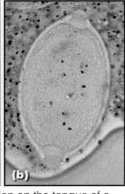

18.7 *Capillaria* sp. **(a)** Infection on the tongue of a Common Buzzard. **(b)** Egg. (© Michael Lierz)

Clinical disease: This is dependent on the *Capillaria* species concerned and the site of infection. It ranges from head or food flicking (with oropharyngeal lesions), to diarrhoea, weight loss, inappetence or lethargy and poor flight performance.

Diagnosis: The characteristic bioperculate lemon-shaped ova (55–70 × 24–35 µm) are found on faecal examination (Figure 18.7b) and on occasions in oropharyngeal scrapings.

Treatment: *Capillaria* commonly demonstrates multiple drug resistance. Typically levamisole, regular doses of benzimidazole and avermectins are ineffective. This author has found fenbendazole, at a dose of 25 mg/kg daily for 5 days, to be efficacious, with repeat faecal testing 3–4 weeks later being indicated. Others recommend avermectins at 0.5–1 mg/kg orally once (Samour and Naldo, 2001).

Control:

- Regular screening (twice a year, i.e. after the flying season and again after the moult, prior to retraining for a new season).
- Environmental parasite control (see later). Treatment without environmental decontamination is meaningless.

Trichinella pseudospiralis

This rare parasite of raptors is distributed worldwide. Adult female worms live in the host's gut, producing larvae, which migrate from the gut and take up residence in skeletal muscle.

- *Clinical disease:* if numbers are great, clinical signs of reduced general activity, diminished competitive success for breeding territory.
- *Diagnosis:* on faecal examination (larvae, rarely seen) or histological examination of skeletal muscle (preferable).
- *Treatment:* fenbendazole (muscle cysts cannot be treated).

Respiratory nematodes

Syngamus trachea

Many free-living as well as captive raptors and quarry species are infected by the 'gape worm'. The adult worms (female 20 mm, male 6 mm) live in permanent copulation, attached to the tracheal mucosa, resulting in a marked inflammatory response. Ova are coughed up from the trachea and are then shed via the gut. The life cycle may be direct (bird to bird), or via a paratenic host such as an earthworm or snail. Encapsulated parasites may remain infective in the paratenic host for long periods of time.

Clinical disease: Birds may show change of voice, inspiratory stridor, or open-mouthed neck stretching (hence the name gape worm) and gasping. Weight loss, inappetence and exercise intolerance may be seen, or even acute respiratory blockage and death in smaller species.

Diagnosis: Infection is confirmed on faecal analysis or tracheoscopy (Figure 18.8).

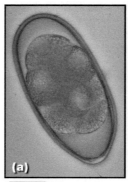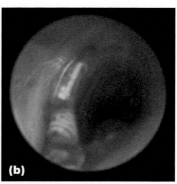

18.8 *Syngamus trachea.* **(a)** Egg. **(b)** Endoscopic view of adult worms within the trachea. (© Michael Lierz)

Treatment: Suspected cases should not be treated prior to confirmation of diagnosis. Therapy with fenbendazole or avermectins is effective. In heavy infections, when worms are treated, dead worms may cause further respiratory embarrassment. Where such circumstances are predicted, concurrent antibiosis should be administered.

Control:

- Regular screening (twice a year, i.e. after the flying season and again after the moult, prior to retraining for a new season).
- Environmental parasite control is essential in view of the direct life cycle (see later).

Serratospiculum spp.

This long thread-like filarial respiratory worm (illustrated in Chapter 20) is found commonly in hot climates (including the Middle East), but rarely in temperate zones, unless the bird is imported. It has recently been reported in New Zealand in a free-living indigenous falcon (Green *et al.*, 2006).

The worm has an indirect life cycle and has been transmitted experimentally via seven different species of beetle (Samour and Naldo, 2001) that live in the environs of captive Saker Falcons and are on occasion ingested by them. Following ingestion the L3 larvae excyst and pass directly to the host's air sac. There they develop into L5 and breed to produce large numbers of thin-walled ova (Figure 18.9), which are coughed up, swallowed and passed via the faeces.

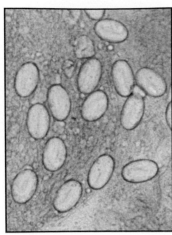

18.9
Serratospiculum eggs. (Courtesy of Jaime Samour)

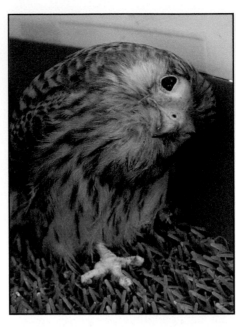

18.10
Severe sinusitis and central nervous system signs in a Common Kestrel with *Cyathostoma* infection.

Clinical disease: Whilst the vast majority of Saker Falcons in the Middle East are infected, few demonstrate clinical signs unless they are subject to concurrent stress or disease. Clinical signs associated with severe infection include air sacculitis, pneumonia and septicaemia (see Chapter 20). Infection may also predispose to aspergillosis.

Diagnosis: The disease may be anticipated based on the patient's provenance, with further suspicion based on radiography, and confirmed by endoscopy or faecal flotation.

Treatment: Historically, treatment with fenbendazole or regular doses of avermectins, followed by endoscopic removal of worms from the air sacs, was recommended. More effective treatment options that are now advised (Samour and Naldo, 2001) use subcutaneous injection of avermectins at 1 mg/kg, repeated 1–2 weeks later. As a higher dosage does have a better effect, the dosage of ivermectin in falcons should be 2 mg/kg to treat this parasite, with a safe dose being up to 4 mg/kg (Lierz, 2001).

Control: This disease is highly prevalent (> 65%) in the Middle East and other warmer climates. Any newly trapped or purchased birds in that area or those imported from that area should be screened for *Serratospiculum* spp. ova in the faeces. Intermediate hosts (e.g. beetles) should be excluded from a bird's environment in those areas of the world where the disease is endemic.

Cyathostoma spp.

These parasites were initially recorded by Simpson and Harris (1992) and have been found in Common Kestrel, Common Buzzard and Eurasian Sparrowhawk. The parasite has a direct life cycle with a facultative paratenic host (earthworm).

Clinical disease: The larvae are located in the trachea, from where they may be coughed up into the nasal passage and sinuses of the host, in which site they then develop to their full size. They may be located in the subconjunctival sac. Within sinuses they tend to cause significant inflammation and sinusitis or neurological signs (Figure 18.10).

Diagnosis: Faecal examination for ova; inspection of the conjunctival sac; endoscopic examination of the affected sinuses; or magnetic resonance imaging.

Treatment: NSAIDs, fenbendazole once with covering antibiosis. Therapy may be unrewarding in the light of the severe inflammation. Surgical access to infected sinuses and debridement is indicated where possible.

Control and prevention:

- Regular screening (twice a year, i.e. after the flying season and again after the moult, prior to retraining for a new season).
- Environmental parasite control (see later). Treatment without environmental decontamination is meaningless.

Cestodes

Tapeworms rarely cause clinical disease. As they rely on intermediate hosts not commonly available in captivity, infection of captive birds is rare and clinical disease is even less common. Even in wild birds clinical signs are rare, as the parasites tend to be well adapted to their hosts, so that few clinical signs are evident.

- *Clinical disease*: rare.
- *Diagnosis*: faecal examination.
- *Treatment*: praziquantel 10mg/kg orally or by intramuscular or subcutaneous injection; repeat after 1 week.
- *Control*:
  - Regular screening (twice a year, i.e. after the flying season and again after the moult, prior to retraining for a new season)
  - Environmental parasite control (see later).

Trematodes

Flukes are typically small (0.5–5 mm in length) and they require from one to four intermediate hosts in order to complete their life cycles. Several species of fluke are found in raptors, but they are not commonly of clinical significance in Europe. *Strigea falconis* is most commonly reported in the Goshawk, Common Buzzard, Saker Falcon and Peregrine Falcon, but others are also reported (e.g. *Clinostomum, Neodiplostomum, Opisthorchis* spp., *Pseudostrigea buteonis*). Eggs are passed in the faeces, developing into miracidia, which infect an intermediate host (typically a snail). In the intermediate host they transform into cercariae, after which they are excreted. The parasite may pass through a second intermediary host (in which they form into metacercariae), after which the definitive host (raptor) ingests them. In the definitive host they develop into a fluke, thereby completing the life cycle. Infection is rare in captivity, due to a lack of the required intermediate host.

Clinical disease
Flukes live primarily in the small intestine, though they have been recorded in the respiratory tract, bile ducts, kidneys, body cavity and circulation (Lacina and Bird, 2000). Diarrhoea, weight loss, inappetence and lethargy may be noted

Diagnosis
Fluke eggs are typically thin walled, dark coloured, oval with a single operculum at one pole (Figure 18.11) and are larger than those of nematodes. Ova are shed intermittently, which means that repeated faecal direct smears are required.

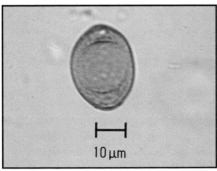

18.11 Trematode egg. (© Michael Lierz)

Treatment
Praziquantel is usually helpful and is administered at 10 mg/kg once, repeated a week later.

Control and prevention

- Regular screening (twice a year, i.e. after the flying season and again after the moult, prior to retraining for a new season).
- Environmental control of parasite and intermediate host (beetles, snails or ants, according to trematode species) is vital (see later).

Protozoa

Trichomonas gallinae
Trichomonas gallinae is a flagellated protozoan that invades the mucosa of the oropharynx, oesophagus and crop, as well as on rare occasions the intestines, orbital sinuses and even viscera. It causes trichomoniasis, often referred to as frounce in raptors.

Raptors are most typically infected after eating fresh (warm) pigeon or other columbiforms. Wild raptors (e.g. Peregrine Falcon and Northern Goshawk) commonly catch and eat pigeons. Young birds, or old birds with other morbidity, may suffer clinical disease; fit and healthy adult birds tend not to.

Clinical disease: The disease may be suspected on clinical appearance (white or yellow necrotic lesions) of the mouth (Figure 18.12). Such birds may be keen to eat (i.e. hungry), but demonstrate oral pain on eating, or may head flick in an effort to clear their mouths during or after eating. These clinical findings may be identical to those seen with candidiasis, capillariasis, or viral or bacterial stomatitis. Diagnosis is not possible without cytology.

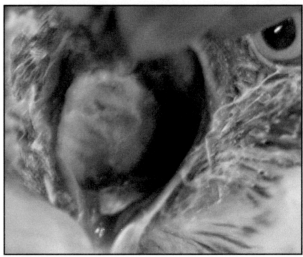

18.12 Trichomoniasis in a Sparrowhawk. (© John Chitty)

Diagnosis: This must always be confirmed by microscopic examination from an oral swab re-suspended in warm saline. Characteristic flagellate ovoid directionally swimming motile protozoa will be seen.

Treatment: The preferred therapy is carnidazole at 30 mg/kg orally as a single dose. If this is not available, metronidazole may be administered at 50 mg/kg orally q24h for 5 days.

Control and prevention: No fresh pigeon should ever be fed to a raptor. Pigeons should first be frozen and then thawed before being used as food. Raptors may become infected subsequent to eating wild-caught avian quarry. If this is a possibility, clinical signs should be monitored on a regular basis.

Coccidia
Four different coccidian genera, *Eimeria, Sarcocystis, Frankelia* and *Caryospora*, have been reported in raptors. Of these only *Caryospora* is of major clinical significance; the others vary in relation to their exact life cycle, but treatment and control are identical. To date *Caryospora* spp. have only been identified in owls and falcons and not in hawks or other raptors.

Caryospora *spp.:* Although reported in two free-living Common Kestrels in Germany and in free-living Red-tailed Hawks in the United States, this infection is found almost exclusively in captive raptors. It constitutes the most prevalent and potentially serious parasitic disease of falcons in captivity. In captive-reared birds in the UK, central Europe, the Middle East and America, 60–65% of all young falcons tested are shown to be infected.

Disease is only of clinical significance in young birds (from fledging to the end of initial training, 30–80 days of age). Adult birds are commonly infected; on occasions disease will occur in adult birds, especially Merlins, if they are naive.

The author has demonstrated a seasonal increase in oocyst shedding immediately prior to the host breeding season (presumably facilitated by a hormone-induced relaxation of immunity). Oocysts become infective when they sporulate 2–4 days after deposition. They remain viable in the environment for 6–12 months. As chicks hatch into the contaminated aviary, they are challenged by the parasite. The clinical response to infection varies with respect to parasite and host species. Due to the nature of captive raptor accommodation, the oocyst concentrations tend to build up within breeding facilities, with clinical disease becoming more and more significant with each successive season.

Clinical disease: If infected juvenile birds remain unstressed until such time as they have developed a solid immunity, they do not typically suffer clinical disease. However, most birds will be removed from the aviary, sold on or trained within the period during which they are susceptible to clinical disease. The latter activities create stress for the bird, with consequent immune suppression and resultant clinical coccidiosis. Merlins tend to be found dead, whilst other species are more likely to be noticed as being off colour and fluffed up, with weight loss and inappetence; they may vomit, they may have diarrhoea (which may contain blood), or they may appear to suffer from extreme abdominal pain or cramps. These clinical signs can be present for 48 hours prior to the shedding of faecal oocysts. Oocysts are of similar or larger size to those of other coccidia and typically one-quarter of the size of most nematode eggs (Figure 18.13).

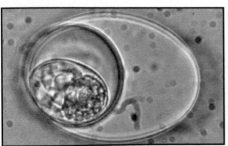

18.13
Sporulated *Caryospora* oocyst.

Diagnosis: Oocysts are most likely to be detected on flotation of faecal samples collected over 3 consecutive days. Whilst low oocyst numbers generally indicate lower clinical disease, this is not universally the case.

Treatment: As treatment is effective in not only clearing oocyst shedding but also coincidentally generating greater immunity than arises naturally in an untreated clinical infection, therapy is indicated even in low infections. A number of therapies have been recommended (clazuril, amprolium, sulphonamides), but by analysis of long-term therapeutic response rates the author has been able to demonstrate a statistically superior response rate when infected birds are treated with toltrazuril at 25 mg/kg orally once weekly on three occasions. Baycox 2.5% is a water-soluble product designed primarily for administration to poultry via drinking water. In order to maintain solubility, it is manufactured as a strongly alkaline solution. This high pH can cause post-gavage vomition, but if the Baycox is diluted 50:50 with a neutral or acid solution (such as certain well known proprietary carbonated soft drinks), immediately prior to application, efficacy will be maintained in the absence of post-administration vomition.

Control: The author advises any owner of new falcons to submit faecal tests for analysis at 30, 50 and 75 days of age. If *Caryospora* spp. have not been detected on the site previously, there is benefit to be gained by keeping the bird in an environment that can be readily cleaned and cleared of oocysts during this risk period. In the author's opinion, once a bird has been shedding oocycts in an aviary or weathering situation, it is unrealistic to think that it is possible to clear the parasite from that environment; indeed it may even be deleterious to do so. In such a scenario, an endemic level of *Caryospora* should be allowed to reinfect falcons naturally on a regular basis so that a solid immunity is maintained. The only risk is for new or young naive birds entering that environment. With such birds, the sooner they become infected the better, and repeated toltrazuril treatment should be targeted to treat infection in the prepatent period.

In a falcon breeding centre, serial faecal analysis may be used to predict at what age each young falcon is likely to be infected. Young birds should all be treated, two to three times, to include the minimum age at which they could be infected, as well as 10 days after the last date when they are likely to be infected and halfway in between. In an ideal situation, young falcons would be vaccinated or infected with a known dose of each species of *Caryospora* (which they might meet in later life), then treated during the prepatent period (say 5–6 days after infection, and again a week later). The duration of the prepatent period varies with respect to host species and the *Caryospora* species involved, ranging from 10 to 16 days. In this way the bird will develop an immunity to any *Caryospora* species of clinical significance, whilst avoiding clinical disease and oocyst contamination of the aviary (Forbes and Fox, 2005).

Cryptosporidium spp.

These are tissue protozoa. Two species that affect avian species are *Cryptosporidium baileyi* and *C. meleagridis*. Cryptosporidiosis has only been reported in three individual falcons (all Gyr or

Gyr-hybrids) (Rodriguez Barbon and Forbes, 2007) and, although a novel clinical disease in this genus, no doubt other cases will be forthcoming. The endogenous phase can be found in the luminal border of epithelial cells of the respiratory, urinary and gastrointestinal tracts. The location has been described as intracellular but extracytoplasmic; there is a structure, formed by the parasite, separating the parasite from the cytoplasm and this structure is considered to have a function in parasite nutrition.

The life cycle is direct and monoxenous. All the forms show sexual and asexual cycles in the same host. The cycle starts with the inhalation or ingestion of a thick-walled oocyst 4–8 μm in diameter and containing four sporozoites, the release of which is temperature-dependent (though bile salts and trypsin are involved in the release), after which the infection occurs in the gastrointestinal tract.

In the respiratory tract the parasite affects the mucociliary function and causes rhinitis, conjunctivitis, tracheitis, sneezing and dyspnoea. In the gastrointestinal tract it has been recorded as affecting salivary glands, small and large intestines and cloaca.

Diagnosis: The disease may be suspected on clinical presentation (Figure 18.14a). Further indications are gained on cytology (Figure 18.14b) and confirmed by positive fluorescence after auramine staining on histopathology. Cray *et al.* (2002) compared the

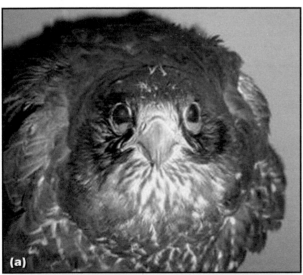

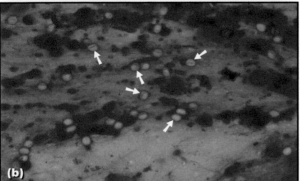

18.14 Cryptosporidiosis. **(a)** Clinical presentation in a Gyrfalcon. **(b)** Cytology reveals the organisms. (b, courtesy of Tom Bailey)

efficacy of different diagnostic tests, namely antigen ELISA kit, acid fast stain, PCR, direct immunofluorescent staining technique and serology. They concluded that the antigen ELISA kit was the most sensitive, but speciation via PCR can be valuable.

Treatment: Treatment is with paromomycin at 100 mg/kg orally q12h for 7 days. This therapy may need to be repeated a week later.

Control: As paromomycin prevents gut shedding but does not eliminate tissue forms, any infected post-treated falcon should be considered potentially infective to other Gyrfalcons and Gyr-hybrids and hence not mixed with such birds. Recrudescence of infection can and does occur. Cryptosporidia survive well in water and so appropriate water hygiene and sanitation is important. Prevention of *Cryptosporidium* infections through environmental control is challenging due to the resistance of the parasite to extreme temperatures and several disinfectants. Direct exposure to sunlight and low levels of humidity decrease the load of *Cryptosporidium* in the environment (Rodriguez Barbon and Forbes, 2007). Peroxygen-based disinfectants have shown high efficacy in inactivating *C. parvum* oocysts. If disinfection is not possible the bird's exposure to the parasite should be reduced by avoiding areas previously occupied by infected animals. In some cases there has been evidence that infection may have arisen subsequent to feeding infected rodents. Sources of food should be screened for this parasite. Overall the indication is that this disease is one that occurs where the host is immunocompromised, and as such is an opportunist parasite. The avoidance or minimization of stress is important as well as strict attention to hygiene during periods when a bird is likely to be stressed (e.g. after transportation or during initial training).

Haemoparasites
These are obligate intracellular parasites that cause disease by destroying host cells. The order Haemosporidae (family Plasmodiidae) includes the genera *Plasmodium*, *Haemoproteus* and *Leucocytozoon*. Most haematozoans are predominantly apathogenic.

Plasmodium spp.: *Plasmodium* is the cause of malaria in humans and other mammals, and in birds. The parasite is transmitted by culicine and anopheline mosquitoes. Eleven different species of *Plasmodium* can be found in birds of prey (Bennett *et al.*, 1993; Telford *et al.*, 1997). Redig *et al.* (1993) found *Plasmodium* spp. in 6.8% of owls and 4.9% of falcons (i.e. a low prevalence compared with other avian haematozoa, which are typically found at 20–30%). *Plasmodium* spp. have been identified in a range of raptor species but they are most prevalent and clinically significant in Gyrfalcons, in which they commonly cause disease ranging from mild depression and anorexia to severe dyspnoea with sudden collapse and death. Restraining suspect malaria-affected patients can prove fatal; preconditioning such birds with oxygen therapy for 20–30 minutes prior to handling and restraint has proved useful (Remple, 1981).

Diagnosis: Diagnosis is by demonstration of *Plasmodium* organisms (which characteristically push the erythrocyte nucleus to one side of the erythrocyte) on blood smears (Figure 18.15).

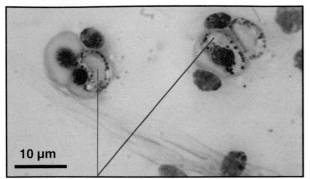

18.15   *Plasmodium* spp. in the erythrocytes of a Snowy Owl's lung tissue.

Treatment: Chloroquine and primaquine or mefloquine hydrochloride alone (Redig *et al.*, 1993).

Control and prevention: Mosquito (vector) control and prophylactic medication with a chloroquine and primaquine combination at 26.3 mg/kg once weekly from 1 month prior to until 1 month post the anticipated mosquito season. Regular screening of blood smears during this period is useful, so that low-grade infections can be detected and treated prior to overt clinical signs.

Haemoproteus *spp.*: *Haemoproteus* is common but clinical disease is reported to be rare (Lacina and Bird 2000), though Mutlow and Forbes (2000) demonstrated a significant incidence of severe disease (PCV dropping to 5–10% and birds dying) in Snowy Owls, Tawny Owls and Harris' Hawks. Disease occurs most frequently in young birds, with severe anaemia, weight loss and typically death by 65–70 days. Transmission may be by hippoboscid flies.

Clinical disease: An alive infected bird will be lethargic and inappetent and will show exercise intolerance. On post-mortem examination there may be white streaks in the leg muscles, enlarged spleen and enlarged liver, with concurrent aspergilloma and *Salmonella* septicaemia. On histopathology, schizonts are found in the liver, spleen, lung, skeletal muscle, heart and brain.

Adult birds carrying an endemic infection will demonstrate higher levels of circulating parasites in the spring, prior to breeding. The life cycle can complete via schizogony with the host being reinfected by itself, or alternatively by gametogony (using a dipteric fly as an intermediate host). Dipteric (biting midges) and hippoboscid flies are known to transmit this parasite.

Diagnosis: Diagnosis is by demonstration of the characteristic halter-shaped gametocytes, which characteristically encircle much of an erythrocyte nucleus (Figure 18.16).

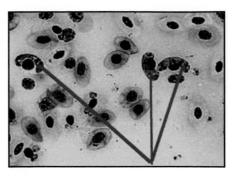

18.16
Haemoproteus noctua in the blood of a Snowy Owl.

Treatment: Treatment can be attempted with chloroquine, or chloroquine with primaquine or mefloquine, but in the majority of cases clinicians fail to eliminate the parasite.

Control: Potential breeding birds of susceptible species (e.g. Snowy Owls) may be screened prior to the breeding season. If birds are found to be infected, they can either be treated in the hope of eliminating the parasitaemia, their eggs taken and hand reared or fostered by a non-infected bird, or breeding prevented. Effective ectoparasite control (e.g. fipronil) should be implemented throughout the breeding season, even in birds where the parasite has not been detected, in the hope of preventing vector (biting insect) spread to young naive birds.

Leucocytozoon *spp.*: These intracellular parasites of both leucocytes and erythrocytes may be transmitted by simulid flies. Ashford *et al.* (1991) believed that *Leucocytozoon toddi* (Figure 18.17) is transmitted by *Culicoides* mosquitoes. The parasite can cause severe disease (weight loss and lethargy) in poultry and reduced clutch size in owls. On post-mortem examination schizonts may be found in muscle, heart, spleen, liver and kidneys, where severe damage can occur. Gametocytes develop in leucocytes and erythrocytes. Infected host blood cells become grossly distorted, generally elongated, with the nucleus of the host cell forming a crescent along one side of the parasite cell.

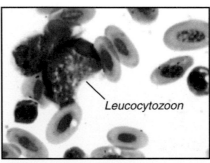

18.17
Leucocytozoon toddi.

Leucocytozoon — Leucocytozoon

Leucocytozoon infections are typically apathogenic. Where clinical disease does occur, it is generally young birds that are affected. Whilst sulphonamide drugs may achieve a reduction in parasite numbers, infection will not be eliminated. Melarsamine at 0.25 mg/kg i.m. for 4 days may be effective.

Babesia: Members of the genus *Babesia* are piroplasms, belonging to the order Piroplasmida. Piroplasms are parasites of birds and mammals, the vector being ticks. *Babesia* spp. are most readily recognized as translucent ovoid structures in the cytoplasm of erythrocytes, approximately one-sixth of the size of the nucleus (Figure 18.18). Disease in raptors due to *Babesia* spp. is rare but can occur when levels of parasitaemia are high (> 25%). No effective therapy for babesiosis in raptors has been described. Imidocarb dipropionate is the drug of choice in companion animals, in which it is given once at 5 mg/kg i.m. or s.c. In the latter situation the drug is reported to have minimal toxic effects (compared with other effective medications) and has been shown to be effective in clinical cases and as a prophylactic agent.

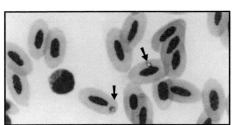

18.18

Babesia shortii in the blood of a raptor. (Courtesy of Gerry Dorrestein)

Advice to clients

Environmental control

In many parasitic situations, control of the environment (intermediate hosts in particular) is an essential part of parasite management. This is only possible if the identity of the parasite is known. If the parasite has a direct life cycle, or an indirect life cycle where the intermediate host lives within the environment of the host, then the environment must be 'decontaminated' and redesigned such that the risk of intermediate host intrusion is minimized or prevented. The majority of intermediate hosts are invertebrates such as earthworms, slugs, snails and beetles.

To prevent re-exposure to a contaminated substrate and intermediate hosts, an aviary should be designed with an impermeable base layer (concrete or a thick plastic vapour membrane), together with a solid barrier at ground level (e.g. at least one layer of breeze blocks or similar, around the perimeter of the aviary). This is readily incorporated when designing a new aviary, but can also be achieved when dealing with a mature but contaminated aviary. By removing the current substrate, laying down a builder's vapour membrane, creating a perimeter barrier and backfilling with sand or gravel, the current contamination is removed and the chances of recontamination are minimized.

Wild or new birds

New or wild (in particular injured) birds should not be admitted into healthy birds' environments until they have been tested for parasites. It is essential to manage any bird's environment to minimize the risk of parasitic disease.

References

Ashford RW, Green EE, Holmes PR and Lucas AJ (1991) *Leucocytozoan toddi* in British Sparrowhawks *Accipiter nisus*: patterns of infection in nestlings. *Journal of Natural History* **25**, 269–278

Bennett GF, Peirce MA and Ashford RW (1993) Avian haematozoa: mortality and pathogenicity. *Journal of Natural History* **27**, 993–1001

Cray C, Miller D, Curtis M, Aiyenimelo O and Clubb S (2002) Comparison of diagnostic assays for the detection of Cryptosporidium. In: *Proceedings of the Annual Conference of the Association of Avian Vets*, pp. 127–129. Association of Avian Vets, Lake Worth, FL

Ferrer D, Molina R, Adelantado C and Kinsella JM (2004) Helminths isolated from the digestive tract of diurnal raptors in Catalonia, Spain. *Veterinary Record* **154**(1), 17–20

Forbes NA and Fox MT (2005) Field trial of a *Caryospora* species vaccine for controlling clinical coccidiosis in falcons. *Veterinary Record* **156**(5), 134–138

Green CH, Gartrell BD and Charleston WA (2006) Serratospiculosis in a New Zealand Falcon (*Falco novaeseelandiae*). *New Zealand Veterinary Journal* **54**(4), 198–201

Lacina D and Bird DM (2000) Endoparasites of raptors – a review and an update. In: *Raptor Biomedicine III*, ed. JT Lumeij *et al.*, pp. 65–99. Zoological Education Network, Lake Worth, FL

Lierz M (2001) Evaluation of the dosage of ivermectin in falcons. *Veterinary Record* **148**, 596–600

Lierz M, Gobel T and Schuster R (2002) Occurrence of parasites in indigenous birds of prey and owls. *Berlin und München Tierärztliche Wochenschrift* **115**(1–2), 43–52

Monks D, Fisher MM and Forbes NA (2006) *Ixodes frontalis* and avian tick-related syndrome in the United Kingdom. *Journal of Small Animal Practice* **47**(8), 451–455

Mutlow A and Forbes NA (2000) Haemoproteus in raptors: pathogenicity, treatment and control. In: *Proceedings of the Annual Conference of the Association of Avian Vets*, pp. 157–163. Association of Avian Vets, Lake Worth, FL

Redig PT, Talbot B and Guarnera T (1993) Avian malaria. In: *Proceedings of the Annual Conference of the Association of Avian Vets*, pp. 173–181. Association of Avian Vets, Lake Worth, FL

Remple JD (1981) Avian malaria with comments on other haemosporidia in large falcons. In: *Recent Advances in Raptor Diseases*, ed. JE Cooper and AG Greenwood, pp. 107–110. Chiron Publications, Keighley, West Yorkshire

Rodriguez Barbon A and Forbes NA (2007) Use of Paromomycin in the treatment of a Cryptosporidium infection in a gyr falcon (*Falco rusticolus*) and a hybrid gyr/saker falcon (Falco rusticolus x *Falco cherrug*). In: *Proceedings European Association of Avian Veterinarians Conference, Zurich*, pp. 191–197

Samour JH and Naldo J (2001) Serratospiculiasis in captive falcons in the Middle East: a review. *Journal of Avian Medicine and Surgery* **15**(1), 2–9

Simpson VR and Harris EA (1992) *Cyathostoma lari* (Nematoda) infection in birds of prey. *Journal of Zoology* **227**, 655–659

Smith SA (1993) Diagnosis and treatment of helminths in birds of prey. In: *Raptor Biomedicine II*, ed. P Redig *et al.*, pp. 21–27. University of Minnesota, Minneapolis

Telford SR Jr, Nayar JK, Forrester GW and Knight JW (1997) *Plasmodium forresteri*, n sp. from raptors in Florida and southern Georgia: its distinction from *Plasmodium elongatum* morphologically within and among host species and by vector susceptibility. *Journal of Parasitology* **83**, 932–937

19

Raptors: infectious diseases

Michael Stanford

Introduction

Captive raptors are frequently exposed to many infectious diseases, especially from their food sources. Perfecting husbandry conditions with particular attention to biosecurity and food preparation will significantly reduce the chance of infections in captive birds.

Viral pathogens are the most common cause of infectious disease in raptors: one post-mortem study demonstrated that 14% of the raptors died from a disease of viral origin and 30% had antibodies to viruses (Heidenreich, 1997).

Although numerous bacteria have been implicated in diseases of captive raptors, caution should always be maintained before diagnosing bacterial disease as faecal, oral or skin swabs may simply reveal bacteria that are part of the normal raptor flora. A combination of clinical signs and the isolation of heavy growths of an individual organism are usually required to indicate bacterial disease.

Fungi are ubiquitous in the environment and normally only cause disease when conditions are not ideal, leading to a compromise in the bird's immune system. This is particularly true for aspergillosis, a common and invariably fatal condition of captive raptors normally caused by *Aspergillus fumigatus* (see Chapter 20). If secondary fungal infections are confirmed, attempts should always be made to identify the primary cause.

Potentially zoonotic infectious diseases and organisms in raptors:

- **Viruses:**
  - **Avian influenza**
  - **Newcastle disease (PMV-1 infection)**
  - **West Nile virus**
- **Bacteria:**
  - ***Chlamydophila* spp.**
  - ***Mycobacterium avium* (avian tuberculosis)**
  - ***Salmonella* spp.**
  - ***Pasteurella multocida* (avian cholera)**
  - ***Yersinia pseudotuberculosis* (pseudotuberculosis)**

Viral disease

Figure 19.1 gives a summary of common viral infectious diseases affecting raptors.

Virus	Clinical signs	Diagnosis	Treatment and control
Influenza A virus*	Respiratory disease of varying severity depending on serotype. Virulent strains can cause high mortality rates	Viral isolation from cloacal swabs or post-mortem tissues; PCR	Supportive therapy. Vaccination. Avoid contact with free-ranging waterfowl
Paramyxovirus 1	Vary from clinically normal to sudden death. CNS signs classic in raptors	Clinical signs; serology; virus isolation; PCR	Inactivated pigeon APMV-1 vaccines annually. Avoid contact with poultry, pigeons and feral birds
Raptor herpesviruses	Anorexia; green urates. 100% mortality	Viral isolation or demonstration of inclusion bodies from liver and spleen; typical yellow foci on liver and spleen	Feed with pigeons that are free of herpesvirus. Vaccine may become available in future
Raptor poxvirus	Nodular lesions develop on featherless areas of skin and drop off within 10 days. May cause septicaemia in immunocompromised birds	Characteristic clinical signs; demonstration of intracytoplasmic Bollinger bodies in biopsy specimens; PCR; virus isolation	Topical antibiosis and cleaning with antiseptics. Pigeon pox vaccines available but effect doubtful. Mosquito control
West Nile virus*	Sudden death. Normally CNS signs followed by death within 48 hours	PCR from oral and cloacal swabs; virus isolation from post-mortem tissues	Mosquito control. Equine vaccine available but effectiveness doubtful
Raptor adenovirus	Haemorrhagic enteritis followed by death	Virus isolation or serology	Avoid feeding racing pigeons to raptors
Rabies virus*	Rarely causes clinical signs but occasionally severe neurological signs	Demonstration of Negri bodies in CNS; virus isolation	Avoid contact with mammals potentially carrying rabies

19.1 Summary of common viral infectious diseases affecting birds of prey. * Notifiable disease in the UK

Avian influenza (influenza A)

Avian influenza is a highly contagious viral disease that affects the respiratory, digestive and neurological systems in many groups of birds, including raptors. Occasionally avian influenza A viruses become highly pathogenic and cause zoonotic infection in humans. At the time of publication, Asian H5N1 influenza virus is of most recent concern in humans.

Aetiology and pathogenesis

Influenza A is caused by an orthomyxovirus. The genome consist of eight segments with a high rate of mutation (antigenic drift). If influenza viruses meet in one host cell they are able to exchange parts of their genome (antigenic shift). This may lead to the occurrence of new highly pathogenic influenza A virus with new biological potential.

Influenza A may be identified on the basis of two schemes. First, the classification is based on differences between haemagglutinin (H) and neuraminidase (N) proteins on the surface of the virus, of which there are 16 and 9, respectively. Secondly, the virus is classified according to its pathogenicity using 6-week-old chickens in an infection trial to obtain the intravenous pathogenicity index. The virus is named according to the type of virus, the initial viral host, location of initial discovery, reference number and year of identification.

Migratory birds, in particular waterfowl, act as reservoirs for the virus and are thought to be responsible for the movement of new serotypes throughout the world (Halverson et al., 1985). Additionally, commercial movements must be considered as transmitters. Although wild birds carry the virus, they rarely succumb to disease; they are, however, responsible for the infection of domesticated birds, especially ducks, chickens and turkeys. An exception is the recent spread of H5N1 which also killed free-ranging waterfowl, a typical virus reservoir.

Clinical signs

The virus is spread by aerosol transmission from respiratory, ocular and gastrointestinal secretions. Morbidity and mortality rates depend on the strain of the virus and the host species. Non-susceptible species may be asymptomatic, whilst susceptible species infected with the same viral serotype may develop severe flu-like clinical signs and die. Clinical signs include respiratory disease of varying severity, anorexia, depression, neurological signs and diarrhoea. In raptors there may be sudden death in the absence of clinical signs. Virulent strains may cause 100% fatality rates in a facility, but with less virulent strains the majority of the birds recover within 10–15 days (Alexander et al., 1986). The recent H5N1 virus from the Asian lineage was shown to be highly pathogenic in falcons within an experimental infection trial without demonstrating any major signs of disease. Only a few days of a reduced food intake prior to death were observed (Lierz et al., 2007a).

Diagnosis

Respiratory signs associated with low pathogenic avian influenza (LPAI) serotypes might suggest influenza A infection but care must be taken to rule out other causes of avian respiratory disease (Ritchie, 1995). Sudden death without clinical signs is common in raptors infected with highly pathogenic avian influenza (HPAI) serotypes. The gold standard diagnostic method in live birds is viral isolation from cloacal swabs or tracheal swabs (preferable for H5N1 diagnostics) within 14 days of the initial infection. ELISA and virus neutralization methods can be used to demonstrate the presence of antibodies to specific influenza A viral strains. The haemagglutination inhibition test is recognized as the gold standard serological assay within the EU, but serological diagnostics are only of use in infections with a low pathogenic influenza virus to allow the bird to survive and develop antibodies. On post-mortem examination, gross changes include air sacculitis, petechial haemorrhage over the lung surface and necrotic debris in the respiratory airways. With H5N1 infection, necrotizing pancreatitis is a common feature even in birds that have died without displaying clinical signs (Tanimura et al., 2006). Pancreatitis has been demonstrated to be a consistent feature in raptors experimentally challenged with HPAI (Lierz et al., 2007a). Viral isolation can be performed from respiratory tissues, liver or spleen.

Treatment and control

In most countries HPAI is a notifiable disease. Treatment of avian influenza outbreaks in birds involves supportive therapy with fluids and antibiotics, although with virulent viral strains an eradication policy is recommended and usually performed by government order. Therefore treatment is only allowed if government advised. Infected birds must be isolated from other birds for 28 days. Vaccines are available for influenza A but, due to the speed of serotype change, they have a limited application. Although vaccinating against the more important H-type viruses would potentially interfere with serological surveillance programmes, vaccines are available that allow for differentiation between field infection and a vaccinated bird. Use of these vaccines is known as the DIVA strategy (Differentiating Infected from Vaccinated Animals).

Influenza A viruses are destroyed rapidly by most detergents and disinfectants or by extremes of pH and heat. Captive birds should have minimal exposure to free-ranging birds but there is no point in culling wild waterfowl, as they simply act as a reservoir for the virus.

Asian H5N1 avian influenza virus

In the last decade a highly pathogenic strain of avian influenza virus with the potential to infect humans (H5N1) has appeared in Asia. At the time of writing, the virus has already been responsible for over a hundred human deaths and large-scale poultry mortality, especially in Asia. All the human cases have involved very close contact between humans and infected birds, but there are concerns that there may be an influenza pandemic if the virus mutates to enable human-to-human spread. The Association of Avian Veterinarians publishes up-to-date information concerning H5N1 avian influenza virus and its control on their website www.aav.org.

Vaccines have been used successfully in exotic bird collections including raptors. A study in Germany demonstrated the effectiveness of protecting raptors from an experimental challenge with H5N1 infection with a H5N2 commercial vaccine (Lierz *et al.*, 2007a) and the significant reduction of virus shedding in vaccinated birds after challenge compared with non-vaccinated birds. Therefore vaccination of such birds is an option, but permitted only with restrictions and special application within different countries. Vaccination is permitted on conservation grounds in UK zoo collections on application to Defra.

Excellent biosecurity is the best method of preventing H5N1 infection in captive raptors. This should include restricting contact with wild birds and having strict disinfection protocols. Up-to-date information on H5N1 may be obtained from the Defra website (www.defra.gov.uk).

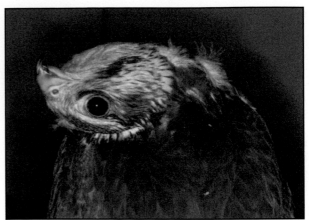

19.2 Classic neurological clinical signs in a Saker Falcon with PMV-1 infection. Falcons typically display a head tilt. (Courtesy of Tom Bailey)

Paramyxovirus 1 infection (PMV-1)

Aetiology and pathogenesis
PMV-1 infection is an acute disease with a high mortality rate in many bird species. In poultry it is more commonly known as Newcastle disease, a name that is also often used by falconers.

Viral strains vary considerably in their virulence and host specificity. Strains causing mild or latent infections in some species of raptor may be lethal to other species, such as poultry, and vice versa. For example, poultry vaccinated with attenuated PMV-1 vaccine, of low pathogenicity to poultry, may be a highly pathogenic food source to raptors. Captive raptors are at risk from the disease due to the practice of feeding potentially infected poultry products or pigeons. Vultures appear resistant to infection (Heidenreich, 1997).

PMV-1 infection may be controlled in poultry and other captive birds by vaccination, good husbandry and quarantine. The pathogenicity of the virus will depend upon the presence of other pathogens and husbandry conditions. In poultry, PMV-1 viruses are classified into three broad groups depending on their virulence: lentogenic (low virulence), mesogenic (moderate virulence) and velogenic (highly virulent). Asymptomatic carriers are also known to exist.

The disease in poultry is notifiable in most countries and in all avian species in the UK (see Chapter 37). It is zoonotic, causing a short-lived conjunctivitis or flu-like symptoms in humans.

Clinical signs
Signs in birds vary widely from subclinical to sudden death, depending on the virulence of the virus strain in addition to the age, species and health of the host. In many cases, in particular in hawks and eagles, clinical signs are relatively non-specific and have varying intensity, with the disease affecting the nervous (chronic central nervous system signs), respiratory (dyspnoea, conjunctivitis and nasal discharge), renal (polyuria) or gastrointestinal (green diarrhoea, anorexia) systems. In falcons the virus causes more severe neurological signs, classically torticollis (Figure 19.2), tremors and ataxia, and is usually fatal within 48 hours of infection. Anorexia for a week might be the only sign in hawks and buzzards, followed by a full recovery (Heidenreich, 1997).

Diagnosis
Ante-mortem diagnosis is often difficult because of the relatively non-specific signs and rapid progression of the disease. Post-mortem changes are also non-specific, with haemorrhage throughout the gastro-intestinal and respiratory systems but no gross pathological changes in the neurological system. A presumptive diagnosis may be made if there is a history of multiple deaths in falcons fed on poultry or pigeons, especially if neurological signs are recognized. In the UK, Defra must be notified on suspicion, not just confirmation of disease. Therefore these tests cannot be requested without reference to the local Divisional Veterinary Manager, who will normally take responsibility for testing and site biosecurity. Viral isolation or PCR tests can be performed on post-mortem tissues (spleen, brain or lung) or on cloacal swabs. Diagnosis may also be confirmed by serology (haemagglutination inhibition test). It may take up to 4 weeks for raptors to demonstrate a titre to PMV-1. In order to differentiate between a vaccine-induced titre and one caused by field infection, it is important to measure rising titres in an outbreak (Ritchie, 1995).

Treatment and control
There is no treatment for PMV-1 infection in raptors other than supportive therapy, which is not usually recommended by the author. Although control is maintained in poultry, with live vaccines administered via intranasal routes or the water supply, the vaccines produce poor serological titres in raptors. Live poultry vaccines may also be potentially lethal to susceptible raptors. Better control is achieved using inactivated vaccines, usually marketed for pigeons but also for poultry, administered by subcutaneous injection. In the United Arab Emirates the use of inactivated pigeon vaccines has been demonstrated to reduce losses from Newcastle disease. In the Middle East inactivated vaccines produced from isolated falcon viral strains have been shown to be effective (Manvell *et al.*,

2000), but as cross-immunity between PMV-1 strains is large, commercially available inactivated poultry/ pigeon vaccines are considered reliable. The use of unvaccinated poultry as a food source may reduce the incidence of infection in raptors. Raptors should avoid close contact with poultry, pigeons and also feral bird populations wherever possible.

Herpesvirus

Aetiology and pathogenesis
Herpesviruses are enveloped pleomorphic viruses ranging from 120 to 200 nm in diameter. Raptors are infected by beta herpesviruses. These are usually host specific and typically cause lifelong latent infections, with intermittent viral shedding. The seroprevalance of herpesvirus in captive falcons in the UK and the differentiation of different herpes serotypes is well researched (Zsivanovits *et al.*, 2004). The viruses result in the formation of intranuclear inclusion bodies (type Cowdry A). Herpesviruses are widespread in both captive and free-ranging raptors including falcons, owls and eagles.

Falcon herpesvirus (falconid HV1)
Falcon herpesvirus has been regularly reported since the early 1970s in the United States, Asia and Europe and causes the condition frequently referred to as inclusion body hepatitis of falcons. The virus has an affinity for hepatocytes and reticuloendothelial cells in falcons. It has not been proven, but it is considered to be transmitted to falcons via feeding infected pigeons. All falcons are susceptible to falcon herpesvirus but Gyrfalcons and their hybrids appear more vulnerable. This may suggest that immunosuppression or stress may be important factors in the development of the disease.

Clinical signs: Falcon herpesvirus is an acute condition, usually fatal within 48 hours of infection. Affected birds are primarily depressed and anorexic. Mutes may contain lime-green urates.

Diagnosis: Ante-mortem diagnosis is usually not possible, due to the rapid progression of the disease. Endoscopic investigation may reveal typical areas of visceral necrosis and blood samples may show a profound leucopenia.

Post-mortem changes include hepatomegaly and splenomegaly, with both organs covered in small yellow-white necrotic foci (Figure 19.3). Due to the rapid progression of the disease, affected birds are often still in good bodily condition. It is important not to confuse these lesions with clinical salmonellosis, which is now thought to be rare in birds of prey. Intranuclear inclusion bodies of type Cowdry A may be demonstrated on histopathological examination of the spleen and liver and these may be considered pathognomonic. Viral isolation or PCR testing should be used to confirm the diagnosis.

Treatment and control: There is no treatment and no commercial vaccine presently available, though an attenuated vaccine has been used successfully in

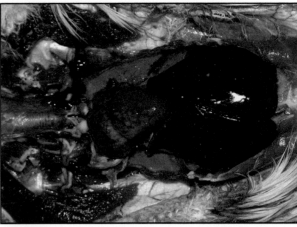

19.3 Typical areas of visceral necrosis on the liver at post-mortem examination of a falcon with herpesvirus infection. (Courtesy of Tom Bailey)

Common Kestrels. Control involves avoiding both use of wild pigeons as a food source and keeping pigeons on the same facility as raptors. The use of domestically reared pigeons that have not been exposed to herpesvirus has been discussed (Redig, 1992), but it is impossible to control as carriers cannot be detected other than by testing every single bird. Therefore pigeons should be avoided as a food source, especially for falcons and, in particular, Gyrfalcons and their hybrids.

Owl herpesvirus (strigid HV1)
Owl herpesvirus has been reported in both captive and wild Strigiformes in North America, Asia and Europe. In captivity affected owls rapidly die, but the demonstration of antibody titres in clinically normal free-ranging owls suggests latent carriers, or birds that have eliminated the infection and are immune. The virus is contracted by ingestion of infected pharyngeal secretions. Clinical signs and pathological changes are similar to falcon herpesvirus and serologically the two viruses are very similar. Some species of owl are more susceptible to owl herpesvirus infection than others; Tawny Owls and Barn Owls appear resistant to infection.

Eagle herpesvirus (acciptrid HV1)
A herpesvirus distinct from falcon herpesvirus has been isolated from both eagles that are clinically normal and eagles demonstrating clinical signs of herpesvirus infection. It is not believed to be of major clinical significance (Kaleta, 1990). In general the occurrence of death due to herpesvirus is rare in accipiters compared with falcons, in which it occurs regularly.

Raptorpox

Aetiology and pathogenesis
Poxviruses are the largest avian viruses (approximately 400 nm diameter) and replicate in the cytoplasm rather than the nucleus. They are species specific and are not considered a zoonotic risk. Poxvirus infections have been reported in free-ranging and

captive hawks, eagles and falcons but not in owls. As poxviruses are considered species specific, it is unlikely that prey animals infect raptors; they are probably spread between the birds directly. Raptor poxviruses are distinct from other avipoxviruses and so raptors cannot be infected by other bird species.

Biting insects, particularly mosquitoes, spread the virus and so the disease is more common in the warmer Middle Eastern states or in the mosquito season in late summer in Europe. Direct contact with open skin lesions also spreads the virus between birds. Outbreaks in Europe have usually involved imported falcons from the Middle East, but the disease has been reported in a released wild Peregrine Falcon in Germany (Cooper, 1993; Krone *et al.*, 2004).

Avipoxviruses are stable in the environment and can survive in mosquito salivary glands for several weeks.

Clinical signs

The disease form depends upon the virulence of the viral strain, the susceptibility of the host and the route of infection (Ensley *et al.*, 1978).

Cutaneous form: This is the most common form of the disease, being characterized by the development of nodular lesions, which bleed when lifted, on the featherless parts of the skin. Nodules appear typically on the commissures of the mouth, eyelids, feet and cere (Figure 19.4; see also Chapter 24). The nodules enlarge over 7–10 days, become crusty and eventually drop off. Healthy birds usually make a full recovery. Immunocompromised birds may succumb to secondary yeast and bacterial infection, which can cause a fatal septicaemia.

Diphtheroid form: This severe form of poxvirus infection is reported in raptors. The virus is transmitted via ingestion and caseous plaques develop on the oropharyngeal mucous membranes. The plaques interfere with eating and even respiration.

Diagnosis

Clinical signs of raptorpox are characteristic, but the condition must be differentiated from trichomoniasis,

capillariasis, candidiasis and vitamin A deficiency (see Chapter 23). Confirmation of diagnosis involves viral culture (from fresh lesions), PCR tests or histopathological examination of biopsy samples to confirm the presence of Bollinger's intracytoplasmatic bodies, which are pathognomonic for poxvirus infection.

Treatment and control

Although there is no specific treatment for poxvirus, the use of topical antibiotics (systemic antibiotics in severe cases) and anti-fungals is essential to prevent secondary infections. Cleaning the pox lesions with a povidone–iodine-based disinfectant is advisable. Vitamin A supplementation has also been recommended to protect epithelial cells (Samour and Cooper, 1993). As the disease is more severe in the immunosuppressed bird, good husbandry limits the severity of infections. In Arab countries the use of pigeon pox vaccines is widespread but as the virus is species specific their effectiveness is in doubt until a raptorpox vaccine is available. The pigeon vaccine is a live vaccine and will potentially cause some clinical signs in birds; it is inadvisable to use it in hunting birds. Control of biting arthropods in the aviary will reduce the spread of the virus. Additionally the burning of pox lesions has been described.

West Nile virus

Aetiology and pathogenesis

West Nile virus (WNV) is a Flavivirus. Biting-insect vectors (usually *Culex* mosquitoes) predominantly spread the virus and birds act as a primary reservoir for the infection. The disease is a notifiable one; it is an important zoonosis that may cause severe encephalitis: 62 people living in New York became infected with WNV in 1999 and seven subsequently died. Since 1999 this virulent strain of WNV has spread rapidly through North America and has now been identified in most states. A serologically identical strain of WNV to that of the US outbreak has recently caused deaths in both humans and birds in Israel.

Following a mosquito's ingestion of blood from a viraemic bird, the virus is amplified in the mosquito salivary glands and the digestive tract. A bird

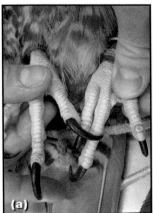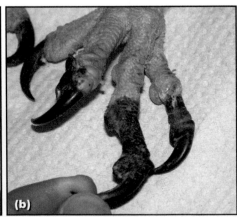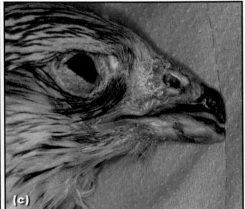

19.4 Raptorpox. **(a)** Early lesions on the feet of a falcon. **(b)** Severe lesions have constricted the blood supply to the distal phalanges, resulting in avascular necrosis. **(c)** Chronic lesions causing severe damage to the beak and cere. The falcon was unable to tear at its food normally. (a, courtesy of Chris Lloyd; b,c, courtesy of Tom Bailey)

subsequently bitten by the infected mosquito will become viraemic for 4–7 days. In addition it is suspected that ingestion of prey infected with WNV could lead to infection in some species of birds and this may be an issue in scavenging raptors. The severity of the viraemia in affected birds depends on the species, with corvids and passerines (House Sparrow in the USA) producing the highest concentration of virus for the longest time. The virus has been demonstrated to cause disease and death in accipiters, Red-tailed Hawks and northern owl species. Poultry appear relatively resistant to the disease. In temperate areas the disease is seasonal, with outbreaks occurring in spring and summer, depending on the size of the insect population.

Clinical signs
Clinical signs vary from sudden death without clinical signs to a neurological disease including ataxia, seizures and twitching. Abnormalities of vision may also be noted. In the majority of cases the disease is terminal in raptors but it has been suggested that some birds may only show mild clinical signs and recover. WNV needs to be differentiated from avian influenza, PMV-1 infection and intoxication.

Diagnosis
Neurological signs combined with a history of WNV in the area aid a presumptive diagnosis. Post-mortem findings include severe haemorrhage of the mucosa and serosa of the gastrointestinal tract. There may also be intraosseous haemorrhage and splenomegaly. Histopathological lesions are pathognomonic, including myocardial inflammation, lymphoplasmacytic encephalitis, ganglioneuritis and pancreatitis (Ellis *et al.*, 2007). Infection is confirmed by viral isolation or PCR tests from oral and cloacal swabs or tissues from a infected bird. Antibodies may be detected by haemagglutination inhibition assays up to 2 weeks post infection in birds not susceptible to the disease.

Control and treatment
There is no treatment for WNV. Since the outbreak in the USA many institutions have used a commercial WNV horse vaccine (Fort Dodge Animal Health, Kansas). In cockatiels it has been shown that two doses of 0.5 ml WNV vaccine manufactured for horses given 2 weeks apart did not produce an antibody response. Higher vaccine doses have been demonstrated to produce some antibody response but with the possibility of side effects. It is useful instead to improve mosquito control in WNV areas until an avian vaccine becomes available. Large-scale surveillance projects are in place in North America to monitor the spread of WNV and involve screening dead wild birds (especially corvids) by PCR and the use of sentinel birds. Elsewhere in the world the disease is rare or unreported at the date of publication. In the UK a surveillance program based on PCR testing of raptors and corvids has failed to produce evidence of disease (Paul Holmes, VLA, Shrewsbury, personal communication).

Adenovirus
Adenoviruses have been associated with clinical signs in several raptor species, including American Kestrels, Goshawks and Merlins and particularly the Mauritius Kestrel, though reports are rare in captive birds. Clinically affected birds exhibit haemorrhagic enteritis rapidly followed by death. Intranuclear inclusion bodies containing adenovirus-like particles have been demonstrated in the liver of affected raptors. Diagnosis can be confirmed by serology or PCR tests. Adenovirus infection is a common problem in racing pigeons characterized by acute enteritis, which is ultimately fatal. It is not known whether this is the same virus causing occasional clinical disease in falcons.

Rabies virus
Many species of raptor, including goshawks, buzzards and kites, have been demonstrated to carry rabies virus, but they do not normally develop clinical signs and simply act as a reservoir for the virus (Gough *et al.*, 1976; Shannon *et al.*, 1988; Gerlach, 1994a). Although the disease in raptors has not been shown to be zoonotic, care should be taken handling wild raptors. Occasionally affected raptors have demonstrated severe neurological signs and death following experimental infection, but affected birds usually mount a rapid antibody response to the virus (Coles, 1997).

Bacterial disease

Figure 19.5 gives a summary of common bacterial infectious diseases affecting raptors.

Avian tuberculosis

Aetiology and pathogenesis
Avian tuberculosis caused by *Mycobacterium avium* is a worldwide problem in captive birds of prey. The disease is a potential zoonosis in immunocompromised individuals, causing respiratory symptoms. The incubation period in humans is not known.

Recently *Mycobacterium genavense* has emerged as a significant pathogen in birds. The source of *Mycobacterium* spp. infection is generally infected birds, such as feral pigeons used as a food source, or contaminated soil. The organism is very resistant in the environment, remaining infectious in soil for many years. It is resistant to disinfectants; decontamination of aviaries is extremely difficult and probably impractical.

Clinical signs
Due to the long incubation period, the disease normally affects adults. Avian tuberculosis is a generalized chronic disease characterized by progressive weight loss despite a ravenous appetite. The disease course last several months and only in the latter stages do birds become disinterested in food. Granulomas forming on the intestinal tract or liver can occasionally be palpated through the abdominal wall. Localized granulomas developing on the bird

Bacterium	Clinical signs	Diagnosis	Treatment and control
Mycobacterium spp. (usually *M. avium* or *M. genavense*)	Chronic weight loss despite good or increased appetite; gastrointestinal granulomas	Endoscopy and biopsy of lesions with histopathological confirmation is the gold standard diagnostic test	Euthanasia as zoonotic and difficult to cure. Avoid food material with potential infection. Decontaminate environment. Avoid contact with free-ranging birds
Yersinia pseudotuberculosis	Sudden death, usually several birds involved	Impression smears of liver granulomas reveal Gram-negative cocci	Rodent control
Pasteurella multocida (avian cholera)	Acute cases get septicaemia and die within hours. Chronic cases suffer from sinusitis and conjunctivitis	Culture from respiratory discharges	Antibiotics for 3 months. Avoid infection from rodents, rabbits and poultry
Escherichia coli	Lethargy with gastrointestinal signs	Culture of overwhelming populations of bacteria from mutes	3-week course of antibiotics. Improve hygiene
Chlamydophila psittaci	Non-specific respiratory and gastrointestinal signs	PCR on pooled mute sample or from tissue samples or swabs (cloacal, eye, choanal slit)	45 days of doxycycline. Consider euthanasia, as zoonotic in collections or with immunosuppressed individuals, but normally good response to treatment
Clostridium botulinum	Flaccid paralysis and death within 48 hours	Clinical signs and history of feeding poor meat	Antibiotics, activated charcoal. Feed fresh food sources
Clostridium perfringens	Gastrointestinal signs with reddish diarrhoea	Culture from food source	Supportive therapy and antibiotics. Correct freezing and defrosting of food
Clostridium novyi and *chauvoei*	Inflamed skin with crepitation	Clinical signs and culture from deep wounds	Wound cleaning and antibiotics
Erysipelothrix rhusiopathiae	Inflamed skin followed by death within 72 hours	Clinical signs; culture from lesions	Urgent penicillin or tetracycline. Rodent control

19.5 Summary of common bacterial infectious diseases affecting birds of prey.

subcutaneously are thought to be in response to talon injuries from infected birds. In contrast to mammals, tuberculous lesions confined to the lungs are rare in birds and so respiratory signs are uncommon.

Diagnosis

A presumptive diagnosis can be made in many cases based on the history and clinical examination. Radiography may reveal enlarged spleen, liver and intestines with the presence of granulomas. The granulomas may be difficult to distinguish from organs. On radiographs opacities may be evident within the skeleton, suggesting mycobacteriosis. Intradermal skin testing has been used in poultry to confirm the disease but this is unreliable in raptors. Blood samples may demonstrate a non-specific leucocytosis, sometimes substantial, often with a monocytosis and raised liver enzyme concentrations. Serological testing (whole blood agglutination) is unreliable, as false negatives are not uncommon. A PCR test is available for both *M. avium* and *M. genavense*. In the author's opinion diagnostic endoscopy is the most useful method of diagnosing avian tuberculosis. It is possible to visualize granulomas and take biopsy samples of suspicious tissues to obtain histopathological confirmation via Ziehl–Neelson staining, which demonstrates numerous acid-fast mycobacteria in positive cases. In some intestinal cases mycobacteria may

be identified in faecal samples, although care must be taken as raptor mute samples may contain non-pathogenic acid-fast rods, leading to false positives. Post-mortem changes include severe emaciation with numerous variously sized yellow nodules, containing yellow caseous exudates, throughout any organ system. Nodules should be differentiated from those caused by herpesvirus or pseudotuberculosis.

Treatment and control

Because of the zoonotic potential of *M. avium* and poor prognosis for successful treatment, humane euthanasia should be recommended once diagnosis is confirmed. Infected birds shed large numbers of organisms into the environment, so all in-contact birds should be screened over 12 months using a combination of blood samples, endoscopy and faecal tests.

Prevention of infection involves prevention of exposure to faeces from potentially infected wild birds, especially waterfowl. All food animals should be examined for evidence of tuberculosis infection prior to feeding. If an aviary is known to be contaminated with *M. avium* the substrate should be removed from the aviary and all furniture destroyed, as disinfection is unreliable. It is best to use non-porous surfaces for aviary floors rather than simply soil, which can easily become contaminated.

Pseudotuberculosis (yersiniosis)

The Gram-negative bacterium *Yersinia pseudotuberculosis* causes yersiniosis. Rodents carry the pathogen and raptors become infected by the faecal–oral route due to food contamination in dirty rodent-infested aviaries. The condition may also be seen in rodent-hunting raptors. Affected birds usually die before diagnosis and post-mortem examination reveals yellow granulomas on the liver and spleen. Impression smears of the lesions demonstrate numerous Gram-negative coccoid rods. Culture of the organism is difficult, requiring cold enrichment, and so it is advisable to inform the laboratory that *Y. pseudotuberculosis* is suspected. Treatment involves antibiosis based on culture and sensitivity results for all in-contact birds.

The disease can be easily prevented by good hygiene and rodent control. Care must be taken using rodenticides, as raptors will ingest the dead rodents. Baits are available that cause no secondary poisoning to raptors (Eradirat, Ilex Organics Ltd, PO Box 158 Market Rasen, UK).

Pasteurellosis

Aetiology and pathogenesis

Avian cholera is caused by *Pasteurella multocida* and is responsible for high death rates in the poultry industry and in wild waterfowl. Raptors may succumb to infection by eating infected poultry, rabbits or rodents. Occasionally cat or rodent bites can transmit the infection, but the disease is normally reported in raptor breeding centres where turkey or duck products are fed. The organism can cause localized infections in humans following talon scratches or bites.

Clinical signs

Affected birds suffer either an acute or chronic form of the disease, depending on the virulence of the organism and the condition of the host. In the acute form, septicaemia develops and the bird dies within hours of the initial infection. In the chronic form, there is classically a watery nasal discharge with swollen eyelids, conjunctivitis and an infraorbital sinusitis. Joints may also be swollen. Although the chronic form of the disease may last several months, death is rare. However, chronically affected birds may become permanently disabled and unfit for falconry.

Diagnosis

Presumptive diagnosis of the chronic form is based on clinical signs subsequently confirmed by culture of *P. multocida* from nasal discharges. The acute form must be diagnosed by blood culture. In smears from heart blood or tissue stained with methylene blue, *P. multocida* demonstrate a bipolar staining, permitting a rapid diagnosis. A serological test can also be used in chronically infected groups to detect antibodies.

Treatment and control

The chronic form is treated using a broad-spectrum antibiotic selected from the results of culture and sensitivity investigations. Birds must be treated for up to 3 months to prevent the formation of a carrier state, so care must be taken not to induce secondary candidiasis or aspergillosis.

Control of the disease involves obtaining food from non-infected sources. In addition, adequate biosecurity to avoid exposure to wild rabbits and rodents is vital.

Clostridium spp.

A variety of clostridia species have been reported in captive raptors, including *Clostridium perfringens, C. botulinum, C. tetani, C. novyi* and *C. chauvoei*.

Clostridium perfringens

Clostridium perfringens is a ubiquitous organism that can contaminate raptor food material prior to freezing. The organism multiplies rapidly during the thawing process, releasing exotoxins. This process is often encouraged by the practice of soaking food in water prior to feeding hunting birds. If excessive exotoxin is consumed, birds suffer a peracute disease, becoming depressed and dying within hours of ingestion. Alternatively if large amounts of bacteria are consumed, birds suffer an acute disease process, becoming depressed with gastrointestinal signs including reddish-brown diarrhoea and regurgitation. The use of antibiotics may lead to an imbalance in gastrointestinal flora, allowing clostridia to multiply.

Clostridium botulinum

Botulism is caused by the neurotoxin produced by *C. botulinum,* which is commonly found on rotting carcasses. Free-ranging raptors do not normally feed on decaying carcasses with the obvious exception of adult vultures, which appear relatively resistant to botulinum toxin. An exception is young vultures, in which botulism is relatively common.

Classical signs include flaccid paralysis of the neck and limbs. Affected birds become recumbent and unable to swallow and exhibit uncoordinated movements. Respiratory paralysis may be fatal within 48 hours. Diagnosis is based on clinical signs and a history of feeding inappropriate meat. Less severe cases recover with supportive therapy, activated charcoal and laxatives, which will help to eliminate the toxin from the body.

Clostridium novyi and *chauvoei*

These clostridia can infect deep puncture wounds, causing a necrotic dermatitis. Affected skin quickly becomes blue–green with evidence of crepitation due to subcutaneous gas formation. Affected birds rapidly die without treatment. All small puncture wounds in raptors should be given prompt attention either by adequate cleansing with a suitable antiseptic or with routine antibiosis.

Clostridium tetani

Tetanus is caused by the release of a neurotoxin produced by *C. tetani.* Raptors are thought to be resistant to tetanus, though one possible infection has been reported in a Saker Falcon following a deep talon wound (Heidenreich, 1997).

Erysipelothrix infection

Erysipelothrix rhusiopathiae, a common pathogen in turkeys, has been reported to cause occasional acute infections in a variety of captive raptors. Rodents act as a reservoir for the organism, which infects wounds usually on the feet. Affected birds present with an inflamed swollen area on infected areas of skin and, if treatment is not immediate, death will occur within 72 hours. Fortunately, *E. rhusiopathiae* is very sensitive to tetracyclines and penicillin, but sensitive tests are required. Adequate rodent control and avoiding feeding turkey poults will prevent the disease. Care must be taken as the disease has zoonotic potential.

Salmonellosis

Clinical salmonellosis is rarely encountered in raptors, even though they are frequently fed pigeons, which are known carriers of *Salmonella* spp., especially *S. typhimurium*. A variety of *Salmonella* species can be identified from a healthy raptor's mutes and these are thought to represent organisms acquired from prey animals. *S. typhimurium* can cause septic arthritis with grossly swollen joints containing purulent exudates. The route of infection is haematogenous. There have been reports about clinical salmonellosis in raptors but the clinical disease seems to be rare, though occasional outbreaks have been reported (Kinne *et al.*, 2007). In this case the source of infection was not identified.

Colibacillosis

Escherichia coli leads to an infectious disease seen in raptors subjected to poor husbandry conditions. It is often associated with secondary *Candida albicans* infections or severe endoparasitism. Colibacillosis is relatively common in overcrowded aviaries; birds becoming infected by the faecal–oral route. It can be common in breeding facilities in the UK.

The main clinical signs are lethargy and gastrointestinal changes such as diarrhoea and regurgitation. Diagnosis is best made by isolation of the pathogen from tissue samples (biopsies) or blood culture. Its isolation from mute samples is normal in raptors and only the complicated determination of pathogen factors would support a diagnosis.

A 3-week course of a broad-spectrum antibiotic, selected on the basis of culture and sensitivity testing, is normally sufficient to treat a colibacillosis outbreak. Aviary hygiene should be addressed.

Chlamydophilosis

Aetiology and pathogenesis

Chlamydophila psittaci infection is commonly reported in a variety of free-living raptors but appears to be of more clinical significance in other birds, such as parrots and pigeons. In one study 74% of a group of free-ranging raptors were demonstrated to be positive for *C. psittaci* by PCR test (Schettler *et al.*, 2003), but another study demonstrated a lower incidence of 16.4% (Lierz *et al.*, 2002). One study showed that *Chlamydophila* antigen was detected in 13.2% of free-ranging raptors, while 85.1% of the same birds tested demonstrated antibodies against *C. psittaci*

(Gerbermann and Korbel, 1993). It is a potentially serious zoonosis, causing severe influenza-type symptoms in humans, and it is important that staff handling wild raptors should be warned about the potential risk of infection. Latent carriers are common in the avian and mammalian world. The organism is spread by aerosol or faecal ingestion and it is suspected that raptors, especially the Common Buzzard, may become infected from their prey animals. Infection has been reported in free-ranging owls and raptors. Stressed birds are more susceptible to infection and shedding of the organism.

Clinical signs

In contrast to other avian species, adult raptors normally demonstrate the chronic form of *Chlamydophila* infection with non-specific respiratory signs, weight loss and diarrhoea, rather than the acute disease. Post-mortem changes typically include a grossly enlarged spleen, hepatomegaly and air sac inflammation.

Young birds may succumb to a fatal acute form of the disease (Gerlach, 1994b).

Diagnosis

Laboratory testing is essential to confirm *Chlamydophila* infection in raptors, although a grossly enlarged spleen seen on radiography or endoscopy (Figure 19.6) should raise suspicions. As with other birds, great care must be taken with diagnosis due to the presence of asymptomatic carriers and the intermittent nature of shedding of the organism. The gold standard test for *Chlamydophila* infection is a PCR test on pooled mute samples (preferably collected over 5–10 days). Additionally a swab taken from eye, choanal slit and cloaca (same swab in that order) is very advantageous for diagnosis, using it within the PCR. There are many antibody and antigen rapid ELISA tests available for blood or faecal samples but it is important to be aware that these are often unreliable. It is possible to demonstrate the organism on impression smears from post-mortem samples, in particular liver, stained with Stamp stain.

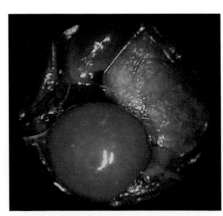

19.6 Classic endoscopic appearance of an enlarged spleen in a Peregrine Falcon with *Chlamydophila psittaci* infection.

Treatment and control

Therapy involves doxycycline or enrofloxacin. Doxycycline should be administered for 45 days at an oral dose of 50–75 mg/kg twice daily in an attempt to eliminate latent carriers. An injectable version of doxycycline (Vibravenos, Pfizer) is available which can be given every 5–7 days by intramuscular injection (100 mg/kg) although it has been associated with muscle necrosis. Unfortunately this drug is no longer available in some countries. The veterinary surgeon must act responsibly with respect to the drug cascade but, in the UK, Vibravenos can be obtained by applying to the Veterinary Medicines Directorate (VMD) for a Special Treatment Certificate. Enrofloxacin has been demonstrated to be effective against *Chlamydophila* infection but doxycycline is still preferred by the author.

Mycoplasmosis

Mycoplasma species are common pathogens in domestic poultry and are responsible for considerable economic losses, but their significance in raptors is unknown, though the presence of mycoplasmas has been frequently reported (Heidenreich, 1997). In one study 32 out of 68 debilitated raptors admitted to a clinic were found positive for *Mycoplasma* spp. but its significance remains unknown (Lierz *et al.*, 2000). More recent studies have demonstrated that nearly all species of raptors, including Common Buzzard, Northern Goshawk and Kestrel, are regularly positive for mycoplasmas despite their origin (whether captive or free ranging). Therefore just the presence of mycoplasmas in a diseased raptor does not lead to the diagnosis. *Mycoplasma* species differentiation is essential to get a further hint that it might be playing a role in the disease process. Some *Mycoplasma* species seem to be commensals in raptors rather than pathogens (M Lierz, personal communication, 2007).

Culture from tracheal swabs is the gold standard method for *Mycoplasma* isolation, but specific culture media and incubation techniques are required. Species-specific PCR tests on tracheal swabs are preferred (Lierz *et al.*, 2007b).

Mycoplasmas are able to be transmitted vertically in raptors but their importance is still not well investigated, as fertile raptor eggs are not available for experimental purposes (Lierz *et al.*, 2007b). A mycoplasmal isolate from a Northern Goshawk egg was shown to be highly pathogenic for chicken embryos, therefore raising concern that it might be important in low hatchability within breeding stock (Lierz *et al.*, 2007c).

Fungal disease

Candidiasis

Aetiology and pathogenesis

Candida albicans is a common commensal found in the oral cavity and upper gastrointestinal tract of raptors. Primary disease, excessive antibiosis or poor husbandry may affect the balance of normal gut flora, and in these situations *C. albicans* acts as an opportunistic pathogen causing the signs of candidiasis. Young birds are very vulnerable to candidiasis. The disease is traditionally known by falconers as soor or thrush in the UK.

Clinical signs

The disease develops significantly prior to demonstration of clinical signs. Food intake may be reduced and affected birds may flick their heads whilst eating, suggesting oral discomfort. Examination of the oral cavity usually reveals yellow plaques on the oral mucosa (see Chapter 23) combined with an unusual odour. The disease normally affects the upper gastrointestinal tract. Intestinal candidiasis has been reported; this causes malabsorption.

Diagnosis

Plaques in the oral cavity are easily visualized. Disease in the oesophagus and crop can be identified by endoscopy. Candidiasis mimics other diseases, especially trichomoniasis (see Chapter 18) and so laboratory identification of the pathogen is vital. The organism is normally identified by a combination of microscopic identification, culture and biochemical reactions. The plaques should be lifted from the oral pharyngeal mucosa with a cotton bud and examined microscopically in a suspension of normal saline for the presence of the oval budding yeast *C. albicans*. This can be stained with Gram's stain to aid identification. Subsequent culture of a plaque at 37°C for 48 hours on Sabouraud's agar will produce a prolific growth of the organism.

Treatment and control

In mild cases involving just the oral cavity, removing the visible plaques with a cotton bud and applying nystatin topically and orally is often sufficient. In severe or chronic cases the use of oral ketoconazole or itraconazole is recommended. It is important to identify and correct any predisposing conditions.

Aspergillosis

Aspergillosis is a common fungal infection of captive raptors caused by *Aspergillus* spp. It is often secondary to other disease or husbandry problems (see Chapter 20).

Control of infectious disease in captive raptors

Although infectious disease is commonplace in captive raptors, the availability of effective commercial vaccines and treatments is poor. Control and prevention of disease outbreaks in raptor facilities should aim to keep the birds in the best condition possible, thus reducing their susceptibility to infection. Biosecurity is the best method to prevent infectious disease outbreaks and written biosecurity protocols should be created for each facility (Figure 19.7).

Many infectious diseases are caused by opportunistic organisms such as *Candida albicans* or *E. coli* and so excellent hygiene should be employed to reduce the load of these organisms. The author recommends the use of F10SC (Health and Hygiene, Johannesburg, South Africa) disinfectant for routine disinfection in raptor facilities. The advantage of this disinfectant is that it may be applied directly over the birds, using a commercial poultry fogging system. It is particularly useful for reducing mycotic spore counts (Temperley and Limper, 2005).

- Apply strict quarantine measures for new additions to centre (30 days minimum)
- Avoid contact with feral populations of birds
- Avoid contact with domestic pigeons and poultry
- Avoid avian-derived food if possible, unless purchased from a disease-free breeder
- Provide excellent nutrition
- Practise adequate vermin control
- Use regular effective disinfection methods
- Avoid environmental stress (no overcrowding, good ventilation, excellent hygiene)
- Isolate sick birds immediately in separate hospital facility
- Always have post-mortem examination of dead birds
- Discourage visitors (consider clothing changes, showering and foot baths)

19.7 Preventive measures for avoiding infections in raptor centres.

Quarantine should employ a strict 'all in, all out' policy, in a building that is completely separate from other birds, for at least 30 days. For economic reasons and convenience it is common practice to feed captive raptors day-old male chicks, which are a by-product of the poultry industry. This food source is potentially contaminated with bacteria (e.g. *E. coli*) due to poor food hygiene and care should be taken to obtain birds from a safe source. An alternative is to feed 'road kill' or 'shot' birds but any feral or wild bird, especially pigeons, could be a potential source of infection. The risk of lead intoxification should never be underestimated when feeding shot food material (see Chapter 26). In the author's opinion it is preferable to feed a non-avian food source such as rabbit or laboratory-sourced rodents. Alternatively, safe avian food material can be obtained from a reputable disease-free breeding unit producing specifically for the raptor market (e.g. Honeybrook Animal Foods, Evesham, UK).

References and further reading

Alexander DJ, Parsons G and Manvell RJ (1986) Experimental assessment of the pathogenicity of eight influenza A viruses of H5 subtype for chickens, turkeys, ducks and quail. *Avian Pathology* **15**, 647–662

Beynon PH, Forbes NA and Harcourt-Brown NH (eds) (1996) *Manual of Raptors, Pigeons and Waterfowl.* BSAVA, Cheltenham

Coles BH (1997) Rhabdoviridae. In: *Avian Medicine and Surgery*, p. 311. Blackwell Science, Oxford

Cooper JE (1993) Avian pox in birds of prey (Order: *Falconiformes*). *Veterinary Record* **85**, 683–684

Ellis AE, Mead DG, Allison AB, Stallknecht DE and Howarth EW (2007) Pathology and epidemiology of natural West Nile infection of raptors in Georgia. *Journal of Wildlife Diseases* **43**(2), 214–223

Ensley PK, Anderson MP, Costello ML *et al.* (1978) Epornitic of avian pox in a zoo. *Journal of the American Veterinary Medicine Association* **173**, 1111–1114

Gerbermann H and Korbel R (1993) Occurrence of *Chlamydia psittaci* infections in free-ranging birds of prey. *Tierärztliche Praxis* **21**, 214–224

Gerlach H (1994a) Viruses. In: *Avian Medicine: Principles and Application*, ed. BW Ritchie *et al.*, pp. 862–948. Wingers, Lake Worth, FL

Gerlach H (1994b). Chlamydia. In: *Avian Medicine: Principles and Application*, ed. BW Ritchie *et al.*, p. 1134. Wingers, Lake Worth, FL

Gough PM and Jorgenson RD (1976) Rabies antibodies in sera of wild birds. *Journal of Wildlife Disease* **12**, 392–395

Halverson DK, Kelleher CJ and Seene DA (1985) Epizootiology of avian influenza: effect of season on incidence in sentinel ducks and domestic turkeys in Minnesota. *Applied Environmental Microbiology* **49**, 914–919

Heidenreich M (1997) *Birds of Prey: Medicine and Management.* Blackwell Science, Oxford

Kaleta EF (1990) Herpesviruses of birds – a review. *Avian Pathology* **19**, 193–211

Kinne J, Joseph M, Sharma A and Wernery U (2007) Severe outbreak of salmonellosis in hunting falcons in the UAE. In: *Proceedings of the 9th Conference of the European Association of Avian Veterinarians and the 7th Scientific ECAMS Meeting, Zürich*, pp. 94–100

Krone O, Essbauer S, Wibbelt G *et al.* (2004) Avipoxvirus infection in peregrine falcons (*Falco peregrinus*) from a reintroduction programme in Germany. *Veterinary Record* **154**, 110–113

Lierz M, Hafez HM, Klopfleisch R *et al.* (2007a) Protection and virus shedding of falcons vaccinated against highly pathogenic avian influenza A virus (H5N1). *Emerging Infectious Diseases* **13**, 1667–1674

Lierz M, Hagen N, Harcourt-Brown N *et al.* (2007b) Prevalence of mycoplasmas in eggs from birds of prey using culture and a genus-specific mycoplasma polymerase chain reaction. *Avian Pathology* **36**(2), 145–150

Lierz M, Göbel T and Kaleta EF (2002) Investigations on the prevalence of *Chlamydophila psittaci*, falcon herpesvirus and paramyxovirus 1 in birds of prey and owls found injured or debilitated. *Tierärztliche Praxis* **30**(K), 139–144

Lierz M, Schmidt R, Goebel T, Ehrlein, J and Runge M (2000) Detection of *Mycoplasma* spp. in raptorial birds in Germany. In: *Raptor Biomedicine III*, ed. JT Lumeij *et al.*, pp. 25–33. Zoo Educational Network, Lake Worth, FL

Lierz M, Stark R, Brokat S and Hafez HM (2007c) Pathogenicity of *Mycoplasma lipofaciens* strain ML64, isolated from an egg of a Northern Goshawk (*Accipiter gentilis*), for chicken embryos. *Avian Pathology* **36**(2), 151–153

Manvell RJ, Wernery U, Alexander DJ and Frost KM (2000) Newcastle disease (avian PMV-1) viruses in raptors. In: *Raptor Biomedicine III*, ed. JT Lumeij *et al.*, pp. 3–6. Zoo Educational Network, Lake Worth, FL

Redig PT (1992) Health management of raptors trained for falconry. *Proceedings of the Association of Avian Veterinarians*, pp. 258–264

Ritchie BW (1995) Orthomyxoviridae. In: *Avian Viruses Function and Control*, ed. BW Ritchie and K Carter, pp. 351–364. Wingers, Lake Worth, FL

Ritchie BW and Carter K (eds) (1995) *Avian Viruses Function and Control.* Wingers, Lake Worth, FL

Samour J (2003) *Avian Medicine.* Elsevier Science, London

Samour JH and Cooper JE (1993) Avian pox in birds of prey in Bahrain. *Veterinary Record* **132**, 343

Schettler E, Fickel J, Hotzel H *et al.* (2003) Newcastle disease virus and *Chlamydia psittaci* in free-living raptors from eastern Germany. *Journal of Wildlife Disease* **39**(1), 57–63

Shannon LM, Poulton JL, Emmons RW, Woodie JD and Fowler ME (1988) Serological survey for rabies antibodies in raptors from California. *Journal of Wildlife Disease* **19**, 244–247

Tanimura N, Tsukamoto K, Okamatsu M *et al.* (2006) Pathology of fatal highly pathogenic H5N1 avian influenza virus infection in Large-billed Crows (*Corvus macrorhynchos*) during the 2004 outbreak in Japan. *Veterinary Pathology* **43**, 500–509

Temperley JP and Limper L (2005) Novel disinfectant for *Aspergillus* control. *International Hatchery Practice* **17**(6), 7–9

Zsivanovits P, Forbes NA, Zvonar LT *et al.* (2004) Investigation into the seroprevalence of falcon herpesvirus antibodies in raptors in the UK using virus neutralisation tests and different herpes isolates. *Avian Pathology* **13**(6), 599–604

20

Raptors: respiratory problems

Tom Bailey

Clinical signs and differential diagnosis

Many predisposing factors to upper and lower respiratory diseases in falcons are management-related. The ideal environment should be well ventilated and free from dust and toxins, while proper nutrition is necessary for a healthy immune system. In raptors the changes associated with falconry (weight reduction, climate changes, taming and training) are important factors that contribute to diseases of the respiratory tract, particularly aspergillosis. The stage in training of the raptor, and the experience of the falconer, should be assessed when the history is taken. The nutritional status of the bird should be considered, because it is well known in psittacine species that hypovitaminosis A is manifested in an increased susceptibility to infections of the respiratory tract (Macwhirter, 1994). Clinical signs associated with the most common respiratory conditions seen in raptors are presented in Figure 20.1. Figure 20.2 presents the differential diagnosis list of respiratory tract diseases in raptors.

Condition	Clinical signs
Upper respiratory tract disease	
Rhinitis and nasal irritation	Nasal discharge, sneezing, staining or discharge in the feathers around the nares, frequent head shaking or yawning to dislodge discharge, choanal discharge and inflammation, plugged nares, open-mouthed breathing, epiphora and conjunctivitis
Sinusitis	Periorbital swelling, chronic or recurrent rhinitis, sunken eyes
Lower respiratory tract disease	
Tracheal disease	Cough, tachypnoea, dyspnoea, open-mouthed respiration, change in vocalization, dilated and inflamed glottis
Pneumonia and air sacculitis	Exercise intolerance, cough, double pump respiratory movement, tachypnoea, dyspnoea and open-mouthed breathing

20.1 Common clinical signs associated with respiratory disease in raptors.

Clinical sign	Differential diagnosis
Nasal discharge	Bacterial infection, particularly by Gram-negative organisms, e.g. *Pseudomonas aeruginosa*, *Proteus mirabilis*, *Escherichia coli* and *Klebsiella* spp. Viral infections, e.g. PMV-1 (note that nervous signs are seen more commonly than respiratory signs in infected raptors) and avian influenza. Avipox infection can result in expansive cere lesions that block the nares and tracheal slit. Fungal infection, e.g. *Aspergillus* spp. Infection with *Chlamydophila* spp. and *Mycoplasma* spp. Non-infectious diseases, e.g. nasal plugs, irritation of the upper respiratory tract with dust, toxins or foreign bodies
Periorbital swelling	Sinusitis caused by bacterial infections, including with *Pseudomonas aeruginosa*, *Proteus mirabilis*, *Escherichia coli* and *Klebsiella* spp. Non-infectious diseases, e.g. subcutaneous emphysema, trauma, subcutaneous haemorrhage, neoplasia and rarely intrasinal or supraorbital trichomoniasis
Acute onset tachypnoea and dyspnoea	Upper respiratory tract infections, e.g. avian influenza, foreign body aspiration, inhaled respiratory toxins, anaemia and aspiration pneumonia
Chronic tachypnoea and dyspnoea	Upper respiratory tract diseases including those causing oral lesions (e.g. granulomas, trichomoniasis, avipox, bacterial stomatitis, capillariasis and candidiasis). Lower respiratory tract diseases, e.g. tracheal disease caused by foreign bodies, granuloma, trichomoniasis, gapeworm infestation (*Syngamus trachea*), aspergillosis, bacterial tracheitis (*Pasteurella multocida*, *Pseudomonas* spp.), pulmonary congestion following trauma. Pneumonia/air sacculitis caused by bacterial, viral, fungal, mycobacterial or parasitic infestation (*Serratospiculum* spp.) Non-respiratory tract disorders including space-occupying masses in the coelomic cavity (granuloma, neoplasia, haemorrhage from trauma, egg binding, hepatomegaly) or including fluid in the coelomic cavity (ascites or egg-related peritonitis)

20.2 Differential diagnosis of clinical signs associated with the respiratory tract in raptors.

Investigation of respiratory disease

Diagnostic procedures for the investigation of respiratory diseases in raptors are listed in Figure 20.3.

Endoscopy (with biopsy and culture) is the most useful technique to diagnose infections of the lower respiratory tract (LRT), particularly aspergillosis and bacterial air sacculitis, in their early stages when treatment may be most effective. In the majority of these early aspergillosis cases radiographic changes will not be apparent, even with digital radiography. Endoscopic images of respiratory tract disease in raptors are shown in Figures 20.4 to 20.7.

Clinical procedure	Comment
Cytology	Of sample exudates (e.g. nares, sinus, choana, glottis and trachea), tracheal washing (0.5–1.0 ml/kg of sterile saline infused into the trachea and aspirated), air sac washing and air sac biopsies
Endoscopy	Of oropharynx, trachea, syrinx, choanal slit, coelomic air sacs, ostium and lung
Endurance test	See text
Haematology and electrophoresis profiles	May indicate inflammatory responses
Histopathology of lesions	Biopsy of cutaneous lesions to confirm avipox infection
Immunology (other)	Rapid avian influenza, PMV-1, *Chlamydophila* kits to test faeces
Microbiology of exudates and any solid lesions	Note that agents isolated may be primary or secondary causes. For viruses use specific transport media
Parasitology of faeces and the oropharynx	Check for eggs of parasites known to infest the respiratory tract (e.g. *Serratospiculum* spp., *Syngamus trachea*)
Radiography	This is helpful to demonstrate both infections of the respiratory tract (e.g. aspergillosis) and other conditions such as space-occupying lesions (e.g. egg binding)
Serological examination	Antibody tests may confirm exposure to *Chlamydophila*, *Aspergillus*, PMV-1, and avian influenza
Virology	For viruses use specific transport media

20.3 Diagnostic procedures for the investigation of respiratory disease in raptors.

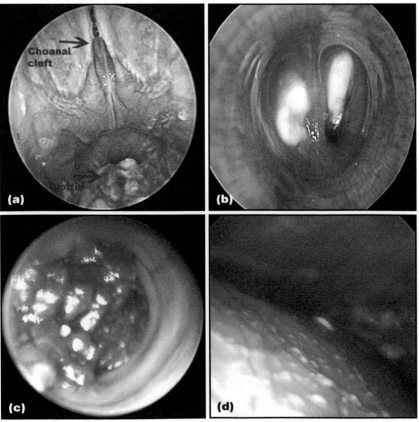

20.4 Endoscopy, bacterial disease. **(a)** Bacterial plaques on the mucous membranes of the oral cavity and the glottis, caused by *Pasteurella* sp. **(b)** The granulomas have blocked the right bronchus completely and the left bronchus by about 90%. **(c)** A piece of meat stuck just above the bifurcation. **(d)** Multiple small bacterial colonies on the air sac membrane covering the serosa of the liver.

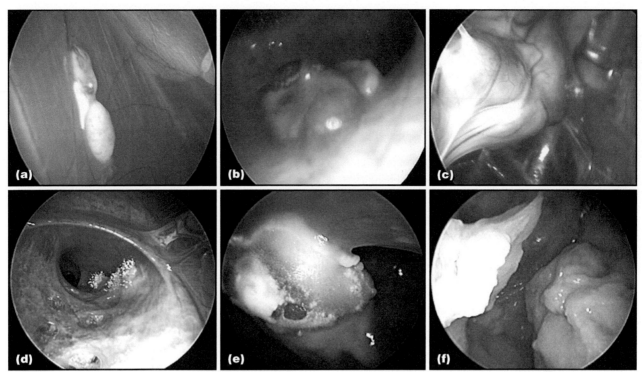

20.5 Endoscopy, fungal disease. **(a)** Fungal granuloma (aspergillosis) with a vascularized capsule. **(b)** Large brownish fungal granuloma adjacent to the ostium of the lung (after biopsy). **(c)** Fungal granulomas can be completely encapsulated within a vascularized capsule. **(d)** Sporulating fungal colonies next to the ostium of the lung. This is a common early location and has to be investigated with special care. **(e)** Large fungal granuloma (aspergillosis). **(f)** If unnoticed or untreated, the fungal infection disseminates throughout the lower respiratory tract and other abdominal organs, filling the air sac completely (together with inflammation products and debris) and possibly breaking through the membrane to spread into neighbouring air sacs. This understandably impedes the breathing of the patient enormously and can make it impossible to perform an endoscopy.

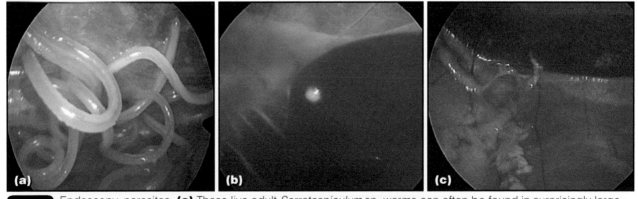

20.6 Endoscopy, parasites. **(a)** These live adult *Serratospiculum* sp. worms can often be found in surprisingly large numbers. **(b)** The *Serratospiculum* nematodes lay their eggs in the air sac, as shown here on the air sac membrane covering the serosa of the liver. **(c)** After parenteral treatment with avermectin drugs, the parasites die and begin to decompose. A few weeks later most of the debris of the worms is already becoming absorbed.

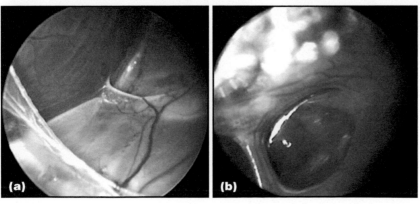

20.7 Endoscopy, lung disease. **(a)** As a result of previous inflammation, adhesions can be seen between different surfaces in the air sac. This interferes with air circulation and may act as a focus for further infection. **(b)** Congestion of the lungs due to infection can occur on different parts of the lung.

Washings and/or biopsy samples from the LRT should be submitted for culture and cytology. In many cases samples from LRT lesions will be culture-negative and cytology is an invaluable tool for providing additional information in these less straightforward cases (Figure 20.8).

Increased respiratory rate at rest and after a controlled endurance exercise (Endurance Test, sometimes called the Stress Test) is considered by some veterinary surgeons to indicate that the respiratory tract is compromised in trained falcons. A high respiratory rate at rest and/or a respiratory rate that does not decrease to the resting value shortly after exercise are indications that further diagnostic tests are necessary. The Endurance Test consists of measuring the respiratory rate per minute at rest and 2 minutes after a 30-second endurance exercise. The exercise is performed by holding the trained raptor on a falconer's glove and moving the hand up and down with slow wide movements in such a way that the bird has to flap its wings continuously in order to keep its balance. After 30 seconds the bird is allowed to rest for two minutes, after which a fit bird is considered to be able to recover a normal respiratory rate (Tully and Harrison, 1994). However, this test must be interpreted cautiously: many factors, including nervous behaviour, nutritional condition and weight in relation to size and breed, will also affect the respiratory rate. Other diseases, not related to the respiratory tract, can also cause respiratory distress (e.g. abdominal pain, ascites, hepatomegaly, cardiac disease).

Upper respiratory tract

Nasal plugs

Falcons often accumulate dust, debris, exfoliated epithelial cells or discharge from episodes of rhinitis in their nares that can harden to become solid plugs. Affected birds can sound as if they have a nasal obstruction and may present with open-mouthed breathing (Figure 20.9). If not removed, such nasal plugs can serve as a nidus for infection. They should be removed by first moistening with swabs and then cleaning with a small bone curette.

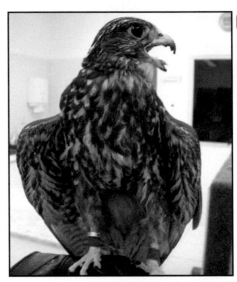

20.9 A falcon showing open-mouthed breathing.

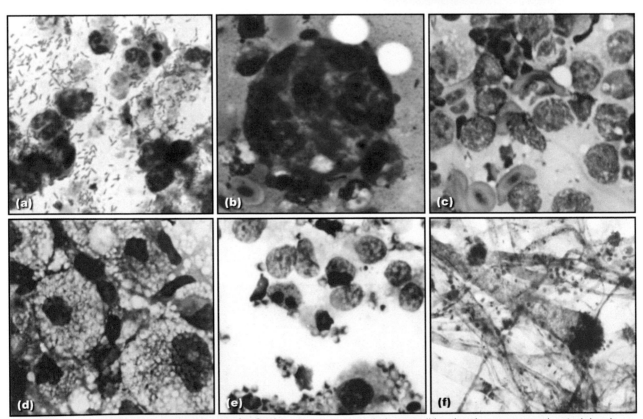

20.8 Cytology smears from the air sac of a Gyrfalcon. **(a)** Bacterial air sacculitis, showing numerous bacterial rods and inflammatory cells. **(b)** Multinucleated giant cell due to fungal infection (aspergillosis). **(c)** Mixed inflammatory cells, including macrophages and heterophils, due to aspergillosis. **(d)** Air sac lining squamous cells showing cytoplasmatic vacuolation, a common finding in fungal air sacculitis and serratospiculosis. **(e)** *Aspergillus* spores and macrophages. **(f)** *Aspergillus* conidiospores, conidiophores and hyphae. (Neat stain, original magnification X1000)

Rhinitis and sinusitis

Rhinitis and sinusitis (Figure 20.10) are usually of bacterial origin. Treatment should be based on isolation and sensitivity testing. Sinus flushing with antibiotic solutions is often necessary to resolve cases of sinusitis (Figure 20.11). Nasal aspergillomas are not infrequently recorded and should be considered in cases of sinusitis that are not responding to antibacterial therapy. Supraorbital trichomoniasis has been reported in Saker Falcons (Samour, 2000a) and should be considered in the differential diagnosis of sinusitis (Figures 20.12 and 20.13).

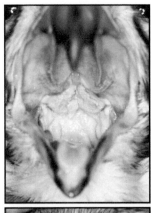

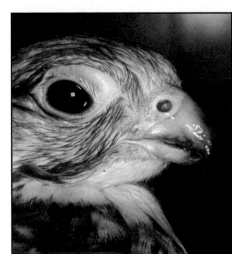

20.13 Choanal necrosis caused by trichomoniasis. Birds with such defects are often more susceptible to upper respiratory tract infections in the future.

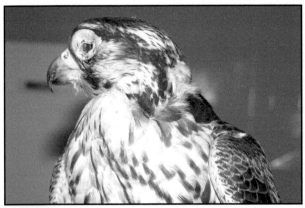

20.10 Sinusitis caused by chlamydophilosis.

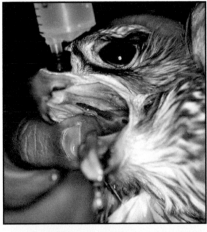

20.11 Flushing the nares of a falcon with sinusitis. (© Michael Lierz)

Pseudomonas sinusitis

Pseudomonas aeruginosa is commonly associated with sinusitis (Figure 20.14), where it is often involved as a secondary invader. *Pseudomonas* produces life-threatening toxins and the organism is resistant to many commonly used antibiotics. Clinical disease is characterized by anorexia, weight loss, unilateral or bilateral sinusitis, and nodular white or yellow caseous lesions in the oral cavity and the tongue. Diagnosis is confirmed by isolation and culture of the organism. Recommended treatment (Samour, 2000b) comprises using a combination of piperacillin and tobramycin, nebulization, debridement of oral lesions, and flushing of sinuses with 5% chlorhexidine gluconate or F10. It is very important to use correctly diluted F10 (see Figure 20.20) as the use of undiluted F10 can lead to a severe inflammatory reaction.

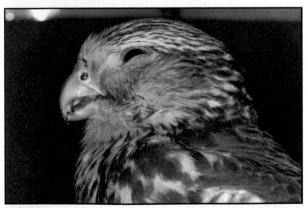

20.12 An advanced case of trichomoniasis that presented with upper respiratory tract signs because of the extensive lesion in the oropharynx, choana and nasal cavity.

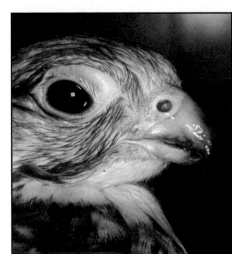

20.14 *Pseudomonas aeruginosa* sinusitis. **(a)** Saker Falcon. (continues) ▶

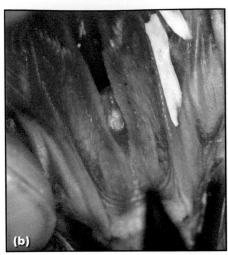

20.14

(continued) *Pseudomonas aeruginosa* sinusitis. **(b)** Abscess in the nasal cavity of a falcon, viewed through the choana.

Other upper respiratory tract disorders

Raptors that present with recurrent upper respiratory signs or chronic signs may have anatomical defects that predispose them to infection. Falcons that lose part of their tongue, often because of severe trichomoniasis, can suffer from recurrent bouts of sinusitis and rhinitis because of food debris impacted in the choana.

Lower respiratory tract

Trachea

Infection with the gapeworm parasite *Syngamus trachea* is the only primarily tracheal disease of raptors. Tracheal foreign bodies are occasionally seen. Otherwise the trachea is affected by other generalized respiratory infections caused by bacteria or fungi. One of the most important fungal disorders of the trachea is the tracheal or syringeal form of aspergillosis, where an aspergilloma obliterates one or both primary bronchi at the level of the syrinx. In these cases the falconer will often notice a change in the voice of the bird. The author has also seen a case of cryptosporidiosis associated with tracheitis and pneumonia.

Cryptosporidiosis

The clinical significance of cryptosporidiosis in raptors is not fully understood. In some bird species it appears to be emerging as a serious disease and the author has seen the enteric form cause severe mortality in juvenile Stone Curlews, and the respiratory form associated with a severe and fatal tracheitis and pneumonia in a hybrid falcon in the Middle East. See Chapter 18 for more details.

Lungs and air sacs

Aspiration pneumonia

Aspiration of food and fluids occasionally occurs following tube feeding of hospitalized falcons that are too weak for the procedure. Very weak birds often regurgitate after tube feeding and ideally such birds should be given fluids and nutritional support by the intravenous or intraosseous routes. The accidental administering of oral medicines by owners, often the commonly administered anti-coccidial agent tolturazol, into the trachea is another cause of aspiration pneumonia. The diagnosis is based on a history of possible aspiration, which includes worsening respiratory distress. Such birds should be hospitalized and given broad-spectrum antibiotics.

Inhalation toxicosis

Inhalation toxicosis can occur in falcons that have been exposed to fumes from domestic fires. While the most common presentation is sudden death, affected birds may be presented with severe acute respiratory signs, typically wheezing and dyspnoea. Endoscopically significant signs include tracheitis, pulmonary congestion and haemorrhage with widespread deposition of inhaled particles throughout the lower respiratory tract. There is no specific treatment for raptors exposed to respiratory toxins and the prognosis is poor. In addition to supportive therapy, affected birds should be given antifungal and antibacterial cover. Also fungal toxins may be inhaled directly, causing a variety of different alterations, such as liver or kidney damage, infertility or embryo toxicity.

Avian influenza

Falcons are susceptible to avian influenza (see Chapter 19).

Bacterial air sacculitis

Bacterial air sacculitis (Figure 20.15) is confirmed following cytology and culture. Endoscopically, bacterial colonies can appear as relatively small white to cream coloured, wet and soft-looking dots with a shiny smooth surface. The bacteria that are commonly isolated from the lower respiratory tract of raptors include *Pasteurella multocida*, *Pseudomonas aeruginosa*, *Escherichia coli* and *Staphylococcus aureus*. Treatment is based on the results of culture and sensitivity testing.

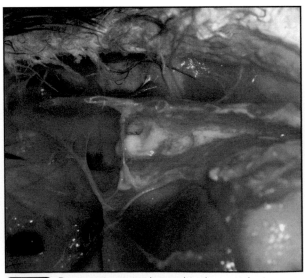

20.15 Post-mortem specimen showing purulent bacterial air sacculitis.

Mycoplasmosis

Many *Mycoplasma* species, including *M. buteonis, M. meleagridis* and *M. falconis*, have been isolated from healthy falcons in Europe and the Middle East. Although *Mycoplasma* spp. are well known pathogens of poultry, causing tracheitis, air sacculitis and chronic respiratory disease, their clinical significance in raptors is unclear. Histological examination of raptor air sacs has shown perivascular infiltration by lymphocytes and plasma cells in some cases and it is possible that these organisms could cause disease in birds with weakened immune systems.

Diagnosis of mycoplasmosis is by isolation and identification of the organism. Selective media are often overgrown by commensals, making isolation difficult. One of the reasons why mycoplasms have rarely been reported from raptors is the difficulty in isolating them. PCR assays have been developed (Lierz *et al.*, 2008) and may be available at diagnostic laboratories. Tetracyclines are recommended because of clinical similarities between mycoplasmosis and chlamydophilosis.

Pasteurellosis

Pasteurellosis affects both captive and wild raptors and is usually caused by *Pasteurella multocida*, although *P. haemolytica* and *P. aerogenes* have been isolated from falcons in the United Arab Emirates. Respiratory infections in raptors generally occur in the respiratory tract, usually following consumption of infected prey (ducks or pigeons). Transmission is via infected aerosols but vectors, particularly wild infected rodents and birds, are important reservoirs of infection. Clinical disease depends on strain, level of exposure and resistance of the raptor. In the acute form, septicaemia and death occur within hours. The chronic form is more commonly seen and is characterized by a watery nasal discharge, swelling of the infraorbital sinuses, inflammation of eyelids and conjunctiva, inflammation of trachea, bronchi and syrinx, pneumonia, air sacculitis and haemorrhagic enteritis. Diagnosis is confirmed following a history of exposure to potentially infected prey and microbial culture (blood culture). Treatment is by appropriate antibiotics (tetracyclines/fluroquinolones) and supportive therapy.

Chlamydophilosis

Chlamydophila psittaci (formerly *Chlamydia psittaci*) is an obligate intracellular bacterial parasite that is sometimes associated with morbidity in raptors. Chlamydophilosis appears to have a multifactorial aetiology in raptors, as clinical disease usually occurs in birds infected with other viral and bacterial agents. Cases often present with a combination of the following signs: anorexia, biliverdinuria, oculonasal discharge, conjunctivitis and sinusitis. The disease is of particular importance in raptor breeding collections, falcon markets and where falconers house a large number of birds together, because this disease can spread widely before it is first recognized and diagnosed.

Radiographic and clinical pathology changes are often suggestive of chlamydophilosis in raptors. Radiographic changes include hepatomegaly, splenomegaly and air sacculitis. Heterophilia and monocytosis are suggestive of active infection. However, while clinical signs and traditional diagnostic assays such as haematology and radiology are helpful, they are generally insufficient to provide a specific diagnosis (see also Chapter 9). Tests for diagnosis of *Chlamydophila psittaci* infection are discussed in Chapters 9 and 19.

Cases are readily treated with a 5-day course of azithromycin at 50 mg/kg orally q24h.

Serratospiculosis

Serratospiculosis is a parasitic disease caused by filarial nematodes of the genus *Serratospiculum* (Figure 20.16). In the Middle East *S. seurati* is the only species that has been identified from captive falcons. In North America *S. amaculata* is considered to be endemic in Prairie Falcons. Raptor species affected include Saker Falcon, Peregrine Falcon, Cooper's Hawk and Northern Goshawk. This author has also found *Serratospiculum* spp. in Desert Eagle Owls (*Bubo ascaphalus*).

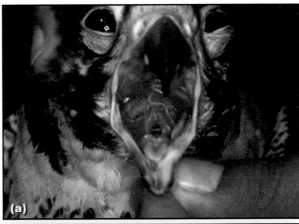

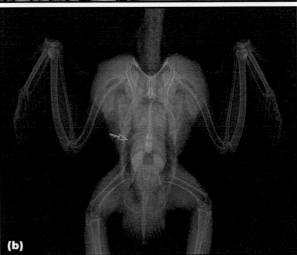

20.16 **(a)** Some *Serratospiculum* infestations can be heavy. In this Peregrine Falcon, the worms were observed in the trachea during clinical examination. **(b)** Focal area of increased radiodensity in the right airspace (arrow). This was a ball of *Serratospiculum* worms, which was removed during endoscopy.

S. seurati is transmitted by ingestion of infected beetles (see Chapter 18) and reinfestation is common in the absence of control of invertebrates in facilities. Adult parasites infest the air sac system. Diagnosis is made following finding of the characteristic eggs in routine faecal flotation or in saline crop swabs (see Chapter 18).

The pathogenicity of this parasite is widely debated. Generally *S. seurati* is considered apathogenic, although severe infestations can be associated with pneumonia, air sacculitis and aspergillosis. Whether heavy infestations of the parasite cause secondary infections is unclear; the parasites may well be innocent bystanders.

Ivermectin and doramectin are routinely used at a dose of 1 mg/kg s.c. and repeated 1–2 weeks later without causing any detrimental effects. The adult parasites can be removed during endoscopy 3–5 days after administration of the first dose of ivermectin. As ivermectin has a wide dose range in falcons, a higher dose might also be chosen, making removal of the parasite unnecessary. Moxidectin is used orally at a dose of 500 µg/kg.

Aspergillosis

Aspergillosis is the most common systemic avian mycosis and is one of the most important causes of mortality of captive raptors. The accounts of an incurable disease of the lungs called *pantas* by the falconer Blome in 1683 may well be the first reference to aspergillosis in hunting falcons.

Clinical disease and pathology: *Aspergillus fumigatus, A. flavus* and *A. niger* typically cause nodular lesions in the trachea, bronchi, lung and air sacs. Aspergillosis in raptors has been classified by Redig (1993) as:

1. An acute form caused by a single exposure to an overwhelming number of spores.
2. A tracheal form.
3. Localized granulomas in the air sacs and lungs.
4. An invasive form that initially affects the respiratory system and then spreads haematogenously and through the air sacs to the rest of the body.

Generally these infections follow a chronic granulomatous course and are often challenging to treat because of the need for potent systemic drugs. In falcons, the most common aetiological agent is *A. fumigatus*, followed in frequency by *A. flavus* and *A. niger*. Most of the *A. fumigatus* strains produce toxins that suppress the immune system. Other fungi can also be isolated (Figure 20.17). Effective treatment can be instituted only in the tracheal and semi-invasive or localized forms. Severe cases, where the patient exhibits cachexia, dyspnoea and vomiting, are beyond the point of treatment.

Clinical signs in falcons with aspergillosis are often non-specific and depend on the organ system involved. Signs include loss of weight, inappetence, tachypnoea, dyspnoea, inspiratory stridor and biliverdinuria, listlessness and anorexia. Inflamed

Fungus	Number of isolates (%)
Aspergillus fumigatus	85 (42.1)
A. flavus	59 (29.2)
A. niger	22 (10.9)
A. terreus	12 (5.9)
Aspergillus sp.	7 (3.5)
Histoplasma sp.	7 (3.5)
Paeciliomyces sp.	3 (1.5)
Scedosporium sp.	2 (0.9)
A. nidulans	2 (0.9)
A. versicolor	1 (0.5)
Candida albicans	1 (0.5)
Mucor sp.	1 (0.5)

20.17 Fungal isolates from air sac biopsies from 202 falcons with lower respiratory tract disease at Dubai Falcon Hospital (Bailey *et al.*, 2005)

air sacs do not produce a respiratory sound and therefore air sacculitis cannot be diagnosed from auscultation.

Diagnosis and control: The history, clinical, radiographic and haematology findings may be suggestive of aspergillosis. Haematological findings include heterophilia, monocytosis and anaemia. Radiographic findings include hyperinflation of the abdominal air sacs, focal densities in the lungs and air sacs (Figure 20.18), and loss of definition of air sac walls. The disease can best be confirmed by endoscopy and cytology/culture of biopsy samples or washings from the lower respiratory tract. Differential diagnoses in a raptor with weight loss, purulent air sacculitis and severe heterophilia would include mycobacteriosis, bacterial air sacculitis and chlamydophilosis.

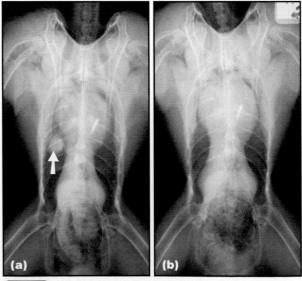

20.18 **(a)** Shadow over the lung in the right airspace caused by an aspergilloma in a falcon. **(b)** After 5 months of voriconazole therapy.

Factors relevant to the investigation of cases of aspergillosis should be identified and corrected, in addition to embarking on medical and surgical intervention. Factors increasing the susceptibility of animals to aspergillosis include:

- Immunosuppression
- Pre-existing diseases (e.g. avipox)
- Treatment with immunosuppressive drugs (e.g. corticosteroids)
- Exposure to respiratory irritants
- Stressful environmental factors (e.g. high humidity, dust, decaying organic matter)
- Malnutrition
- Other causes of physiological stress (e.g. recent capture)
- Long-term antibiosis.

Other lower respiratory tract disorders

Histoplasma is a rare cause of lower respiratory tract disease in falcons in the Middle East. *Histoplasma capsulatum* occurs naturally in soil in warm humid areas of the world and lives as a soil saprophyte, particularly where animal faeces accumulate. Infection of the respiratory tract occurs when dust containing spores is inhaled. Clinically apparent histoplasmosis can be a localized benign pulmonary disease, or a disseminated, progressive and potentially fatal disease. Treatment involves the same antifungal agents used to treat aspergillosis.

Marked pulmonary congestion and air sacs filled with blood clots can occur secondary to trauma in falcons, often as a result of colliding with the side of an aviary or with vehicles during training. Long-term exposure to dust can lead to anthracosis.

Treatment

Nebulization

Inhalation is a practical route of administration to treat diseases of the upper and lower respiratory tract, skin or feathers. The nebulizing equipment for birds must be able to deliver particles <3 μm if they are to enter the lung and caudal air sacs. Particles of 3–7 μm are deposited in the trachea. A great advantage is that handling and resulting stress are minimized, as birds can be left hooded in a nebulization chamber (Figure 20.19). Suitable doses for nebulizing raptors are given in Figure 20.20.

Aerosol therapy/atomization

While nebulizing is useful for individual and less nervous raptors that can be confined to a purpose-built chamber, fogging (Figure 20.21) may be considered as another means of delivering aerosol therapy to birds in avicultural settings.

Fogging groups of birds in aviaries using a commercially available 'smogger' unit and F10 has been used as part of the treatment protocol for a variety of conditions, including chlamydophilosis and other bacterial upper respiratory tract infections, and even as part of a treatment strategy to control the spread of an outbreak of cutaneous pox. Verwoerd

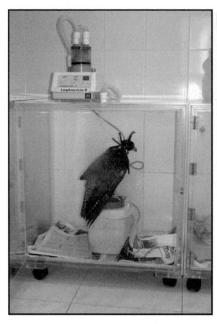

20.19 Nebulization of antibacterial and antifungal agents is an important part of the therapy of respiratory diseases in raptors.

Drug	Dilution	Administration
Antifungals		
Amphotericin B	10 mg in 20 ml normal saline solution	30 min q12h
Enilconazole	50 mg drug in 25 ml normal saline solution	30–45 min q12h
Torbinafine	Use 1 mg/ml solution	30 min q8h–q12h
Clotrimazole	Use 10 mg/ml (1%) solution	30–45 min q8h–q12h
Voriconazole	Use 2 ml (20 mg) of prepared solution in 20 ml saline	30 min q12h
Antibacterials		
Amikacin	100 mg in 20 ml normal saline solution	15–30 min q12h
Enrofloxacin	200 mg in 20 ml normal saline solution	15–30 min q12h
Gentamicin	100 mg in 20 ml normal saline solution	15–30 min q12h
Piperacillin	200 mg in 20 ml normal saline solution	15–30 min q6h–q12h
Tylosin	200 mg in 20 ml normal saline solution	15–30 min q12h
Other		
Acetylcysteine 20%	1 ml in 9 ml of normal saline solution	
F10 disinfectant	1 ml F10 disinfectant in 250 ml normal saline solution (1:250 dilution)	30–45 min q8h–q12h

20.20 Suitable drugs and doses for nebulizing raptors.

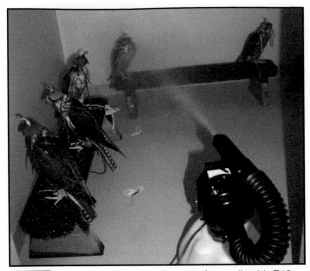

20.21 Falcons being atomized, or 'fogged', with F10 administered with a commercial fogger unit.

(2002a,b) discussed the application of F10 in the biosecurity, preventive health and treatment of clinical avian cases.

Fogging units can be used to treat individual birds either within their breeding aviaries or within a 'treatment' or hospital room. Birds can be given one or two 30-minute atomization sessions daily, in addition to parenteral treatment with whatever antibiotic or antifungal agents are indicated. Surprisingly, while atomization units are noisy, raptors do not appear to be disturbed when they are used, and they seem to enjoy standing in the mist produced by the foggers. The ability to treat a bird within its environment is a tremendous advantage, particularly in breeding establishments where catching and medicating birds is an unwanted inconvenience for avicultural staff.

In addition to treating birds, a fogger unit is used with F10 to disinfect hospitalization chambers and quarantine wards.

Antiparasitic and antibacterial therapy

These are discussed in Chapters 18 and 19, respectively.

Antifungal therapy

If diagnosed in the early stages, aspergillosis can be successfully treated with oral itraconazole or voriconazole, and nebulization with amphotericin B or F10. Because of the slow onset of action of azole antifungals, it is recommended to use initial amphotericin B therapy for serious systemic fungal infections followed by an azole agent (Papich et al., 2001).

Itraconazole can be administered as beads or as a suspension. The suspension is easier to administer, because the correct volume can be injected into the meat. In addition to medical intervention the factors relevant to cases of aspergillosis being investigated should be corrected. The success of treatment depends on location and extent of the lesions. Treatment goals for aspergillosis are: (i) removal of lesions that restrict airflow; (ii) killing and elimination of the fungus; and (iii) provision of supportive care. Unless the lesions are detected early, drug therapy

alone is unlikely to be effective because of the thick caseous encapsulation that develops in the air sacs.

Surgery and topical therapy
In advanced cases it is necessary to remove granulomas surgically from the air sacs, or lesions that are blocking the trachea or syrinx. Tracheal aspergillomas are best treated with surgical debridement via endoscopy. Depending on their size and extensiveness, air sac granulomas can either be removed surgically using a lateral laparotomy approach, or more discrete and detachable lesions can often be removed in piecemeal fashion using biopsy forceps. Such granulomas, as well as those in the air sac, can also be debrided using a diode laser via an endoscopic working channel (see Chapter 13).

Direct application of antifungal agents on to the lesions is an important therapeutic adjunct in birds. Studies in dogs with nasal aspergillosis have shown that, while systemic therapy is successful in 50% of cases, systemic therapy and local irrigation of nasal lesions is successful in 90% of cases (Clark, 1999). Topical application of diluted enilconazole, voriconazole and F10 on to lesions during endoscopy is performed by some avian veterinary surgeons.

Caseous masses can sometimes develop in the supraorbital region following infections in the infraorbital sinuses. Surgery to remove such masses is usually necessary to remove the caseous purulent material that acts as foci for new infections (Samour, 2000a).

Placement of a caudal air sac tube
The avian flow-through system means that artificial ventilation can be achieved by giving fresh oxygen down the trachea or via an air sac tube (see Chapter 10) if the trachea is obstructed. The tube may be used for topical treatment of air sacs as well as assisting with respiration.

Supportive therapy
Supportive therapy includes fluids (intravenous, subcutaneous or intraosseous), tube feeding, antibiotics, anti-emetic drugs, immune stimulants and vitamin A supplementation, according to the needs of the case. The use of immunosuppressive drugs (steroids) in birds is controversial and should be avoided (Chitty, 2001). Indeed cortisone-treated animals (rabbits) are more susceptible to invasive aspergillosis. Immune stimulation may have a role in the future.

Duration of therapy
Recommendations for antifungal treatment duration vary from 2 to 6 months, and one month past the resolution of the disease. Jones et al. (2000) reported that 3–6 months of treatment with itraconazole in raptors at 10 mg/kg once a day did not result in any sign of toxicosis.

Response rate and susceptibility to reinfection
Despite numerous published treatment protocols, few data have been published on the response to treatment so that the efficacy of different regimens can be objectively assessed. Similarly, little has

been published on the susceptibility of recovered animals to rechallenge with aspergillosis. Recrudescence of aspergillosis infections in falcons that have received treatment for aspergillosis is not uncommon in the Middle East and many birds succumb to amyloidosis after recovering from aspergillosis. Falcons that have recovered from the disease have successfully bred and so treatment of breeding birds should be attempted.

Prophylactic itraconazole is recommended for captive-held birds undergoing a change in management, especially high-risk species and during times of stress such as trauma. *Aspergillus* spp. can colonize damaged airways (Richardson, 1998), so probably prophylactic antifungal medication should be considered as part of the therapy of many respiratory tract infections of susceptible species. Daily fogging with F10 of susceptible birds is used to lower the environmental load of respiratory pathogens such as *Aspergillus* spp. in the Middle East. Recommendations to prevent aspergillosis in captive avian collections are presented in Figure 20.22.

- Maintain high standards of hygiene to maintain a healthy environment (reduce exposure to mouldy vegetation in litter and feed)
- Environmental screening of avicultural facilities
- Increase ventilation within facility
- Spray litter and facilities with disinfectant
- Fogging facilities in the presence of live animals/birds with F10 disinfectant
- Reduce stress (especially newly captured birds)
- Ensure that any weight reduction in birds being trained that have been freshly trapped from aviaries is done gradually
- Prophylactic antifungal medication during periods of stress and particularly for susceptible species hospitalized for serious conditions (e.g. following fracture repair)

20.22 Recommendations to prevent aspergillosis in captive avian collections (Redig, 1993).

Amyloidosis

Amyloidosis is an emerging and significant disease in falcons in the Middle East (McKinney, 2002) and is associated with chronic inflammatory or infectious stimuli such as aspergillosis in falcons. Gyrfalcons appear to be very susceptible to this disease, which commonly occurs in birds that are being treated for or have had a history of treatment for aspergillosis. Amyloidosis refers to the deposition of amyloid A, a fibrillar protein derived from immunoglobulins within the body. Amyloid A is a degradation product of an acute-phase protein and amyloidosis denotes a pathological tissue change due to the deposition of amyloid proteins. Amyloid is relatively insoluble and is resistant to proteolysis, so when it is deposited in tissues it cannot be eliminated, resulting in tissue destruction.

Clinical signs vary according to the organ most affected by amyloidosis. Clinical signs of amyloidosis in raptors include exercise intolerance, weight loss with normal appetite (in falcons the mutes are normal until the terminal stages), abnormal feather moult and lime-green discoloration of the urates. Endoscopic examination shows a green-tinged swollen liver with a waxy appearance and an enlarged spleen. Diagnosis is based on liver biopsy with special stains to confirm the presence of amyloid. Histological examination demonstrates the amorphous, eosinophilic nature of amyloid that is stained red by Congo red and shows a green birefringence when viewed under polarized light. Apart from biopsy, there is no other test available to diagnose this condition ante-mortem. Progressive amyloidosis is ultimately fatal. Therapy is aimed at correcting the underlying infection. Colchicine and vitamin C therapy may be helpful (Hoefer, 1997).

References and further reading

Anderson AA and Vanrompey D (2003) Avian chlamydiosis. In: *Diseases of Poultry, 11th edn*, ed. YM Saif, pp. 863–882. Iowa State University Press, Ames

Bailey TA and Sullivan T (2001) Aerosol therapy using a novel disinfectant to treat upper and lower respiratory tract infections in birds. *Exotic DVM* **3**, 17

Bailey TA, Silvanose C, Pesci E and Di Somma A (2005) *Histoplasma* sp. – incidental finding, underdiagnosed, or occasional opportunistic pathogen of falcons in the Middle East? In: *Proceedings of the European Association of Avian Veterinarians Conference, Arles*, pp. 479–481

Bauck L (1994) Mycoses. In: *Avian Medicine: Principles and Application*, eds BW Ritchie *et al.*, pp. 997–1006. Wingers, Lake Worth, FL

Burek K (2001) Mycotic disease. In: *Infectious Diseases of Wild Mammals*, ed. ES Williams and IK Barker, pp. 518–520. Iowa State University Press, Ames

Chitty JR (2001) Use of corticosteroids in birds. *Veterinary Record* **149**, 499

Clark WT (1999) Diseases of the respiratory system. In: *Textbook of Small Animal Medicine*, ed. JK Dunn, pp. 345–350. WB Saunders, London

Cooper JE (2002) *Birds of Prey: Health and Disease*. Blackwell Science, Oxford

Dalhausen B, Lindstrom JG and Radabaugh S (2000) The use of terbinafine hydrochloride in the treatment of avian fungal diseases. In: *Proceedings of the Association of Avian Veterinarians, Portland, Oregon*, pp. 35–42

Di Somma A, Bailey T, Silvanose C and Garcia-Martinez C (in press) The use of voriconazole for the treatment of aspergillosis in falcons. *Journal of Avian Medicine and Surgery*

Flammer K (1997) Chlamydia. In: *Avian Medicine and Surgery*, ed. RB Altman *et al.*, pp. 364–379. WB Saunders, Philadelphia

Forbes NA (1996) Respiratory problems. In: *BSAVA Manual of Raptors, Pigeons and Waterfowl*, ed. P Beynon *et al.*, pp. 180–188. BSAVA, Cheltenham

Forbes N and Altman RB (eds) (1998) *Self Assessment Colour Review of Avian Medicine*. Manson Publishing, London

Fox NC (1995) *Understanding the Bird of Prey*. Hancock House, Surrey, British Columbia

Heidenreich M (1995) *Birds of Prey: Medicine and Management*. Blackwell Science, Oxford

Hoefer HL (1997) Disease of the gastrointestinal tract. In: *Avian Medicine and Surgery*, ed. RB Altman *et al.*, pp. 419–453. WB Saunders, Philadelphia

Jones MP, Orosz SE, Cox SK and Frazier DL (2000) Pharmacokinetic disposition of itraconazole in red-tailed hawks (*Buteo jamaicensis*). *Journal of Avian Medicine and Surgery* **14**, 15–22

Jones MP and Pollock CG (2000) Supportive care and shock. In: *Manual of Avian Medicine*, ed. GH Olsen and SE Orosz, pp. 17–47. Mosby, St Louis

Lierz M (2001) Evaluation of the dosage of ivermectin in falcons. *Veterinary Record* **148**, 596–600

Lierz M, Hagen N, Harcourt-Brown N *et al.* (2007) Prevalence of mycoplasmas in eggs from birds of prey using culture and a genus-specific mycoplasma polymerase chain reaction. *Avian Pathology* **36**(2), 145–150

Lierz M, Hagen N, Lueschow D and Hafez M (2008) Species-specific polymerase chain reactions for the detection of Mycoplasma buteonis, Mycoplasma falconis, Mycoplasma gypis and Mycoplasma corogypsi in captive birds of prey. *Avian Diseases* **52**, 94–99

Lierz M, Schmidt R, Goebel T, Ehrlein J and Runge M (2000) Detection of *Mycoplasma* spp. in raptorial birds in Germany. In: *Raptor Biomedicine III*, ed. JT Lumeij *et al.*, pp. 25–33. Zoological Education Network, Lake Worth, FL

Lierz M, Schmidt R and Runge M (2002) Mycoplasma species isolated from falcons in the Middle East. *Veterinary Record* **151**, 92–93

Lumeij JT (1994) Hepatology. In: *Avian Medicine: Principles and Application*, ed. BW Ritchie *et al.*, pp. 522–537. Wingers, Lake Worth, FL

Macwhirter P (1994) Malnutrition. In: *Avian Medicine: Principles and Application*, ed. BW Ritchie *et al.*, pp. 842–861. Wingers, Lake Worth, FL

Magnino S, Fabbi M, Moreno A *et al.* (2000) Avian influenza virus (H7 serotype) in a saker falcon in Italy. *Veterinary Record* **146**, 740

Manvell RJ, McKinney P, Wernery U and Frost K (2000) Isolation of a highly pathogenic influenza A virus of subtype H7N3 from a peregrine falcon (*Falco peregrinus*). *Avian Pathology* **29**, 635–637

McKinney PA (2002) Amyloidosis in falconiformes. In: *Proceedings of the Australian Chapter: American Association of Avian Veterinarians, Surfers Paradise Conference*, pp. 257–264

Morishita T, Lowenstine LJ, Hirsh DC and Brooks DL (1996) *Pasteurella multocida* in raptors: prevalence and characterization. *Avian Diseases.* **40**, 908–918

O'Malley B (2005) *Clinical Anatomy and Physiology of Exotic Species.* Elsevier Saunders, Edinburgh

Ofner W, Bailey T, Silvanose C and Di Somma A (2005) Common endoscopic and cytology findings of respiratory tract diseases in falcons in the Middle East. *Exotic DVM* **7**, 35–43

Oh S, Martelli P, Hock OS *et al.* (2005) Field study on the use of inactivated H5N2 vaccine in avian species. *Veterinary Record* **157**, 299–300

Orosz SE and Frazier DL (1995) Antifungal agents: a review of their pharmacology and therapeutic indications. *Journal of Avian Medicine and Surgery* **9**, 8–18

Papich MG, Heit MC and Riviere JE (2001) Antifungal and antiviral drugs. In: *Veterinary Pharamacology and Therapeutics*, ed. RA Adams, pp. 918–932. Iowa State University Press, Ames

Phalen D (2006) Preventive medicine and screening. In: *Clinical Avian Medicine*, ed. G Harrison and T Lightfoot, pp. 573–586. Spix, Palm Beach, FL

Philippa JDW, Munster VJ, Van Bolhuis H *et al.* (2005) Highly pathogenic avian influenza (H7N7): vaccination of zoo birds and transmission to non-poultry species. *Vaccine* **23**, 5743–5750

Powell FL (2000) Respiration. In: *Sturkie's Avian Physiology, 5th edn*, ed. GC Whittow, pp. 233–264. Academic Press, San Diego

Prescott JF (2000) Antifungal chemotherapy. In: *Antimicrobial Therapy in Veterinary Medicine*, ed. JF Prescott *et al.*, pp. 367–395. Iowa State University Press, Ames

Redig P (1993) Avian aspergillosis. In: *Zoo and Wild Animal Medicine: Current therapy 3*, ed. ME Fowler, pp. 178–181. WB Saunders, Philadelphia

Redig PT and Ackermann J (2000) Raptors. In: *Avian Medicine*, ed. TN Tully *et al.*, pp. 180–214. Butterworth Heinemann, Oxford

Richardson MD (1998) *Aspergillus* and *Penicillium* strains. In: *Microbiology and Microbial Infections: Volume 4 Medical Mycology*, ed. L Collier *et al.*, pp. 281–312. Arnold, London

Ritchie BW (2003) Management of avian infectious diseases. *Proceedings of the Association of Avian Veterinarians European Committee and European College of Avian Medicine and Surgery, Tenerife*, pp. 417–438

Ritchie BW and Harrison GJ (1994) Formulary. In: *Avian Medicine: Principles and Application*, ed. BW Ritchie *et al.*, pp. 457–478. Wingers, Lake Worth, FL

Samour JH (2000a) Supraorbital trichomoniasis in two saker falcons (*Falco cherrug*). *Veterinary Record* **146,** 139–140

Samour JH (2000b) *Pseudomonas aeruginosa* as a sequel to trichomoniasis in captive saker falcons (*Falco cherrug*). *Journal of Avian Medicine and Surgery* **14**, 113–117

Samour JH (2006) Avian influenza in Saudi falcons. *Falco, Newsletter of the Middle East Falcon Research Group* **27**, 21

Samour JH and Naldo J (2001) Serratospiculiasis in captive falcons in the Middle East: a review. *Journal of Avian Medicine and Surgery* **15**, 2–9

Schmidt RE, Reavill DR and Phalen DN (2003) *Pathology of Pet and Aviary Birds*. Iowa State University Press, Ames

Tully TN and Harrison GJ (1994) Pneumology. In: *Avian Medicine: Principles and Application*, ed. BW Ritchie *et al.*, pp. 556–581. Wingers, Lake Worth, FL

Van Borm S, Thomas I, Hanquet G *et al.* (2005) Highly pathogenic H5N1 influenza in smuggled Thai eagles, Belgium. *Emerging Infectious Diseases* **11**, 702–705

Verwoerd D (2002a) F10 and veterinary clinical usage. In: *Proceedings of the British Veterinary Zoological Society, Edinburgh*, pp. 55–58

Verwoerd D (2002b) F10 with individual and population examples/case studies. In: *Proceedings of the British Veterinary Zoological Society. Edinburgh*, pp. 59–61

Walsh TJ, Mitchell TG and Larone DH (1995) Histoplasma, blastomyces, coccidioided, and other dimorphic fungi causing systemic mycoses. In: *Manual of Clinical Microbiology*, ed. PR Murray, pp. 749–764. ASM Press, Washington, DC

Wernery U and Kinne J (2002) Pasteurellosis in falcons. *Falco, Newsletter of the Middle East Falcon Research Group*, 19

21

Raptors: reproductive disease, incubation and artificial insemination

Michael Lierz

Normal reproduction

Pair behaviour

Raptors tend to be monogamous and pairs are more or less in close contact throughout the year; most have well demarcated territories, which are defended most strongly in the breeding season. The migratory species have less out-of-season contact and return to their territories just prior to breeding. Most raptors use the same breeding territory and nest every year. A change of partners can occur if one dies; sometimes another bird displaces one of the partners and occasionally this can even occur during the breeding season.

Most European non-migratory raptors tend to have a lesser display season in autumn that reinforces the pair bond for the next breeding season. With the increase in day length (temperature is less important), the main display seasons starts between February and April, preparing both sexes for reproduction. Polygyny, where a male pairs with two females, is reported in falcons, as is colony nesting in harriers.

Usually males are about a third smaller than females. The female protects the nest, eggs and young birds and also broods the eggs for almost their entire incubation. The male is mainly responsible for hunting and provides food to the brooding female, only occasionally relieving her on the nest. As part of courtship, the male offers food to the female, which together with special sounds ('kazick') and behaviour ('bowing') (Figure 21.1) proves his ability to take care of the family. As the male is smaller, this procedure is dangerous for him and in some instances he can be caught by the female. This needs to be kept in mind when breeding in a confined space in captivity. The

male is unable to escape from the female when he feels himself in danger; he needs to know exactly how to approach the female. It is very common for captive male goshawks to be killed by their mate, even when they have bred compatibly in previous years.

The male is the key factor in 'natural' reproduction in captivity. The female is generally prepared for reproduction by the increasing day length but needs the display behaviour of the male to complete her cycle. It is essential to use a male that is not afraid of the female. Usually females show some aggression towards the male when first introduced into an enclosure. The male can reduce this aggression by avoiding the female when she is aggressive but also by approaching her to make his courtship display. Brave males are of special importance.

It is of great advantage to use males for breeding that have been used successfully for falconry. These birds are used to humans and are calmer in the enclosure during feeding time. They are not distracted by human noises and can concentrate on courtship and reproduction. Having been successful hunters appears to increase their assertiveness. It is also of advantage to pair an experienced male with a young female. After successful breeding, the female can be paired the next year with a young male; experienced females are usually not as aggressive as young females. Some females with a high potential for aggression (mainly due to mismanagement during rearing and partial imprinting on humans) require very experienced males or cannot be used for pair reproduction in captivity.

During the breeding season it is important to feed the pair several times a day with small amounts of food. This enables the male to present the female regularly with food, increasing the pair bond and decreasing any aggression. It also confirms that the male is able to provide regular food for the female and her young.

Outside the breeding season aggression from the female increases, the level varying between species. Falcons can be kept as pairs throughout the year, but goshawks need to be separated. In nature male goshawks maintain contact with the females throughout the year but fly off when the female gets too close. This is not possible in captivity and males are regularly killed by the females if they are not separated after the chicks are raised. Goshawk pairs are usually kept in a double enclosure, with the male and female separated by wooden bars. This allows

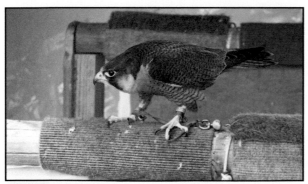

21.1 Display behaviour of an imprinted male Peregrine Falcon, demonstrating 'bowing'. (© Michael Lierz)

them to see each other and in spring enables courtship displays to be developed relatively safely. When the breeder judges the birds to be compatible the bars are opened. In addition some primaries of one wing of the female can be cut, to reduce speed and manoeuvrability within the cage.

Exceptionally, the Harris' Hawk is a social group-living raptor. Aggression between the partners is low and pairs can usually be kept together all year around. In this species one male might also be paired with two or more females, which is almost impossible in other species.

Breeding enclosures

Breeding enclosures for raptors should be closed on all sides. They are known as 'skylight and seclusion' aviaries. The open top is covered with two layers of plastic-coated mesh (at least 15 cm apart) to avoid direct contact between wild raptors and the breeding pair. The nest sites should be protected by a small roof to keep them dry. Each enclosure (or breeding chamber) should have at least two nesting sites (Figure 21.2), allowing the birds to select their nest and to change the nest if the first clutch is removed. To minimize human contact, the birds are observed through small holes or better still with closed-circuit television (CCTV); opening hatches are used for feeding and water. The ground should be covered with large-grade gravel laid down on an easily drained substrate, allowing the rain to wash excrement away but also excluding earthworms (potential paratenic hosts for parasites). Nest material is chosen according to the species: small-grade gravel for falcons and branches (preferably coniferous wood) for accipiters.

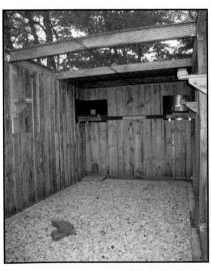

21.2 Breeding chamber for falcons with two nesting sites (covered), gravel on the floor, sides closed and perches with artificial turf. (© Michael Lierz)

Copulation, eggs and chicks

Display behaviour results in copulation, which may occur only a few times in the morning and evening or frequently throughout the day, depending on the pair. During copulation the female crouches submissively and the male flies on to her. This can be misinterpreted as aggression by inexperienced females, preventing copulation.

Evidence of display behaviour does not guarantee fertile eggs. Copulation usually starts about 14–21 days before the first egg is laid. The female becomes

inactive about 2 days before the first egg is laid and will often be seen near the nest. It may be possible to see abdominal distension. If there is any disturbance, such as feeding by the breeder, the bird appears to be normal. Display behaviour is still present. It is important to differentiate this physiological behaviour from pathological signs of egg binding or systemic diseases. CCTV observation is of advantage as it can be difficult for breeders to predict what is happening and to differentiate between illness and normality without this accessory.

Some males can be abnormally keen to brood the eggs, stopping copulation after the second egg is laid and thereby causing the fourth and subsequent eggs to be infertile.

Larger falcons and goshawks lay 3–5 eggs (usually 4) and eagles and vultures lay two eggs in a clutch. The eggs are laid 2 days apart and brooding usually starts with the second or third egg (or the first with eagles and vultures). Incubation is mainly carried out by the female but the male broods the eggs when the female is preening or feeding. The incubation period is species-dependent (Figure 21.3).

Species	Incubation period (days)	Clutch size
Peregrine Falcon	31–33	3–5
Gyrfalcon	32–33	3–5
Saker Falcon	31–33	3–5
Lanner Falcon	31–33	3–5
Merlin	28–30	3–4
Northern Goshawk	32–34	3–5
European Sparrowhawk	32–34	3–6
Common Buzzard	33–38	3–5
Harris' Hawk	32–34	3–5
Golden Eagle	43–45	2
White-tailed Sea Eagle	34–42	2
Bald Eagle	35–36	2
Red Kite	31–32	3–5
Black Kite	31–32	3–5
Griffon Vulture	48–54	2
Cinereous Vulture (European Black Vulture)	50–55	2

21.3 Incubation periods and clutch size of selected birds of prey.

Some breeders want a second clutch. This is especially important for pairs with inexperienced partners, who tend to have infertile eggs in the first clutch. However, the eggs are not removed until after 10 days of incubation. This causes better pair bonding, as the male brings food to the brooding female and the birds often take turns brooding the eggs. In addition, for eggs incubated artificially the percentage that hatch is higher if they have already been incubated naturally by the female.

Display behaviour usually resumes a couple of days after the eggs have been taken away. Experienced pairs start copulating after that time. The first egg of the second clutch is usually laid 12–14 days after removal of the first clutch.

Artificial incubation allows more control over the hatching process and also prevents siblicide. The second clutch is removed and replaced by artificial eggs, which allows them to be exchanged for the chicks when they are old enough for the parents to be allowed to rear them. If the first clutch was fertile, the eggs of the second clutch can be removed by changing them with chicks from the first clutch.

Chicks returned to parents should be at least 5 days old (preferably 6–8 days) as by this age they can hold their heads up for some time. Chicks need to be ringed at 10–11 days old and some breeders put the chicks back with the parents after ringing. Unfortunately, by this age the imprinting process has already started and can be directed towards humans rather than birds. It can also be dangerous to put the chicks into the nest, as their sudden movements stimulate aggressive responses from the parents. If the chicks are hungry, their insistent begging noises override parental aggression and the parents will feed the chicks. If the parents are inexperienced, only one chick should be placed in the nest. If it survives, the other chicks can be added. It is useful to leave one artificial egg in the nest as this encourages the female to continue incubating, ensuring that the chicks also remain covered – out of sight and out of harm.

Using imprinted females, the basic procedures are similar; the breeder takes the part of the male. With imprinted females 'egg pulling' is possible. After the second egg is laid, both eggs are taken out and the female is given one artificial egg. Subsequent eggs are taken away as well. Females stop laying when they have completed their clutch, which they assess by the number of eggs they are incubating rather than the number they have laid. Females whose eggs are removed keep laying and can produce up to 20 eggs. This method is also possible with breeding pairs, but the stress caused by the owner entering to remove an egg every 2 days causes egg production to stop.

Manipulating the females to produce an abnormal number of eggs in a series is not recommended: it is impossible for the female to replace all the nutrients that she puts into each egg and she will become seriously weakened. Many of the later eggs will be so nutrient-poor that they will have poor hatchability and the young birds that manage to hatch will often suffer from vitamin and mineral deficiencies.

Artificial insemination

Artificial insemination has been used to avoid the above-described problems in pair bonding, especially aggressive females injuring or killing their partners. Artificial insemination also allows hybridization between species that would not reproduce under natural circumstances.

Semen donation

It is possible to obtain semen from nearly every sexually mature male. The requirements are that the male is not stressed and experiences a natural daylight cycle. Semen production occurs and the semen is stored in the paired receptacles of the ductus deferens next to the cloaca. It is very difficult to collect semen from males in copulating pairs, as they empty the receptacles continuously by natural copulation. Parent-raised males (including wild birds) usually provide semen for a few donations and it is usually only a small volume, as the stress of catching reduces semen production.

Imprinted males make much better semen donors. The breeder acts as the bird's partner, offering food as well as crouching and chirping. The semen is collected by massage techniques or by using a special hat. The hat covers the breeder's head, including neck and ears; there is usually a rim for the bird to perch on and a gutter into which the semen drains (Figure 21.4). The hat technique requires a specially trained bird and contamination of the semen sample is more likely.

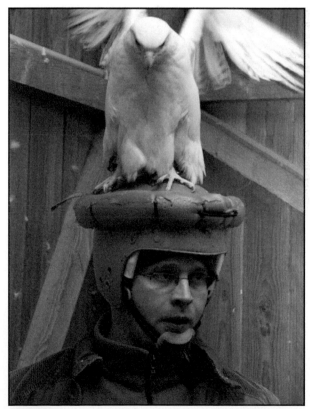

21.4 Imprinted Gyrfalcon male copulating on a special hat to collect its semen from the hat's border. (© Michael Lierz)

The massage technique is more commonly used. It is vital that the bird has passed mutes prior to the massage, to avoid contamination of the semen with urine or faeces. The bird is hooded and placed in dorsal recumbency. The body wall is gently massaged towards the cloaca with a little pressure left and right of the cloaca. The drop of sperm is collected into a plain capillary tube (Figure 21.5).

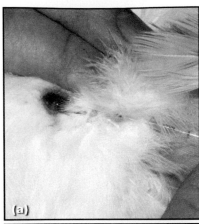

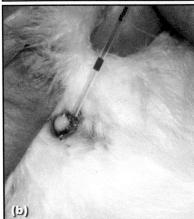

21.5
Sperm collection using the massage technique.
(a) Collection of semen (watery appearance).
(b) The white colour shows that it has been contaminated by urine. (© Michael Lierz)

Semen quality

After the semen has been collected, its quality should be evaluated under the microscope (Figure 21.6). Where semen quality is poor or vital spermatozoa are absent, artificial insemination does not make much sense and there is no need to stress the female. It is important to investigate each semen sample for the number of sperm, the percentage of viable and motile sperm, the percentage of deformed sperm heads and the orientation of the sperms' movements. In good quality semen, more than half of the sperms are moving towards the air/semen border in the capillary tube. It is important to use warmed tubes and to examine the semen in a warm environment. Evaluation of avian semen can be based on the same parameters as those used for evaluating mammalian semen.

Insemination

Any female raptor can be artificially inseminated, but the stress of the procedure leads to problems in parent-reared or wild females. Usually only one or two inseminations are possible in such birds and the quality of the eggs following the procedure can be poor, with thin-shelled or depigmented eggs being regularly observed. In human-imprinted females the procedure is well tolerated.

The semen is sucked into a small flexible tube connected to a syringe for transmission. The female is wrapped in a towel and fixed in dorsal recumbency. The cloaca is spread by a rabbit-mouth spreader. The oviduct opening is easily visible and the flexible tube containing the semen can be introduced (Figure 21.7). In well trained imprinted birds direct cloacal insemination is possible, avoiding restraint of the bird for each insemination, but this leads to a reduced fertility rate compared with direct uterine insemination.

Insemination is usually performed daily 3–5 days before the first egg is expected. This is judged by behaviour, abdominal distension and previous laying date, as many birds lay around the same day each year. Subsequent insemination is done immediately after the egg is laid. One insemination is able to fertilize a maximum of two consecutive eggs and so several inseminations are necessary to fertilize the whole clutch.

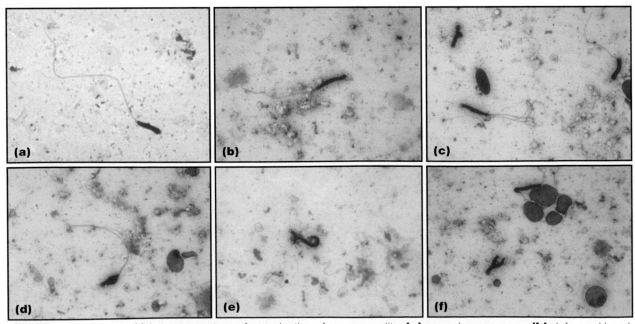

21.6   Giemsa stain of falcon spermatozoa for evaluation of semen quality: **(a)** normal appearance; **(b)** deformed head; **(c)** multiple tail; **(d)** deformed body and double tail; **(e)** double head, deformed body, no tail; **(f)** deformed sperm and a granulocyte indicating an inflammatory process within the testis or deferens duct. (© Michael Lierz)

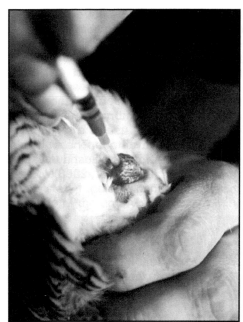

21.7

Insemination of a female falcon. (© Michael Lierz)

Incubation techniques

Many breeders favour artificial incubation, as it lowers the risk of egg damage compared with natural incubation. Poultry eggs have been artificially incubated for centuries. Eggs and chicks affected adversely by artificial incubation did not hatch; this selection process has resulted in high hatching rates. Raptors have not evolved under domestication; each egg laid has to be considered as an individual and need its own attention, which involves far more work per egg.

Incubator systems

Several types of incubator are available for raptor breeding. Incubators with a heating loop on top without ventilation are inexpensive but have a poor hatch rate. Automated incubators ventilated by warmed circulating air are very popular, especially if the rotation of the ventilator is slowed to reduce vibration. Contact incubators are a new type in which a warmed latex-bag heating system comes down on to the eggs, simulating the brooding female; the heating bag is lifted off the eggs and the eggs are then turned, mimicking the normal behaviour of the parent. The increased success of such incubators compared with the ventilation system has yet to be fully evaluated.

Eggs need regular turning or the embryo and its membranes will attach to the shell. An automated turning system is recommended, turning the egg every 2 hours and needing one hour for the turn. This also avoids vibration of the egg, which is especially important during the first half of the incubation period.

Using several incubators at the same time enables the breeder to have a range of humidity, allowing the rate of weight loss to be tailored to individual eggs.

Incubator hygiene is vital for breeding success. The warm moist incubation climate encourages fungal and bacterial growth. To reduce this, egg shells should be disinfected prior to incubation and regular disinfection of the incubator is recommended.

Temperature and humidity

Raptor eggs are incubated at a lower temperature (37.2–37.4°C) than poultry eggs. The room temperature outside the incubator must be more or less stable as this influences the climate inside the brooding room. It must always be kept in mind that the incubator cannot regulate the temperature downwards, therefore optimal room temperature is 20–22°C.

Egg weight management

For successful incubation and hatching, eggs must lose a certain amount of water over the incubation period. In raptors, the egg must lose 13–15% of its weight between laying and pipping. Too little water loss causes an oedematous chick, but too much water loss causes dehydration. Weight loss of the egg in an incubator is dependent on the humidity. Raptor eggs are incubated without additional water supply.

Where egg pulling is practised, the fresh weight of the egg is known and the total weight lost is calculated at 15%. A graph of weight loss is made where the weight lost is divided by the days of incubation until pipping (e.g. falcons have 32 days incubation time, but pipping occurs at day 30). The egg is weighed daily and compared with the graph. Where instead of being pulled the eggs are incubated artificially after being brooded for 10 days by the parents, the original weight is unknown. Recommendations to multiply egg size (width × length) by a species-specific factor are unreliable. In such cases the weight of the eggs must be estimated, but the days of brooding by the females must be known (Figure 21.8).

Egg weight on day 9 of incubation: 44.79 g.

Peregrines brood for 32 days but pipping occurs on day 30.

Weight loss in 30 days of incubation = 15%.

Average weight loss per day (15/30) = 0.5%.

9 days of incubation = 4.5% weight lost so far, i.e. egg still 95.5% of original weight.

44.79 g = 95.5% of original weight.

Estimated original weight = (44.79/95.5) ×100 = 46.9 g.

15% of 46.9 g = 7.036 g weight lost in 30 days (0.2345 g/day) (weight at pipping: 39.86 g).

This egg was incubated without additional humidity and interference and pipped at 39.64 g.

21.8 Calculation of the daily weight loss of a Peregrine Falcon egg after 9 days of incubation by the parents.

Eggs losing too much weight must be transferred to an incubator with higher humidity. If the weight loss is insufficient (which is more common), it is possible to lower the humidity using air-drying systems but this is often unsuccessful. To increase water loss it is useful to grind the egg shell at the blunt end with sandpaper. This will remove the relatively waterproof protein cuticle, but, more importantly, it will thin the shell and open the pores, allowing increased water loss (Figure 21.9). If the egg loses too much weight after this procedure, the ground area can be reduced with paraffin wax or water-resistant tape (Figure 21.10). Such manipulations should not be performed before day 20 of incubation.

oviduct. Reasons include inflammation of the oviduct, sometimes due to contaminated semen used in artificial insemination, or systemic infection with an acute onset of severe clinical disease.

In most cases the egg is fully developed and stays in the lower part of the oviduct. Although oviduct inflammation might be a reason, hypocalcaemia or stress due to disturbance is more likely. Artificially inseminated untrained or non-imprinted females in particular may develop egg binding due to the stress of insemination. If eggs are removed before the clutch is complete, the female may leave the nest and egg binding might result if she does not accept an alternative.

Hypocalcaemia may be a cause if egg pulling (see above) is practised or with one of the later eggs of a clutch. Due to the massive demand on calcium for shell production, commonly used food may not meet the requirements.

Rarely, reproductive neoplasms or skeletal deformities may also be reasons for egg binding, such as deformed or (very rarely) over-large eggs.

Clinical signs: These include reduced activity by the female. She stays on the nest with eyes closed for several hours. It is very difficult to distinguish between egg-laying lethargy, which may occur before the first egg, and real egg binding. If the inactivity occurs after the first egg has been laid, egg binding is more likely. In egg binding, leg weakness may also occur due to increased pressure on vessels and nerves. Urinary or intestinal obstructions may also result.

Diagnosis and therapy: The history is of great importance in distinguishing an unwell bird not laying the egg from a case of egg binding. Questions should cover how many clutches the female laid during the last and the present season, how many eggs are now expected, whether any problems occurred with eggs laid previously, and what the bird's diet is and whether it has been supplemented, especially with calcium and vitamin D.

The first step is radiography (both body views; see Chapter 11) to evaluate the egg shell, form and size as well as the bird's pelvic bones and the occurrence of medullary bone deposition (Figure 21.17a). If the egg shell has developed but no medullary bone is present (Figure 21.17b), calcium deficiency is likely.

The use of patient-side devices to assess plasma ionized calcium levels is also highly recommended to assess the need for calcium as part of the therapy and for monitoring response to dosing.

In such cases calcium and vitamin D are supplemented by direct application followed by a supplemented diet and the bird is placed back in the breeding chamber. The application of oxytocin is questionable as it increases the blood pressure of the female and might lead to circulatory problems. It has been observed that the egg is laid quickly after oxytocin application but the female may die a few hours later. Therefore the use of oxytocin should be avoided.

Some authors suggest the use of prostaglandin E2 gel applied topically per cloacum to the uterine sphincter as an aid to dilating this sphincter and inducing uterine contraction.

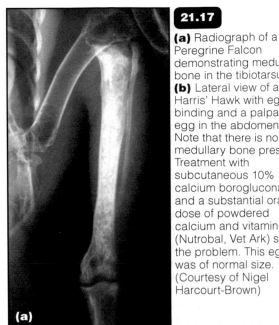

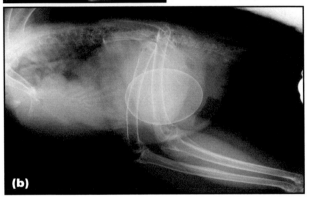

21.17
(a) Radiograph of a Peregrine Falcon demonstrating medullary bone in the tibiotarsus. **(b)** Lateral view of a Harris' Hawk with egg binding and a palpable egg in the abdomen. Note that there is no medullary bone present. Treatment with subcutaneous 10% calcium borogluconate and a substantial oral dose of powdered calcium and vitamin D (Nutrobal, Vet Ark) solved the problem. This egg was of normal size. (Courtesy of Nigel Harcourt-Brown)

Calcium deficiency is unlikely in cases where the bird does present sufficient medullary bone, and it must be determined whether the egg can be laid naturally (malformed pelvic bones, egg-shell deformation, no shell present) or if other reasons are present (Figure 21.18). If so, manipulation of the egg within the abdomen is quite possible using *lateral* pressure through each side of the bird's body (downward pressure can cause damage to the kidneys and also can reduce their blood supply). Gentle pressure will cause a shelled egg to present at the exit to the oviduct and it can be removed with sustained pressure, lubrication and gently easing the oviduct over the egg. These eggs invariably have no cuticle: without the cuticle, the egg's surface is relatively rough and the egg does not slide out as easily as a normal egg.

If the egg shell is very thin, the egg can be collapsed by aspiration of its contents after the shell as been punctured with a large needle and then delivered through the cloaca. Once the egg is out a blood sample for CBC is useful, but application of antibiotics (to prevent infection of the oviduct), fluids (subcutaneously and orally), calcium and warmth are always recommended.

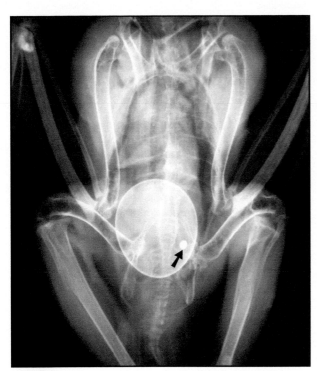

21.18 Ventrodorsal view of a Goshawk with egg binding and with a palpable egg. The egg was shelled and adequate medullary bone was present. Note the piece of lead (arrowed) in the gizzard. The bird was given edetate calcium disodium by intramuscular injection and laid the egg within 12 hours. Further treatment for the lead poisoning was required. The egg was of normal size. (Courtesy of Nigel Harcourt-Brown)

Surgery: If the egg cannot be presented at the exit to the oviduct, surgical intervention is necessary as a uterine torsion may be present (see Chapter 14). All manipulations are performed under general anaesthesia. If the bird is already very weak, the owners must be informed that anaesthesia does have an increased risk. After any intervention, it is advisable to keep the bird away from the breeding pen and its partner, to interrupt the laying cycle for some days.

In a very few cases an egg may have been prolapsed into the urodeum. These eggs are difficult to remove and also the egg obstructs the ureters, which means that the bird may start to go into renal failure. This should be borne in mind after removal of the egg.

Infection and thickening or scarring of the vent may prevent an egg from being laid. An episiotomy may be needed. After such intervention some birds will not be able to lay reliably and should be removed from the breeding programme, as should birds with a recurrence of egg binding or detected irreversible abnormalities (e.g. malformed pelvic bones, repeated laparatomy).

Salpingitis

Bacterial infection of the oviduct may occur after artificial insemination. Semen contamination with faeces/urine or the introduction of a contaminated tube into the oviduct results in such infections and so it is more common if the procedure is performed by untrained people. Cloacal infections may lead to ascending infection of the oviduct, as will ruptured eggs or undetected egg binding. Such infections are often fatal as they are recognized too late for treatment. In some cases alterations of the egg shell (depigmentation, rough or irregular shell) might be detectable. If the bird is only used for breeding, intensive antibiotic treatment may be tried. The treatment of choice is ovidectomy, which is not a loss as most cases of salpingitis result in infertility of the female. An experienced breeding bird can often be used for crèche-rearing young birds, even if she is unable to lay eggs herself.

Prolapse

Prolapse of the oviduct is sometimes difficult to differentiate from a cloacal prolapse (the proctodeum or urodeum, or both, can prolapse) and often both occur. Oviduct prolapse is very rare outside the breeding season, as the oviduct is too small. Prolapse of the oviduct can occur due to egg binding as the bird increases abdominal pressure to lay the egg. It may also be present in older females after laying an egg, as suspensory ligaments of the oviduct can be stretched or weakened and torn. Also, oviduct neoplasms or infections may be causes.

First, the bird requires intensive fluid therapy and antibiotic treatment, but a prolapse of the oviduct requires immediate surgical intervention (see Chapter 14). Because the reproductive, urinary and intestinal tract all empty into the cloaca, pushing a prolapse 'back inside' and retaining it with a purse-string suture, instead of making a diagnosis, frequently condemns the bird to death.

Egg peritonitis

Egg peritonitis is rare in raptors compared with other birds that lay more eggs, such as chickens. Yolk material in the abdominal cavity causes inflammatory reactions and may be absorbed without any further problems. A larger amount of yolk material, or bacterial colonization of the foreign material, leads to a rapid and extensive inflammatory process resulting in severe illness. Untreated it is usually fatal. Yolk material enters the abdominal cavity by oviduct rupture or if the infundibulum fails to gather the yolk at the time of ovulation.

Clinically the signs may be associated with egg laying but they sometimes occur after the breeding season; the owner reports that the female has laid no eggs, or fewer eggs than expected. Radiography shows the presence of an amorphous mass and fails to demonstrate an egg. An increased white blood cell count and elevated serum fibrinogen confirm an inflammatory process. Ultrasonography can be useful. A fine-needle aspirate of the abdominal contents is very informative and can also be used for bacteriology (often *Escherichia coli*). If possible the bird should be stabilized first; it will require surgical removal of the egg yolks and probably hysterectomy. Prognosis is guarded.

Egg pathology and hatching problems

Eggs that do not develop are known as clear eggs: candling shows no blood vessels. Examination of clear eggs is important in detecting early signs of problems in a breeding facility.

The first step is to differentiate between an infertile egg and one where early embryonic death has occurred, which cannot be done by candling. The examination is performed using sterile gloves, instruments and dishes.

1. The egg shell is disinfected with a formalin-based solution.
2. The egg is opened at the blunt pole at the border of the air cell (Figure 21.19) and the contents are emptied on to a sterile Petri dish.
3. Using a microscope, the blastoderm at the top of the egg yolk is examined for embryonic development.
4. A sample of the yolk is streaked on blood agar and incubated aerobically and anaerobically.
5. The empty shell is filled with peptone solution, used for *Salmonella* enrichment (Figure 21.20), and closed by gauze soaked in paraffin wax.

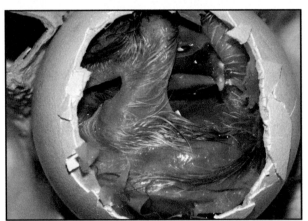

21.19 At the blunt end, the egg is opened at the air bulb border for investigation. This demonstrates the correct position of the embryo in the egg immediately prior to pipping. (© Michael Lierz)

1. The freshly emptied egg shell is filled with peptone broth up to the former air bulb border for pre-enrichment.
2. The whole egg is closed using paraffin gauze to prevent further contamination and incubated at 37°C for 24 hours.
3. Afterwards pre-enrichment broth is transferred into Rappaport–Vassiliadis broth (1:100) and further incubated at 41°C for 48 hours as a selective enrichment.
4. A sterile loop is dipped into the selective broth and streaked on to *Salmonella*-selective agar medium (Gassner, Rambach) for further incubation at 37°C for 24 hours.
5. *Salmonella* colonies show a specific growth (colour) according to the selected agar medium and can be further differentiated using rapid plate agglutination with commercially available antisera.

21.20 *Salmonella* enrichment.

If embryonic development is present:

- The time of death should be estimated. Helpful tools are the Homberger and Hamilton stages and a poster demonstrating the development of a kestrel embryo produced by Pisenti *et al.* (2001)
- With larger embryos, samples of the amniotic fluid should also be taken for bacteriological investigation, followed by a full examination of the embryo, taking samples of liver and yolk for bacteriology
- There is evidence that mycoplasmas might also play a role in embryo mortality, as occurs in poultry, and the occurrence should be investigated by isolation or preferably PCR examination (Lierz *et al.*, 2007a)
- Additionally the embryo is opened along the ventral midline and placed into a good volume of 10% buffered formalin solution for histopathological examination to detect any abnormal signs leading to the problem.

Embryo problems

Reasons for infertility have been described above.

- It must always be considered that, after the egg is laid, nothing can be added to the embryo's nutrition and this nutrition must last the embryo for 30 days plus. The diet of the parents, in particular the female, is very important, and supplementation must start weeks before the egg is laid.
- The egg can be contaminated by pathogens within the ovary and the oviduct, a common occurrence with *Mycoplasma* and *Salmonella* infections. After being laid, the warm egg cools, contracting the contents and absorbing air (forming the air cell at the blunt end) and pathogens into the egg through the pores. Therefore hygiene is essential. Bacterial contamination can prevent embryonic development and leads to embryonic death in the first half of incubation.
- When incubated eggs are removed from the parents to the incubator they are very vulnerable to vibration, especially during the first 3 days of incubation. Also, cooling (or any climate change) during transport causes rapid death of the embryo.
- Improper artificial incubation (e.g. wrong temperature) can cause embryo death at any stage of incubation. Slightly too cool a temperature slows embryonic development and causes death at the end of incubation. Slightly too warm a temperature can cause abnormal development of the embryo; for instance, it has been suggested as a cause of eye deformities (Harcourt-Brown, 2003) or late embryonic death. Failure to retract the yolk sac (Figure 21.21), skeletal deformities and torticollis can be temperature-related.
- Deficiencies in the egg (vitamin E, selenium, iodine) usually cause late embryonic death; this occurs later because vital nutrients will be used up as the embryo grows.

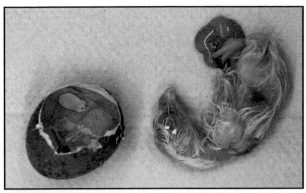

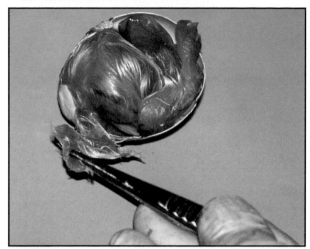

21.21 Peregrine Falcon chick that failed to retract the yolk sac. (© Michael Lierz)

Hatching problems

Hatching problems often have the same causes as late embryonic death.

- Deficiencies are a common cause.
- Poor incubator hygiene causes late embryonic death and hatching problems, especially after pipping. When the chick has made the first hole in the egg shell, the external barrier is breached. If infection, especially fungal, is present in the incubator, the chick breathes in spores or toxin-contaminated air, with fatal consequences.
- A common hatching problem is oedema of the neck (Figure 21.22). Although the egg shell can be breached, oedema prevents the chick from opening the egg further because repetitive neck movements are impossible. In most cases this occurs if the eggs do not lose enough fluid (weight) during incubation (see above); however, calcium deficiency causes sufficient muscular weakness to prevent hatching. Renal failure or

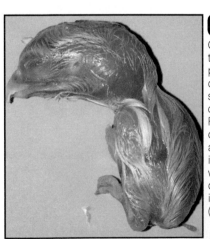

21.22

Gyrfalcon embryo that died directly prior to pipping, demonstrating severe neck oedema. Frequently the cause of this alteration is insufficient loss of water/weight during the incubation period. (© Michael Lierz)

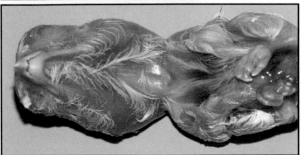

general infection (bacterial, *Mycoplasma*) of the embryo can lead to similar signs.

- Malpositioning of the embryo in the egg also leads to a failure of hatching as the embryo cannot enter the air sac and turn to break the egg shell (Figure 21.23).

21.23 Post-mortem examination of a Peregrine Falcon egg that failed to pip. It shows that the embryo's position made it impossible to move its beak into the air cell. (Courtesy of Nigel Harcourt-Brown)

Often overlooked are environmental toxins that can accumulate in the female and be transferred to the egg yolk and developing embryo. Toxins may originate from pesticides, paints or metals or may be of fungal origin. Depending on the type and amount of toxins, they may cause embryonic death at any stage of development, hatching problems or deformities. A more detailed overview is provided by Romanoff (1972).

Figure 21.24 summarizes possible causes of hatching failure in raptors.

Neonatal mortality

Neonatal mortality might in reality be a late embryonic death and therefore have the same causes. This is particularly true for incubation abnormalities causing dehydration or oedema or even malposition within the egg.

- Nutritional deficiencies of the parents will produce weak chicks. Such chicks are unable to swallow food or to lift their head for begging and die within a few hours of hatching. Investigation into the parents' nutrition is vital (see Chapter 17).
- Hatching is a big effort for the chick. Keeping the newly hatched chick warm and dry is essential and mistakes are often made (see above). If chicks hatch under the parents their movements may make inexperienced birds nervous so the female leaves the nest. In addition to chilling, the chicks can be injured or killed.
- The newly hatched bird is also very vulnerable to infections. Again, incubator hygiene is most important.

Egg pathology	Possible causes
Infertile egg	Both birds female; pair too old; no copulation (one inexperienced partner, male afraid, stress for the pair); asynchronized display (pair of different subspecies); extreme climate; male infertile; parent nutrition
Early embryonic death	Improper incubation (temperature) (disturbance of the pair); extreme climate; inexperienced partner; nutritional deficiency; hybridization of one partner; infection; inadequate transport of incubated eggs; egg storage prior breeding too long
Late embryonic death	Improper incubation (temperature, weight lost, insufficient turning, poor ventilation) (disturbance of the pair); extreme climate; inexperienced partner; nutritional deficiency; infection; rough handling of eggs (e.g. for candling); environmental toxins
Death during pipping (head in air bulb)	Nutritional deficiencies; improper incubation (weight lost, poor ventilation, insufficient turning); infections; incubation hygiene; malposition of the chick; environmental toxins
Chick oedema (see Figure 21.22)	Humidity too high (insufficient weight lost); temperature too low; kidney failure due to environmental toxins
Weak chicks	Nutritional deficiency of the parents (vitamin E, selenium, iodine, calcium); temperature too low or high; humidity too low (exsicosis)
Failure of yolk sac retraction (see Figure 21.21)	Insufficient weight lost; temperature too low
Umbilical infections	Poor incubation hygiene; vertically transmitted pathogens
Curled toes	Infections; temperature too high
Skeletal deformities	Nutritional imbalances of the parents; infections; temperature too high; genetic
Eye disorders	Environmental toxins; temperature too high; genetic; nutritional deficiency
Extended hatching time	Weak chick; nutritional deficiency; temperature too low; humidity too low (dried egg membranes)

21.24 Possible causes of hatching failure in birds of prey.

- During development the embryo seeks a large portion of its calcium from the egg shell. Poor shell quality may lead to a calcium-deficient embryo with muscle weakness, resulting in difficulties with hatching or begging.

Failure of yolk sac retraction

The yolk sac is usually retracted into the abdominal cavity during the 48 hours from pipping to hatch. Failure might be related to suboptimal incubation conditions, infections or may be accidental. The first two reasons have a poor prognosis, as usually other abnormalities are present as well. The last can be treated: the part of the yolk sac protruding from the abdomen can be sealed by closing the abdominal wall over the sac (using a 2 metric (3/0) nylon suture) followed by disinfection of the stump using povidone–iodine. The prognosis of such cases is guarded and the chicks need intensive care. With the yolk sac they will have lost a large amount of nutrition and vitamins that would have been used during the first few days of life. This must be replaced with higher than usual amounts of vitamins, minerals and energy supplements. In addition antibiotic treatment (e.g. amoxicillin) after such a procedure is recommended.

Inflammation of the navel, including bacterial septicaemia

Inflammation of the navel occurs regularly with poor incubation hygiene or with bacterial contamination of the egg. Usually *Escherichia coli* or staphylococci are the cause. Immediate disinfection of the navel after hatching using povidone–iodine solution is strongly recommended. An infected navel appears to be slightly red, progressing into a large red area on the abdomen. Within a few hours it can change to a greenish-blue colour. The infection ascends, involving the retracted yolk sac followed by the liver and ending in a fatal septicaemia. At first the chick becomes inactive, followed by severe depression, loss of appetite and vomiting. The complete process may need only a few hours until death occurs. Aggressive antibiotic and fluid treatment is required when the first signs of navel infections are present, but even then the majority of cases die.

Deformities

Deformities of the extremities may be genetic or related to breeding climate or infections. *Mycoplasma lipofaciens*, isolated from an egg of a Northern Goshawk, was able to cause curled toes in chicken and turkey embryos as described for various *Mycoplasma* species in poultry (Lierz *et al.*, 2007b).

Osteodystrophy might also occur in neonates due to a deficiency in the parents.

Splay legs occur during the first 2 weeks of life and the condition is often caused by insufficient nutrition of the chick, too cool a temperature (the chick stands up and tries to reach the heat source) or inadequate nest material. Placing such chicks in small cups to assist the correct placement of the legs under the chick's body is of great help.

Hypoglycaemia and stargazing

If the chick is kept too cold after hatching or if it gets too little food, signs of hypoglycaemia (incoordination followed by convulsions and death) can occur rapidly. Raising the ambient temperature along with oral and subcutaneous administration of glucose solution will reverse the early clinical signs quickly.

Stargazing usually occurs in older chicks but can also occur in younger birds. Vitamin E, thiamine and selenium deficiencies are supposed to be the cause, though this has not been proven on a regular basis. In the neonate they are related to a poor diet for the parents; in older chicks the signs relate to an insufficient supply to the chick itself.

References and further reading

Anderson Brown AF and Robbins GE (2002) *The New Incubation Book: Revised Millenium Edition*. Oxford University Press, Oxford

Anderson Brown AF (1988) *Kunstbrut – Handbuch für den Züchter* [*The Incubation Book*]. M & H Shaper, Hannover

Deeming DC (ed.) (2002) *Avian Incubation: Behaviour, Environment and Evolution*. Oxford University Press, Oxford

Hamberger V and Hamilton HL (1951) A series of normal stages of development in the chick embryo. *Journal of Morphology* **88**, 49–92

Harcourt-Brown N (2003) Microphthalmia, cataracts, and microphakia in artificially incubated and reared hybrid falcons (*Falco* spp.). In: *Proceedings of the 7th European AAV conference and 5th ECAMS scientific meeting, 22–26 April 2003, Tenerife, Spain*, pp. 197–203

Harvey R (1993) *Practical Incubation*. Hancock House Publishers, Surrey, British Columbia

Heidenreich M (1997) *Birds of Prey: Medicine and Management*. Blackwell Science, Oxford

Lierz M, Gooss O and Hafez HM (2006) Noninvasive heart rate measurement using a digital egg monitor in chicken and turkey embryos. *Journal of Avian Medicine and Surgery* **20**(3), 141–146

Lierz M, Hagen N, Harcourt-Brown N *et al.* (2007a) Prevalence of mycoplasma in eggs from birds of prey using culture and a genus-specific mycoplasma-PCR. *Avian Pathology* **36**, 145–150

Lierz M, Stark R, Brokat S and Hafez HM (2007b) Pathogenicity of *M. lipofaciens* (Strain ML64), isolated from an egg of a Northern Goshawk (*Accipiter gentilis*), for chicken embryos. *Avian Pathology* **36**, 151–153

Pisenti JM, Santolo GM and Yamamoto J (2001) Embryonic development of the American kestrel (*Falco sparverius*): external criteria for staging. *Journal of Raptor Research* **35**, 194–206

Romanoff AL (1972) *Pathogenesis of the Avian Embryo*. John Wiley, New York

22

Raptors: paediatrics and behavioural development and disorders

Michael P. Jones

Rearing strategies

Parent-rearing

Raptors that are parent-reared are raised in aviaries with limited to no visual stimulation from the outside world except for the sky above and ambient sounds. These types of aviary, also termed skylight or seclusion aviaries, are designed to provide an environment in which raptors may reproduce with minimal interruption and that only allows the growing chicks interaction with their parents or siblings. Human contact is usually kept to a minimum but windows may be provided to allow the chicks to see and become somewhat accustomed to the presence of humans. Parent-reared chicks may stay with the parents from the time the egg hatches until the young chick fledges (Figure 22.1).

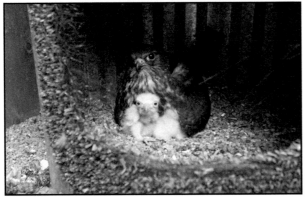

22.1 A female Black Merlin brooding Gyrfalcon × Merlin. (Courtesy of Danny Erstgard, Pacific Northwest Falcons)

Advantages

Allowing the parents or foster parents to raise chicks is less time-consuming for the breeder or falconer. The chicks learn proper social interaction with the parents and siblings, which is preferred by most falconers. This is especially true for gregarious species such as Harris' Hawks, which should preferably stay with the parents until approximately 16 weeks. Some large buzzards such as the Red-tailed Hawk should also be parent-reared as they are less likely to develop aggressive behaviour or excessive screaming than if they are hand-raised and mal-imprinted. Even the Common Buzzard, which is not considered to be aggressive, can become aggressive towards humans if mal-imprinted (Fox, 1995a).

Disadvantages

Limited contact with humans means a reduced ability to evaluate the health of the young raptors. Parent-reared raptors are more likely to resemble wild-caught hawks and will be wild with an intractable disposition when they are initially caught up for training. The young raptors will also be fearful of humans and anything else that is not a sibling or a parent, so the training and manning process may take slightly longer (a few days) and be more intensive. Training for falconry, especially of accipiters, is geared towards taming and recovery as these birds can easily be lost when flown free.

Hand-rearing

Hand-rearing young raptors creates imprinted or, more correctly, mal-imprinted birds. These birds are reared exclusively by humans and develop a filial–maternal bond with their human caregiver. Depending upon the method(s) used, the process of hand-rearing a young raptor can be an extremely time-consuming endeavour. Some falconers/trainers will attempt to habituate young raptors to as many sights and sounds as possible during the initial stages of rearing. Others, perhaps the majority, hand-rear their birds in closed rooms. In the latter case the birds are primarily in contact with their keeper, and contact with other people and exposure to other sights and sounds are kept to a minimum.

When choosing a rearing strategy the future purpose of the raptor must be considered. For example, if the raptor will be used as a future natural breeder with conspecifics it is better if it is parent-reared. If artificial insemination is to be used, the bird should be hand-reared.

The imprinting process naturally occurs at an early age in the life of most altricial birds such as raptors and is species- and time-dependent. This sensitive time period is most likely longer than in precocial birds, which seem to imprint for life within the first few hours of hatching. McElroy (1977) suggested that imprinting the Cooper's Hawk to be used in falconry is best when the young are taken from the nest between 12 and 18 days of age. Afterwards, attempts at imprinting the Cooper's Hawk will leave the falconer frustrated at the lack of tameness of the hawk and may result in moments of intense and seemingly unexplainable fear or aggression. McDermott (1998) suggested that taking the eyas Cooper's Hawk at the much younger age of 7–10 days is ideal. It has been reported that the imprinting of Sparrowhawks to humans optimally

250

occurs between days 1 and 8 (Jones, 1980). At this formative period the Sparrowhawk will most likely accept the human as a parent as well as a future sexual partner. This acceptance may continue if the hawks are taken from the nest between days 10 and 14; however, they will most likely not accept the human as a sexual partner later on. Large falcon species react impartially until around 14 days of age, at which point they become firmly imprinted on the person or bird feeding them (Heidenreich, 1997).

Most of the literature involving raptor imprinting seems to focus on diurnal birds of prey. Nocturnal birds of prey (owls) are different in that they do not become imprinted on humans until later during fledgling development, since their cues for identification with a species or object are determined more by sight and to a lesser degree sound (Jones, 1980). McKeever (1979) suggested that the sensitive time period lasts from 14–21 days up to 42 days in these species.

An alternative to complete hand-raising is to 'dual imprint' young hawks or falcons (see crèche-rearing, below). Many breeders wishing to increase production of falcons may prefer hand-rearing chicks in that it allows them to produce two clutches of eggs or young from the female during a single breeding season (see Chapter 21).

Advantages
Depending upon the degree to which an imprinted hawk or falcon is socialized, they are usually extremely tame (Figure 22.2) and show little or no fear of humans, dogs, automobiles, planes flying overhead, passing trains, and other sights and sounds that would otherwise frighten a non-imprinted raptor. The high degree of tameness of imprinted raptors used in falconry allows for greater field control without having to dramatically reduce the bird's weight to get desired behaviour and responses.

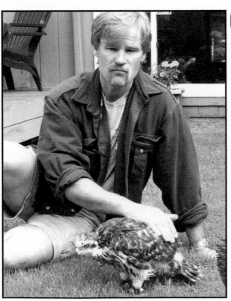

22.2
A young North American Goshawk going through the imprinting process. (Courtesy of Don Hunley)

At an appropriate age, imprinted raptors often accept the human surrogate parent as a mate, which facilitates semen collection from the males and artificial insemination of females (see Chapter 21).

Disadvantages
The process of imprinting a raptor is long and tedious, often requiring several months of moderate to intense daily socialization of the bird to new and unfamiliar people, animals, objects and situations. One major drawback is the potential for the development of behavioural problems (e.g. screaming and aggression) if food is limited to adjust the bird's weight. Due to the potential for aggression, imprinting is better left to experienced falconers/trainers and is not recommended for large raptors such as the Golden Eagle.

Crèche-reared or cohort-reared
Crèche-reared or cohort-reared raptors are groups of chicks of similar age that are raised with human contact. The degree of human contact and interaction may be limited to just feeding time or may be as involved as the imprinting process, where the chicks become dually imprinted on their cohorts as well as humans.

Advantages
Cohort- or crèche-reared chicks will typically accept human interaction, are acceptably tame and have few of the vices of excessive screaming or unacceptable behaviours seen in imprinted raptors. Since these birds are also socialized with conspecifics, crèche- or cohort-reared raptors may also make breeders because they are able to recognize their own species and can be bred by natural or artificial means.

Disadvantages
Crèche-rearing can be just as time-consuming as hand-rearing. These birds may also become noisy and aggressive during weight management.

Diet and nutrition

In order to ensure proper growth and development, young raptors must be fed food of the highest quality regardless of whether the food is home-produced or purchased from a reputable source (see Chapter 16).

Casting material (feathers or fur) is not offered to the young chicks during the first 6–10 days of age. This is more a matter of convenience, as it allows handlers to follow a tighter feeding schedule if they do not have to keep track of whether the young chick has cast or not. After 10 days of age, casting is encouraged. As the chicks age they are offered diets that meet their nutritional needs for maximum musculoskeletal and feather growth. After 10 days of age chicks may be successfully raised on freshly killed or frozen chickens or quail. Heck and Konkel (1991) also recommended skinning the carcass and removing the head, neck, crop, wings, feet, tail and digestive tract, while leaving all other organs within the coelomic cavity. The quail is then ground in a meat grinder and immediately fed to the chicks or placed in a sealed container and refrigerated for use later. It is not recommended to store food overnight; instead the amount needed for 24 hours should be prepared fresh daily. At feeding time only the amount of food that is necessary is warmed to room temperature in a covered dish for 15–30 minutes or by placing the meat in a plastic bag and dipping the bag in warm water (Heck and Konkel, 1991). It is important to remember to check the crop prior to feeding and only feed a newly hatched chick when the crop is empty. Chicks are normally fed every 3–4 hours except during the evening (Heck and Konkel, 1991). Haak (1992) suggested feeding eyasses under 2 weeks of age every 3 hours between 6 am and 10 pm; chicks aged 2–4 weeks should receive four to six meals. Eyasses aged 4–6 weeks eat three large meals daily, while chicks 6–10 weeks old eat two meals a day and those older than 10 weeks will consume a single meal a day (Haak, 1992).

Vitamins and mineral supplements may be added to the food prepared for feeding young chicks (see Chapter 17).

Growth and development

Young raptors grow exponentially and rapidly progress through various stages of development that are probably similar for most raptor species. Figure 22.3 summarizes the normal maturation process of young raptors from the time of hatching into adulthood.

Stage 1	Newly hatched chick is offered food by parents
Stage 2	Downy chick begs for food from the parent
Stage 3	Newly fledged chick chases parent(s) for food; when satisfied it plays with and chases objects resembling prey, but does not catch live prey
Stage 4	Chick physically attacks parents for food
Stage 5	Parent drops dead prey for chick, which chases and catches it; chick search image reoriented from parent to the prey
Stage 6	Parent drops live prey, reinforcing connection of pursuit with food
Stage 7	Chick has increasing difficulty in obtaining food from its parents and is left unattended for longer periods of time; it becomes more successful in catching its own live prey and begins to stray away from the nest area, hunting
Stage 8	Chick is completely weaned to independence

22.3 The normal stages of development as young raptors mature from hatchlings to adults. Data from Sherrod (1983).

Immediate post-hatching period

Physical development
When raptor chicks hatch they are covered with a sparse white natal down in most species, but this is not always the case. Harris' Hawk and Brown Falcon chicks, for example, hatch with a slightly buff-coloured down.

Behavioural development
Shortly after hatching, a chick assumes a C-shaped posture (Figure 22.4) when not being fed by a parent, but will quickly crane its head and neck upward and 'chirp' for offered food. The initial posture is due in

part to the pronounced hatching muscle on the dorsal aspect of the neck but this disappears after a couple of days. Once the female begins to feed the chicks they readily beg for food and grow very rapidly. Moss (1979) described the weight gain of nestling Sparrowhawks as being slow for the first 4–6 days, then a period of rapid weight gain for 10 days, followed by a return to slow weight gain thereafter.

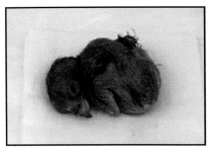

22.4 A recently hatched falcon chick; note the chick's posture. (Courtesy of Danny Erstgard, Pacific Northwest Falcons)

Days 1–7 post hatching

Physical development
Diurnal raptors may hatch with their eyes open or closed, but usually by day 2 their eyes have begun to open and they are fully open by day 6. Nocturnal species such as owls hatch with their eyes closed; their eyes begin to open at 4–6 days of age.

Behavioural development
By day 3 chicks are able to sit on their tibiotarsal–tarsometatarsal joints, pant and exhibit the first signs of grooming.

Days 7–14 post hatching

Physical development
At approximately one week the first down begins to give way to a thicker and often darker down. For larger species such as eagles this thicker down may not come in until nearly 20 days of age. Within the first 2 weeks chicks are becoming more mobile (using their wings for balance) and are able to move for short periods. These movements are directed toward the edge of the nest to defecate (as in the case of accipiters) as well as to position themselves to receive food. As chicks become more mobile they also begin to feed themselves.

Days 14–21 post hatching

Physical development
In general the first sign of pin feather development occurs about a third of the way through the fledgling period and the first feathers to grow are the primaries (remiges) followed closely by the tail feathers (retrices). In some smaller raptor species remiges may already emerge early in the second week (approximately day 9) post hatching. In the Peregrine Falcon the growth of the flight feathers is first noted around days 14–16, and in the North American Goshawk between days 14 and 17. Also at this time most chicks have visual capabilities comparable to adult raptors. Their auditory system is developing rapidly and they have developed a very thick coat of secondary down.

Between 2 and 4 weeks of age the feet of Peregrine Falcon chicks are nearly full sized and appear disproportionately large for their body size.

Behavioural development

The imprinting of the young raptor to its parents and siblings (and thus to future mates) and its surrounding environment and the development of fear responses are well underway at this age. This process is rather lengthy and continues throughout the time the young bird is in the nest with its parents, as well as through social interactions between the young raptor, its siblings, the parents and conspecifics. As the young raptor grows it begins to recognize its siblings as competitors for food and it will mantle, i.e. spread the wing and tail feathers over food to keep other raptors from seeing and possibly stealing whatever it possesses.

Days 21–28 post hatching

Physical development

Feathers are beginning to emerge around the auricular region and along the nape and breast region. Greater coverts, upper tail coverts and scapular feathers are also starting to emerge, while remiges and retrices are erupting from their sheaths. However, the crown of the head is still downy at this time. Goshawk chicks are approximately one-half their adult size (Figure 22.5).

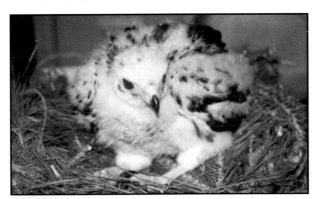

22.5 A juvenile North American Goshawk at approximately 22–26 days of age. This Goshawk was imprinted and used for falconry.

Behavioural development

At approximately 3 weeks of age goshawk chicks begin flapping their wings for short periods of time (3–5 seconds) and may attempt to peck food from the parent's mouth when being fed. Falcon and hawk chicks have the ability to attempt to escape from handlers and defend themselves with their feet, rolling on their back to do so.

Days 28–35 post hatching

Physical development

At 4 weeks of age the chicks are beginning to lose their downy feathers, especially around the eyes, and stand more upright without having to use their wings for balance as much as before. The feathers continue to emerge along the nape while covert and scapular feathers continue to fill in the upper wing, back and breast area and the chick continues to look visibly darker with each passing day. This time period represents the midpoint of the chick's transition from a down-covered chick to the juvenile-plumaged fledgling; chicks are nearly full grown in terms of body size and weight. Within a short time the chicks may actually outweigh their adult parents. At approximately 30 days in falcon chicks and 32 days in goshawk chicks, dark feathers are beginning to emerge on the crown of the head and at the commissure of the mouth. The chicks are beginning to lose much of their down on the breast, except for the centre and on the coelomic cavity, while breast feathers are beginning to fill in. Meanwhile, the back and dorsal side of the wings are nearly 90% feathered, the under-tail coverts are filled in and feathers begin to emerge over the femoral regions. Although there are genetic and environmental factors that govern the final size of the chick, size will vary between species (Springer and Osborne, 1983).

Behavioural development

During this period the chicks are also very attentive to their surrounding environment, even intently observing parents exchanging food near the nest. Sleeping while standing is also observed at this time. At this age, the chicks continue to beg the parents for food, but are readily able to feed themselves and may become very aggressive towards siblings and parents over food. The chicks may be very vocal at this age and continue to flap their wings vigorously.

Days 35–42 post hatching

Physical development

At 5 weeks in Peregrine Falcon chicks and approximately 6 weeks in North American Goshawks the chicks are nearly fully feathered save for a few tufts of down on the crown (Figure 22.6) and under the wings.

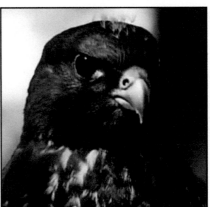

22.6 A juvenile Black Gyrfalcon at approximately 6 weeks of age. Feathering is complete except for a few tufts of down on the crown.

Behavioural development

Some chicks, particularly males, may even begin to 'branch' (walk along the branches) at 33–35 days of age in the case of goshawks. Tiercel Peregrine Falcons may fledge at this age and make their first flight as young as 35 days of age. Goshawk chicks may begin to fledge from the nest at approximately 36–38 days.

It should be noted that the above times are guidelines, as smaller falcons and accipiters may fledge at approximately 25–32 days, while larger raptors such as Golden Eagles and Griffon Vultures may not fledge until 70–80 days and 80–115 days of age, respectively. At this time the bird should be fully grown, including feather growth. In Peregrine Falcons withdrawal of blood from the growing feathers (hard-penning) occurs around day 70 and it is at this time that breeders will remove them from the chamber away from their parents. Among the accipiters, hard-penning occurs around day 60 in the Northern Goshawk and days 47–50 in the smaller Cooper's Hawk (McDermott, 1998). Species such as the Eurasian Sparrowhawk may have similar hard-penning times to the Cooper's Hawk.

Post-fledging period

In several species there is an extended post-fledging period (between fledging and complete independence) that allows the bird to mature while still receiving some benefits of parental care. There is still much to be learned about this period in wild raptors, and it may take years to complete in some species (eagles). Although both males and females will remain in the immediate vicinity of the nest it is believed that the smaller males tend to develop more rapidly than the females in all measures of behavioural development. Perhaps this allows the males to survive in the presence of their larger female siblings, as fledging times between males and females may be separated by several days (Johnsgard, 1990). The males mature faster, become more proficient hunters earlier than their female siblings and are more likely to disperse from the nest site sooner.

In most species the oldest and most recently fledged chicks may stay in close proximity to the nest while the younger siblings are still being cared for. During this time the young may take short 'test flights' to nearby structures and then return to the nest when the parents return with food. As their powers of flight improve, the young may actually put themselves in such a position as to intercept the parent bird(s) (usually the male) as they return to the nest with food. The immediate post-fledging period is also a dangerous one for the young hawk, falcon or eagle as they are often very noisy (screaming) and conspicuous enough to draw attention to themselves or their siblings still in the nest (Johnsgard, 1990).

The duration of the post-fledging period varies among raptor species; it may be as short as 2–3 weeks in species such as harriers and kites to as long as 10–12 weeks in species such as the Red-tailed Hawk and Bald Eagle (Johnsgard, 1990). Complete 'weaning' of young raptors from the parents may be rather sudden and may be related to the problems the young may have as they become independent, in terms of the amount of prey available and the proficiency of the young raptors.

Predatory behaviour is instinctive in young raptors and they will attempt to chase and capture prey even in the absence of parent birds. In some species of accipiters (Eurasian Sparrowhawk) and falcons the parents may release prey that is still alive in order to encourage the young to become proficient predators.

For most wild raptors the post-fledging period ultimately leads to dispersal and a solitary lifestyle. The most notable exception to this rule amongst birds of prey is the Harris' Hawk. A linear hierarchy exists within groups of Harris' Hawks, which number around five individuals or more and consist of an alpha male and female (breeders), a beta male and several immature hawks that are usually, but not necessarily, related to the alpha hawks (Jim Dawson, Raptor Biologist, Sonora Environmental Consultants, Inc., personal communication). The group will cooperatively hunt prey as well as assist in the care of the current year's nestlings. Cooperative hunting has its advantages in that much larger prey can be captured than by a single hawk, allowing more for all the 'pack' (Weidensaul, 1996). The same cooperative hunting behaviour is seen in birds of this species used for falconry, making the Harris' Hawk a favourite of falconers who like to 'socialize' during hunting trips.

Paediatric diseases

Nutritional and non-infectious diseases
Figure 22.7 gives information about nutritional and non-infectious diseases in young raptors.

Hypothermia
Shortly after hatching chicks are covered with a sparse natal down and are therefore unable to maintain their own body temperature. This is a critical time as poor brooding by inexperienced adult birds (for parent-reared chicks) or inadequate brooder temperatures may lead to hypothermia. The brooder temperature should be set at 36°C (97°F) and then reduced by 0.3–0.6°C (0.5–1°F) per day until the chick can be moved to room temperature, which occurs 10–14 days post hatching (Joseph, 1993). Alternatively, the newly hatched chicks may be maintained at incubator temperatures for the first 48 hours and then kept at brooder temperatures of 32–35°C for the first week (Cooper, 2002). Young chicks should be given a temperature gradient and allowed to choose the temperature most comfortable to them (see Chapter 21). Chicks that are too warm will pant, while chicks that are too cold will often huddle together and shiver. If at all possible, no chick should ever be placed in a brooder alone. Brooding chicks as cool as comfortable appears to improve their down condition and overall health (Joseph, 1993).

Infectious diseases

Viral diseases
Avian poxviruses and herpesviruses may affect raptors of all ages. Chapter 19 gives information regarding clinical signs, pathology, diagnosis and treatment of viral diseases that affect birds of prey.

Disease	Aetiology	Clinical signs	Diagnosis	Treatment and prevention
Retained yolk sac	Failure to retract yolk sac prior to hatching	Small or large yolk sac which has not fully absorbed	Physical examination	*Small yolk sac:* maintain chick in a brooder for 4–5 days on clean, dry surface while yolk is absorbed and yolk sac dries up *Large yolk sac:* amputation of yolk sac is required before it ruptures; a single sterile ligature is placed around the stalk and the yolk sac is amputated distal to the ligature. A small amount of iodine may be used to disinfect the remaining stump; these chicks must be supplemented with vitamins for the first few days of life
Nutritional osteodystrophy (leading to osteomalacia)	Improper Ca:P Overfeeding of meat and viscera by parents	Inability to stand or walk, skeletal (spraddle-leg) and beak malformations, poor growth, polyuria, polydipsia, fractures of long bone	History, clinical signs, physical examination, clinical pathology (total plasma calcium and ionized calcium). Radiology demonstrating decreased bone density, fractures and skeletal malformations	Important to offer chicks bone by day 5. Increasing calcium intake through administration of oral (calcium lactate, bone meal or whole prey) or parenteral calcium. Euthanasia may be necessary in severe cases
Rickets	Inadequate dietary vitamin D₃	Similar to clinical signs seen with osteodystrophy	Same as osteodystrophy. Radiology will demonstrate widened, deformed and abnormally mineralized growth plates	Vitamin D3 supplementation with multivitamin and mineral supplement
'Stargazing'	Thiamine (vitamin B1) deficiency	Seizures, incoordination and opisthotonus in raptors of various ages	History, clinical signs and physical examination	Vitamin B complex (10–30 mg/kg) daily until signs resolve. Harris' Hawks suffering from repeated seizures may require long-term administration of vitamin B complex
Vitamin E deficiency	Excessive storage and rancidity of food	Clinical signs may be similar to thiamine deficiency Poor hatchability of chicks, splayed legs and incoordination	History, clinical signs, physical examination. May result in white muscle disease	Improve diet and administer 0.5 mg selenium plus 1.34 IU vitamin E s.c.; repeat in 72 hours
Splay legs	Chicks kept on slick surfaces and therefore unable to support their weight	Legs splayed outwards and development of valgus deformities	History, clinical signs and physical examination	Quick recognition of the problem. Provide rough non-slippery substrates or padding that allow chicks to sit with legs underneath them in a normal position. Affected birds may be hobbled with medical tape or maintain legs in normal position by placing them in foam padding for 2–3 days. Severely affected chicks with concomitant osteodystrophy should be euthanased

22.7 Nutritional and non-infectious diseases of young raptors.

Bacterial diseases

The environment in which young raptors hatch and grow, regardless of whether the egg is naturally or artificially incubated and the chicks are parent- or hand-reared, may contain any number of bacterial organisms. Some of these may be considered normal or transient flora in immunocompetent birds of prey yet may also cause embryonic death or severe disease in young growing raptors. Ultimately, diagnosis is dependent upon the presence of a lesion or appropriate clinical signs and isolation of one or more bacterial organisms in substantial enough numbers for them to be considered pathogenic.

Bacterial organisms in raptor systems: Bacterial organisms cultured from the upper gastrointestinal tract (oropharynx) (e.g. *Staphylococcus aureus*, *Bacillus*, *Corynebacterium*) and the lower gastrointestinal tract (e.g. *Escherichia coli*, *Enterococcus*, *Proteus*) most likely represent normal flora, but given the right conditions (immunocompromised host, poor nutrition, concomitant disease) these same organisms can become highly pathogenic.

Bacterial organisms more commonly associated with disease of the gastrointestinal tract include *Escherichia coli*, *Salmonella*, *Mycobacterium*, *Clostridium*, *Pasteurella* and *Proteus*. Although *E. coli* is a constituent of the normal flora of the gastrointestinal tract, it may become highly pathogenic (Needham, 1980).

Staphylococcus (but not *S. aureus*) and *Streptococcus* may be considered normal flora of the respiratory tract in raptors but still have the potential to cause disease. Bacteria more commonly considered to be pathogenic and that have been isolated from birds of prey with respiratory disease include *E. coli* and *Staphylococcus aureus*, as well as species of *Pasteurella*, *Acinetobacter*, *Moraxella*, *Aeromonas*, *Pseudomonas*, *Klebsiella* and *Mycoplasma* (Richter, 1980; Joseph, 1993; Lierz, 2000, Cooper, 2002; Lierz, 2002).

Bacterial skin infections in raptors are uncommon. However, traumatic wounds that are self-inflicted or result from prey, collisions with stationary/moving objects or arise from improperly fitted falconry equipment (jesses and anklets) may develop secondary infections from *Staphylococcus*, *E. coli*, or *Proteus*. Granulomatous lesions of the skin may also be associated with mycobacterial infections (Cooper, 2002). Infection of the tissues of the eye and its adnexa may involve *S. aureus*, *E. coli*, *Mycoplasma* or any number of other bacterial organisms.

Clinical signs and diagnosis: Clinical signs associated with bacterial infections in young raptors often include lethargy, dehydration, poor appetite, poor weight gain or weight loss, poor feather growth, vomiting or regurgitation and sudden death. If illness is not addressed immediately, young raptors may succumb to septicaemia with multiple organ (kidney and liver) failure.

Diagnosis of bacterial diseases in paediatric raptors requires a thorough evaluation of the patient, including complete blood count, biochemical analysis and bacteriological culture of suspected lesions.

Treatment and prevention: Treatment must be instituted quickly and involves correcting dehydration though fluid support, appropriate topical or systemic antibiotic therapy based on clinical experience and culture and sensitivity results, and other supportive care as needed.

Prevention of bacterial infections in young raptors is most effective if breeders follow a closed aviary concept similar to those adopted by psittacine aviculturists. For example:

- Latex gloves should be used when handling chicks and hands should be thoroughly washed between chicks and groups of chicks
- Chicks raised in an incubator should be raised separately from chicks hatched in the nest
- Personnel caring for adult birds should not feed chicks without taking appropriate measures to minimize passage of bacterial organisms to the chicks
- Adult raptors should never be allowed into the nursery area
- Chicks removed from the nursery due to illness should not be allowed to return (Clubb *et al.*, 1992).

Parasitic, protozoal and fungal diseases

Coccidiosis: Coccidian parasites that affect raptors include *Caryospora*, *Cryptosporidium*, *Eimeria*, *Frenkelia*, *Sarcocystis* and *Toxoplasma gondii*. Coccidia are generally considered to be non-pathogenic in adult raptors and as such they tend to remain asymptomatic. In juvenile raptors clinical signs are usually vague but may include lethargy, depression, diarrhoea (with or without blood in the stool), poor body condition, slow weight gain or weight loss and even death (see Chapter 18).

Aspergillosis: Young raptors, especially those that are stressed or debilitated, are very susceptible to fungal infections, the most common of which is caused by *Aspergillus fumigatus* (see Chapter 20).

Candidiasis: Candidiasis is seen in young and adult raptors alike; however, young raptors with relatively naive immune systems are commonly affected. *Candida* most commonly affects the gastrointestinal tract and this results in either plaque-like lesions on the mucosa of the tongue, pharynx and crop or a deep-seated infection of the gastrointestinal tract with or without oral lesions. When not systemically affected, clinical signs in young raptors associated with candidiasis may include reluctance to swallow, decreased appetite, swelling within and around the oropharynx, weight loss, vomiting, regurgitation and depression. Diagnosis is usually made by demonstrating *Candida* spp. in Gram stains of lesions in the oral cavity, oesophagus, cloaca and faeces or by culture. Any raptor with candidiasis, regardless of its age, should be thoroughly evaluated for the possibility of concomitant underlying diseases that compromise the immune system. Prolonged antibiotic therapy should be avoided in young raptors if possible as this may contribute to the development of candidiasis. Dietary management, including food source, storage and preparation (especially for chicks that are hand-reared), must be evaluated thoroughly.

Behavioural problems in juvenile captive raptors

Behavioural problems in young captive raptors are often the result of improper handling of chicks as they mature or errors in judgement during the training process. More specifically, behavioural issues arise due to the formation of familial pair bonds in mal-imprinted raptors, or arrested behavioural development. Unfortunately, these problems are reported in the veterinary literature either infrequently or not at all, but are common in the falconry literature. Just as in pet birds, it is important to remember that changes in behaviour may be an indication of the presence of disease in a raptor and should be evaluated appropriately.

Infantile behaviours

Infantile behaviour is quite common in juvenile captive birds of prey and may often be exhibited by adult raptors that have recently been introduced to captivity.

Without being too anthropomorphic, regression to infantile or juvenile behaviour may be seen in human children as a way of dealing with stressful situations; a defence mechanism, if you will, that allows the child to regain the security and carefree world of childhood (Jones, 1980). The same may be true for raptors. Most likely, the root cause is inappropriate bonding (imprinting or strong food association) between the handler and the raptor, with cessation of the normal development and dispersal process.

Food begging

Food begging behaviours (screaming, lowered body posture with slight flapping of the wings or even aggression) are extremely common in human mal-imprinted raptors. Most often food begging is the result of a hunger response, but this is not always the case. Young raptors may also demonstrate food begging behaviours even when satiated. Similar begging behaviours are also seen in wild raptors of varying ages that have recently been introduced to captivity. In many instances birds that are receiving prolonged treatment for medical or surgical problems or maintained in rehabilitation centres for extended periods will revert to juvenile behaviours once they begin to recognize humans as a source of food. This process may occur within only a few days of captivity. Caution must be used when handling these raptors as they lose most but not all fear of humans and will treat their caregiver just as they would a parent, sibling or competitor. As a result, captive raptors should not be allowed to see food in the bare hand, and every attempt should be made to conceal the food as it is being placed into the enclosure or cage. Some falconers/trainers place the food in the empty cage while the raptor is away for training, and then allow the raptor to 'discover' the food upon its return to the enclosure. Another option is to use PVC tubing that will allow food to be placed in the enclosure on a platform. However, feeding raptors through a tube may not completely prevent or remove food-associated begging as raptors are intelligent enough to recognize the sequence of events (including sounds) leading up to the placement of food in the enclosure through a tube.

Screaming

Screaming is a normal behaviour in juvenile raptors as they interact with parent birds and siblings. Excessive non-stop screaming for prolonged periods, often for hours and in the absence of food association or the presence of a parent raptor or surrogate, is not normal. Young raptors will scream in recognition of their parents and in anticipation of being fed. In captivity juvenile as well as older raptors that recognize the human handler as the source of food may scream. The problem is intensified by the rather loud screams that some raptors can emit; large falcons in particular.

Screaming is a difficult problem to deal with and can try the patience of any falconer, handler or trainer. Unfortunately, this behaviour is one that is easily, and often unintentionally, rewarded in an effort to get the bird to stop, if only for a moment. For example, offering food to a raptor that is screaming out of hunger may get it to stop momentarily but only further reinforces that behaviour. This is especially true if the raptor sees the caretaker only when it is to be fed. McDermott (1998) suggested that screaming will decrease with the increase of non-food oriented time spent with the raptor in its caregiver's presence. There is also some thought that screaming may result from frustration experienced by a raptor that is unsuccessful when hunting or not allowed to catch prey.

Given time, screaming may diminish or cease as the raptor matures. If it does not resolve, the raptor may need to be placed in a different environment (short term or long term) away from the individual who raised it. In the author's experience, some vices such as screaming and aggression may diminish significantly or disappear altogether when raptors are rehomed. 'Decrowing' procedures to reduce the volume of screaming are never an option.

In captive raptors, especially falconry birds, the orientation of the raptor away from the human as the provider of food and towards the catching of prey can have a dramatic influence on the degree and duration of screaming. The sooner the young raptor is catching prey, the less likely it is to scream and remain oriented to the falconer or trainer as the sole source of food; the raptor is allowed to go through the normal maturation process. Species that are not used for falconry may benefit from use of a swung lure (falcons), or a lure machine that drags a lure for species more oriented to ground quarry (hawks and eagles) may help the raptor's transition from dependence upon the trainer to 'catching' prey.

Aggression

Aggression is a common problem in mal-imprinted raptors, especially in accipiters, eagles and some owl species. Aggression is normal when it is directed towards the intended quarry. However, in captivity this aggression is often misdirected towards other raptors or even people, resulting in potentially dangerous situations.

Intraspecies aggression

In certain species, such as Harris' Hawks, it is important to understand that there is a hierarchy which affects relationships within the group and between individual birds. The most dominant to least dominant in a group of wild or captive Harris' Hawks is as follows: mature females, mature males, immature females and then immature males. Most displays of aggression between Harris' Hawks are just that – displays, with dominance being determined with minimal physical contact. However, on occasion physical contact may lead to serious injury.

A 'Cain-and-Abel' syndrome is seen in several species of raptors such as Greater Spotted Eagle, Spanish Imperial Eagle, Red-tailed Hawk, Golden Eagle, Long-legged Buzzard and other species where the older and stronger sibling kills the younger (Meyburg and Pielowski, 1991). Interestingly, the adults make no attempt to interfere with this process.

It is possible that the older sibling kills the younger as a consequence of perceived competition for food and the attention of the adults. Most likely it is the result of one chick hatching earlier than the others so that there is a considerable difference in size (Heidenreich, 1997). In captive raptors, human intervention may be necessary to prevent injury or death to younger smaller siblings.

Intraspecies aggression may be considered normal in raptors that are not kept as pairs together and may even occur outside the breeding season between birds that are paired together as breeders (see Chapter 21).

Interspecies aggression

Interspecific aggression most often involves confrontation within a captive situation, because aggressive tendencies cannot be channelled toward natural activities such as foraging for prey. In group-reared raptors or mixed aviaries, placing different species together can be disastrous if evasive movements used by one species trigger the hunting instinct of a larger species. Removal of troublesome or unsociable raptors from the enclosure may be the only way to resolve aggression problems in mixed aviaries.

At falconry gatherings or other situations in which there are two or more raptors tethered in close proximity to each other, it is imperative to make sure that they cannot reach each other. If two birds are unexpectedly able to reach each other they may inflict serious injuries or potentially kill each other. The equipment (see Chapter 2) should be thoroughly checked before placing a raptor into a weather yard with other raptors so that there are no accidental escapes. Should one raptor break its equipment or pull its perch from the ground while in a weathering yard, the results can be quite disastrous, with one or more birds being killed or eaten.

Aggression towards humans

Aggression towards humans is most likely the result of arrested development at a stage where the young bird of prey would physically attack the 'parent' for food. In this situation familiarity leads to aggression, as the raptor treats the handler as it would another raptor and lacks the fear response that would normally cause the bird to divert its aggressive tendencies away from a human. It has been suggested that aggression, at least in imprinted accipiters such as the Northern Goshawk, is a symptom of a larger more complex issue stemming from improper handling and socialization during the imprinting process, especially during the immediate post-hatching period (McDermott, 1998). The problem may also be cumulative as multiple unrelated events or similar events (unrecognizable to the falconer or handler) build upon themselves, ultimately triggering an aggressive reaction. Events that could trigger an aggressive reaction include: wearing an offensive article of clothing, not allowing the raptor to consume all food offered on the glove, towering over a raptor as it eats, or even weight reduction that is too fast or too slow. The aggressive reaction may then become a behavioural pattern.

Harris' Hawks, which are easily socialized and trainable, can become quite aggressive towards humans. In some instances the human handler unknowingly becomes subordinate. There are many anecdotal reports of Harris' Hawks (more commonly females) attacking people because they consider them to be subordinates, or as they protect their mates in the breeding chamber (Jim Dawson, personal communication). In some situations the arrangement of the perches in the mews or chamber in which the Harris' Hawk is kept allows the eyes of the hawk to be above those of the owner or trainer – a dominance issue. This may be more of a problem in wild-caught Harris' Hawks in captivity (Jim Dawson, personal communication).

Feather plucking, chewing and self-mutilation

Feather plucking, feather destructive behaviour and self-mutilation are commonly documented in companion avian species, especially psittacids. Psychological reasons are commonly involved; however, aetiologies of feather plucking vary and may range from infectious diseases (bacterial, viral, fungal, protozoal and parasitic) to trauma, neoplasia and behavioural issues (boredom, frustration, lack of hunting or exercise and aggression). Similarly, raptors can and do show feather-destructive behaviours, though they are reported with less frequency than in psittacine species. Often, raptors that are feather pickers or self-mutilators are birds that have been in captivity for long periods, those in stressful situations (e.g. housed next to busy roads, construction, barking dogs) or those deprived of social interaction (human or otherwise) (Jones, 2001). Feather plucking seems to be more commonly reported in captive-bred Harris' Hawks, which seem to get bored rather easily: they are by nature a gregarious species and lack of socialization, including human interaction, may influence the degree of boredom or frustration the hawk experiences. Commonly, feather plucking is noted on the legs (Figure 22.8) and pectoral regions but the shoulder regions and dorsal antebrachium can also be affected. Usually, the primary and secondary flight feathers are left untouched.

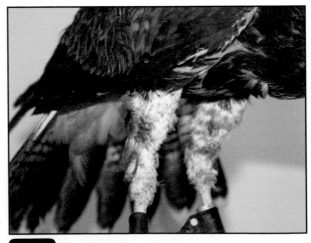

22.8 Feather plucking in an adult Harris' Hawk.

Self-mutilation is relatively uncommon in raptors. In many instances trauma to a limb may be the inciting cause. Interestingly, species such as the Merlin and American kestrels will mutilate their own feet. In the author's experience, self-mutilation has been noted in Screech Owls following the placement of external coaptation (figure-of eight bandage) and a Black Vulture with self-inflicted wounds to one shoulder.

Although the motivation for inappropriate feather damaging behaviour or self-mutilation may be difficult to understand in birds of prey, the objective of management to identify and treat the underlying cause is the same. A minimum database for case work-up should include a detailed history and a complete physical examination with laboratory diagnostics (complete blood count, biochemical analysis, heavy metal screening and faecal examination for parasites). Ancillary diagnostic tests may include cytology of the skin and feather pulp, histopathology of skin and feathers, as well as culture and sensitivity testing of any affected areas of skin. A muscle biopsy may help to delineate aetiologies for mutilating of the skin and underlying structures. If the results of the diagnostic tests are sufficient to explain the clinical signs, then the bird should be treated appropriately (see Chapter 24). If not, behavioural causes for feather plucking or self-mutilation should be considered.

Feather plucking is not an easy problem to resolve in raptors. In those cases involving diagnosed disease entities (infectious, inflammatory or neoplastic conditions) specific therapy can be instituted. However, in cases of feather plucking or self-mutilation due to behavioural issues, treatment should centre around providing adequate stimulation in the form of hunting if the bird is a falconry bird, environmental enrichment during long periods of inactivity, adequate exercise, numerous opportunities to bathe (sun and water) and controlled exposure to the elements. Small species that are easily stressed (Screech Owls and small accipiters) should have every opportunity to hide from perceived predators. Environmental enrichment during periods of inactivity may be very helpful in preventing boredom. The use of psychotropic chemotherapeutics may be beneficial, but more scientific evidence needs to be collected demonstrating the effectiveness of these therapies.

References and further reading

Beebe FL (2002) *The Compleat Falconer*. Hancock House Publishers, Blaine, Washington

Boal CW (1994) A photographic and behavioral guide to aging nestling Northern goshawks. *Studies in Avian Biology* **16**, 32–40

Butterworth G and Harcourt-Brown NH (1996) Neonate husbandry and related diseases. In: *BSAVA Manual of Raptors, Pigeons and Waterfowl*, ed. PH Beynon *et al.*, pp. 216–223. BSAVA, Cheltenham

Clubb SL, Clubb K, Skidmore D, Wolf S and Phillips A (1992) Psittacine neonatal care and hand-feeding. In: *Psittacine Aviculture: Perspectives, Techniques and Research*, ed. RM Schubot *et al.*, pp. 11.1–11.12. Aviculture Breeding and Research Center, Loxahatchee, FL

Cooper JE (2002) *Birds of Prey: Health and Disease*. Blackwell Sciences, Oxford

Coulson JO and Coulson TD (1995) Group hunting by Harris' hawks in Texas. *Journal of Raptor Research* **29**, 265–267

Dierenfeld ES, Sandfort CE and Satterfield WC (1989) Influence of diet on plasma vitamin E in captive peregrine falcons. *Journal of Wildlife Management* **53**, 160–164

Forbes NA and Flint CG (2000) *Raptor Nutrition*. Honeybrook Farm Animal Foods, Evesham, Worcestershire

Ford E (1992) *Falconry: Art and Practice*. Blandford, Sterling Publishing, New York

Fox N (1995) *Understanding the Bird of Prey*. Hancock House Publishers, Blaine, Washington

Haak B (1992) *The Hunting Falcon*. Hancock House Publishers, Blaine, Washington

Hardaswick VJ (1984) Growth and behavioral development of peregrine x prairie falcons. *Journal of North American Falconer's Association* **23**, 13–21

Heck WR and Konkel D (1991) Incubation and rearing. In: *Falcon Propagation: A Manual on Captive Breeding*, ed. JD Weaver and TJ Cade, pp. 34–76. The Peregrine Fund Inc., New York

Heidenreich M (1997) *Birds of Prey: Medicine and Management*. Iowa State University Press, Ames

Johnsgard PA (1990) *Hawks, Eagles & Falcons of North America; Biology and Natural History*. Smithsonian Institution Press, Washington DC

Joseph V (1993) Raptor pediatrics. *Seminars in Avian and Exotic Pet Medicine* **2**, 142–151

Jones CG (1980) Abnormal and maladaptive behavior in captive raptors. In: *Recent Advances in the Study of Raptor Diseases, Proceedings of the International Symposium of Diseases of Birds of Prey, London*, pp. 53–59

Jones MP (2001) Behavioral aspects of captive birds of prey. *Veterinary Clinics of North America Exotic Animal Practice* **4**, 613–32

Lierz M, Schmidt R, Brunnberg L and Runge M (2000) Isolation of *Mycoplasma meleagridis* from free-ranging birds of prey in Germany. *Journal of Veterinary Medicine Series B* **47**, 63–67

Lierz M, Schmidt R and Runge M (2002) Mycoplasma species isolated from falcons in the Middle East. *Veterinary Record* **151**, 92–93

McDermott M (1998) *The Imprint Accipiter*. Michael McDermott Publisher, Cedar Hill, MO

McDonald PG (2003) Nestling growth and development in the brown falcon, *Falco berigora*: an improved ageing formula and field-based method of sex determination. *Wildlife Research* **30**, 411–418

McElroy H (1977) Hand raising the Cooper's Hawk from the early stages of withdrawal. In: *Desert Hawking*, pp. 9–14. Cactus Press, Yuma, AZ

McKeever K (1979) *Care and Rehabilitation of Injured Owls*. WF Rannie, Lincoln, Ontario

Meyburg BU and Pielowski Z (1991) Cainism in the greater spotted eagle (*Aquila clanga*). *Bulletin Birds of Prey* **4**, 143–148

Moss D (1979) Growth of nestling sparrowhawks (*Accipiter nisus*). *Journal of Zoology* **187**, 297–314

Needham JR (1980) Bacterial flora of birds of prey. In: *Recent Advances in the Study of Raptor Diseases*, ed. JE Cooper and AG Greenwood, pp. 3–9. Chiron Publications, Keighley

Richter T and Gerlach H (1980) The bacterial flora of the nasal mucosa of birds of prey. In: *Recent Advances in the Study of Raptor Diseases*, ed. JE Cooper and AG Greenwood, pp. 11–14. Chiron Publications, Keighley

Samour J (2000) Appendix VIII. In: *Avian Medicine*, ed. J Samour, pp. 388–418. Mosby, Philadelphia

Sherrod SK (1983) *Behavior of Fledgling Peregrines*. The Peregrine Fund Inc., Ithaca, NY

Springer MA and Osborne DR (1983) Analysis of growth of the red-tailed hawk. *Ohio Journal of Science* **83**, 13–19

Weidensaul S (1996) *Raptors: the Birds of Prey*. Lyons and Burford, New York

Peregrine Falcon development age guide. Online URL: www.peregrine-foundation.ca/info/ageguide1.html. Last accessed October 2006

23

Raptors: gastrointestinal tract disease

Chris Lloyd

Clinical history, examination and diagnosis

An accurate history is important to arrive at a diagnosis in a bird with possible gastrointestinal (GI) disease (see Chapter 7). Questions related to recent weight changes and training methods will help to establish the kind of stresses being placed on the bird. The food type, source, feeding methods and any recent changes in diet are also of vital importance. The owner should be questioned on how the bird eats and the quality of the casting and mute. Soiling about the cloaca and a foul smell from the mutes or mouth should be looked for during the examination. Further diagnostic techniques are described in Figure 23.1. Differential diagnosis and treatment of clinical signs associated with GI tract disease are outlined in Figure 23.2.

Diagnostic technique	Description	Clinical application
Direct wet crop swab	Saline-soaked swab used to sample mouth and upper GIT. Hanging drop from swab is examined microscopically	Diagnosis of upper GIT pathogens such as *Trichomonas* spp. trophozoites and *Capillaria* spp. ova
Faecal examination: direct and flotation	See Chapter 18	Detection of faecal parasites
Proventricular wash	A lubricated feeding tube or catheter is directed into the proventriculus in the conscious or anaesthetized animal. Warm sterile saline (1–2% of body weight) is infused and retrieved for culture and cytology. This technique can also be performed using an endoscope with operating channels	Useful method for obtaining more representative cytological and bacteriological pictures from the upper GIT in cases of regurgitation or malabsorption
Cytology	Faecal stains: faeces smeared thinly on slide with cotton bud Smears can be stained with Gram, Rapid ('Kwik Diff', Thermo Electron Co, USA) or Ziehl–Neelson stain	Rapid assessment of microbial flora. The presence of only one type of bacterium or a very high proportion of sporulating Gram-positive bacilli may be significant and warrant culture. Results must be interpreted in the light of other clinical signs
	Rapid stain or Gram stain of oropharynx/crop	Detection of yeast, bacteria, inflammatory reactions, squamous metaplasia of stratified squamous epithelium
Bacterial/fungal culture	Blood agar used for aerobic bacteria; McConkey agar for anaerobes and Sabouraud's agar for yeast and fungi	Findings must be interpreted in light of other clinical findings. Mixed bacterial commensals common on culture and transient bacterial contaminants may also be cultured. Pure growth may be abnormal. Birds with normal crop cytology may have heavy *Candida* spp. growth on cultures
Viral culture	For isolation of viruses shed via gastrointestinal tract	See Chapter 19
Endoscopy	See Chapter 13	Visualization of organs, mucosal surfaces. For specimen, culture and biopsy collection. Foreign body retrieval
Radiography	See Chapter 11	Assessment of organ size, detection of foreign bodies and lead shot, detection of impactions/obstructions of stomach or small intestine, cloacal atony/distension/uroliths. Presence of gas in intestine is abnormal and may indicate ileus, bacterial, viral or parasitic gastroenteritis or obstruction. A uniformly distended GIT may indicate viral or bacterial enteritis, septicaemia, peritonitis, parasitism, heavy metal poisoning or neoplasia. Aerophagia may occur in severe dyspnoea

23.1 Gastrointestinal diagnostics.

Clinical sign	Diagnostics	Differential diagnosis	Treatment
A: White/ yellow spots or diptheritic membranes in upper GIT. Blood in casting or from mouth	**A1:** Examination of mouth under anaesthesia including base of tongue. **Endoscopy** of choanal slit, cervical and thoracic oesophagus, crop and proventriculus (see Chapter 13) **Cytological examination** of faeces, casts, swabs from upper GIT **Radiology** Involvement of skeletal structures with deep necrotic lesions of the oral cavity especially caused by *Trichomonas* spp. **Blood haematology and biochemistry** Gouty tophi in the mouth (Figure 23.4) associated with high levels of uric acid in the blood	**A2: Bacterial stomatitis** (Figure 23.3a) *Pseudomonas* spp. appear as small white caseous lesions of the oropharynx or tongue Gram stain will confirm Gram-negative rods, bacterial cultures required. *Pasteurella*. Bipolar staining of smear with methylene blue may give diagnosis	Antibiosis based on culture and sensitivity results Curetting of caseous abscesses and topical application of iodine or chlorhexidine mouthwashes. Treatment of primary cause, e.g. *Trichomonas* spp., foreign body, parasite, hypovitaminosis A, stress/ immunosuppression. Tube feeding may be required
		A3: Parasitic stomatitis *Capillaria* spp. Bi-operculate eggs found on wet preparation	Fenbendazole 25 mg/kg orally daily for 5 days
		A4: Parasitic stomatitis *Trichomonas* spp. (Figure 23.3b). Motile protozoal trophozoites seen on microscopic wet preparation (see Chapter 9)	Carnidazole 25 mg/kg orally for 1–2 days. Metronidazole 50 mg/kg daily for 5 days. Careful debridement of caseous material in severe case follows treatment of parasites. Eliminate reinfection. Prognosis good in early cases and guarded in advanced cases with deep tissue damage
		A5: Fungal *Candida albicans:* white-grey to green-grey diptheritic membranes (Figure 23.3c). Microscopically after Gram stain appears as purple–blue oval, round or budding cell 3.5–6 × 6–10 µm (see Figure 23.7). Parent cells and buds joined by narrow base. Pseudohyphae (resembling septate hyphae) can form on animal tissue	Nystatin 300,000 IU/kg orally q12h for 7 days. Itraconazole 10 mg/kg orally q12h for 5 days. Topical miconazole gel
		A6: Viral (owl herpesvirus, poxvirus (Figure 23.3d)) PCR of swabs from affected tissue may be diagnostic	Supportive treatment. Prognosis very guarded See Chapter 19
		A7: Visceral gout Crystals appear as very sharp white spots just under epithelial layer of mucosa. Often most evident at back of oropharynx	Aggressive IV continuous infusion fluid therapy, but prognosis usually hopeless
		A8: Hypovitaminosis A Squamous metaplasia of epithelial cells lining mouth and crop seen on cytological preparation of crop swab	Vitamin A supplementation. Attention to diet quality (see Chapter 17)
B: Dysphagia/ anorexia	**B1:** Examination of mouth as for A1. Also pay attention to tongue. Tracheal rings of prey items (Bailey, pers. comm.) or string foreign bodies can cause constricting lesions **Radiology** As for A1. Radiology also used to detect fractures of skull and mandible **Endoscopy** May be required to eliminate aspergillosis, air sacculitis **Cytology** See Figure 23.1 **Haematology and biochemistry** **Viral cultures** **Blood lead**	**B2:** Stomatitis. See A1–A8	See A1–A8
		B3: Foreign body in choana or penetrating wounds to the roof of the mouth. Abscess formation is common. Linear foreign body trapped at tongue base	Detection and removal of foreign body. Caseous abscess drainage and curettage/flushing. Suitable antibiotic based on culture and sensitivity
		B4: Trauma of hyobranchial apparatus leading to tongue paralysis (Heidenreich, 1997)	Euthanasia
		B5: Systemic disease	See Chapters 18–26
		B6: Ingluvitis (bacterial, fungal, parasitic, nutritional)	Treatment of underlying cause. See stomatitis as described in A1–8
		B7: Gastrointestinal foreign body	See main text section 'Gastrointestinal foreign bodies'
		B8: Toxicity	Lead/ammonium nitrate poisoning. See Chapter 26
		B9: Overfed/overweight	Slowly reduce weight to flying weight
		B10: Bird unaccustomed to food type	
		B11: 'Over-training' with dehydration and cachexia	Rest bird, rehydrate orally, offer small amounts food with no casting or institute forced feeding

23.2 Differential diagnosis and treatment of clinical signs associated with gastrointestinal tract disease in raptors. (continues) ▶

Clinical sign	Diagnostics	Differential diagnosis	Treatment
C: Vomiting/ regurgitation	**C1:** Examination and procedures as for A1 and B1	**C2:** See B5–B8	Vomiting birds should be treated with bolus intravenous fluids and metoclopramide (1–2 mg/kg i.m. or i.v. q8–12h) until aetiology is established. Birds that continue to vomit can be placed on continuous intravenous infusion until vomiting is controlled
		C3: Air sacculitis and aspergillosis	See Chapter 20
		C4: Enteritis (bacterial fungal, parasitic, viral)	See main text sections 'Bacterial enteritis', 'Viral enteritis', 'Candidiasis'
		C5: Motion sickness	Travel with starved bird
D: Delayed crop emptying/ crop stasis	**D1:** Examination and procedures as for A1 and B1	**D2:** See B5–B8	
		D3: Overtraining, dehydration, cachexia	
		D4: Overfeeding hungry, weak or underweight bird	
		D5: Displaced coracoid fracture	
		D6: Crop abscess/burn (see Figure 23.9)	
E: Diarrhoea	**E1: Faecal aerobic/ anaerobic culture, direct exam and cytology Radiology**	**E2:** Viral, bacterial, parasitic, fungal enteritis	See Chapters 18, 19 and main text sections 'Bacterial enteritis', 'Viral enteritis', 'Candidiasis'
		E3: Dietary changes	Probiotics
		E4: Systemic disease such as liver disease or amyloidosis	
		E5: Lead poisoning	See Chapter 26
F: Blood in faeces	**F1: Faecal examination** (see Figure 23.1) **Cloacal endoscopy** (see Chapter 13)	**F2:** Parasitism: coccidia, *Capillaria* spp.	See Chapter 18
		F3: Cloacal disease	See main text section 'Peritonitis'
		F4: Clostridial enterotoxaemia	See main text section 'Bacterial enteritis'
		F5: Neoplasia	
		F6: Lead poisoning	See Chapter 26
		F7: Reproductive disease	See Chapter 21
G: Green faeces		**G1:** Starvation	Green colour of faeces and urates is due to bile staining
		G2: Falcon herpesvirus	Lime-green faeces and urates are very poor prognostic sign for bird and are often seen in cases of hepatic amyloidosis and advanced aspergillosis
		G3: Amyloidosis	
		G4: Lead poisoning	
H: Voluminous, clay-coloured or undigested food in mutes		**H1:** Malabsorption, stress, 'sterile' gut post antibiosis, pancreatic insufficiency	
J: Yellow/red faeces and urates		**J1:** Multivitamin preparations Renal disease	

23.2 (continued) Differential diagnosis and treatment of clinical signs associated with gastrointestinal tract disease in raptors.

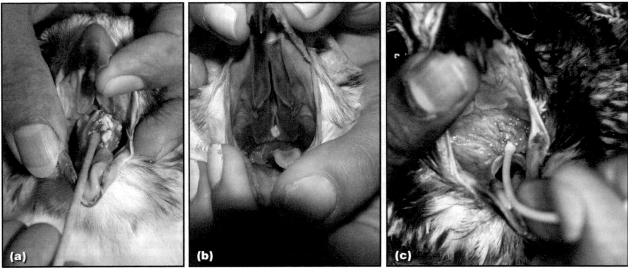

23.3 Stomatitis. **(a)** Bacterial, affecting the laryngeal mound in a falcon. **(b)** *Trichomonas* can cause highly destructive lesions. This infection had affected the Eustachian tube, causing middle ear disease. **(c)** *Candida*. (a,c, courtesy of Tom Bailey)

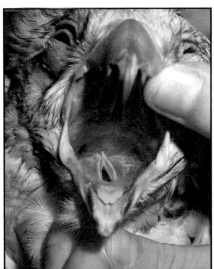

23.4 Gout crystals are visible in the oropharynx of this falcon. Despite aggressive fluid therapy, the falcon died within 24 hours.

Examination of mutes

Mutes collected by the falconer should be taken from a clean surface, wrapped in cling film or silver foil and cooled until examined. Most falcons will defecate in the surgery on being unhooded and this can be collected on a paper plate before it contacts the ground. Trained falcons can be encouraged to produce a mute if the face is lightly sprayed with water whilst the bird is unhooded. Raptors transported to the surgery in a carrier box will often have passed a mute in transit. Birds kept in aviaries or on blocks should have plastic sheeting or wax paper placed under or around the perch to collect mute samples. The client should be encouraged to submit multiple faecal samples, either pooled or separately, to maximize the chances of detecting parasites such as *Capillaria* spp. or ascarids that may shed low numbers of ova, or coccidian oocysts that are shed irregularly during the day.

The faeces should be examined for consistency, colour and foreign material. Heidenreich (1997) recommended washing a faecal sample in a fine sieve to identify foreign material such as sand or grass.

Microscopic examination for parasites is described in Chapter 18. Healthy mutes should have a well formed faecal pellet and white urates with a clear liquid component (see Chapter 7). The form and colour of normal stools can vary with the diet fed; for example, birds fed red meat may pass a dark or black stool while those on white fatty meat can produce yellow stools.

Examination of casts

All raptors will egest the non-digestible material from the meal (a casting). The digestive efficiency of raptors varies and owls produce larger casting than diurnal raptors because the less acidic proventriculus is unable to digest smaller bones. Normal pellets are usually a well formed oval, odourless and may be covered in a thin layer of mucus that quickly dries (see Chapter 7). Abnormal pellets are misshapen, wet, have a strong odour and may contain undigested foods. Blood on a pellet may suggest some oesophageal, crop or proventricular inflammation. If upper gastrointestinal tract bleeding is suspected but cannot be seen in the cast material, it may be worth offering white rodents; this will result in a white cast being produced, enabling blood to be visualized more easily. Microscopic examination of casting may reveal parasites.

In the Middle East birds are rarely fed casting and will sometimes produce soft wet foul-smelling pellets. This problem has a dietary cause and can be reversed if the bird is given food items with feathers or fur.

Viral enteritis

Enteritis is a feature of a number of viral diseases, including paramyxovirus 1 and falcon adenovirus (see Chapter 19). In practice these viral diseases cause other more severe clinical diseases than enteritis. Proventricular dilatation disease has been described in a Peregrine Falcon although no cause could be identified (Shivaprasad, 2005).

the mouth, oesophagus and crop. The condition may start slowly with few clinical signs, but progress to a disease characterized by pseudomembranous necrosis and thickening of the upper alimentary tract. The birds may be anorexic and dysphagic and may food flick, vomit or lose weight. A common sign is an 'itchy crop' where the bird constantly moves to 'pass the crop over' despite there being no food in it.

Diagnosis

Diagnosis is usually easily made by visualizing typical *Candida albicans* blastospores on a cytological sample from the upper GI tract after rapid or Gram stain (Figure 23.7). Typical white colonies will develop when swabs are inoculated on to Sabouraud's agar. Lesions in the crop and oesophagus can be visualized by endoscope. If the lesions are swabbed, normally *Candida* spots are easily removed without bleeding while *Trichomonas* and *Capillaria* lesions often bleed on removal of the spot. Wet pox lesions may not bleed but leave a mucosal erosion.

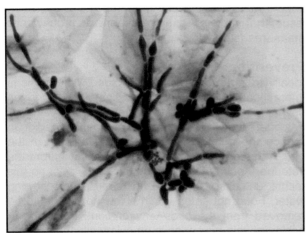

23.7 *Candida* cells and pseudohyphae from the crop of a falcon (Gram stain). (Courtesy of Renata Padrtova, Nad Al Shiba Veterinary Hospital)

Treatment

Treatment with antifungals such as nystatin (300,000 IU/kg orally q12h for 7 days) or itraconazole (10 mg/kg orally q12h for 5 days) together with probiotics is effective. Samour *et al.* (2002a) described the successful use of miconazole gel applied directly to the crop and oesophagus twice daily for 5 days. In curing and preventing this disease it is important to consider predisposing factors, including incorrect husbandry and nutrition.

Pancreatic disease

The pancreas has an endocrine and an exocrine function: over 99% of the avian pancreas is devoted to producing digestive enzymes; as an endocrine organ it secretes glucagon, insulin and somatostatin. While in most birds it is thought that glucagon is the major glucose regulating hormone, studies in carnivorous birds have suggested that they are more insulin-dependent (Rae, 2000).

Diabetes and pancreatic atrophy have been reported in raptors (Wallner-Pendleton *et al.*, 1993; Samour *et al.*, 2002b) while pancreatic lesions have also been reported in association with *Chlamydophila* (Mirande *et al.*, 1992), West Nile virus (Wunschmann *et al.*, 2005) and avian influenza (Lierz *et al.*, 2007). In the case described by Samour *et al.* (2002b) the affected bird was polyphagic, losing weight and passing voluminous mutes. Serum amylase was considered elevated by the author. Specific diagnostics usually require pancreatic biopsy.

Crop stasis (sour crop)

This condition occurs when food is retained in the crop after feeding and fails to pass into the proventriculus. The food then putrefies in the crop, causing toxaemia and ultimately death.

Starvation of a raptor, proventricular impactions or systemic diseases that cause general dehydration or debilitation can lead to an episode of crop stasis or 'sour crop'. Commonly the syndrome occurs when a hungry raptor is fed to excess after hunting, especially with fresh-caught or novel food items, or when a falconer simply wishes to increase the bird's weight rapidly.

Clinical signs

Birds are often presented with non-specific signs of illness such as depression, ruffled feathers and closed eyes. A distended crop is often visible and a foul smell emanates from the mouth. The mucous membranes appear cyanotic and the bird displays signs of endotoxic shock. The condition will rapidly progress to collapse and death if left untreated.

Treatment

Food retained in the crop for longer than expected for the particular bird warrants action by the veterinary surgeon. Emptying the crop is the priority in such cases. If the crop is emptying slowly and the veterinary surgeon is confident there is no obstruction, warmed fluids (s.c. or i.v. bolus) plus metoclopramide (0.5–1 mg/kg i.m. or orally) can be effective in moving the food into the proventriculus. Oral fluids (1–3% of body weight) can also help in passage of food. Intravenous Duphalyte at 5 ml/kg mixed 50:50 with 0.9% saline will induce vomiting (TA Bailey, personal communication) within minutes in falcons, as will enrofloxacin injected intramuscularly, and both can be used in mild cases of crop stasis when the bird is still strong and alert.

If this is not successful, general anaesthesia with isoflurane, intubation and manual emptying of the crop is required. The author prefers to gavage the crop with warm isotonic saline (10–20 ml/kg) whilst clamping the cervical oesophagus with the fingers and gently massaging the crop. The bird is then inverted and pressure on the oesophagus released. Food can then be 'milked' back into the oral cavity and removed by forceps or long cotton buds. It is essential that the crop is emptied in its entirety and that clear saline is retrieved before the procedure is stopped. Birds that suffer from this condition are often hypovolaemic and intravenous fluids via an indwelling catheter may be required. Fluids can be given as a single bolus according to indirect blood pressure measurements, which should not fall below 150 mmHg in Peregrine, Gyr and Gyr-hybrid falcons (Lloyd, 2007). Samour (2006) recommended instilling the proventriculus with a 0.1% chlorhexidine solution to reduce the bacterial load in the upper GI tract. Antibiosis and treatment of underlying conditions will be required. Tube feeding of these birds with increasing viscosities of liquid feed should be undertaken until motility of the crop has been re-established.

Crop fistulae and abscesses

Penetrating foreign bodies, sharp bones, fight injuries, *Capillaria* spp. or *Trichomonas gallinae* are common causes of this condition. The position of the lesion in the crop will determine if an abscess or fistula forms (Figure 23.8). Chicks hand reared on feeds heated in a microwave can suffer from thermal crop burns if the food is unevenly heated. Heidenreich (1997) considered that a distended crop is at risk of damage or tearing if traumatized.

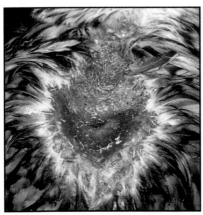

23.8 Crop fistula secondary to *Trichomonas* spp. in a Peregrine Falcon. (Courtesy of Tom Bailey)

Treatment
Fistulae and abscesses usually require surgical treatment. The latter must be removed together with the capsule and appropriate antibiosis administered (Figure 23.9). The surgical treatment of crop fistulae is described in Chapter 14.

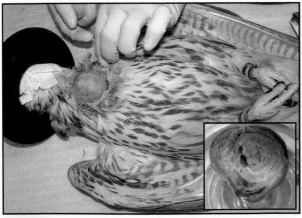

23.9 Crop abscess *in situ* and (inset) after removal. (Courtesy of Mirjam Hampel, Nad Al Shiba Veterinary Hospital)

Gastrointestinal foreign bodies

Various foreign bodies have been reported in birds of prey. One of the most important is lead, which can result in a toxicosis (see Chapter 26). Other foreign bodies include sand (Figure 23.10), grit (usually ingested when the bird is fed from an unsuitable surface), grass, synthetic matting materials and excessive casting/bone. Samour (2006) suggested that such foreign bodies can significantly reduce the volume of the proventriculus or ventriculus but they can also cause impaction at these sites or in the small intestine, often at the duodenal loop.

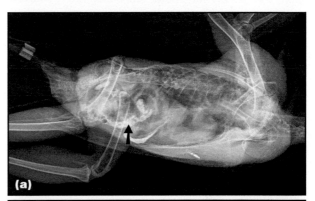

(a)

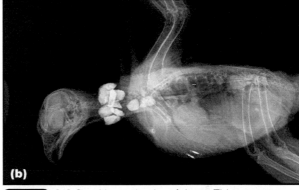

(b)

23.10 **(a)** Sand ingestion in a falcon. This a common problem in falcons in the Middle East. **(b)** Crop foreign body: this bird had ingested stones. (Courtesy of Tom Bailey)

Clinical signs and diagnosis
Reduced appetite, anorexia, regurgitation, vomiting or delayed crop emptying are common clinical signs. A reduction or absence of faeces may suggest obstructions. Radiology will show radio-opaque foreign bodies, such as sand in the GI tract, while gaseous dilatation of the intestines or proventriculus may be present. McMillan (1994) stated that any gas visible on radiography in the raptor GI tract was abnormal. Proventricular impactions caused by radiolucent material may be harder to identify without barium contrast. The barium will permeate the casting material and surround foreign bodies but little will progress to the small intestine.

Endoscopy of the upper GI tract and proventriculus may be useful while laparoscopy may locate impactions of intestines and assess gut viability or rule out peritonitis. Perforating foreign bodies are not uncommon, especially from sharp splinters off long bones.

Treatment

Impactions of the proventriculus/ventriculus can be relieved by gentle ventricular irrigation with warm fluids. A lubricated lamb-feeding tube is useful for this procedure and the bird should be anaesthetized and intubated. This procedure could also be performed with a rigid endoscope within a working channel with valves. This allows the clinician to manage the amount of water being used (see Chapter 13), enabling the proventriculus to be flushed while simultaneously removing portions of impacted material with grasping forceps. Proventricular/ventricular foreign bodies such as stones or metal can also be retrieved endoscopically. Alternatively, birds in good condition and without impactions can be given fibrous casting, such as feathers (a pigeon or quail skin turned inside out), which should enable the foreign body to be expelled with the casting.

Sand impactions of the small intestine are common when birds are fed directly off a sand floor. If the obstruction is not complete, it can be relieved with oral fluids and liquid paraffin ± metoclopramide. It is important that the bird continues to pass mutes. Failure to produce mutes within a few hours of oral fluid administration may suggest a complete obstruction of the small intestines/ventriculus requiring surgical correction (see Chapter 14). It is important to prevent access to the item responsible for impaction, to avoid recurrence.

Intestinal volvulus and intussusception

Forbes (1996) described signs of inappetence, tenesmus and fresh or digested blood in the faeces with these conditions, which are rare and generally occur secondary to another intestinal disorder. These cases will require supportive fluids and surgery (see Chapter 14). Intestinal volvulus is rare in birds but does occur. The birds may still be eating, with a reduced appetite and they pass faeces, usually diarrhoea. Volvulus may be difficult to see on radiographs, though gas within the intestine may be visible (Figure 23.11) and contrast radiography can be helpful. The only diagnostic approach is intestinal surgery with end-to-end anastomosis (see Chapter 14). The prognosis following intestinal surgery in raptors is extremely guarded.

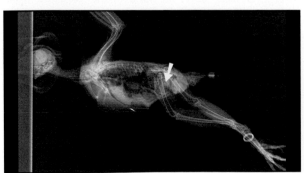

23.11 Gaseous dilatation of the intestine in this case was associated with a *Salmonella* spp. enteritis. (Courtesy of Tom Bailey)

Peritonitis

Peritonitis often follows penetrating or perforating injuries. Shotgun injuries, intestinal foreign bodies or necrotizing systemic diseases such as aspergillosis and trichomoniasis are common causes (Figure 23.12). Severe intestinal impactions can also lead to peritonitis. Egg peritonitis is described in Chapter 21.

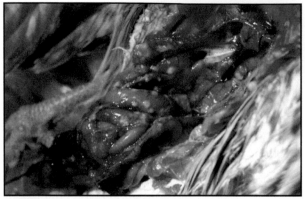

23.12 Peritonitis. In this case trichomoniasis had led to a secondary *E. coli* peritonitis.

Birds with acute peritonitis die quickly, often within a few days, and will show signs such as vomiting, diarrhoea and collapse. Early diagnosis is important, but the disease carries a very poor prognosis.

Cloacal disease

Cloacal prolapse

The origin of cloacal prolapse must be correctly identified. Oviduct, intestine and cloacal tissue can all prolapse through the cloaca secondary to abdominal straining. It may be associated with intestinal impactions or infections, salpingitis, egg binding, cloacitis or intra-abdominal masses. The surgical treatment of cloacal prolapse is discussed in more detail in Chapter 14.

Cloacal calculi

These calculi are caused by the accumulation of urates in the cloaca and may lead to partial or complete cloacal obstruction (Figure 23.13). The author has commonly seen cases occurring secondary to

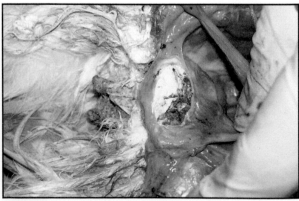

23.13 Cloacal urolith, preventing normal defecation in this bird.

cloacal atony in recumbent birds. The bird is often soiled around the vent and the calculi may be palpable digitally or visible on radiographs or via cloacoscopy. Large calculi may lead to post-renal obstruction and intestinal obstruction. The calculus can often be manually expressed from the cloaca. Large stones may require surgical removal (Best, 1996).

Cloacitis

Cloacitis may present as soreness and soiling of the vent. There may be fresh blood in the mute. Cloacitis occurs secondary to trauma, egg laying or cloacoliths and is often associated with *Pseudomonas* or *E. coli* infection. Appropriate antibiosis either locally or systemically and treatment of the underlying cause are usually effective.

Cloacal atony

Cloacal atony occurs when the cloaca fails to expel faecal and urinary waste. The cloaca becomes markedly distended, often displacing the intestines cranially on lateral radiographs. Most cases seen by the author have been secondary to spinal damage or neuromuscular disease. The cloaca and motor muscle for the tail are innervated from the pudendal plexus and so any damage to, or cranial to, the synsacrum will result in both tail and cloacal paralysis. The birds are invariably recumbent due to leg paresis. The close association of this plexus with the kidney should ensure that nephritis is listed as a possible cause of this problem, in the author's opinion.

References and further reading

Bangert RL, Ward AC, Stauber EH, Cho BR and Widders PR (1988) A survey of the aerobic bacteria in the feces of captive raptors. *Avian Diseases* **32**(1), 53–62

Barnes JH and Gross WB (1997) Colibacillosis. In: Calnek BW (Ed) *Diseases of Poultry, 10th edn*, ed. BW Calnek, pp. 131–141. Iowa State University Press, Ames, Iowa

Battisti A, Di Guardo G, Agrimi U and Bozzano AI (1998) Embryonic and neonatal mortality from Salmonellosis in captive bred raptors. *Journal of Wildlife Diseases* **34**(1), 64–72

Cooper JE (2000) Avian microbiology. In: *Laboratory Medicine: Avian and Exotic Pets*, ed. AM Fudge, pp. 90–98. WB Saunders, Philadelphia

Cooper JE (2002a) Infectious diseases, excluding macroparasites. In: *Birds of Prey: Health and Disease*, ed. JE Cooper, pp. 84–104. Blackwell Science, Oxford

Cooper JE (2002b) Miscellaneous and emerging diseases. In: *Birds of Prey: Health and Disease*, ed. JE Cooper, pp. 185–216. Blackwell Science, Oxford

Denbow DM (2000) Gastrointestinal anatomy and physiology. In: *Sturkie's Avian Physiology, 5th edn*, ed. GC Gittow, pp. 299–325. Academic Press, San Diego

Forbes NA (1996) Chronic weight loss, vomiting and dysphagia. In: *BSAVA Manual of Raptors, Pigeons and Waterfowl*, ed. PH Beynon et al., pp. 189–196. BSAVA, Cheltenham

Fudge AM (2000) Avian liver and gastrointestinal testing. In: *Laboratory Medicine. Avian and Exotic Pets*, ed. AM Fudge, pp. 47–55. WB Saunders, Philadelphia

Gerlach H (1997) Bacteria. In: *Avian Medicine: Principles and Application* (abridged edition), ed. BW Ritchie et al., pp. 520–536. Wingers, Lake Worth, FL

Heidenreich M (1997) *Birds of Prey: Medicine and Management*. Blackwell Science, Oxford

Lloyd CG (2007) Measurement of indirect arterial blood pressure in anaesthetised falcons. In: *Proceedings of the 9th Conference of the European Association of Avian Veterinarians and the 7th Scientific ECAMS Meeting, Zurich*, pp. 441–444

McMillan MC (1994) Imaging techniques. In: *Avian Medicine: Principles and Application*, ed. BW Ritchie et al., pp. 246–326 . Wingers, Lake Worth, FL

Mirande LA, Howerth EW and Poston RP (1992). Chlamydiosis in a Red Tailed Hawk (*Buteo jamaicensis*). *Journal of Wildlife Diseases* **28**, 284–287

Rae M (2000) Avian endocrine disorders. In: *Laboratory Medicine: Avian and Exotic Pets*, ed. AM Fudge, pp. 76–89. WB Saunders, Philadelphia

Samour JK (2006) Management of raptors. In: *Clinical Avian Medicine, Vol. II*, ed. GJ Harrison and TL Lightfoot, pp. 915–956. Spix, Palm Beach, FL

Samour JK and Naldo JL (2002a) Diagnosis and therapeutic management of candidiasis in falcons in Saudi Arabia. *Journal of Avian Medicine and Surgery* **16**(2), 129–132

Samour JK and Naldo JL (2002b) Pancreatic atrophy in a Peregrine falcon (*Falco peregrinus*). *Veterinary Record* **151**(4), 124–125

Samour JK and Naldo JL (2004) Radiographic findings in falcons in Saudi Arabia. *Journal of Avian Medicine and Surgery* **18**(4), 242–256

Schrenzel M, Oaks JL, Rotstein D et al. (2005) Characterisation of a new species of Adenovirus in falcons. *Journal of Clinical Microbiology* **43**(7), 3402–3413

Shivaprasad HL (2005) Proventricular dilatation disease in a Peregrine falcon (*Falco peregrinus*). In: *Proceedings of the Association of Avian Veterinarians, Monterey*, pp. 107–108

Wallner-Pendleton EA, Rogers D and Epple A (1993) Diabetes mellitus in a red tailed hawk (*Buteo jamaicensis*). *Avian Pathology* **22**, 631–635

Wernery U, Kinne J, Sharma A, Boehnel H and Samour JH (2000) Clostridium enterotoxaemia in Falconiformes in the United Arab Emirates. In: *Raptor Biomedicine III*, ed. JT Lumeij et al., pp. 35–42. Zoological Education Network Inc., Florida

Wunschmann A, Shivers J, Bender J et al. (2005) Pathological and immunohistochemical findings in goshawks (*Accipiter gentilis*) and Great Horned Owls (*Bubo virginianus*) naturally infected with West Nile Virus. *Avian Diseases* **49**(2), 252–259

Zucca P (2002) Anatomy. In: *Birds of Prey: Health and Disease*, ed. JE Cooper, pp. 13–27. Blackwell Science, Oxford

24

Raptors: feather and skin diseases

John Chitty

Anatomy and physiology

The anatomy of the skin and feathers is discussed in Chapter 5. As with all species, an understanding of what is normal, and what is not, is essential (Figure 24.1).

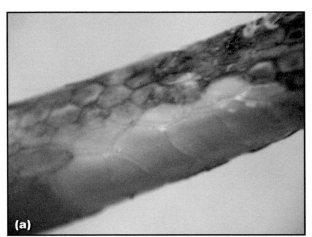

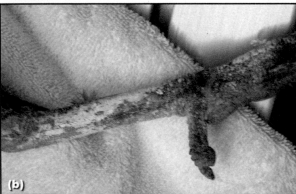

24.1 **(a)** Scaled skin of a Common Buzzard. Note that the superficial layer has been lost over part of it. This is *not* a pathological lesion. **(b)** White 'crusts' over the leg of an American Black Vulture. These are urate deposits caused by the bird urinating over its legs. This is a normal behaviour in New World vultures, and is believed to be linked to thermoregulation. (© John Chitty)

Skin physiology is similar to that of other birds, but the moult does have an impact on the working raptor.

In the wild the moult is, basically, a regular phenomenon where all feathers are renewed. The interval varies between species. It is an energy-expensive process and so its timing is generally governed by events such as nesting, rearing and migration. It usually starts at the end of the breeding season so that it is completed before the start of winter. In some species (e.g. female Northern Goshawk) it is timed to coincide with breeding such that the bird is moulting while incubating eggs.

Moulting can be considered in two stages (Edelstam, 2001):

1. Body feathers: moulted first, in a wave from head to tail.
2. Rectrices and remiges: start to be moulted after the body moult. Feathers are lost in ones or twos from each side in a symmetrical pattern. The primaries are moulted in a sequence from innermost to outermost (falcons P4–P10; other falconiform species P1–P10). Secondary flight feathers are more complicated, but still have a fixed and symmetrical moult sequence.

The stimuli for the start of moult are poorly understood and almost certainly vary between species and between different environments. However, timing and pattern of moult is designed to allow the raptor to maintain itself during a period of flight compromise.

In captivity the needs are different. The working falconer cannot afford for a raptor to be moulting when it is naturally stimulated, which may occur during the flying season and compromise hunting ability. Therefore management (see Chapter 2) is designed to encourage moult in the 'close season' when the bird is in either the breeding aviary or the moulting aviary. Falconers usually provide a flush of nutrition in the belief that it will stimulate moult. They may also add supplements to enable rapid feather replacement.

In the wild the moult is a gradual cyclical replacement of feathers stimulated by seasonal changes, whereas in captivity a rapid replacement is required at a time dictated by the keeper. It is not surprising that problems with moult – whether too slow, not occurring, or not occurring at the right time – are often reported.

There is often a request to stimulate moult. Stimulation and 'speeding' of moult are summarized by Cooper (2002), where various techniques are described along with their varying degrees of success. They include: light cycles; warmth (i.e. indoor housing); and drugs (progesterone, thyroxine).

This summary also highlights the need for great care when using drugs to stimulate moult. Both thyroxine and progesterone may be associated with severe systemic side effects and should be discontinued if these become apparent. In addition, thyroxine supplementation has been associated with feather dystrophies (Van Wettere and Redig, 2001). This is particularly the case where the pharmacological form is used rather than the traditional feeding of thyroid gland (often impossible since the recognition of spongiform encephalopathies). It is safer not to use drugs to induce moult unless a clear deficiency or hormonal syndrome can be recognized.

To this end, a poorly moulting bird should be thoroughly investigated with respect to systemic disease, endoparasitism, management and diet, and imping history (see Chapter 8). However, it is often the case that the falconer may just have to cope with the situation.

Approach to feather and skin cases

As with all species, it is important to consider the whole bird, not just the integument. Therefore a full management and clinical history, clinical examination and investigation (haematology/biochemistry with or without radiography, endoscopy, etc.) is mandatory in all but the simplest cases. Sampling techniques are described in Figure 24.2 and are discussed fully in the *BSAVA Manual of Psittacine Birds*.

Feather diseases

Ectoparasites

A variety of ectoparasites may colonize the feathers of a raptor (Figure 24.3). Their life cycles and biology are discussed more fully in Chapter 18. Few have any direct pathological effect on the feathers, though lice and mites may occasionally cause direct feather damage if present in very heavy numbers. Some may act as disease vectors. Their presence in large numbers may also indicate underlying health problems in the bird.

Both feather mites and lice should be considered host (or genus) and site specific. The latter aspect is emphasized by differences in shape (especially lice) depending on the feathers on which they are found. The bird controls their numbers by preening and by wing flapping (moulting of feathers will also cause 'moult' of parasites, though many have evolved ways of detecting the loosening of the feather and will move to a neighbouring feather). Therefore the presence of large numbers of feather parasites indicates debility of the bird, prompting investigation of systemic disease rather than simply ectoparasite control.

Feather damage

Usually feather damage does not result from parasites; other causes are much more common (Figure 24.4). Generalized feather loss appears to be very unusual.

Technique	Indications	Notes
Skin scrape	Crusts; hyperkeratotic lesions	Performed as for dogs and cats. Note that cells tend to present in sheets or 'rafts'
Feather digest	Feather damage; changes in calamus	Digest feather in warmed 10% potassium hydroxide, then centrifuge
Pulp cytology	Feather chewing; feather damage	Techniques as for parrots. Rectrices or remiges may be removed, the calamus incised and contents scraped on to a slide. For smaller body feathers, a drop of pulp may be extracted by squeezing (remove the first drop as this will be blood contaminated) or by needle aspiration
Skin acetate	Excessive scale; hyperkeratosis/crusts; exudative lesions	Technique as for dogs and cats. Romanowsky-type stains are normally used
Biopsy	Unusual lesions. Cases that fail to respond to rational therapy, or where other diagnostic tests indicate the need for biopsy	Should always include a feather follicle, but *do not* sample a flight feather follicle as this will result in permanent loss of that feather. The skin should not be aseptically prepared as this will remove surface cells. Avian skin contains a mesh of muscles linking feather follicles. The consequence of this is that on removing a section of skin the muscles contract, resulting in a tiny curled biopsy and a very large hole especially if excisional biopsy is used. A piece of adhesive tape may be placed over the skin and a sample taken through this using a biopsy punch. This should be done with care to avoid damaging underlying tissues. The sample with adhesive tape attached is placed in formol saline and submitted for histopathology

24.2 Specific dermatological sampling techniques.

Parasite	Signs/significance
Feather lice/mites	May result in feather damage. A heavy infestation may be a sign of ill-health
Louse flies (also known as flat flies or hippoboscid flies)	May cause anaemia in a very young or very weak bird. Otherwise of little clinical significance but act as vectors for important blood parasites (*Haemoproteus* spp., *Leucocytozoon* spp.) as well as poxvirus
Quill mites (*Harpyrhynchus* spp.)	Colonize the pulp of growing feathers. Damage may result in abnormal feathers and 'pinching off'

24.3 Ectoparasites of raptor feathers. (See Chapter 18 for more details.)

Cause	Appearance	Notes	Therapy
Stress marks ('fret' marks; see Chapter 7)	Lines across feathers. Sometimes feathers may snap at these places. On the wings these may then appear as if the feathers have been trimmed	Stress marks result from interruption of feather growth at a certain point in time. Marks on single or small localized groups of feathers may be due to localized damage or folliculitis. Where many feathers are affected (or symmetrical marks on rectrices/remiges) systemic causes should be investigated, e.g. disease, endoparasitism, malnutrition. However, it should be remembered that these marks represent events during the feather development, i.e. they may be historical	No specific therapy other than treatment of the specific cause
Physical damage	Bent or broken feathers may result from collisions or from poor handling techniques. Fraying of rectrices or the outer remiges may result from perching that is too close to the ground or to walls of e.g. aviary or bay	Falconers become very annoyed when feathers are damaged during clinical therapy. They have good reason, as damaged feathers will not be replaced till the next moult and may compromise flight. Careful handling and careful positioning of perches in aviary, bay or hospital unit will reduce the chances of damage. Tail guards will protect the rectrices of birds unable to perch (see Chapter 6)	Small numbers of broken feathers may be replaced by imping (see Chapter 8). Slightly bent feathers may be steamed and re-shaped
Pinching-off (see Figure 24.5)	Feathers are shed prematurely with the calamus shortened and 'pinched' in appearance	Although the loss of the feather stimulates new feather growth, the problem often continues. Causes include folliculitis and *Harpyrhynchus* mites	Treat cause of folliculitis. Ivermectin may be effective against quill mites
Broken blood feathers	Often heavy blood loss with blood splashed around the enclosure. The broken feather is usually easy to find		The feather should be pulled out. Tying-off or cautery may result in further damage. Removal of the feather stimulates growth of a new feather
Dystrophy	A variety of shapes possible. It is important to distinguish dystrophy from damage	May be localized or generalized. Investigation will be based on this. See 'Stress marks' (above). Localized causes include folliculitis. Generalized causes include systemic illness, endoparasitism, malnutrition and use of thyroxine as a moulting aid	Depends on cause

24.4 Causes of feather damage.

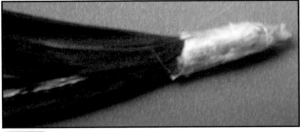

24.5 Pinched-off feather. (© John Chitty)

In the few cases seen by this author, it tends to result from extreme debility or malnutrition and the breaking-off of malformed feathers. Localized feather loss may result from folliculitis or localized damage.

Folliculitis

This is generally a localized problem. It may present as:

- Feather loss
- Feather damage/dystrophy
- Feather chewing.

Typically, examination will reveal inflammation and swelling centred on feather follicles (Figure 24.6). Swabs may be taken from the follicle and submitted for cytology and culture/sensitivity tests. Bacterial infections appear much more common than yeast.

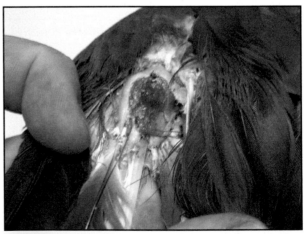

24.6 Advanced folliculitis with a granulating ulcerated lesion centred on the feather follicle. (© John Chitty)

Therapy involves systemic antibiosis or antimycotic therapy. Underlying causes should be identified if possible. Often folliculitis involves the primary feathers and trauma appears to be an important cause.

Most cases resolve successfully and future feather regrowth is normal. However, in some cases (especially in aviary birds) where the lesions have not been detected at an early stage, there may be scarring or even loss of the follicle, resulting in abnormal or no feather regrowth.

Feather destructive disorders

Feather plucking (Figure 24.7) and chewing have only recently been described in captive raptors, but appear to be increasing problems. As with feather destruction in parrots, there may be many underlying causes, both medical and behavioural (see Chapter 22). Most cases occur in 'social' raptors such as the Harris' Hawk and (in the author's experience) kites and American Black Vultures. Hand-rearing may be an important underlying factor. Many cases appear to occur during training, which is a particularly stressful period.

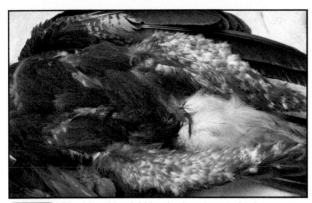

24.7 Plucking Harris' Hawk showing typical distribution of plucking. (© John Chitty)

Feather pulpitis also appears to be important, as all cases seen by the author have shown this on cytology and responded fully or partly to antibiosis. It is not known whether pulpitis is a primary, secondary or perpetuating factor. In one Brahminy Kite, cyclical feather plucking appeared to be associated with pulpitis and appeared to recur on a seasonal basis, prompting concerns of an underlying allergic condition. However, it should also be borne in mind that many husbandry systems are altered on a seasonal basis and allergy is yet to be confirmed as a cause of plucking in raptors.

Chewing of remiges does appear to be linked to bacterial folliculitis, which in the author's experience is a primary cause of this sign (Figure 24.8). No evidence of feather or skin mites as a cause of feather destructive disorders has been seen by the author.

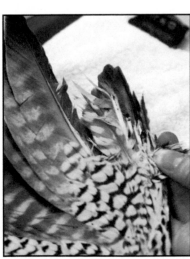

24.8 Feather-chewing Northern Goshawk. Folliculitis was the cause after a crash-landing into dirty water during a hunting trip. *Pseudomonas aeruginosa* was cultured from the follicles and the bird responded well to antibiosis. (© John Chitty)

Investigation of these cases should be similar to that undertaken in plucking parrots:

- Full history
  - Signalment, management, diet
  - History of the condition: when started, area originally plucked or chewed, spread to other areas, when it occurs, vocalizations during plucking, association with human or bird presence
- Clinical examination
  - Including dermatological examination and thorough search for ectoparasites
  - Cytological sampling of feather pulp; skin scrapes, impression smears and acetates of skin lesions; skin biopsy (including feather follicle) as necessary
- Blood sampling: full haematogical and biochemical profile
- Faecal examination for endoparasites
- Full body radiography
- Laparoscopy if deemed necessary following other tests.

Therapy depends on the determined cause. Generalized therapies should be avoided. In particular, Elizabethan or extension collars (as used in parrots) will probably result in excessive stress to the bird. Modified hoods (see Chapter 16) designed to prevent damage to bandages may be effective in preventing further feather damage, but should only be employed in the short term and alongside rational therapy.

Skin diseases

Ectoparasites
Skin ectoparasites are summarized in Figure 24.9.

Parasite		Signs/significance
Mites	*Cnemidocoptes*	Unusual. Signs as in other species with burrowing mites causing hyperplastic reactions on legs or cere/beak
	Epidermoptid mites	Unusual, but more common than *Cnemidocoptes*. Burrowing mites cause skin hyperplasia, crusts, pruritus and feather loss (Figure 24.10)
	Dermanyssus	Not truly a skin mite as the bulk of their life cycle is spent free-living (up to 5 months between feeds). They will emerge at night and suck blood – resulting in pruritus and, in severe infestations, anaemia. They are particularly associated with raptors housed in or near former poultry sheds
	Ornithonyssus	Rare. Similar to *Dermanyssus* except that the entire life cycle is spent on-bird. This means that clinical signs (pruritus and anaemia) are more intense

24.9 Ectoparasites of raptor skin (see also Chapter 18). (continues) ▶

Parasite		Signs/significance
Flies	Myiasis	Invasion of diseased tissue by larvae of Calliphoridae (blowflies), e.g. *Calliphora* (bluebottle) and *Lucilia* (greenbottle). This is uncommon in UK birds as most will nest and fledge before the main fly season (Malley and Whitbread, 1996). It is therefore only seen in extremely debilitated birds
	Gnats/ mosquitoes	Biting insects transmit various diseases. Mosquitoes: *Haemoproteus* spp., avipox virus (USA: equine encephalomyelitis, West Nile virus). Gnats – *Leucocytozoon* spp.
Ticks		Hard ticks (Ixodidae) may feed on birds in the UK; soft ticks may be found on newly imported birds Large numbers may cause irritation, debility, anaemia and death. Transmit haemoprotozoa (e.g. *Aegyptionella* spp.), arboviruses (e.g. louping ill (grouse)), *Borrelia* spp. (Kurtenbach *et al.*, 1999)

24.9 (continued) Ectoparasites of raptor skin (see also Chapter 18).

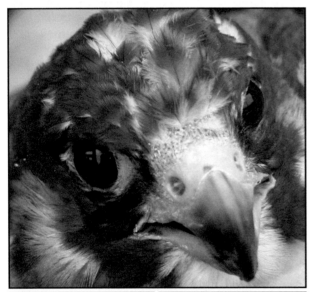

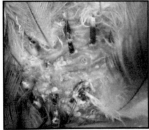
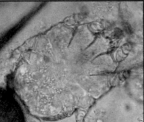

24.10 Epidermoptid mite infestation of a Peregrine Falcon. A topical solution of 1:50 invermectin:propylene glycol was applied to the lesions twice at monthly intervals. (© John Chitty)

Tick reactions

Tick reactions are a major problem in captive raptors (see Chapter 18). The first sign is normally an extremely sick or collapsed bird with extensive haemorrhagic swelling of the face or head (Figure 24.11). The tick is normally associated with this swelling. In a recent study (Monks *et al.*, 2006), the major or sole tick associated with lesions was identified as *Ixodes frontalis*. This study failed to show a link with tick-borne pathogens. It is therefore likely that this syndrome may be associated with a tick saliva toxin or a hypersensitivity reaction.

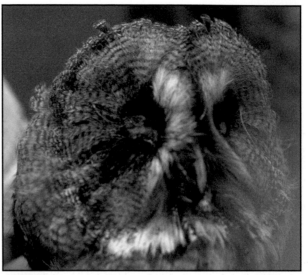

24.11 Tick reaction around the right eye of a Great Grey Owl. (© John Chitty)

Interestingly, the reaction is only associated with tick attachment around the head. In some cases seen by the author there have also been ticks on the body that have not had an associated reaction. It is possible that these body ticks may have been of another species.

Chastel *et al.* (1991) showed that reactions were more common in unusual hosts or with multiple engorged adult female ticks. This may suggest a novel infection or, more likely, a host–parasite intolerance.

Birds showing tick reactions should be treated as emergencies. Fluids, broad-spectrum antibiosis and short-acting corticosteroids (e.g. dexamethasone) should be administered as quickly as possible. Monks *et al.* (2006) described a therapeutic success rate of 75%. In this author's experience, provided birds are presented quickly enough, survival rates can be much higher.

Wounds

Surgical management of skin wounds is discussed in Chapter 14. However, some wounds may not be amenable to immediate surgical intervention, due to any of the following:

- Infection
- Not enough tissue to close the wound after debridement (e.g. on distal limb)
- Chronic wounds where granulation is already progressing.

In these cases medical management is essential, either to prepare the wound prior to surgical closure or to allow healing by second intention.

Principles of wound healing and methods available are similar to those in mammals, except that the rate of healing in avian patients is much faster. Many raptors will tolerate dressings well, although Harris' Hawks appear more likely than most to remove dressings and bandages. A modified hood may be used to prevent the bird from traumatizing the wound or dressings during healing (see Chapter 16).

When managing this type of wound it is vital to debride any infected or damaged tissue. Bacteriological swabs should be taken and antibiotic therapy should be based on these results. Typically *Staphylococcus* spp. or environmental Gram-negative rods (e.g. *Escherichia coli*) will be found. Amoxicillin/clavulanate is a useful first-choice antibiotic. Systemic antibiosis should be maintained until the wound has healed completely.

The wound can then be managed using hydrophilic dressings that encourage granulation (e.g. OpSite, Smith & Nephew; Granuflex, Convatec; Aquacell Ag, Convatec; Collamend, Genitrix). These should be changed regularly. Where there are large defects, VetBioSIST (Global Products) is extremely useful in either granular or sheet form. Choice of dressing is generally made on the basis of lesion type, size and position as well as the bird's tolerance of dressings. For example, dressing sheets that need holding in place with a bandage are excellent for wounds of the legs and feet. Where the wound is on the body, bandages are hard to keep in place and dressings that may be sutured over the wound, or gels, are more appropriate.

If the bird will not tolerate a dressing or if it is desirable to manage the wound in open fashion, daily bathing using povidone–iodine or chlorhexidine followed by application of Intra-Site gel (Smith & Nephew) appears to work well. The wound can be further protected by an application of OpSite spray (Smith & Nephew) or, if in an area likely to be heavily contaminated, the gel can be mixed with a little silver sulfadiazine cream.

Puncture wounds (e.g. from another raptor's talons) should not, in general, be sutured or dressed, as regular bathing and irrigation are essential. It is important to start systemic antibiosis as soon as possible and 'grabbed' birds should always be seen as a matter of urgency. There may also be considerable bruising to skin and underlying organs; many birds are presented in shock. Fluids and non-steroidal anti-inflammatories may also be indicated initially. Surgical closure is indicated as soon as the wound has healed sufficiently.

Wounds of the feet and scaled legs are discussed more fully in Chapter 16. These can be much more tricky to deal with as there is less skin available for repair, hence the need for some degree of medical management in almost all cases.

Squirrel bites appear to be of particular importance. The typical wound is on the foot or leg, a couple of millimetres long, and appears innocuous. It is often left untreated other than staunching blood flow and initial cleaning. Unfortunately, these bites tend to introduce bacteria (possibly mixed aerobe and anaerobe) and erosive infections will result. These may not be apparent for a few weeks, by which time there may be osteomyelitis or tenosynovitis. Post-infection tendon rupture is not unknown. It is therefore recommended that squirrel bites should be seen as a matter of urgency, the wound thoroughly irrigated, and antibiosis instigated. The author typically uses a 14-day course of amoxicillin/clavulanate in the first instance.

Pyoderma

The best known example of pyoderma in raptors is bumblefoot. This, along with other abscessing infections of the skin of the foot, is discussed fully in Chapter 16.

Pyoderma of the feathered skin seems to be becoming more common in Harris' Hawks (Figure 24.12). It is generally seen over the propatagium or the precrural fold. The infection can become very deep and may result in complete skin breakdown.

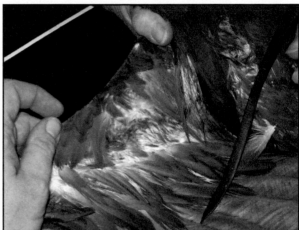
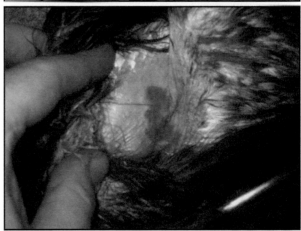

24.12 Pyoderma in two Harris' Hawks. (© John Chitty)

In general these infections are bacterial, though yeast infections with *Malassezia* spp. have been reported. Primary causes are rarely, if ever, discovered and this has an impact on therapeutic success. Injury and self-trauma may be important. Hypersensitivity has also been proposed.

The lesions present as feather loss with crusting and excoriation of the skin. Cytological sampling enables distinction between bacterial and yeast infections. Culture and sensitivity tests are used to choose appropriate drug therapy.

It is also recommended that skin biopsy is performed in all cases along with systemic investigations in order to attempt to elucidate the primary cause. Biopsy can be frustrating in the early stages as changes may be 'swamped' by the secondary infection. It may therefore be deferred until after the start of antimicrobial therapy.

Topical antimicrobials may also be used, including F10SC (Health & Hygiene Pty; 1:250 dilution applied daily), chlorhexidine (dilute 1:50 and apply daily) or chlorhexidine–miconazole shampoo (Malaseb, Leo Animal Health). Some clinicians find dietary essential fatty acid supplementation useful.

It is likely that therapy will be required for several months. Resection and repair may be possible if lesions become small enough (especially in the precrural fold), but wound breakdown is common.

Therapy should be continued while healing is occurring. Failure to improve or relapse must be aggressively investigated; in particular, the identity of colonizing microbes and antimicrobial sensitivity should be re-checked along with skin biopsy. The author has had two cases in raptors that progressed to squamous cell carcinoma, presumably as a result of continuous skin irritation.

Poxvirus

This is discussed in Chapters 16 and 19. Lesions (nodules or crusts) may be seen over the scaled areas of skin, i.e. face and feet. Occasionally they are seen on feathered skin. They are pruritic and readily become secondarily infected. Lesions may also become established on the oral mucous membranes and eyelids, resulting in difficulty in feeding and consequently debility.

Neoplasia

Squamous cell carcinoma appears to be quite common, probably as a consequence of chronic skin irritation (Figure 24.13). A wide range of other

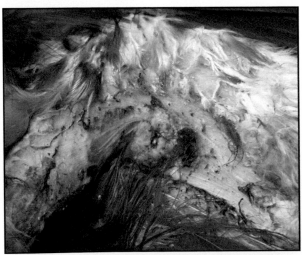

24.13 Squamous cell carcinoma in a Harris' Hawk. This was secondary to long-standing pyoderma that initially responded to antibiosis. The lesion was located at the top of the leg. It is presumed that it resulted from chronic irritation from the skin infection, as biopsy samples taken early in the condition showed no evidence of neoplasia. (© John Chitty)

neoplasms have also been identified (Forbes *et al.*, 2000) (see Chapter 26). Neoplasia should be considered as a differential for any case of nodular/macular, proliferative or ulcerative skin disease as well as non-healing conditions.

Diagnosis is made by biopsy or cytology. Ideally neoplasms should be surgically resected and submitted for histopathology for diagnosis and assessment of adequacy of removal, as well as likelihood of recurrence or spread. Where this is not possible, prognosis is poor, but chemo- or radiotherapy may be possible in some cases.

Adnexa

Diseases of the beak and talons are discussed in more detail in Chapters 8, 15 and 16. As with other birds, systemic diseases affect the adnexae.

Uropygial gland

Impaction of this gland is less common in raptors than in other species. The appearance of impaction is similar to that in other species. Gentle massage may resolve blockage. If not, hot-water compresses may be applied and a gentle 'milking' massage applied. Should this also fail, surgical lancing and flushing (with iodine or diluted F10SC) of the impacted gland should be employed. Systemic antibiosis may also be required, especially where regular infections are seen. Adenocarcinomas of the gland have also been described (Malley and Whitbread, 1996).

Specific disorders

Subcutaneous emphysema

This is an occasional consequence of trauma and damage to the air sacs. It will often present as a generalized swelling. The sensation of crepitus on palpation gives a tentative diagnosis. Radiography will confirm and may assist in determining cause. Most cases resolve with time and birds often appear unaffected even in severe cases. However, if it is a problem, drainage of the air is simple and recommended. In some cases a stent or drain should be fitted, but most will only require a single drainage.

Wingtip oedema and necrosis syndrome

WTONS is a curious disease where blood flow to the wingtips appears to be reduced, resulting initially in oedema then dry necrosis until the wingtip and associated primary feathers are lost (Figure 24.14). It should be distinguished from 'blaine' (a traumatic carpitis that is normally unilateral, centred on the carpus and warm to the touch).

The prognosis is good if caught early. Therapy involves broad-spectrum antibiosis and vascular stimulants (isoxsuprine orally and 'Preparation-H' topically). All cases should be radiographed as in the advanced stages erosive lesions may be seen developing in the second phalangeal bone. This is a poor prognostic sign, as is passage to dry necrosis.

The disease appears to be limited to this region. Once the wingtip is lost, there does not appear to be progression into more proximal parts of the wing.

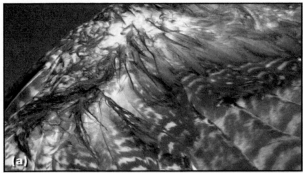

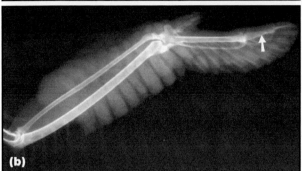

24.14 **(a)** Wingtip oedema and necrosis syndrome in a Harris' Hawk. Note the oedematous fluid *between* the feather follicles. **(b)** Radiograph of WTONS in a different Harris' Hawk. This is a very unusual case, as the swelling occurs around secondary as well as the primary feathers. The position of the fluid accumulations is obvious. The arrow indicates the position on P2 where erosive lesions may be found; this is an indicator of a poor prognosis, as this is where the necrotic wingtip will break off. (© John Chitty)

The aetiology is still unknown, but low ground temperatures may be involved. To prevent its occurrence, no young raptor should be tethered within 45 cm of the ground in winter unless heat is supplied. Wet birds should not be left out at night in winter (tethered or in aviaries) and access to water should not be allowed after noon in winter in order to allow drying before nightfall. However, attribution to 'frostbite' appears simplistic. While it is fair to say that most cases occur in warm-climate birds (e.g. Harris' Hawk, Lanner Falcon), cases have also been reported in other species. Similarly, although most cases occur immediately following cold weather, some do occur at other times. It is therefore likely that cold is the final trigger for a condition that may have its origins in vasculitis due to infection or toxin. In some seasons no cases are seen, but the advent of one case normally precedes others.

Elucidation of underlying causes is hampered by the success of therapy of early cases. Sampling or biopsy of the wingtips in these cases is very likely to compromise a case that can be expected to recover. In the later stages biopsy will not further hinder the (now) hopeless case but, by this stage, primary lesions are long gone.

The author has carried out some preliminary investigation of serum protein electrophoresis in this disease. In the early stages alpha-globulins appear raised, with lowered levels of beta- and gamma-globulins. As the condition progresses all protein fractions increase. This tends to suggest an underlying inflammatory component.

Otitis

Otitis (Figure 24.15) is unusual in raptors. In some cases it appears to be linked to sinusitis and upper respiratory infections. It may also be linked to epidermoptid mite infestation causing skin proliferation and hyperkeratinization around the entrance to the external auditory meatus. However, most cases appear to be idiopathic bacterial infections and are frequently bilateral. The author has not seen birds with recurrent problems as is common in small animal cases.

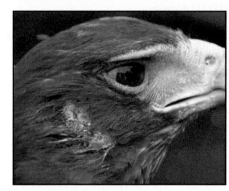

24.15 Otitis in a Harris' Hawk. Bacterial infection was apparent but the underlying cause was never established. (© John Chitty)

Therapy includes treatment of underlying causes, systemic antimicrobials and gentle cleaning with dilute chlorhexidine or F10SC. Polypharmacy products used for treatment of otitis in dogs should never be used, as the corticosteroids may be absorbed and cause problems or lead to ischaemic necrosis due to the reduced vascularization of the internal skin.

References and further reading

Chastel C, Guiguen C, Chastel O and Beaucournu JC (1991) Pathological effects, vector role and new host of *Ixodes Pari* (= *Ixodes frontalis*) Acari Ixodoidea Ixodidae. *Annales de Parasitology Humaine et Comparée* **66**, 27–32
Chitty JR (2000) Ectoparasites of raptors. In: *Proceedings of the British Veterinary Zoological Society Spring Meeting 2000 (Cotswold Wildlife Park)*, pp. 30–31
Chitty JR (2005a) Feather and skin disorders. In: *BSAVA Manual of Psittacine Birds, 2nd edn*, ed. N Harcourt-Brown and J Chitty. BSAVA, Gloucester
Chitty JR (2005b) Feather plucking/chewing in raptors. In: *Proceedings of the 26th Conference of the Association of Avian Veterinarians. Monterey*, pp. 91–93
Cooper JE (2002) *Birds of Prey: Health and Disease*. Blackwell Publishing, Oxford
Edelstam E (2001) Raptor moult patterns and age criteria. In: *Raptors of the World*, ed. J Ferguson-Lees and I Christie, pp. 50–53. Helm, London
Forbes NA and Simpson GN (1993) Pathogenicity of ticks on aviary birds. *Veterinary Record* **133**, 532
Forbes NA, Cooper JE and Higgins RJ (2000) Neoplasms of birds of prey. In: *Raptor Biomedicine III*, ed. JT Lumeij *et al.*, pp. 127–145. Zoological Education Network, Lake Worth, FL
Heidenreich M (1997) *Birds of Prey: Medicine and Management*. Blackwell Science, Oxford
Jones MP (2001) Behavioral aspects of captive birds of prey. *Veterinary Clinics of North America: Exotic Animal Practice* **4**, 613–632
Knott CIF (1993) Ticks on aviary birds. *Veterinary Record* **133**, 376
Kurtenbach K, deMichelis S and Sewell H-S (1999) The role of wildlife in the epidemiology of Lyme disease. *BVA Congress Seminar Day 23/9/99 (Bath, UK) 'Zoonotic Diseases of UK Wildlife'*
Malley AD and Whitbread TJ (1996) The integument. In: *BSAVA Manual of Raptors, Pigeons and Waterfowl*, ed. PH Beynon *et al.*, pp. 129–139. BSAVA, Cheltenham
Monks D, Fisher M and Forbes NA (2006) *Ixodes frontalis* and avian tick-related syndrome in the United Kingdom. *Journal of Small Animal Practice* **47**, 451–455
Philips JR (1990) What's bugging your birds? Avian parasitic arthropods. *Wildlife Rehabilitation* **8**, 155
Van Wettere A and Redig PT (2001) A review of methods used to induce molting in raptors. *Hawk Chalk* **30**(2), 46–56

25

Raptors: ophthalmology

David L. Williams

Anatomy and physiology

Anatomy of the avian eye is well covered by Martin (1985), to which the reader is directed for further information; see also Chapter 5. The avian eyelids are mobile, the lower more so than the upper. No meibomian glands are present but a lacrimal gland, varying in size between species, is present inferior and lateral to the globe. The Harderian gland acts as a second lacrimal gland at the base of the nictitating membrane. The nictitating membrane actively moves over the cornea during blinking and in the menace response. Inferior and superior nasolacrimal puncta at the medial canthus drain lacrimal secretions into the nasal cavity.

The orbit is open but, since the globe occupies the vast majority of the space, the rectus and oblique muscles are not well developed and torsional movements of the globe are limited in many species to between 2 and 5 degrees. A key point in the anatomy of the avian orbit is the close approximation of the tightly packed orbit with the infraorbital diverticulum of the infraorbital sinus. Sinusitis and enlargement of this diverticulum will therefore lead to periorbital or orbital compression and signs of periorbital swelling, conjunctivitis and sometimes intraocular disease, though such findings are far rarer in raptors that in columbiforms and anseriforms.

The globe may be anterioposteriorly flattened with a hemispherical posterior segment, as in psittacids and the majority of birds, or rounded in diurnal raptors and tubular in owls. The sclera immediately posterior to the cornea contains scleral ossicles and through its full circumference the sclera has a support of hyaline cartilage. The cornea is similar to that of mammals except that it is obviously considerably thinner, exact thickness depending on the size of bird, and it has an acellular anterior Bowman's layer. The anterior segment is relatively shallow compared with the posterior segment but again anatomical differences occur between species, with many owls having an unusually deep anterior chamber facilitating observation of the iridocorneal angle through which the aqueous humour drains from the eye.

The iris is thin and contains striated dilator and constrictor muscles and chromatophores, giving a great variety of colours in different species. Iris colour can vary between the sexes and at differing ages of bird within one species, though this is less the case in raptors than in other avian species. One American report showed variation in iris colour in kestrels with age, gender and PCB intoxication (Bortolotti et al., 2003). Pupillary light reflexes do occur but are complicated by the fact that voluntary constriction and dilation is also possible even in the absence of retinal stimulation. The complete decussation of the optic nerves means that no true consensual pupillary light reflex can be elicited. The striated muscles of the iris mean that mydriasis, whether diagnostically for fundoscopy or therapeutically in uveitis, must be achieved by the use of muscle relaxants rather than the anticholinergic mydriatics such as atropine and tropicamide used in mammals. Vecuronium has been shown to be an effective mydriatic agent in kestrels and in other raptors (Mikaelian et al., 1994).

The lens is soft, either almost spherical in nocturnal birds or with a flattened anterior face in diurnal species. The fundus varies considerably in colour between species, but a constant feature is the pecten, a comb-like black or brown projection of choroidal tissue into the vitreous. The small regular torsional movements of the avian eye sweep the pecten through the relatively fluid posterior vitreous, dispersing a serum filtrate of nutrients and oxygen from the pecten blood vessels even as far as the peripheral retina (Pettigrew et al., 1990). Most avian species have no ophthalmologically distinct fovea with a higher photoreceptor concentration giving high visual acuity, but many raptors have one and diurnal raptors have two. It is suggested that in bi-foveate birds, one fovea is placed for near vision and prey-devouring, the other for distance accommodation and prey capture. The fovea of many raptors is funnel-shaped, giving a very high acuity in this area with vision an order of magnitude more acute than that of humans (Tucker, 2000).

As their sight is such a key sense, it is all the more important to be able to evaluate, diagnose and treatment ophthalmic problems accurately, successfully and quickly. However, before evaluating the avian eye, it should be asked exactly what birds do see. Their colour vision is markedly different from that of humans, as they see not only in the three colours perceived by humans but also in the ultraviolet. Vision of light at ultraviolet wavelengths is well recognized as important in behavioural traits ranging from territorial aggression in blackbirds to fish catching in gulls, but even in raptors (as in many other species) appreciation of ultraviolet cues is important in mate selection. Their ability to perceive a flickering light is markedly more acute than most mammals, including humans. With a higher flicker fusion frequency than the human eye, they see a standard mains light or strip bulb as flickering, which may have substantial welfare implications for birds housed indoors (Nuboer *et al.*, 1992; Maddocks *et al.*, 2001)

Clinical examination

Ophthalmic evaluation of the avian eye differs little from that of its mammalian counterpart. Given the small size of many raptor eyes and the prevalence of anterior segment disease, magnification using a head loupe and good illumination are sufficient for many ophthalmic cases. Examining the retina can be more taxing: use of the direct ophthalmoscope (Figure 25.1a) allows examination of the eye in a routine

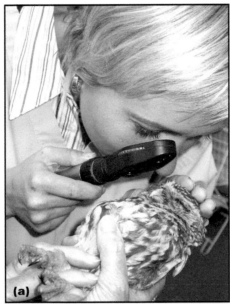

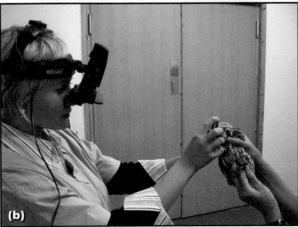

25.1 **(a)** Use of the direct ophthalmoscope for examination of the raptor eye. This relatively simple technique, which gives a magnified image of the retina but can also be used for evaluation of the iris and cornea, does place the examiner's face perilously close to the bird's beak – as can be seen here. **(b)** Use of the indirect ophthalmoscope. This requires a reasonably dilated pupil and gives a wide field of view of the retina. The disadvantage is that the image is inverted, so this technique requires practice. (© David L. Williams)

manner and evaluation of the fundus at a setting of zero dioptres, while the indirect ophthalmoscope (Figure 25.1b) can give much improved fundoscopic images where size of the pupil allows: the Tawny Owl has a wide pupil, while the Barn Owl has a pupil sufficiently miotic that evaluation of the retina can be difficult. Use of non-depolarizing muscle relaxants such as vecuronium applied topically can yield sufficient mydriasis to allow fundoscopy even through these normally miotic pupils.

Care must clearly be taken when examining these birds closely: the danger of the proximity of the examiner's nose to the beak of the examinee cannot be over-stressed (Figure 25.1a). Indeed effective mydriasis and akinesia for ophthalmic examination can both be produced in birds by use of a general anaesthetic using the standard endotracheal technique or via cannulation of the caudal thoracic air sac. The author considers that the benefits of such an examination technique are outweighed by the potential risks where ophthalmic evaluation can readily be carried out in the conscious bird.

Ancillary tests such as evaluation of lacrimation with the Schirmer tear test (STT) and measurement of the intraocular pressure by tonometry can provide valuable additional clinical information in diseased eyes. In the only major study of its kind, Korbel and Leitenstrofer (1998) evaluated tear production in normal birds of prey using a modified STT strip giving values of 4.1 ± 2.7 to 14.4 ± 7.2 mm/min and 2.0 ± 1.7 to 4.2 ± 3.1 mm/min (using 4 mm strips) in Falconiformes and 10.7 ± 4.0 to 11.5 ± 5.4 mm/min and 3.6 ± 1.7 to 5.9 ± 3.1 mm/min (using 4 mm strips) in Accipitriformes. Due to the lack of a lacrimal gland, Strigiformes showed STT levels below 3 mm/min. The wide differences between species mean that assessment of a normal bird of the same age, gender and species is to be recommended.

Tonometry has been investigated in normal individuals of various raptor species. The normal intraocular pressure, as measured by applanation tonometry can vary quite considerably between different raptor species, being 20.6 mmHg in Red-tailed Hawks in one report and 10.8 mmHg in Great Horned Owls in the same study (Stiles *et al.*, 1994). Concurrent evaluation of non-affected birds of the same species in the same environment must be undertaken when assessing intraocular pressure changes in an individual raptor.

Ocular disease: diagnosis and treatment

Adnexal and globe defects

Congenital abnormalities of the globe have been described in raptors (Buyukmihci *et al.*, 1988), mostly involving microphthalmia (Figure 25.2) but also cataract and retinal dysplasia.

Trauma

The majority of ocular lesions seen in raptors are as a result of trauma. In a large survey of birds admitted to a raptor rehabilitation centre in the USA, 14.5% of

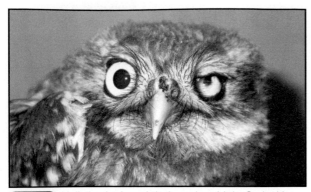

25.2 Unilateral microphthalmos in a Little Owl with abnormal pupil shape and concurrent corneal opacity. (© David L. Williams)

birds had an ocular defect, 90% of these being traumatic (Murphy *et al.*, 1982). A smaller study in the UK specifically of Tawny Owls noted ocular lesions in 75% of birds, with 60% of these being post-traumatic (Cousquer, 2005). A study of chronic ocular lesions in Tawny Owls after road traffic accidents showed similar prevalences of lesions in the cornea, lens and retina to humans with high-speed blunt ocular trauma (Williams *et al.*, 2006). Clearly the majority of such birds are unsuitable for release into the wild and the ethics of their maintenance in captivity is questionable.

Conjuctival disease

Conjunctival disease is generally not considered a problem in raptors, though in one study the ocular irritation provoked by grass seeds was considered sufficient to lead to death of affected individuals (McCrary and Bloom, 1984). In pigeons the disease is much more concerning, with mycoplasmal infection leading to the conjunctivitis and sinusitis of 'one-eyed cold' (Loria *et al.*, 2005). Although mycoplasmas have been isolated from falcons (Furr *et al.*, 1977) and buzzards (Bolske and Morner, 1982), the organism does not cause the severe ocular lesions seen in pigeons. Conjunctivitis with subsequent symblepharon formation has been noted in a group of septicaemic Snowy Owl chicks (Figure 25.3) (Williams and Flach, 2003) and may be related to more general inflammatory processes in generalized infection.

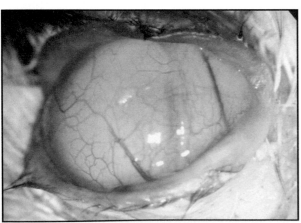

25.3 Symblepharon following septicaemia in one of a brood of Snowy Owl chicks. (© David L. Williams)

Corneal lesions

The large palpebral apertures and wide corneal surface of many raptors render corneal trauma common, and lesions from sharp penetrating corneal injury to persistent ulceration can be treated with techniques similar to those used in the dog and cat, be they immediate closure of penetrating wounds, superficial keratectomy for persistent corneal ulceration or conjunctival flaps for non-healing ulceration (Andrew *et al.*, 2002; Park and Gill, 2005; Gionfriddo and Powell, 2006). This is an area where the standard treatments in companion animal species can be extrapolated to the avian sphere. Persistent ulceration can occur in older birds even without trauma (Figure 25.4) and these defects can be very difficult to heal. Keratitis can occur following long-term ocular surface exposure (Figure 25.5) and with little likelihood of return to normal vision in these birds. Debridement of persistent ulcers in raptors can be valuable, as can grid keratotomies with subsequent protection of the ocular surface with a third eyelid flap, but the thin nature of the raptor cornea should alert the veterinary surgeon to the risks involved in a surgery such as grid keratotomy.

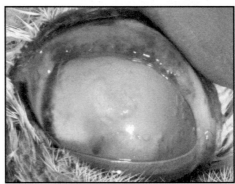

25.4 Chronic non-healing ulceration in an aged Snowy Owl in captivity. (© David L. Williams)

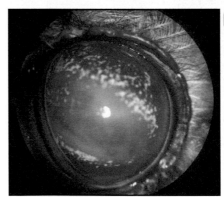

25.5 Ulcerative keratitis with calcium deposition following exposure after trauma and eyelid paralysis in a Tawny Owl. (© David L. Williams)

Anterior segment disease

Uveitis is a common sequel to injury but may occur as an apparently primary disease or secondary to cataract formation. Preventing and resolving miosis in such cases can be very difficult with non-depolarizing muscle relaxants as the only effective mydriatics available. Topical anti-inflammatories such as the steroids prednisone acetate or dexamethasone alcohol, or non-steroidal anti-inflammatories, such as ketorolac or flurbiprofen, are important in reducing the inflammation in these eyes, which may present as a dark swollen iris with synechiae or frequently as a turbid fibrinoid aqueous (Figure 25.6).

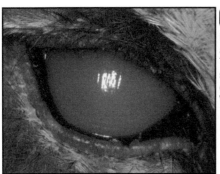

25.6 Fibrinoid aqueous in a Tawny Owl with severe uveitis. (© David L. Williams)

Lenticular disease

Whether post-traumatic or as a primary disease, cataract is all too common in raptors (Figures 25.7 and 25.8) and cataract surgery is frequently performed. Phacoemulsification is a successful technique in producing a comfortable visual eye (Kern *et al.*, 1984) although the acute vision of raptors probably means that a fully successful surgery should include the placement of an intraocular lens (Carter *et al.*, 2007), a technique requiring the construction of a suitably sized lens and calculation of the appropriate lens power after retinoscopy and keratometry of the individual's eye – clearly not a task to be undertaken lightly. Postoperative inflammation and opacification of the posterior capsule are commonly seen postoperative complications (Figure 25.9).

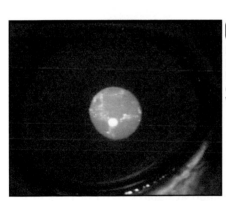

25.7 Mature cataract in a young Harris' Hawk. (© David L. Williams)

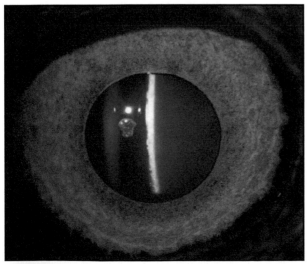

25.8 Slit-lamp examination of a cataract in an Eagle Owl. (© David L. Williams)

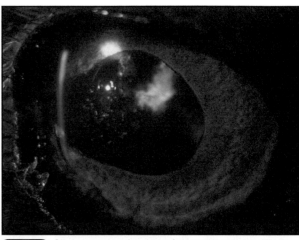

25.9 Slit-lamp examination of a cataract in an Eagle Owl after phacoemulsification. While the procedure was successful in returning vision to the bird, iridal inflammation, here manifest as dyscoria (abnormal pupil shape), as well as posterior capsular opacification are seen. (© David L. Williams)

Another condition of the lens seen relatively regularly after trauma is that of lens luxation (Figure 25.10). Surgical removal is the preferred therapeutic option (Brooks *et al.*, 1983).

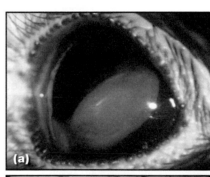

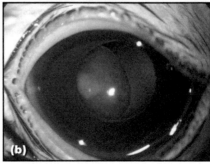

25.10 **(a)** Post-traumatic lens luxation in a Peregrine Falcon. **(b)** Microphakia in a falcon. (a, courtesy of Keith Barnett; b, courtesy of Ingrid Allgoewer)

Glaucoma

Increased intraocular pressure can occur after separation of the iris root from the sclera during trauma, but glaucoma has also been noted as a presumed primary condition in Snowy Owls (Rayment and Williams, 1997). Gonioscopy in this case demonstrated an abnormal iridocorneal angle (Figure 25.11). Here a Barkan goniolens was used, but in many raptors the anterior chamber is deep enough and the cornea sufficiently steeply curved that simple slit-lamp biomicroscopy (Figure 25.12) or direct ophthalmoscopy is sufficient to see the iridocorneal angle.

26

Raptors: systemic and non-infectious diseases

Richard Jones

Poisoning

Birds of prey have become well known for their susceptibility to environmental contaminants. A dramatic drop in the populations of some raptor species during the 1960s and 1970s alerted the world to this problem and since then many of the substances responsible, especially DDT, have been banned from use in many countries. More recently the veterinary use of diclofenac has been specifically implicated in the decline of the critically endangered Oriental White-backed Vulture in Asia.

Raptors in captivity are also vulnerable to a number of toxins via ingestion, inhalation or direct contact, and may present with a variety of clinical signs as a result. A detailed history is therefore paramount in the investigation, including detailed questioning on recent food items, possible exposure to aerosols or any medications and preparations applied either topically or parenterally. Any products suspected of causing toxic effects should ideally be brought with the patient at time of presentation.

Figure 26.1 outlines a general approach to the treatment of toxicoses.

Poison information centres
In cases of suspected toxicosis, it is worth contacting national poison information services. In the UK, for example, the Veterinary Poisons Information Service (VPIS) is a subscription service that provides advice on all aspects of the treatment of acute toxic exposures. Information provided may also help to increase their database. Veterinary practices registered with the VPIS may use its numbers to obtain advice 24 hours a day. For information on toxic emergencies, contact:

- UK: (Leeds) +44-(0)113 245 0530; (London) +44-(0)20 7635 9195
- Germany: Erfurt: +49-(0)361 730730; Berlin: +49-(0)30-19240
- Austria: +43-1-4064343
- Switzerland: 0041-44-251-5151
- International: World Directory of Poison Centres, www.who.int/ipcs/poisons/centre/directory/en/

Step	Action
Prevent exposure to further toxins	1. Remove bird from source of exposure to toxin 2. Remove any toxins from feathers, skin and eyes: • Flush eyes with saline; wash feathers with mild warm detergent • Rinse thoroughly with water • Flush acid or caustic alkali with water (do *not* try to neutralize with sodium bicarbonate or vinegar – exothermic reactions cause more damage!) 3. Decrease absorption from GI tract: • Repeated gavage of crop/proventriculus (must intubate bird to avoid aspiration; best carried out within 3 hours of exposure, using saline) • Removal of solid objects via gavage or surgery • Use activated charcoal, sodium or magnesium sulphate as cathartics if toxin in lower GI tract
Institute supportive therapy	Heat; oxygen; fluids; reduce stress
Provide specific antidote if available	

26.1 General approach to the treatment of toxicoses.

Ingested toxins

Lead poisoning
Lead ingestion is a relatively common cause of poisoning in captive raptors. Lead is usually ingested in the form of shotgun pellets or fragments of rifle rounds present in the tissues of an animal that was either shot (Figure 26.2) or had ingested the pellets. It is common practice in falconry to feed with care any prey species caught by a hunting hawk, but the fact that the food item was caught by the hawk does not rule out a previous non-fatal shot injury. Another common misconception is that the carcasses of head-shot rabbits are safe to feed to captive raptors. Radiographs of such carcasses have revealed the dissemination of metallic fragments throughout the body, therefore still posing a risk.

Raptors have a built-in defence mechanism against lead poisoning by virtue of the act of casting (regurgitating indigestible portions of their meal) within

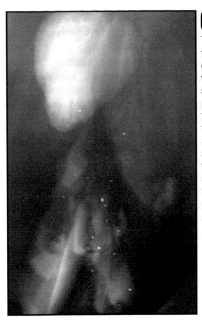

26.2
This radiograph of the heart and lung of a roe deer shot with a single bullet shows multiple lead pieces distributed throughout its tissues. Thus, animals killed by shooting, of whatever type, should not be used to feed raptors. (Courtesy of A. Valentin)

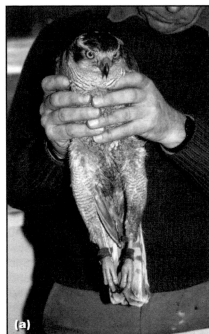

26.3
(a) Goshawk demonstrating hind limb paresis due to lead poisoning.
(b) Lead toxicity in a Peregrine Falcon. Note the posture, sitting on the 'hocks' with feet clenched. (a, courtesy of Neil Forbes; b, © John Chitty)

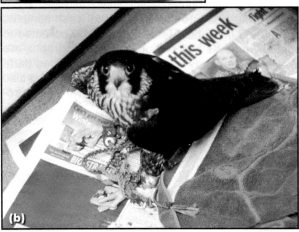

12–18 hours after eating. If the hawk has not been fed any such material (i.e. feather, fur) the problem will be exacerbated with the bird unable to expel the offending lead pellets. Lead also appears to reduce stomach motility, further exacerbating its effects.

Particles that remain in the digestive tract are exposed to corrosive stomach acids. Lead is therefore released, absorbed into the systemic circulation, and deposited throughout the body. Lead competes with calcium, interfering with many of its important functions. It is also taken up into the bone and in cases of chronic intoxication clinical signs may become obvious in laying females during calcium mobilization. It also produces anaemia in affected animals by interfering with the action of enzymes (alpha-aminolaevulenic acid), especially those involved in haemoglobin synthesis.

Lead particles not exposed to stomach acid, such as those lodged in muscle or bone (from a previous non-fatal shot injury for example), remain intact and pose minimal threat to the bird. As such, unless particles are very superficial or associated with an active inflammatory response, surgical removal is generally not indicated.

Raptor species vary greatly in their sensitivity to lead intoxication. The amount ingested and its rate of passage through the digestive tract also influence the range and severity of clinical signs in affected birds. Initial clinical signs of lead intoxication include depression, anorexia, crop stasis and weight loss, leading to a number of neurological deficits including hind limb paresis (Figure 26.3), visual disturbances and convulsions. Green diarrhoea with biliverdinuria (see Chapter 7) is also characteristic of the disease.

Diagnosis: The two main diagnostic aids for lead toxicosis are radiography and blood lead levels. Lead pellets are extremely radiodense and thus easily visualized radiographically (Figure 26.4). Both lateral and ventrodorsal views are recommended to ensure that any metallic fragments are in the intestinal tract

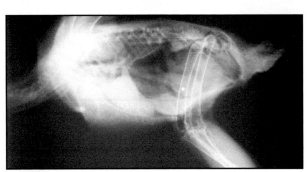

26.4 Radiograph demonstrating lead in the proventriculus of a Saker Falcon. (Courtesy of Jaime Samour)

and not incidental fragments in soft tissue/bone or radiographic artefacts. Radiology alone, however, is not reliable: in one study (Redig, 1993) only 15% of raptors diagnosed with lead poisoning had pellets still retained in the intestinal tract at time of admission. Furthermore, given the current use of non-toxic steel/bismuth-based shot, radiodense objects present in the stomach may not necessarily be lead.

wall. Endoscopic examination of crop and proventriculus revealed marked inflammation of the mucosa. Haematology in all cases revealed a severe leucopenia. In a number of cases secondary intestinal and crop candidiasis was apparent. Successful treatment of such cases involved broad-spectrum antibiotics, fluconazole (2–5 mg/kg q24h), metoclopramide (2 mg/kg i.m. q12h) fluid therapy and tube feeding directly into the proventriculus, bypassing the crop, over a period of 3–5 days until appetite returned. Obviously with the widespread use of this formulation in a variety of avian species with no apparent adverse effects, the above cases may have been species-specific idiosyncratic reactions or overdoses. However, the author is of the opinion that it should be used with caution in raptors and only if deemed appropriate following faecal parasitology at a maximum dose of 25 mg/kg with the 2.5% suspension (where overdosage is less likely).

Ivermectin: Fatalities have occurred in birds following ivermectin injection. They can be due to overdosage of the ivermectin but in smaller psittacines, for example, propylene glycol (used to dilute the ivermectin) has been implicated. Blindness, seizures and death can occur. Intensive nursing and administration of dexamethasone have been successful in the treatment of suspected cases of toxicity.

Metronidazole: Tremors, convulsions and extensor rigidity have been observed in birds following overdosage with dimetronidazole/metronidazole and deaths have occurred in psittacids. Toxicity is usually reversible with withdrawal of medication and supportive therapy.

Other preparations: Nephrotoxicity may be seen with aminoglycoside antimicrobials, parenteral amphotericin B and injectable amoxicillin/clavulanate (NA Forbes, personal communication). Other preparations implicated in toxic episodes in raptors include a variety of vitamin/mineral supplements (usually from exceeding manufacturer's recommendations). Toxicoses generally arise with over-supplementation of the fat-soluble vitamins D, E, A and K. In raptors the most common presentation involves vitamin D3 which, in excessive levels, causes mobilization of calcium from bone, resulting in soft tissue calcification and in some cases renal failure. There have been reports of vitamin B6 intoxication in raptors, a problem that was previously described only in pigeons.

Oncology

Historically the diagnosis of neoplasia in birds of prey has been a relatively rare occurrence but the likelihood of neoplasia may well increase with longevity, inbreeding and exposure to potential carcinogens.

Relatively little is known about the aetiology, pathogenesis, incidence and behaviour of neoplasms affecting captive and free-ranging raptors (Forbes *et al.*, 2000). Neoplasms can be classified according to their tissue origins (e.g. connective tissue, fibrous or muscle) or by their cellular composition and activity (e.g. benign or malignant). They may present as obvious palpable masses (e.g. some cutaneous tumours) or may occur within major organs (e.g. liver) where their presence may be more difficult to diagnose at an early stage. Neoplasms affecting raptors are described in Figure 26.6.

Tumour	Species	Behaviour	Treatment
Tumours of connective tissue			
Fibrosarcoma	Peregrine Falcon, Northern Goshawk, Red-tailed Hawk, miscellaneous owls, falcons, eagles	Sites include head, neck, wings, legs, flanks and feet. Described as locally invasive with potential to metastasize	Prompt surgical excision usually curative. Intratumoral cisplatin and orthovoltage radiotherapy has been used successfully on fibrosarcoma in a macaw
Myxofibroma	Cape Griffon Vulture	Site: plantar aspect of foot. Locally invasive, regrowth likely	Surgical excision
Fibroma	European Kestrel	Rare. Firm masses with predilection for skin/subcutaneous tissues of wing, leg, face, beak, neck or sternum	Surgical excision
Histiocytic sarcoma	Great Horned Owl	Multicentric distribution. Large highly pleomorphic tumours. Retrovirus involvement suspected but not confirmed	Euthanasia if extensive
Tumours of adipose tissue			
Lipoma (Figure 26.7)	Northern Goshawk, American Kestrel, Saker Falcon, Gyrfalcon	Sites included feet, dorsal wing and adjacent to preen gland. Rare benign neoplasm of raptors	Surgical excision

26.6 Neoplasms in raptors. (Data courtesy of NA Forbes, JE Cooper and RJ Higgins) (continues) ▶

Tumour	Species	Behaviour	Treatment
Tumours of bone, cartilage and muscle			
Osteosarcoma	Hybrid falcon, Eurasian Buzzard	Sites were radius and sternum. Slow growing but destructive	Euthanasia usually indicated
Osteoma/chondroma	European Kestrel and miscellaneous owls	Sites include radius, frontal bone and tibiotarsus. Benign	Such tumours are curable if complete surgical removal is practical
Rhabdomyosarcoma	Lappet-faced Vulture	Site was myocardium found at necropsy	
Leiomyoma	Golden Eagle	Site was digit of foot although more typically arise from smooth muscle of gut, female reproductive tract	Surgical excision was curative in the described case
Mixed cell tumour	Seychelles Kestrel	Multiple lesions were found on the chest and head at necropsy. Tumour showed a mixture of tissues including lymphangiomatous, epithelial and chondromatous	
Tumours of glandular tissues			
Adenocarcinoma	Common Buzzard, Red-tailed Hawk, Peregrine Falcon, Bearded Vulture, Ayres Hawk Eagle, Mauritius Kestrel, Merlin, Lanner Falcon, Golden Eagle, Northern Goshawk, Little Owl, Great Horned Owl	Primary tumour involved a variety of glandular organs (oviduct, liver, preen gland, kidney, salivary gland, skin) with secondary tumours in many other tissues, particularly liver and lung. Most cases fatal though for those where lesion was confined to preen gland surgical excision was curative	Surgical excision where possible (preen gland)
Adenoma	Hybrid falcon, Long-crested Eagle, Red-tailed Hawk	Nasolacrimal duct and kidney	Surgical excision where practical but majority found at necropsy
Carcinoma	Merlin, Red-tailed Hawk, Augur Buzzard	All cases found at necropsy. These aggressive neoplasms (some with marked necrosis) were found in kidney and air sac with secondary tumours in the liver	
Endocrine tumours (all incidental findings at necropsy)			
Thyroid follicular cystadenoma, thyroid cystic fibroadenoma	Crested Caracara, Black-chested Buzzard Eagle	Benign proliferation of areas of thyroid follicles	
Adrenal cortical carcinoma	Long-crested Eagle	Neoplastic transformation of adrenal cortical cells	
Integumental tumours			
Squamous cell carcinoma	Peregrine Falcon, Lanner Falcon, Red-tailed Hawk, European Eagle Owl, Harris' Hawk, Bald Eagle, Montague's Harrier	Affected sites were predominately flank or thigh with single cases affecting palate, metatarsal skin, cloaca and tail base. Classed as locally invasive with potential to slowly metastasize. Ulceration of overlying skin with secondary infection is common feature	Surgical excision or the topical use of 5-fluorouracil has been described in other species and so may have merit in raptors
Epidermoid carcinoma	Red-tailed Hawk	Sites include pharynx and membrane nictitans	Surgical excision of nictitating membrane
Papilloma	Peregrine Falcon, King Vulture, Northern Goshawk, Tawny Eagle, Lanner Falcon	Sites include crop, glottis, cloaca and digit. Lesions proliferative, often with fibrovascular stalks. In psittacids, hepatic and bile duct carcinoma lesions may be secondary to cloacal or choanal papilloma and in other birds cutaneous papillomatosis has been shown to be virus-induced	Digital, cloacal and glottal cases were cured by surgical excision although all cases not treated by surgery appeared to be self-limiting
Haemangioma	Peregrine Falcon	Site: skin of dorsal cranium	Surgical excision was curative
Mast cell tumour	Burrowing Owl, Great Horned Owl, Short-eared Owl	Lesions limited to oral cavity and head and demonstrated proliferation of mast cells that contained granules that stained well with toluidine blue or Giemsa stain	Wide surgical excision can be curative but regrowth common

26.6 (continued) Neoplasms in raptors. (Data courtesy of NA Forbes, JE Cooper and RJ Higgins) (continues) ▶

Tumour	Species	Behaviour	Treatment
Tumours of eye and neural tissue			
Melanoma	Great Horned Owl, Striped Owl, Red-tailed Hawk	Clinical cases affected eye; incidental findings at necropsy of such neoplasms included lung and adrenal gland	Enucleation should only be considered in extreme circumstances in raptors and cannot be recommended in falconry or wild hawks
Astrocytoma	Great Horned Owl	Single case detected in brain stem	
Lymphoid tumours			
Malignant lymphoma	Peregrine Falcon, Gyrfalcon, Snowy Owl	Lesions seen in bone marrow, lungs, liver, pericardium, kidney, spleen, small intestine, testes and fat. Postulated viral origin but to date virus isolation unsuccessful	
Malignant thymoma	Saker Falcon	One case reported at necropsy. Lesions found in lungs, suggesting metastatic spread from thymus	
Lymphoid leucosis	Merlin, Grey Kestrel, Harris' Hawk, European Eagle Owl	Lesions found in liver and other viscera. Retroviridae have been shown to cause neoplasms in poultry and possibly other species. In raptors virus isolation where attempted was negative	
Erythroblastosis	Gyrfalcon	Form of erythrocytic leukaemia	
Lymphosarcoma	Harris' Hawk, Great Horned Owl, miscellaneous hawks	Neoplastic lymphocytic cells infiltrating a variety of tissues, including the bone marrow. Immature (neoplastic) lymphocytes may be observed in blood film	
Marek's disease	Eurasian Sparrowhawk, Great Horned Owl, Little Owl (all cases were free ranging)	Sites included sciatic nerve, liver, spleen, kidney and pancreas	
Miscellaneous tumours			
Teratoma	Eurasian Buzzard	Abdominal mass	
Xanthoma	Eurasian Buzzard, Bateleur, Merlin	Sites included infraorbital sinus, abdomen, spleen and liver. Xanthoma not a true neoplasm but inflammatory intumescence resulting from lipid-laden macrophages, giant cells, free cholesterol and fibrosis and appears as yellow subcutaneous nodules or thickenings which may be featherless and ulcerated. Often found at sites of chronic trauma/inflammation	Clinical cases can be managed with surgical excision where possible
Mesothelioma	Ferruginous Hawk	Lesions (papillomatous branching tumours) found at necropsy were in triosseum, pneumatic humerus and lung	

26.6 (continued) Neoplasms in raptors. (Data courtesy of NA Forbes, JE Cooper and RJ Higgins)

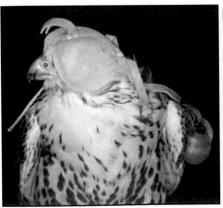

26.7 An infiltrating lipoma involving the carpus of a Saker Falcon. (Courtesy of Jaime Samour)

Diagnosis

When presented with a possible case of neoplasia it is advisable to carry out a thorough examination, assessing the bird as a whole and then concentrating on the tumour itself. In this way intercurrent disease and any additional tumour lesions may be detected. These may influence the overall outcome of the case. Although fine-needle aspiration and cytology may be of use in such cases, a definitive diagnosis is only obtained through biopsy and histopathological examination by an experienced avian pathologist. For internal neoplasia, radiography, clinical chemistry and endoscopy-guided biopsy may all need to be employed.

Therapy

Although there is some historical information on the diagnosis and treatment of avian neoplasms, clinicians should be aware of the great advances in comparative oncology in recent years and consider using therapeutic regimes that have proved to be effective in other species. Treatment of neoplasia in birds has relied largely on surgery. The use of chemotherapy and radiation is a new and relatively unexplored field. A number of chemotherapeutic agents have recently been used in birds, including prednisolone, doxorubicin, cisplatin, chlorambucil, cyclophosphamide, vincristine and alpha-interferon, often with good responses (Forbes *et al.*, 2000). When confronted with a confirmed case of neoplasia a current literature search is warranted due to the rapid advances and changes in treatment recommendations. Most reports of treatment protocols are either anecdotal or involve a single patient. Many are not published but are to be found in avian discussion groups on the internet, which can be an extremely useful source of information on such topics. In addition, consultation with a veterinary oncologist will increase the likelihood of selecting an appropriate treatment regime and properly administering the chosen therapy.

Cardiovascular disease

Cardiovascular disease has traditionally been underdiagnosed in the raptor patient. In the majority of cases, disease involving the heart or vascular system is discovered incidentally at necropsy. Ischaemic heart disease, pericardial effusions, vegetative endocarditis and aortic ruptures have been identified this way in raptors. In contrast, *in vivo* diagnosis is comparatively rare, due to the non-specific clinical signs and accompanying disease overlying the cardiac signs.

Cardiovascular examination can be challenging, since the rapid heart rate can make detection of murmurs and arrhythmias difficult and there is often difficulty in peripheral pulse detection. Clinical signs of heart disease are similar to those in mammals. Exercise intolerance, dyspnoea, hepatic congestion and ascites are seen, but coughing is generally not a feature in the avian patient.

Diagnosis is based on history, physical examination and auscultation. A complete haematology and biochemistry analysis together with radiography, electrocardiography (ECG; see Chapter 12), endoscopy and ultrasonography are indicated in suspected cases of heart disease and are probably best performed under isoflurane or sevoflurane anaesthesia.

Peripheral blood pressure can be measured using a sphygmomanometer and appropriately sized small animal cuff. A Doppler unit is used for the audio pulse. Sites for placement of the cuff are the upper humerus or thigh. The Doppler is placed distal to the cuff. Systolic blood pressure is considered elevated above 180 on either the wing or leg site.

As well as being able to visualize the heart and major vessels directly, endoscopy provides the opportunity to collect fluid present in the pericardial sac for bacteriology, cytology and clinical chemistries.

Atherosclerosis

Atherosclerosis has been described in birds of prey. It affects primarily the brachiocephalic trunk and abdominal aorta and is characterized by degenerative changes and the deposition of collagen, cholesterol and calcium in the arterial wall, decreasing the diameter of the vessel (Figure 26.8).

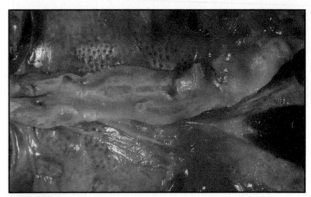

26.8 Atherosclerotic lesions in the aorta of a Peregrine Falcon. (Courtesy of Pat Redig and Arno Wunschmann)

Clinical signs of atherosclerosis are rarely reported and it is often associated with sudden death, but subtle and intermittent signs that include dyspnoea, weakness and neurological signs may be present. Blood chemistry (see Chapter 9) may reveal elevated plasma cholesterol (in particular the low density fraction). In some cases radiographs indicate a prominent aortic arch. Overfeeding and lack of exercise are associated with this condition in birds and generally such patients are over 5 years of age. Risk factors such as elevated blood cholesterol and high serum lipids probably play a role, as in mammals. Raptors easily become overweight under captive conditions and those that do are at a much higher risk of developing the disease. In birds fed *ad libitum* and not exercised regularly, it is advisable to have at least one fasting day per week as a preventive measure.

Endocardial disease

Vegetative endocarditis of the aortic and mitral valve may cause vascular insufficiency, lethargy and dyspnoea. Valvular endocarditis is most common in birds with chronic infections (e.g. salpingitis, hepatitis or bumblefoot) and has been described in raptors. Factors that have been associated with endocardial or valvular lesions include chronic bacterial septicaemia and degenerative myocarditis (in which cases blood cultures are used to identify and thus properly address a causative agent), frostbite and congenital lesions that alter blood flow. Frequently implicated bacteria include streptococci, staphylococci, *Escherichia coli*, *Pasteurella*, *Pseudomonas aeruginosa* and *Erysipelothrix rhusiopathiae*. Lesions consist of yellow irregular masses on any of the heart valves.

Myocarditis and cardiomyopathy

In mammals myocarditis can occur secondary to many common viral, bacterial, mycotic and protozoal infections. Cardiomyopathy has been associated with thyroid diseases, anaemia, malnutrition, metabolic disorders, neoplasia and toxaemia. The pathogenesis of myocarditis and cardiomyopathy in birds is similar to that described in mammals.

Sarcocysts (muscle cysts containing bradyzoites, the asexual generation of *Sarcocystis* spp.) have been reported in the myocardium of European Sparrowhawks. A degenerative condition of the myocardium has been reported in Bald Eagles in association with lead toxicity. Dilated cardiomyopathy has been described as a cause of mortality in captive bearded vultures.

All conditions that lead to cardiomyopathy or myocarditis may result in increased myocardial irritability and cardiac arrhythmias that can be detected by ECG. Radiographs and echocardiography may reveal cardiomegaly in such cases.

Pericardial disease

Pericardial effusion is a relatively common finding in birds. Transudates occur with congestive heart failure and hypoproteinaemia. Exudates may be present in a variety of infections (e.g. *Escherichia coli*, *Strepto-coccus*, *Salmonella*). Tuberculous and mycotic pericarditis have been described in raptors, as has pericarditis urica in birds with visceral gout (see later). Haemopericardium may occur as a result of trauma or neoplasia-induced rupture of the myocardium.

Principles of therapy

Before deciding on a treatment regime when dealing with the performance falconry bird or wild raptor, careful consideration must be given to the prognosis and likelihood of recovery to full fitness. Although certain conditions such as bacterial endocarditis may respond well to treatment, in many cases of advanced cardiac disease in raptors euthanasia is indicated on humane grounds. Falconers often develop a very strong bond with their hunting hawks and, although cardiac disease may spell the end of a bird's hunting career, in exceptional circumstances the falconer may wish to manage the condition medically and retire the bird to an aviary to live out its life.

Pharmacokinetic information is only available on a small number of drugs in a small number of avian species, so much is extrapolated from mammalian medicine.

Cardiac glycosides

These improve contraction and relaxation of the heart muscle and decrease the beat frequency. This leads to a reduction of oxygen need and an improvement of circulation of blood in the coronary vessels. Resorption of ascites and/or oedema increases. Digoxin is the most commonly used and indications include emergency situations and cardiac diseases that involve volume overload, e.g. valvular insufficiency. Its therapeutic margin is very small and side effects can be similar to the initial presentation for cardiac failure, i.e. lethargy, anorexia, emesis, diarrhoea, ascites and oedema. Elimination times vary significantly between species. Contraindications are ventricular tachycardia, AV block, hypercalcaemia and hypokalaemia. It may be best used initially to stabilize a bird in an emergency rather than for long-term therapy. Initial doses are suggested at 0.02–0.05 mg/kg q12h for 2–3 days, then decreased to 0.01 mg/kg q12–24h.

Antiarrhythmics

Prior to treatment, causes of arrhythmias due to electrolyte imbalances need to be excluded. To date these drugs have only been investigated in turkeys to protect against the development of atherosclerotic plaques, so their role in the raptor patient needs further investigation. Oxprenolol has been used at 2 mg/kg orally daily. Other potential uses, such as for supraventricular or ventricular arrhythmias, have not been described.

ACE inhibitors

Angiotension-converting enzyme inhibitors seem to be of greatest value in many types of avian heart disease and appear fairly safe. The mechanism of ACE inhibitors is based on inhibition of angiotensin II, which is responsible for contraction of arterial and venous vessels and subsequent retention of sodium and water in the kidneys. Inhibition leads to improvement of kidney function and increased diuresis, and it decreases blood pressure. It decreases pre- and after-load on the heart, allowing cardiac muscle cells to recover. A suggested dose of enalapril in birds is 5 mg/kg/day with reduction in dose down to 1 mg/kg/day with improvement in clinical signs. It can be combined initially with diuretics as well as glycosides.

Calcium sensitizers

Calcium sensitizers (e.g. pimobendan) are substances with a positive inotropic effect that also improve myocardial oxygen economy and contribute to peripheral arterio- and venodilation. They are indicated in mammalian cases of congestive heart failure and so may have merit in similar avian cases. To date, however, as with so many other agents, scientific reports of their use in the avian patient are lacking.

Diuretics

While the exact pharmacodynamic mechanisms of furosemide are not known in birds, it does appear to effect diuresis. Indications for use include oedema, ascites and pericardial effusion. Dosage is usually 0.1–2.0 mg/kg/day orally or i.m. (Harrison and Lightfoot, 2006). As in mammals, long-term treatment can lead to potassium deficiency, and hydration must be monitored closely.

Nephrology

Renal disease in raptors is often difficult to diagnose because clinical signs are generally non-specific and frequently complicated by secondary changes caused by renal dysfunction. When compared with mammalian counterparts, the avian urogenital system has many structural and functional differences, which need to be considered. One of the most unique features of the avian kidney is the presence of two types of nephron: those with a loop of Henle (mammalian type) and thus able to concentrate urine; and those without (reptilian type). Since birds have primarily 'reptilian'-type nephrons, which produce isosmotic urine, urine concentration is limited. It does occur, however, via the coprodeum and rectum, which are capable of both water and electrolyte resorption. Birds, unlike mammals, also have a renal portal system which works by either directing blood to or shunting it past the kidney as directed by the renal portal valve (see Chapter 5). This of course means that blood may pass through the kidneys prior to any other organ and therefore has implications when drugs are administered into the hind limbs. This may therefore increase the effects of nephrotoxic drugs and/or enhance the elimination of medication by taking the compound directly to the kidney (see Chapter 8).

Clinical signs

Clinical signs of renal disease are generally non-specific in the avian patient as most are part of multi-systemic disease.

Lethargy, anorexia, regurgitation, weight loss, polydipsia/polyuria and changes in colour or consistency of the urine fraction are all typical of renal disease in raptors. Lameness can also be a feature of renal disease, due to pressure on the ischiadic nerve by the swollen kidney.

Diagnosis

To diagnose renal disease accurately a thorough clinical investigation, including haematology, biochemistry, radiography and biopsy, is required.

Urate examination

Urinalysis is not routinely performed in avian medicine because of the difficulty in separating the urine from the urate and faecal portion. Changes in colour or consistency of urates, however, are often an indication of disease. A green-tinged urate portion often indicates renal haemorrhage or hepatic disease due to reduced capacity to conjugate biliverdin pigments (see Chapter 7). Haemolysis (e.g. due to *Plasmodium* infection) may also lead to excess amounts of biliverdin being passed by the affected bird. The identification of casts in urinary sediment is strongly suggestive of renal disease.

Radiography

Radiography is useful for visualizing kidney size and density. A reduction in size and increase in density generally accompany dehydration, with swelling evident in cases of nephritis, gout or neoplasia.

Haematology and biochemistry

Changes in haematology parameters with suspected renal disease are again relatively non-specific and can include heterophilia and anaemia. Selected plasma biochemistries may provide useful information with regard to renal function and pathology. Plasma uric acid can be a useful screening tool for renal disease, but filtration must decrease by 70–80% before plasma uric acid is elevated. It has been demonstrated that a significant postprandial increase in plasma uric acid and urea concentration occurs in clinically normal raptors, including

Peregrine Falcon and Red-tailed Hawk. It is therefore recommended that raptors are fasted for at least 8 hours prior to sampling.

Endoscopy, biopsy and CT scanning

Endoscopy is extremely useful in the investigation of renal disease, as size can be assessed together with the possible identification of cysts, neoplasia, gout or granulomas (see Chapter 13).

A definitive diagnosis can only be obtained via biopsy. The preferred site is the cranial pole of the kidney via a lateral approach through the caudal thoracic air sac.

A more detailed description of renal disease and its diagnosis may be found in Lierz (2003). Recently CT scanning has been of use in the investigation of renal disease in the avian patient (see Chapter 12).

Renal diseases

Viral infection

A number of viruses can affect the raptor kidney, including herpesvirus, adenovirus and paramyxovirus. However, they are usually part of a generalized infectious process.

Bacterial infection

Bacterial infections of the kidney are most commonly acquired via the haematogenous route, resulting in both interstitial nephritis and glomerular nephritis. They often occur secondary to septicaemia but may also result from bacteria that ascend from the cloaca. Because of the renal portal system and possible shunting of blood from the intestines directly to the kidneys, alimentary tract organisms may contribute to kidney infections and should be considered when using antimicrobial therapy. Diagnostically, white blood cell count evaluation, total protein measurement and blood/urine cultures may reveal the causative organism.

Fungal infection

Infection of the kidney by fungal agents is generally as a result of direct spread from air sac granulomas caused by *Aspergillus* spp. Because the infection is localized, specific renal signs are unlikely to be seen.

Congenital defects

Renal agenesis, hypoplasia and polycystic kidneys have been reported in a number of avian species, including raptors, and are believed to be hereditary in nature (Styles and Phalen, 1998). Affected birds may be asymptomatic or present in acute renal failure, depending on the severity of the lesion.

Toxicity

Many nephrotoxins cause renal tubular necrosis in raptors, including lead, aminoglycoside antibacterials, mycotoxins from *Aspergillus* spp. and non-steroidal anti-inflammatory drugs. The veterinary use of diclofenac has been specifically implicated in the decline of the critically endangered Oriental White-backed Vulture in Asia.

Amyloidosis

Renal, splenic and hepatic amyloidosis have been described in falcons usually in association with chronic inflammation including bumblefoot, aspergillosis or severe crop trichomoniasis. It may also arise without evidence of an inflammatory focus, believed to be a primary immune-mediated syndrome, or as a single disease entity without a prominent underlying cause, possibly due to a chronic immune system response.

Nutritional disorders

Fatty liver/kidney syndrome has been described in captive Merlins and was thought to be associated with obesity and a high-fat diet consisting solely of day-old chicks.

Neoplasia

Renal carcinoma, adenocarcinoma, lymphosarcoma and malignant lymphoma have all been described in raptors.

Ureteral obstruction

Displacement or obstruction of ureteral orifices can occur due to intestinal or cloacal prolapse or cloacal obstruction caused by egg binding, faecoliths, uroliths, foreign bodies, tumours or inflammatory conditions. A bilateral obstruction will rapidly lead to visceral gout. Unilateral obstructions will lead to atrophy and compensatory hypertrophy of the contralateral kidney. Cloacal uroliths appear to be over-represented in Barn Owls and can be removed with care under general anaesthesia.

Articular and visceral gout

Hyperuricaemia is defined as any plasma uric acid concentration higher than the calculated limit of solubility of sodium urate in plasma and is an indication of nephrosis or impaired renal function. Prolonged hyperuricaemia can result in urate precipitation in joints (articular gout) and in visceral organs or other extra-visceral sites (visceral gout) (Figure 26.9). Gout should not be regarded as a disease entity but as a clinical

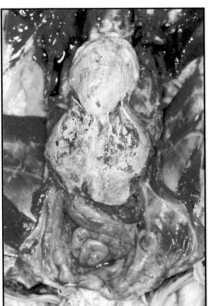

26.9

Visceral gout: urate crystals on the pericardium and liver capsule on post-mortem examination of a hybrid falcon. (Courtesy of Jaime Samour)

sign of any severe renal dysfunction that causes a chronic moderate hyperuricaemia. The joints and synovial sheaths may be predilection sites because of a lower temperature than the rest of the body. Articular gout is rare but has been reported in raptors (mainly Strigiformes) and presents as pasty white deposits in a variety of articulations. Visceral/renal gout will rapidly lead to death of the affected animal.

Therapy

Treatment options for renal disorders in birds depend upon the cause and type of kidney disease and secondary complications present. Most renal patients are medically managed. Surgery may be indicated in cases of articular gout, where small incisions are made over the lesions under general anaesthesia and the pasty material is expressed manually. This procedure is often bloody and so a tourniquet may be placed proximal to the foot, with postoperative bandaging to control haemorrhage and prevent secondary infection. Cloacoliths and other cloacal masses may be easily removed to relieve a potential ureteral obstruction. Although not yet reported in raptors, successful extra-corporeal shockwave litho-tripsy for removal of uric acid concrements in the urinary tract has been described in birds (Machedo et al., 1997). Renal masses can be biopsied or even removed/debulked via endoscopy and/or diode laser.

Diuresis and fluid therapy

As in other animals with renal disease, maintaining hydration is essential in birds with most kidney disorders.

Anuric and oliguric patients require diuresis. Clinically, providing parenteral fluids often induces diuresis in birds, even those suffering from most forms of renal disease. Until acid–base and electrolyte disorders have been better evaluated in birds with renal disease, balanced electrolyte solutions should be used to maintain hydration, replace fluid losses and induce diuresis as needed.

The estimated daily fluid requirement for most birds is approximately 50 ml/kg/day. In addition, it has been recommended that 10% of the bird's body weight should be given in fluids when the patient shows renal compromise. Once a dose has been determined, warmed fluids should be given via the intravenous, intraosseous, subcutaneous or oral (tube/syringe feeding) route. The intravenous and intraosseous routes are the most appropriate for critically ill patients (see Chapter 8).

Fluid therapy (in combination with other necessary medication) is generally continued until uric acid levels drop to within normal limits and clinically the bird is showing signs of improvement (e.g. eating, more active, improvement in urate colour and consistency).

Antibiotics

Antibiotics are indicated in patients with known or suspected bacterial nephritis. Drug choices are based on an isolated renal organism (i.e. identified via kidney biopsy) or a suspected infectious agent (blood, salpinx, or cloacal/faecal cultures) and their ability to enter the nephron via the glomerulus. Clinical consideration of potential antimicrobial-induced toxicities is important. Although mammalian literature warns of potential nephrotoxicity with amphotericin B, cephalosporin, fluoroquinolone, trimethoprim/sulphonamide and tetracycline use, only aminoglycosides and injectable potentiated amoxicillin have been definitively associated with renal disease in raptors. The author presently favours marbofloxacin at a dose of 10 mg/kg q24h for cases of suspected bacterial nephritis as a first line antibiotic, unless cultures suggest otherwise.

Managing hyperuricaemia

In Psittaciformes and Columbiformes, allopurinol has been recommended as an adjunct therapy in cases of renal disease and has been shown to decrease uric acid production. Specifically, allopurinol inhibits xanthine oxidase, which is required to convert hypoxanthine to xanthine and subsequently to uric acid. However, in Red-tailed Hawks allopurinol has been shown to be toxic at higher doses (see Chapter 7) and its use in raptors is controversial.

Urate oxidase (Uricozyme), a drug that metabolizes uric acid and is used in human cancer therapy, might also prove useful for the treatment of hyperuricaemia in birds. Urate oxidase catalyses the conversion of urate and oxygen into allantoin and hydrogen peroxide, which is further degraded and excreted as allantoic acid. In one promising study urate oxidase was given to pigeons and Red-tailed Hawks; when compared with controls, a number of dosing regimes caused a significant decrease in plasma uric acid concentration within 2 days of the first dose.

In humans, colchicine is known for its anti-gout activity. Clinical use of colchicine suggests possible benefit in reducing hyperuricaemia in birds.

Hepatic disease

Physical findings associated with liver disease are often non-specific and so their diagnosis can present a significant challenge. Clinical signs are often the classic 'sick bird' signs of fluffed-up oval-eyed appearance, anorexia, depression and occasionally polydipsia and polyuria. In chronic cases poor feather, beak and talon quality may be a feature. Vomiting, coelomic swelling and dehydration may be observed. Coelomic swelling due to hepatic enlargement may cause tachypnoea or dyspnoea by exerting pressure on the air sac system. Weight loss despite polyphagia can be a feature of chronic disease. Apparent hepatic encephalopathy has been observed as a sign of advanced liver disease in birds (M Stanford and K Eatwell, personal communication) but its pathogenesis is not well understood.

Green urates are suggestive of liver disease (see Chapter 7). Icterus or jaundice caused by hyperbilirubinaemia is not a feature of avian hepatic disease.

Avian plasma may be coloured yellow by carotenoids (in the case of captive raptors, ingested from food items, especially yolk from day-old chicks) and this normal colour should not be misinterpreted

as icteric plasma. However, following haemolysis (due to *Plasmodium* infection, for example) the plasma may become green due to biliverdinaemia.

Diagnosis

A detailed history is required, covering all aspects of husbandry (housing, recent food items, drugs administered, any recent trauma), together with clinical examination. Palpation of the enlarged liver is possible just beyond the caudal edge of the sternum. Blood sampling (full haematological and plasma biochemical analysis), radiography and laparoscopic examination should be performed as part of the investigation, but a definitive diagnosis can only be obtained following biopsy (via either midline laparotomy incision or laparoscopy). Ultrasonography may also have merit in cases of suspected liver disease to evaluate hepatic architecture (especially if the bird is ascitic) (see Chapter 12).

Haematology

Estimation of the packed cell volume, haemoglobin and leucocyte counts should give some indication of the degree of dehydration, anaemia or the presence of an infectious agent. The presence of blood parasites (*Plasmodium*, *Leucocytozoon*) can also be noted.

Plasma biochemistry

Plasma biochemical parameters are rarely specific for liver disease in birds. Elevated aspartate aminotransferase (AST) alone does not establish liver disease, as levels are also raised following muscle cell damage. To differentiate liver from muscle damage, bile acids and creatine kinase (CK) (elevated in muscle damage but not in liver damage) should also be measured. AST is not necessarily increased in chronic hepatic conditions and levels may be normal in birds with relatively severe liver pathology. Moderate to severe elevations in bile acids (250–700 μmol/l) indicate a marked loss of hepatic function and a poor prognosis (e.g. severe hepatic fibrosis, advanced hepatic lipidosis and active infections). Minimally elevated levels (50–150 μmol/l) suggest discrete liver lesions with some normally functioning liver remaining (hepatic neoplasia, e.g. lymphoma, or granulomatous inflammation, e.g. mycobacteriosis). It should be noted that haemolysis and lipaemia might falsely elevate results. Cholinesterase is synthesized in the liver and therefore a decreased level indicates liver malfunction (see Chapter 9).

Imaging

Both hepatomegaly and ascites due to liver disease may be diagnosed radiographically (Figure 26.10).

Endoscopic examination and biopsy

The laparoscopic approach to the liver and biopsy technique is described in detail in Chapter 13. Endoscopy of the liver can provide valuable information regarding change in colour or consistency of the liver parenchyma (e.g. in hepatic lipidosis, neoplasia) or the presence of granulomas or microabscesses (e.g. tuberculosis, yersiniosis, aspergillosis).

295

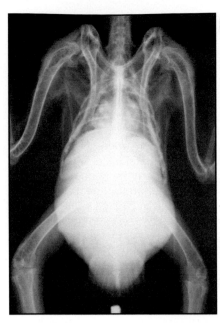

26.10

Radiograph demonstrating marked hepatomegaly/ascites and loss of the normal hourglass shape of the cardiohepatic silhouette. (Courtesy of Jaime Samour)

Liver biopsy, however, is required for a definitive diagnosis of hepatic disease. Although relatively easy to perform, the procedure does carry a degree of risk, since blood-clotting ability may be compromised in birds with liver disorders. Birds that have prolonged bleeding times following venepuncture or evidence of thrombocytopenia are not good candidates for liver biopsy. Indications for biopsy are in patients where there is hepatomegaly or gross pathology evident on laparoscopic examination.

Hepatic lipidosis

Lipids are normally transported to the liver from the gastrointestinal tract and adipose tissue in the form of chylomicrons and free fatty acids, respectively. Within hepatocytes, free fatty acids are esterified to triglycerides that are complexed with apoproteins to form low-density lipoproteins, which are released into plasma as a readily available energy source. Hepatic lipidosis, or fatty liver, occurs when the rate of triglyceride accumulation within the hepatocytes exceeds either their rate of metabolic degradation or their release as lipoproteins.

Hepatic lipidosis is not a specific disease entity but can occur as a sequel to a variety of disturbances of normal lipid metabolism. Excessive dietary intake of fat or increased mobilization of triglycerides from adipose tissue subsequent to increased demand, such as starvation or endocrine abnormalities, may be responsible. A fatty liver and kidney syndrome has been described in captive Merlins (see Chapter 17).

Hepatotoxins

The liver is the most common site for toxic injuries. It receives the majority of its blood supply from the portal vein, draining blood from the gastrointestinal tract. Therefore ingested toxic substances, including bacterial products (clostridial toxins), heavy metals (e.g. lead from contaminated food items), pharmaceuticals and other chemicals absorbed into the portal blood, are transported to the liver. The liver possesses enzymes capable of metabolizing a variety of endogenous and exogenous substances for elimination from the body. This metabolic process may alter some substances such that they become toxic. Toxin production may result in necrosis of hepatocytes, which may be replaced by fibrotic cells or infiltrated with lipids. This process can be self-perpetuating, even if the inciting agent is no longer present.

Neoplasia

Liver tumours can be primary or metastatic and include hepatic carcinoma, adenocarcinoma, bile duct carcinoma and lymphosarcoma (see above).

Amyloidosis

Hepatic amyloidosis in raptors generally occurs as a consequence of prolonged inflammation resulting from chronic infection or tissue destruction (e.g. bumblefoot, aspergillosis, mycobacteriosis) but can occur as a primary immune-mediated event.

Trauma

Rupture of the liver is most likely to occur secondary to liver diseases such as hepatic lipidosis, amyloidosis and neoplasia, but in the hunting falcon collision with prey or an obstacle can result in significant hepatic trauma/haemorrhage. Generally this is not fatal provided that bleeding is contained by the liver capsule or confined to one of the hepatic peritoneal cavities.

Therapeutics

Supportive care for birds with hepatic disease includes fluid therapy, nutritional support and treatment of ascites, coagulopathies and encephalopathy.

Fluid therapy and nutritional support

Aggressive fluid therapy (see Chapters 7 and 8) will flush toxins and toxic by-products through the metabolic pathways and from cells, organs and blood. Nutritional support with gavage tubing should be provided three to four times daily to the anorectic patient. A high-quality balanced formula with appropriate levels of vitamins and minerals should be chosen based on individual requirements. For the raptor patient, the author favours liquidized Hill's a/d given at a volume of 10–20 ml/kg per feed.

Therapy for encephalopathy, ascites and coagulopathies

The exact pathogenesis of hepatic encephalopathy in birds is poorly understood; however, it is assumed that, as in mammals, it is in part due to elevated blood ammonia levels. In suspected cases, lactulose may be used orally at 0.5 ml/kg q12h; it is fermented in the gut by bacteria into acetic acid and lactic acid, which reduces the pH. The acidification causes ammonia (NH_3) to migrate from the blood into the colon where it is trapped as an ammonium ion (NH_4^+) and expelled with the faeces. These acids also increase osmotic pressure, drawing water into the bowel and causing a laxative effect. Lactulose has minimal side effects and is therefore considered safe to administer to birds during gavage feeding for hepatic disorders.

Removal of a large volume of ascitic fluid from a patient with advanced liver disease can cause severe protein loss. Removal is only indicated if the ascites is associated with respiratory embarrassment or anorexia. Diuretics may be useful in controlling fluid retention but, in the author's experience, in such cases hepatic pathology is so advanced that prognosis for a falconry bird or wild raptor is generally hopeless and euthanasia should be considered on humane grounds.

Cholestasis can cause impaired production of coagulation factors as well as vitamin K malabsorption. Coagulopathies may be observed as petechiae, haemorrhage or melena. Blood component therapy and vitamin K supplementation may be considered in such cases. Vitamin K administration may also be a useful consideration prior to liver biopsy.

Pharmacological therapy

As well as concurrent supportive therapy as described above, the proper choice of pharmacological therapy depends on a definitive diagnosis, ideally by liver biopsy/culture and sensitivity. In cases of hepatitis, broad-spectrum antimicrobials (marbofloxacin, potentiated amoxicillin) are indicated based on the results of culture and sensitivity tests. Anecdotally prednisolone has been used in the treatment of chronic active hepatitis of unknown aetiology in Grey Parrots. Corticosteroids may therefore have merit in the raptor patient but are contraindicated in cases of infectious hepatitis. Antifibrotics (e.g. colchicine) may also be of use where there is evidence of hepatic fibrosis. Colchicine is believed to inhibit fibrosis and may also protect the liver from further damage by stabilizing the hepatocyte plasma membrane.

Integrative therapies

Once labelled as 'alternative', there is currently an increasing interest in the complementing of traditional regimes with herbal remedies, nutraceuticals and acupuncture. Advice of an avian veterinary surgeon experienced in such practices should obviously be sought prior to treatment, but hepatoprotectants (e.g. vitamin E, milk thistle and urodeoxycholic acid) have been used in the treatment of liver disease in birds and numerous anecdotal reports support their use in therapy.

Thyroid disease

Disorders of the thyroid in raptors are rare but hypothyroidism (thyroid hypoplasia/dysplasia due to dietary iodine deficiency) has been reported in a White-backed Vulture and a Southern Caracara. Thyroid neoplasia (follicular cystadenoma, cystic fibroadenoma) has been described in raptors at post-mortem examination, but not apparently associated with clinical disease.

Incoordination and fits

The causes of fits and incoordination in raptors are summarized in Figure 26.11.

Nutritional and metabolic	Hypoglycaemia; calcium/phosphorus/vitamin D3 imbalances (neonates, egg-laying females); thiamine deficiency (Harris' Hawks, Goshawks, fish-eating raptors); hyperglycaemia (Goshawks); hepatic encephalopathy; heat stress, hyperthermia; idiopathic epilepsy
Toxic	Heavy metal (lead); pesticides (organophosphates, organochlorines); strychnine; alpha-chloralose; clostridial toxins
Infectious	Bacterial (*Listeria*, *Salmonella*, *Staphylococcus*, *Pasteurella*, *Clostridium*, *Mycobacterium*); viral (paramyxovirus, influenza virus); fungal (aspergillosis) or parasitic (sarcocystis, toxoplasmosis; meningitis or encephalitis
Traumatic	CNS trauma or haemorrhage
Neoplastic	Astrocytoma; melanoma

26.11 Causes of fitting and incoordination in raptors.

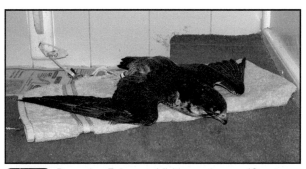

26.12 Peregrine Falcon exhibiting seizures. (Courtesy of Tom Bailey)

Often the seizure or episode of incoordination may occur 'in the field' and emergency advice must be given over the phone prior to travelling to the surgery. Immediate care should include getting the bird into a warm, dark, padded environment and keeping any external visual, auditory or noxious stimuli to a minimum (this is often aided by hooding the bird in question). If the bird is recumbent it should be propped up in sternal recumbency with its head supported, which can be achieved with a rolled-up towel (Figure 26.13). The bird must be carefully monitored to ensure that its airway remains clear at all times, particularly if any vomiting or regurgitation occurs.

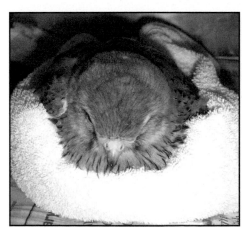

26.13 A rolled-up towel is used to support this collapsed European Kestrel.

If hypoglycaemia is suspected (most common in a young or inexperienced hawk following a period of physical exertion, particularly in cold or wet conditions), a small amount of glucose powder may be rubbed on to the mucous membranes of the oral cavity. The exception is in Goshawks, which appear to be prone to episodes of hyperglycaemia associated with stressful events (Forbes, 1995).

Another important aspect to stress to the owner at this point is under no circumstances should the bird be fed solids prior to its visit to the surgery, as this may lead to regurgitation during subsequent anaesthesia or a potentially fatal sour crop. For further details on critical care, see Chapter 7.

Diagnosis and treatment

A fitting raptor demands prompt diagnosis in order to instigate appropriate therapy. In the short term, seizures can be controlled with midazolam (0.5–1 mg/kg i.v. or i.m., q12h or q8h) or diazepam at the same dose. The latter, although effective, is less rapidly absorbed by the intramuscular route and more irritant to muscle and soft tissue. If the bird fails to respond to the above, further sedation or light anaesthesia is warranted with isoflurane, sevoflurane or ketamine (5–10 mg/kg i.m.). At this point intubation and ventilation are indicated. Hyperthermia should be addressed by soaking the plumage (e.g. by spraying with a plant mister), placing feet in a cold-water bath and cloacal lavage.

A detailed history is imperative and should include careful questioning on diet (appropriate calorific, mineral and vitamin content; recent contaminated food items), activity prior to event (egg laying, exercise, trauma), other clinical signs (weakness, unexplained weight loss, regurgitation), concurrent medications, toxic exposure (inappropriate ectoparasite application, environmental exposure to pesticides) and possibility of heat stress (e.g. no access to shade).

A minimum database should include a complete blood count, biochemical analysis including blood glucose and ionized calcium (though often misleading unless taken during or immediately following seizure activity) and radiographs to assess cranial or spinal injuries, to screen for metallic particles and to evaluate bone quality and density.

Further diagnostics may include endoscopy, blood cultures, virology (PMV, influenza isolation), intestinal contents analysis (e.g. for clostridial toxins) and MRI. Whole-blood acetylcholinesterase activity (if organophosphate toxicity is suspected) and lead values should be measured.

Following diagnosis, specific treatment modalities can then be instigated and these are covered in detail in the appropriate chapters of this manual.

Acknowledgements

The author would like to thank the following for their assistance in the preparation of this manuscript: Alistair M Lawrie BVMS MRCVS, Professor Patrick T Redig DVM PhD, N Gallagher and Dr Cathy A Johnson-Delany DVM DipABVP.

References and further reading

Cooper JE (2002) *Birds of Prey: Health and Disease, 3rd edn.* Blackwell Science, Oxford

Forbes NA (1995) Differential diagnosis and treatment of fitting in raptors with particular attention to the previously unreported condition of stress induced hyperglycaemia in Northern Goshawks. In: *Proceedings of the European Association of Avian Veterinarians Conference, Jerusalem, 1995,* pp. 128–131. AAV, Lake Worth, FL

Forbes NA, Cooper JE and Higgins RJ (2000) Neoplasms of birds of prey. In: *Raptor Biomedicine III,* ed. JT Lumeij *et al.,* pp. 127–145. Zoological Education Network, Lake Worth, FL

Harrison GJ and Lightfoot TL (eds) (2006) *Clinical Avian Medicine.* Spix, Palm Beach, FL

Heidenreich M (1997) *Birds of Prey: Medicine and Management.* Blackwell Science, Oxford

Lierz M (2003) Avian renal disease: pathogenesis, diagnosis and therapy. *Veterinary Clinics of North America: Exotic Animal Practice* **6,** 29–53

Lumeij JT, Remple JD, Redig PT, Lierz M and Cooper JE (2000) *Raptor Biomedicine III.* Zoological Education Network, Lake Worth, FL

Machedo C *et al.* (1987) Disintegration of kidney stones by extra corporeal shockwave lithotripsy in a penguin. In: *Proceedings 1st International Conference on Zoological and Avian Medicine, Oahu, September 1987,* pp. 343–349

Redig PT (1993) *Medical Management of Birds of Prey.* Raptor Center, University of Minnesota Publications, Minneapolis

Redig PT, Cooper JE, Remple JD and Hunter, DB (eds) (1993) *Raptor Biomedicine.* Chiron Publications, Keighley

Samour J (2000) *Avian Medicine.* Harcourt Publishers, London

Styles DK and Phalen DN (1998) Clinical avian urology. *Seminars on Avian Exotic Pet Medicine,* **7(2),** 104–113

Pigeons: nutrition

René Becker

Basic principles of pigeon nutrition

Apart from fruit pigeons, the pigeon is a typical granivore. Its diet basically consists of seeds from different cereals, legumes and oilseeds. These are supplemented with minerals, plants and to some extent animal feeds.

Feeding behaviour

Pigeons select seeds both visually and by touch through nerve endings at the tip of the beak. The food is then rapidly carried to the pharynx by the tongue. With bigger grains, quick movements of the head help to pass on the food.

The oesophagus leads into the crop, which consists of two parts and serves both to store and to soak the food. From here, the food is transported to the proventriculus, which functionally is comparable to the mammalian stomach. Thence to the gizzard (consisting of several compartments), where the mechanical maceration of feed takes place so that the digestive enzymes secreted from the mucosa of the proventriculus can come into effect. After further maceration and assimilation of nutrients in the intestine, the chyme (partly digested food) eventually accumulates in the cloaca, where it is mixed with uric acid from the kidneys and both are excreted together in the faeces (see Chapter 7).

For drinking, almost the whole beak is dipped into water, which is sucked into the oral cavity by creation of a negative pressure. Therefore some of the water that entered the oral cavity goes back into the water bowl, causing possible contamination with pathogens (e.g. trichomonads).

Equipment

Pigeon feed is put into long feeding troughs that allow several pigeons to eat simultaneously. For drinking water, a trough with a storage volume of about 4 litres is most commonly used (Figure 27.1). The majority of commercially available drinking troughs are designed for four pigeons per trough. They are manufactured from material that is easy to clean, such as glass or plastic. This is important since the drinking trough is one of the most important transfer routes for disease. Many breeders use two separate drinking troughs, used alternately in order to permit each trough to dry out completely when not in use. It is also advisable that feed troughs should be maintained hygienically (Figure 27.2). Easy-to-clean plastic or metal inserts are available for feed troughs.

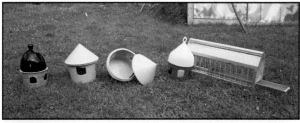

27.1 Water containers for pigeons. The ceramic pots on the left are preferable to the plastic pots (right) as the surface is smoother, allowing them to be cleaned more easily and bacteria and algae removed. Far right: this drinking system is used to train pigeons to drink through the bars, which they need to learn before being transported. (Courtesy of E and R Schmölz)

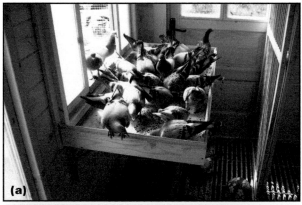

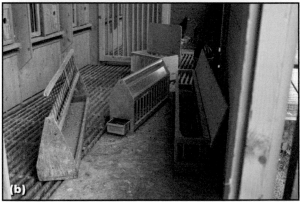

(a)

(b)

27.2 **(a)** Feeding tables such as this one are often used by fanciers for young pigeons, to allow all the birds to feed at the same time and encourage them into the flock more quickly. However, faecal contamination of the food is more likely using this system and so good hygiene is essential. **(b)** A range of feeding systems (a roof is preferable). It is important to ensure that the birds cannot defecate on the food. (Courtesy of E and R Schmölz)

Feeding routines

Pigeons are usually fed twice daily. The total amount of feed per pigeon and per day averages about 30 g, split into two portions. This is only a general guideline and it is very important that the exact amount of feed is adjusted to the current demands of the bird. For instance, higher energy demands and therefore larger amounts of feed are necessary if the ambient temperature is low, or during rearing and racing seasons.

Ad libitum feeding, by which the pigeon can choose the amount and time of feeding, is usually not advisable, especially during the racing season.

Water intake

Water uptake is closely related to the ambient temperature. The average water uptake is 50 ml/pigeon/day. The amount of water drunk decreases if drugs or feed additives are added (see later). Many products affect the taste of the water and require habituation of the birds. This aspect must be considered, especially in times of high demand (e.g. during the racing season in summer), in order to avoid subclinical dehydration resulting in a decrease of racing performance.

Feed mixtures

Commercially available mixtures of grain are commonly used for pigeons. Different mixtures are adapted to the varying amount of stress a pigeon is subjected to over the year and many animal feed suppliers offer appropriate mixtures for different circumstances.

Cereals

Cereals are a compact, nutrient-rich and high-energy feed that is ideal for pigeons. On average, cereals contain 58–70% carbohydrates, 7–14% crude protein and approximately 5% crude lipids. The germ bud contains varying amounts of vitamins, minerals, amino acids and fats. Figure 27.3 gives the composition of a commercially available standard feed mixture that can be used during the breeding and racing season.

Component	Proportion
Yellow maize	30%
Wheat	20%
Mixed peas	31.5%
Milo	8%
Dari	8%
Striped sunflower seeds	1%
Kardi seed	1%
Australian peas	3.5%
Buckwheat	1%

27.3   Standard feed mix.

As well as its composition, the quality of the grain mixture is of major importance. Cereals should only contain fully mature grains, i.e. with a high percentage of potential germination. The feed should not be dusty and must be free from contamination, including fungal organisms and pests (e.g. corn weevil).

Supplements

Supplementation with minerals and grit is indispensable for optimal digestion. Commercially available grit mixtures consist of small indigestible stones that are necessary for mechanical maceration of the feed in the gizzard. Pigeon stones are offered in the form of little cubes or baked in clay pots. Well balanced grit mixtures or pigeon stones should also include all the major and trace elements that are essential for maintaining the body's physiological processes. A wide range of grits and mineral powders is available. Since pigeons prefer a salty taste, grit stones containing high amounts of salt are eagerly ingested, but acceptability should not be the only guideline. The daily provision of such supplements is crucial for achieving excellent health status and high capacity in the birds and there is an increased requirement for these substances during times of high energy demand.

Pellets

Modern feed mixtures often contain artificially produced components in the form of pellets, extruded corn or so-called coated corn. The classic pellet is made by pressing whole grains and special pelleting binders together. In the extrusion process maceration of ingredients occurs during a short period of heating. In 'coated' corn a special layer of mashed feed surrounds a single grain (e.g. sorghum). The coated grain still has its natural shape, making it acceptable to the bird. This kind of feed is thought to upgrade basic grain mixtures. Minerals, vitamins, essential amino acids and herbal components are added according to need (breeding season, racing period, moult; see below). Thus the deficits of pure grain diets are compensated for and the requirement for food additives is reduced.

Forage

The provision of forage in modern pigeon breeding is nearly obsolete, even though pigeons avidly ingest green plant matter when offered. Many breeders still feed self-made mixtures of garlic and onion in order to enhance their birds' metabolism, and food mixtures for the resting period during the winter often contain vegetables such as carrots, celery and beetroot, which the breeders hope will provide a purging and gut-cleansing effect. However, the proportion of vegetables should not exceed one-third of the total daily ration, to avoid indigestion due to ingluvial atony.

Feeding according to energy demands

The feeding of high-performance pigeons for breeding and racing is matched to varying energy demand over the 'pigeon year', which can be divided into four phases: moult; breeding; racing season; and resting period.

Moult

The main moult comprises complete displacement of the contour feathers (see Chapter 24), and ranges from September to the end of November in Central Europe for example. It requires supplementation of all essential substances for the new growth and the diet has to be diverse and rich in energy and protein. Specialist feed manufacturers offer prefabricated 'moult mixtures', some of which are supplemented with extruded corn to balance the deficits of ordinary grain mixtures. Additionally, a number of commercial food additives contain the essential substances (methionine, lysine, tryptophan, biotin, zinc, polyunsaturated fatty acids and lecithin) for new feather formation. Iodine is also recommended for supporting the bird's metabolism in this highly active phase.

Breeding

The pigeon's reproductive period, from the beginning of egg production to the weaning of the offspring, is comparatively short.

A unique feature of the pigeon is the ability to produce 'crop milk' to feed the squabs. Under the influence of prolactin, the crop lining thickens (10–20 × normal thickness) during incubation and the holocrine crop glandular tissue begins to secrete the cream-coloured crop milk (Figure 27.4). Sheets of lipid-filled epithelial cells are also desquamated into it and become part of the secretion. Concentrated crop milk production ceases about 10 days post hatching, but may continue in a less concentrated form for about 3 weeks. Crop milk is mainly composed of fat (5–7%), protein (11–13%) and minerals (1.5%), with no carbohydrate. It is low in vitamins A and C and has a low calcium and phosphorus content but contains essential amino acids, fatty acids and immunoglobulins.

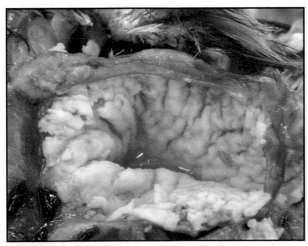

27.4 Production of crop milk. (Courtesy of Gerry Dorrestein)

A young pigeon can only develop into a successful high-performance racing pigeon if its nutrition (Figure 27.5) is optimally matched with actual demand at every stage during the maturation process.

During the breeding period the diet should contain an increased protein content of 17%. Other essential substances such as minerals and trace elements must also be provided. Grit mixtures (see above) are

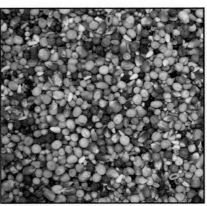

27.5 Food for rearing young pigeons, rich in protein (peas and soya). (Courtesy of E and R Schmölz)

of major importance for egg shell formation and optimal growth. Vitamin supplementation is equally important. Fat-soluble vitamins have a great influence on fertility (vitamin E), rate and quantity of lay (vitamin A) and calcium uptake (vitamin D3). There are several commercial products that meet the requirements for optimal breeding results. These mostly include extruded or coated grains containing all the essential compounds needed for breeding. The addition of water-soluble minerals completes an optimal diet.

Racing season

During the racing season a systematic feeding programme is the basis for successful results. The performance demands on the racing pigeon every week are extremely high and demand-based feeding is especially vital in this period. Since pigeons usually undergo one race every week with a 7-day interval, there is a special feeding programme for the days between flights (Figure 27.6).

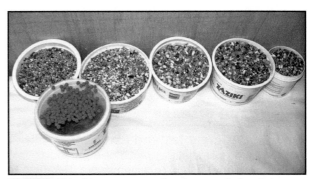

27.6 Weekly programme for pigeons during the racing season, changed daily starting from the day after the race (left to right): return feed; maintenance; recreation with increased energy and protein until the next race. The pieces of dried carrot in the front are for vitamin A. (Courtesy of E and R Schmölz)

Directly after the race, electrolytes and high-quality and highly digestible energy sources, such as glucose, are given in order to shorten the period of time for recovery. The diet on the day of return and the first few days thereafter should also include a high amount of carbohydrates and fat, but at the same time be highly digestible through lower protein content.

At the beginning of the week the diet should consist of a higher fibre fraction, which accelerates the purging of the intestine. During the phase of recovery and reconstruction of lost body tissues in the middle of the week, the protein content of the diet must be elevated. Towards the end of the week the diet should be high in fat to restore the pigeon's energy sources.

Modern feed mixtures contain very low protein concentrations, resulting from the almost complete absence of legumes. It is common for food additives containing highly digestible proteins and amino acids to be added to the normal diet to satisfy the need for these substances. Since the pigeon gains most of its energy supply during the race from burning fats, seeds with high fat contents are included in high proportions in modern feed mixtures (see above). Moreover, several compounds containing different kinds of oils for the provision of extra energy are also added. The demands for vitamins (especially B), minerals and trace elements are equally increased during this phase and many food additives are available to counterbalance possible deficiencies.

Feedstuff and food-additive manufacturers offer complete packages for total care during the racing season. As well as specialized feed mixtures and food additives, these also include preparations to support the bird's metabolism in order to increase the racing pigeon's fitness level in general.

Resting period
During the resting period in winter, an adequate diet is comparably low in protein content and fibre and the energy content must not be too high. The goal for this period of comparatively low exercise is to avoid over-feeding and excessive weight gain. However, if the ambient temperature is very low the energy level of the diet must be increased, e.g. by adding extra maize. There are various commercial products available.

It is important not to switch to a different type of feed too abruptly. Approximately 3 weeks before the start of the breeding season the diet for the resting period should steadily be replaced by the breeding diet.

Nutritional disease

Vitamin deficiencies and toxicosis
A long-lasting complete absence of a particular vitamin in the diet can lead to avitaminosis. Because of modern husbandry conditions, with only restricted free flying or even complete housing in aviaries, the birds no longer have any access to natural vitamin sources. The vitamin content of diets based on grain is generally not sufficient to meet the bird's demands, especially as its content varies depending on the quality of the grains and method of storage. Furthermore, demand is increased during the breeding, racing and moulting periods and so deficiencies may be observed more often. Therefore pigeons require vitamin supplementation during these periods of high demand in particular.

Vitamin B deficiency
In pigeons only vitamin C can be synthesized endogenously. Vitamin K and the B vitamins can be obtained from intestinal flora, but B vitamins, as major promoters of metabolism, should still be supplemented during the racing season. Food-additive manufacturers offer a broad selection of vitamin preparations to satisfy all vitamin needs. From experience, the administration of B vitamins exhibits the greatest effect when given at the end of the week, i.e. the last two days before the day of the race.

It is important to ensure that all compounds are of high quality and are stored under adequate conditions, as B vitamins in particular are extremely sensitive to high temperatures.

An inadequate supply of B vitamins is followed by a general decrease of the bird's metabolic capacity and thus decrerased vitality. This leads to unsatisfactory breeding, moulting and racing results.

Beriberi, the classic disease resulting from vitamin B deficiency, is known in pigeons. It is characterized by a dysfunction of the nervous system; the birds show opisthotonos and are unable to stand (Figure 27.7). If this stage is reached, birds usually die. The disease is caused by sole feeding of predominantly unpeeled grains. This is now hardly ever seen, since modern commercial feed mixtures contain vitamin-enhanced extruded or coated corns. Prophylaxis is most important.

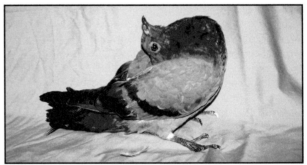

27.7 Signs of vitamin B1 deficiency. (© Michael Lierz)

Vitamin D deficiency
Lipid-soluble vitamins are closely related to crucial functions in the pigeon's metabolism. Vitamin D functions as a regulator for calcium–phosphorus homeostasis and is of major importance during the breeding period, as it directly influences egg shell quality and the skeletal development of young birds. Even if the mineral supply is optimal, skeletal malformation can occur if vitamin D is deficient. Vitamin D precursors are found in germ buds and converted to the active form through the influence of ultraviolet light, which is why access to natural sunlight is vital. Nevertheless, vitamin D should be supplemented during the breeding season to avoid diseases such as rickets. This disease particularly occurs in undersupplied nestlings. The typical signs are growth retardation, a misshapen sternum and poor feathering in young birds.

Adult birds lacking vitamin D can show paralysis during laying, since the bird's calcium demand exceeds the amount that can be absorbed from the intestine. Consequently calcium is mobilized from endogenous storage in the bones. In most cases this disease is not simply vitamin D deficiency but a consequence of inadequate mineral supply and insufficient access to sunlight.

Vitamin D dosages must always be measured out accurately, since lipid-soluble vitamins are stored in the body and oversupply can lead to irreversible damage, e.g. calcification.

Mineral/electrolyte deficiency or overdosage

For undisturbed metabolism, reproduction, growth, moulting and high racing performance an adequate supply of minerals and electrolytes is essential. Otherwise decreased performance ability and an enhanced susceptibility towards diseases will occur. Major elements/electrolytes are required in higher doses and include calcium, phosphorus, potassium and chloride, of which calcium is the most important. Of the trace elements, iodine is of highest significance.

Calcium and phosphorus

Calcium is involved in bone development, cell metabolism, muscle activity, blood coagulation and egg shell production. Since the calcium content of grain mixtures is usually not sufficient, pigeons must be provided every day with grit mixtures, which generally contain calcium-rich clamshells.

Calcium deficiency during the reproductive period results in a reduced quality of the egg shell (which is about 90% calcium carbonate). It may also lead to paralysis in laying birds as a consequence of the mobilization of huge amounts of calcium from endogenous storage for egg shell production. In young pigeons, calcium deficiency leads to 'rickets' (see also vitamin D deficiency, above) of which a typical sign is a deformed sternum. Adult pigeons with calcium deficiency show osteomalacia.

Phosphorus is abundant in legumes and cereal germ buds and therefore a deficiency seldom occurs. In general, common mineral and grit mixtures contain calcium and phosphorus in the optimal ratio of 2:1. Regular *ad libitum* supply with such feed additives on a daily basis is important, but it is also important that excessive dietary phytates do not bind calcium, thus reducing its bioavailability.

Sodium, potassium and chloride

Sodium, potassium and chloride are responsible for the maintenance of the cell's osmotic pressure and are also required for absorption and transportation of nutrients. Furthermore they are involved in the conduction of electric potentials from cell to cell. Sodium and chloride are usually sufficient in feed mixtures. Higher contents can be found in mineral and grit mixtures, in which salt (NaCl) is often used to make the mixtures more attractive for the pigeon. Mixtures with a high salt content are usually ingested eagerly, but the breeder should only offer them in a restricted manner, to avoid sodium poisoning or dehydration.

Magnesium

Magnesium is vital for conducting electric potentials and for muscle activity. During times of high performance there is an increase in demand for magnesium. Many electrolyte mixtures that are added to the normal diet after a race contain magnesium to prevent deficiency signs.

Iodine

Both during the growth period and for high performance metabolism during racing, an adequate supply of iodine is essential. Iodine-containing preparations are included in nearly every nutritional concept for pigeon breeding as well as racing to increase the pigeon's performance. These preparations have a clear positive effect on the pigeon's general condition. Iodine has several other important functions. If added to the drinking water it functions as a disinfectant. Moreover, it decelerates the growth of spores of yeast and bacteria in the intestinal tract. Therefore, iodine should be administered after every antimicrobial treatment. Iodine is contained in higher amounts in grit mixtures, especially if they contain clamshells. During periods of high performance the additional supplementation of such preparations may well be required. With iodine deficiency, hyperplasia of the thyroid gland will occur. This has been documented in pigeons several times but no longer plays a major role today, thanks to the general provision of high-quality feed. Provision of this trace element is by regular feeding of iodine-containing mineral mixtures. Therapy involves administration of commercially available iodine-containing drugs over several weeks.

Malnutrition and loss of performance

Modern feeding techniques and an increasing professionalism in the sport of pigeon racing have helped to make the occurrence of classic nutritional diseases such as those described above a rare event. During the breeding season there are sporadic cases showing clinical signs resulting from the undersupply of certain nutrients, but in many cases this is more often the result of poor health status and consequently inadequate utilization of nutrients than a true undersupply.

High demands are made on pigeons concerning their physical fitness. The birds can only meet these demands if they have been properly supplied with all essential nutrients from the egg. The basis for high performance during the racing season (which is the most important time for the breeder) is the optimal provision of nutrients at *all* times of the year. All too frequently breeders only worry about their pigeons' health status just as the racing season is about to start. At this point it is too late to compensate for neglect during the rest of the year. As explained above, special commercial feeds with a protein content matched to the demands of the breeding period, the moult and the racing season, along with a generous supply of minerals and the regular administration of vitamins (especially lipid-soluble vitamins), are required.

Nutritional deficits are likely to express themselves in poor feathering during breeding and moulting. Dry and rough feathers with poor pigmentation and so-called 'fret marks' (translucent lines in the feather) indicate undersupply or poor utilization of nutrients. Deficits can also be apparent in growth retardation and general poor development of the bird. Well developed birds have dense and smooth feathering that is rich in pigmentation, whereas undernourished birds are skinny and badly feathered.

Successful pigeon racing depends on many factors. Quality of the bird, health status and the environment of the housing are key points. Optimal nutritional provision during the racing season is an additional factor and this is where many breeders make elementary mistakes. Breeders offer homemade pigeon feeds and mix feed additives to compile their own provision plan that is often mismatched with the actual demands of the pigeon. The result of inadequate nutrition during times of high stress will be exhaustion, which in the majority of the cases can be seen from midway through the racing season. Malnutrition also decreases the pigeon's defence system against infection. Therefore a well balanced diet and short periods of recreation between the flights are crucial. Since with increasing flight distances the demand for essential nutrients also rises, the bird's diet must be formulated accordingly.

Intoxication with feed or medication

Severe intoxications associated with clinical signs have become rare in modern husbandry, but there can still be huge differences in the quality of grain mixtures and they might also be stored inadequately. This can lead to contamination of the feed and, depending on the kind of contaminant involved, can result in clinical signs very similar to those for toxicosis.

Despite the high quality of commercial feed mixtures, there are still occasional occurrences of feed pests such as various corn weevils and flour mites. Feed mites, which grow optimally in feed that is stored in warm damp conditions, can lead to digestive problems in the pigeon if ingested, and also promote secondary growth of mould fungi.

Mycotoxins

Unclean feed stored inadequately (i.e. in warm and damp conditions) often results in the growth of putrefactive bacteria and mould fungi, especially *Aspergillus*. As well as loss of nutritional quality in spoiled feed, mycotoxins can lead to disease. Toxins produced by *Aspergillus.* in particular may lead to disorders of the bird's general condition, anorexia, severe liver disease and even death, or simply poor breeding and racing performance, depending on the dosage of the toxin. It requires only a very low content of toxins in the feed to influence the pigeon's performance. It is essential that feed is stored in dark, dry and airy conditions and that there is a high throughput of feed.

Feed contamination with fungal toxins has become very rare. The classic problem is contamination with ergot, which grows as a corn-like structure on the ear of cereals. The toxins cause vessels to constrict, which can cause extremities to die off.

Plant toxins

Plant toxins only sporadically affect pigeons as birds have limited time for flying outdoors. Toxic plants are also often rejected due to their bad taste and are only ingested in case of deficits in the usual diet. Young pigeons are the most affected. This is because the young birds are allowed more time for free flying and spend a lot of time exploring the aviary's nearby surroundings, especially during the first few weeks. A typical toxic plant is the yew tree (*Taxus baccata*), parts of which contain the alkaloid taxin, which causes respiratory paralysis and impairment of cardiac function.

Mineral toxicosis

The administration of mineral supplements can also cause signs of intoxication. Especially during the rearing season, young pigeons develop a real hunger for salts to match their high demand. Mineral and grit mixtures and 'pigeon stones' are often picked up eagerly. In cases where the sodium chloride content of these feed additives is too high, intoxication expresses itself in watery to mucoid faeces. With severe NaCl intoxication massive withdrawal of water leads to the death of the bird. A short withdrawal of *ad libitum* feeding of the mineral mixture is helpful and mineral drinks or less attractive mixtures should be given instead.

Drug overdosage

Intoxications can be associated with the application of drugs via drinking water or feed. In most cases this is because the breeder has used the wrong dosage. Low dosages in the range of few grams cannot be measured precisely with measuring spoons. Also most pigeon breeders are well provided with all the very common drugs and often use them without due care. Another factor of vital importance is the amount of water uptake, since this varies depending on the ambient temperature. As a general rule for the administration of drugs via drinking water, it is assumed that the intake of drinking water is 1 litre/day for 20 pigeons. If the ambient temperature is very high, this intake can easily double. This would lead to an increased intake of the drug if the dosage remains the same. The problem is often seen with nitroimidazole, a drug that is commonly used for the treatment of trichomoniasis. Young pigeons in particular are extremely sensitive to overdosage and develop clinical signs such as torticollis, resembling a paramyxovirus infection. Clinical signs mostly disappear when the administration of nitroimidazole is stopped.

Another common sign of intoxication is a problem with moulting, which may be caused by the administration of sulphonamides and antiparasitic drugs (e.g. fenbendazole).

The administration of fenbendazole is very difficult, due to the need for exact dosing; overdosage leads to severe liver and kidney failure that results in the death of the bird.

There have been instances of overdosage of streptomycin, which causes reversible paralysis but may also lead to death.

28

Pigeons: the poor performance bird

Alistair Lawrie

Introduction

This chapter focuses on the performance of racing pigeons, but also applies to exhibition and game pigeons as they, too, have to be in excellent health to compete successfully.

The aim of the pigeon fancier is to have a flock of healthy birds that regularly outperform their competitors. Winning races can only be achieved by having a healthy flock that contains exceptionally high-performance individuals. 'Poor performance' in the racing pigeon may be due to unrealistic expectations on the part of the owner or to genuine deterioration in the performance of an individual bird.

Performance relates to the genetics and quality of the individual bird. Other factors affecting performance may be the relative resistance of the flock to certain diseases, the fitness of individual birds through proper conditioning and training, and even a bird's innate better-than-average ability to navigate successfully.

Factors affecting performance

Poor performance of the individual bird can be multifactorial. Factors that contribute to this may be genetic, the presence of subclinical or clinical disease, parasitism, poor condition or fitness, physical injury or feather loss.

Genetic selection

Without having good quality stock, outstanding success cannot be achieved and this will become a major limiting factor. Purchase of good foundation stock is essential, but the ability to select and pair up individual birds to improve the quality of the loft is dependent upon the talent of the flock owner. Some strains of birds may also have greater genetic resistance to certain infections.

Most breeding pigeons are selected on the basis of their past performance in races. Many of the birds that do not perform well will simply be culled by the fancier. Young birds are watched carefully in their early days within the loft and are assessed by watching their interaction with and even dominance over other youngsters and also by observing how well they perform on trial flights.

Subclinical disease

The existence of clinical or, more often, subclinical disease is a common reason for poor racing performance (see Chapter 3). Subclinical problems may be suspected if a bird shows a delayed recovery after a race.

Respiratory diseases are probably the most important diseases at the subclinical level and these may be exacerbated by stress and overcrowding in lofts and racing baskets. Poor loft ventilation and hygiene also have marked effects upon the spread and severity of respiratory conditions (see Chapter 30).

The nature of pigeon racing means that there is contact between individual birds from different lofts brought together in cramped and unhygienic conditions. Contact with wild and stray birds also affords the opportunity to contract disease. Thus the greatest health risk to a racing pigeon is from another pigeon.

Parasitism

Parasites (see Chapter 29), which may be protozoa, nematodes or cestodes, will not only have a direct effect on the bird but will also reduce its general health status and immune system so that subclinical conditions may persist or become clinically apparent. Large coccidial or *Spironucleus* burdens in young birds and *Trichomonas* infections at any age will have a debilitating effect. Heavy external parasite burdens are more commonly seen in ill or debilitated birds.

Condition and fitness

If pigeons are not in peak condition, or are lacking in fitness, this will result in less racing success and will also contribute to some birds returning from races in an exhausted condition or not returning home at all.

Poor condition may result from poor management, inappropriate husbandry or disease. Feeding and nutrition (see Chapter 27) can have profound effects on the pigeon's general health, wellbeing and endurance and thus its racing performance.

Fitness and training are also management issues and depend partly upon the skill and experience of the fancier. Unfit or debilitated birds should never be sent to race, not only because they may not perform well but also because they may contract diseases more easily from other pigeons. They may then introduce these conditions to their own lofts when they return. As with all animals, fit healthy unstressed individuals are less likely to succumb to infectious disease.

Physical injury

Physical injury or pain will reduce a bird's flying efficiency and obviously any signs of injury should preclude that bird's inclusion in a race. Similarly, birds that have lost or damaged feathers or are moulting will not perform as well as they should.

The approach to the poor performance bird

History

In common with most other investigations, a good history is imperative and one must determine at the outset whether it is a symptom of a flock problem or just the problem of that individual bird. Figure 28.1 gives a checklist of matters to be investigated in poor-performance flocks.

What is the owner's complaint? Are all the birds underperforming or is it just one individual that has a disappointing racing history? Is it just this season and have race times deteriorated since the season began? Answers to these questions can help to determine whether it is a recent or chronic problem.

Knowledge of the genetics and breeding history of the flock is useful as is an assessment of the skill, knowledge and aspirations of the fancier (which may sometimes be unrealistic).

The age group of birds that are affected is significant, since some problems will affect mainly young birds, and it is also important to know the bird's sex.

Loft disease history

The disease history of the loft must be investigated with regard to any disease outbreaks and their treatment. Some diseases may have been treated inappropriately or with inadequate doses and treatment courses, enabling them to become chronic or subclinical.

There may be prophylaxis of certain diseases by vaccination and it is important to know who vaccinated the bird, which vaccine was used and whether the application and vaccine storage were according to the manufacturer's instructions. Vaccine failure may occur, especially if vaccination is done by owners themselves after acquiring the vaccine from unreliable sources.

It should also be ascertained whether other 'prophylactic treatments' have been given by the fancier (e.g. antibiotics before the racing season). Fanciers often give non-prescribed antibiotics 'prophylactically' to 'prevent' respiratory disease, but these are often used for inadequate times and at subtherapeutic doses. Are routine anti-protozoals and anthelmintics used? If so, when, how often and for how long?

Post-mortem examination results for birds that died or were culled are always valuable but it is not often carried out on a routine basis, unless there are significant problems in the loft with overt illness. When dealing with lack of performance due to infection, once clinical signs are seen the infection, and thus damage, has already occurred. Any treatment will limit damage to the birds but will not necessarily let them return to full fitness for the rest of that racing season.

Loft husbandry

Where the problem is poor flock performance, it is essential that the veterinary surgeon visits the loft to see what the husbandry conditions and standards are like (see Chapter 3). Diets, supplements, food storage and appetites can be discussed along with training methods while visually assessing the loft hygiene, stocking density and ventilation. Pigeons do not like draughty conditions. Light levels may be inadequate, or there may be extreme temperature fluctuations due to inadequate insulation, positioning of the loft or having too many windows. Condensation problems may also ensue. Gross examination of droppings is important, as is estimating the water consumption of the birds (polydipsia often being associated with illness). Training methods and the loft's daily routine must be known. Do the birds mix with other birds, do they go 'fielding' (i.e. eating in farmers' fields) and do they eat roof moss?

Subject	Check
Husbandry, feeding and housing	Visit loft and check stocking density, hygiene, ventilation, separation of age groups, feeding and supplements, training methods, fancier's experience
History	Previous success and success of related/neighbouring flocks; quality and genetics of birds; previous illness; beginning and duration of the problem; any new birds introduced or stray birds appeared?; number of birds not returning home after races
Disease monitoring	Routine parasitological and bacteriological (*Salmonella*) screening in place?; anthelmintic and anti-protozoal treatments; antibiotic treatments (prescribed or unprescribed). Duration of treatment courses and dosages given. Diagnosis made? Deaths? Any signs of respiratory disease seen in the loft recently?
Culling policy	How many birds culled and reasons for doing so. Post-mortem examinations performed?
Racing systems used	Widowhood, natural, darkening, etc.; class and age of stock affected; post-race recovery of birds and their after-race nursing or treatment; any 'doping' used (e.g. corticosteroid eye drops)
Examination of individual birds	Physical check; diagnostic samples
Diagnosis	Specific treatment of diagnosed disease or advice on improving husbandry and management, quarantine, etc.
Start a flock health plan	Routine screening, veterinary visits and post-mortem examination of all culled or dead birds

28.1 Checklist for investigation of poor flock performance.

The culling policy within the loft must be discussed since the keeping of 'poor doers' can contribute to maintaining chronic infections within the loft. Similarly, enquiring whether any stray birds have appeared in the loft or whether any new birds have been purchased recently may indicate possible routes of introduction of new diseases.

Loft performance

Comparing previous years' racing and breeding performance is necessary and it is also useful if the veterinary surgeon has some knowledge of performance in other lofts in the same locality. It can be difficult to assess loft performance without referring to the performance of birds from nearby lofts, since racing speeds will be dictated by prevailing weather conditions at the time. Speed will also depend on the length of the race. A loft average speed can be calculated over a number of races and is usually calculated on a distance-per-minute basis. An average speed of approximately 1300–1400 yards/min (1200–1300 m/min, or about 80 km/h) might be considered a good result. Maximum speeds of winning pigeons with the benefit of back winds range up to 110 km/h (approximately 2000 yards/min) averaged over the whole race.

Clinical examination

The most important thing to bear in mind when examining a pigeon is that poor performance may be due to subclinical illness and therefore, by definition, there will be no obvious physical signs. It may also be due to a combination of factors, such as disease, poor nutrition and poor husbandry. Signs of health and disease in pigeons are listed in Figure 28.2.

Initial assessment

The bird's demeanour should be assessed in the carrying box if possible, bearing in mind that any sick bird will try to mask its clinical signs of illness.

Normal stance, brightness and alertness should be observed and whether there is any abnormality of wing carriage. A bird that is fluffed up, has abnormal head carriage or is dull has significant clinical signs. Evidence of respiratory distress (e.g. tail bobbing, tachypnoea or mouth breathing) should be obvious but other signs such as weight loss and cloacal staining will not be apparent until the bird is handled.

Pigeons are generally very easy, calm birds to handle and the veterinary surgeon must learn to handle them properly and gently (see Chapter 6).

The pigeon should be sat gently in the palm of one hand while the pectoral muscle mass is assessed. This may be less than expected in diseased or dehydrated birds but may be quite normal in a bird that is not ill but is just underperforming.

A detailed clinical examination from beak to tail should then be carried out as outlined in Chapter 7. Signs specific to lack of condition in racing pigeons or to those with respiratory infections are changes in the cere from the normal white, powdery appearance in the healthy pigeon to a grey, greasy appearance with sometimes dampness about the nostrils. In addition there may be slight swelling of the head (sinusitis), epiphora (conjunctivitis) or fluffing up of the feathers around the head, giving it a swollen look. If there is any nasal or ocular discharge, the shoulders and back feathers may be wet due to the bird wiping its beak and eyes on them and affected birds may scratch at their heads, ears or nares. Beak breathing is seen in cases of severe respiratory distress but can also be observed in birds that are overweight, poorly trained or hot.

Body part	Healthy	Signs of illness/problems
Cere	Clean, white and chalky/dusty	Grey or greasy. Nasal discharge or staining
Eyes	Bright and alert. Good eye colour and normal pupillary responses	Swelling of eyelids or epiphora. Periorbital/sinus swelling or rubbing eyes. Crusty lesions around eyes
Head	Tight feathering over head area and alert demeanour	Fluffing of head feathers. Scratching at ears. Abnormal head posture or nervous signs
Feathers	Feathering smooth and with a powdery 'bloom'. All feathers present and lying in correct orientation	Feather loss. Dampness on feathers (shoulders and wings from beak wiping). Soiling with faeces (vent). External parasites. Feather damage
Feet	Usually red, clean, smooth and shiny	Crusting or scaling
Body	Good pectoral muscle bulk and tone	Muscle wasting. 'Hard feeling' pectoral muscles (dehydration). Obesity
Abdomen	Slightly concave. Clean cloaca	Swelling of abdomen or cloaca
Mouth and pharynx	Pink, clean and 'dry'	Diphtheresis or intraoral plaques. Large numbers of white salivary tissue 'spots' on hard palate. Sour smell. Bubbles of moisture
Respiration	Inaudible. 20–35 breaths/minute	Mouth breathing, tachypnoea, adventitious respiratory sounds. Sneezing, coughing
Legs and wings	Normal stance and wing posture	Drooping wing. Swollen joints. Lameness
Faeces	Bulky, fairly firm faeces with cap of white solid urates	Faeces watery, scanty or with mucus. Urates discoloured, absent or polyuria

28.2 Signs of health and disease in the racing pigeon.

Oral cavity: Examination of the oral cavity should establish the presence or absence of diphtheritic plaques (possibly indicative of trichomoniasis, herpesvirus, poxvirus or candidiasis).

Small white spots on the hard palate of pigeons are usually interpreted as being indicative of a cellular immune reaction with accumulation of cellular debris in the mucus glands there.

Crop: Crop palpation will reveal the presence or absence of food or thickening of the crop lining (trichomoniasis or feeding young).

Respiratory and cardiac systems: In severe respiratory conditions, adventitious lung sounds may be heard by auscultation. The cardiac rate and rhythm can also be assessed. The heart rate varies from 180 to 250 beats per minute and the respiratory rate is usually between 20 and 35 breaths per minute.

Respiratory problems are probably the most important cause of disappointing performance and they can be a diagnostic challenge. Very slight or minor problems can influence performance.

Respiratory function will, of course, be affected by abdominal conditions that constrict air sac and lung function, such as hepatic enlargement, ascites, salpingitis/egg binding, abdominal tumours or obesity. Obese birds will not only be unfit but will also be carrying excess weight and be poor athletes.

Wings and legs: Wing and limb function must be assessed, including examination of long bones for signs of fractures or distortions. Joints and associated structures must be given especially close examination in pigeons, since swelling of them may be symptomatic of infection (e.g. salmonellosis, gout or other septic or traumatic arthritis). Muscle trauma and bruising will temporarily affect performance but peak muscle activity is only going to be achieved in fit, trained birds on good diets (see Chapter 27). Leg bands should be examined since they may become tight on the limb if there is any foot or joint swelling associated with diseases, or thickened skin from poor diet.

Injuries may be present because of accident or territorial fights with other birds.

Plumage: Feathers must be in perfect condition for maximum flying and aerodynamic efficiency. Feather quality must be good with no signs of 'fret marks' (indicting previous stress, illness or malnutrition) or parasite damage (lice and mites), and a bird in good condition should show an overall 'bloom' with plenty of powder down. Integrity, condition and presence or absence of individual feathers applies to the contour feathers as well as the remiges and retrices.

Diagnosis

The aim of examination and investigation is to establish a specific diagnosis. Subclinical disease in a flock is common and this may explain the 'tonic' effect of antibiotic courses administered by the fancier without any diagnosis having been made. Some possible causes of weight loss are outlined in Figure 28.3.

Aids to diagnosis are discussed in detail in Chapters 7 to 13. They include the following.

Cause	Examples
Endoparasites	Nematodes – *Ascaridia columbae, Capillaria obsignata, Orithostrongylus quadriradiatus, Syngamus trachea.* Cestodes – *Hymenolepis, Raillietina.* Trematodes – *Echinostoma revolutum.* Protozoa – *Trichomonas, Eimeria labbeana, E. columbarum, Spironucleus, Toxoplasma*
Bacterial infection	Acute or chronic enteric infection or those causing granulomas in the liver, e.g. *Salmonella, Mycobacterium, Escherichia coli.* Air sac granulomas
Viral infection	Viral hepatitis, e.g. adenovirus, herpesvirus, circovirus
Major organ dysfunction	Hepatic disease (tumours or parenchymal disease), chronic salpingitis, nephritis, diabetes, poisoning
Malnutrition	Poor feeding, starvation, dehydration
Other conditions	Traumatic ventriculitis from foreign body ingestion and penetration
Stress	Bullying, overcrowding
Dehydration	After hard racing or disease (e.g. enteritis)

28.3   Some causes of 'going light' in pigeons.

Crop swabs and crop/oesophageal endoscopy: Crop sampling is performed using swabs moistened with saline or by carrying out a warm saline crop wash. Immediate microscopic examination is imperative since the motility of *Trichomonas* organisms decreases rapidly with time. Samples can also be examined with rapid or Gram stains for the presence of yeasts or bacteria. Direct (endoscopic) examination of oesophageal and crop mucosa can show the presence of diphtheritic plaques.

Faecal examination: Information can be obtained by gross examination of colour, form and consistency of both the faecal portion and the urates/urinary portion. Polyuria, a common sign, should be differentiated from diarrhoea. Appropriate parasitological examinations should be carried out by McMaster flotation and counting method for helminths, cestodes and protozoans. The time of day may be important for sample collection (e.g. *Coccidia* counts may be different in the afternoon compared with early morning and are usually highest between 0800 and 1600 hours). Investigation for the presence of *Salmonella* is also highly recommended on a regular basis, at least two or three times a year.

Haematology and biochemistry: In the racing pigeon, haematological parameters such as packed cell volume (PCV) and leucocyte counts can be estimated fairly rapidly and can be used (together with other measurements) to indicate dehydration, anaemia and infection. Blood samples in pigeons are normally taken from the ulnar or metatarsal veins (the jugular and associated venous plexus should be avoided) with red cell parameters being at the top end of most avian reference ranges, PCV being about 50%, haemoglobin 160 g/l and RBC approximately 3.5×10^{12}/litre.

Impression smears: Impression smears from the eye and conjunctiva can be stained with modified Ziehl–Neelsen (Stamp) for evidence of *Chlamydophila psittaci* infection. In case of suspicion, the diagnosis should be made using the more sensitive PCR method.

Serology: Serology can be used to detect the presence of antibodies to *Salmonella* infection if a flock investigation is being performed. Acute salmonellosis in a flock will be accompanied by clinical signs (see Chapter 29).

Radiography and ultrasonography: In the individual bird these can be used for examination of the respiratory tract and hepatic swelling, and to investigate some aspects of cardiac function and reproductive tract dysfunction.

Electrocardiography and blood pressure: ECG examination, together with radiography and ultrasonography, is essential for the assessment of any suspected cardiac dysfunction. Blood pressure measurement can be performed using an appropriate-sized cuff around the humerus and a Doppler/pressure gauge instrument over the radial artery. However, this technique is probably more useful for measurement of trends of blood pressure whilst pigeons are undergoing anaesthesia than for interpretation of specific values in the conscious bird.

Hormonal investigation: Underperformance has sometimes been attributed to endocrine abnormalities, e.g. hypothyroidism. Thyroid function is very difficult to assess in birds because of difficulties in measuring their very low and fluctuating levels of thyroid hormones. Thyroid stimulating hormone is also very difficult to obtain. Empirical administration of thyroid supplements is not recommended.

Post-mortem examination: Any bird that is being culled for underperformance should be subjected to a full post-mortem examination (see Chapter 9). If this is done routinely, useful information can be gained about the health status of the flock. It is imperative that this is carried out on birds that die due to illness.

Analysis of diets: A dietary investigation should be carried out if there appears to be a flock problem of loss of performance or associated poor condition without signs of diseases. Good quality feed should be fed, and diets high in fat and protein are needed for maximum performance (see Chapter 27). The addition of vitamins and minerals to the diet should be discussed, as should the storage and procurement of the food.

Veterinary involvement in improving performance

Infectious disease is not necessarily the main factor affecting performance in a flock. Disappointing performance of the loft as a whole requires a review of the entire management system and the health status of the flock. Assuming that there is found to be good health and management, good racing results will then depend upon the quality of the birds. Figure 28.4 gives a summary of veterinary advice aimed at improving the flock's overall health and racing performance.

Subject	Advice
Husbandry and housing	Adequate ventilation, stocking density level, adequate hygiene, sufficient lighting, humidity and positioning of loft
Diet	Composition, suitability for racing, quality and supplements
Prophylactic vaccinations	Types of vaccine, timing and administration
Routine monitoring	Health checking of birds and routine faecal monitoring
New birds	Quarantine, health check and disease screening
Different ages of birds	Keep young stock separate from adults
Culling	Any young birds with severe respiratory disease or those not thriving
Monitor breeding results and look for signs of disease in young birds	Actively look for predisposing factors such as circovirus infection
Prophylactic treatments	Establish regimens as a result of parasite monitoring and disease surveillance and breeding times. Timing of anthelmintic treatment (e.g. not during moult) and being careful with dosing rates and lengths of courses when using fenbendazole (Howard *et al.*, 2002)
Training	Training advice and treatment of birds after races to avoid after-flight stress (especially with young birds), e.g. high energy foods, soya milk and vitamins
Post-mortem examination	On all culled birds or those that die
Records	Keep performance and non-return rate records. Compare with other lofts and with previous season's results
Racing birds	Ensure that fancier only races pigeons that are in 'fit' or 'top' condition. Unfit birds or those in poor condition will not win and are more susceptible to picking up disease whilst being transported with other pigeons
Therapy	Prescribe and dispense treatments for diagnosed conditions at appropriate doses and for adequate lengths of time if disease outbreaks occur

28.4 Summary of veterinary advice to improve overall health and racing performance.

Treatment

Since the cause of poor performance is often multi-factorial, a broad approach is usually necessary rather than one specific 'cure'.

Improved management and quality of birds

Management can be improved by education of the flock owner and encouragement to adopt routine disease control measures. Nutrition can be changed easily and quickly, as can environmental conditions within the loft. Particular attention needs to be paid to hygiene, ventilation and stocking density.

In some cases, the quality of the birds in the loft can be gradually improved by selective breeding and buying in 'new blood' from other successful fanciers. There will be occasions, where the original birds are of poor quality and performance, when the quickest route to success will be by buying in new breeding stock and starting afresh. This, of course, takes time since a whole new season's birds must be bred before racing can take place (only pigeons born and trained from a particular loft are likely to return to it when raced). The pigeon keeper must have faith in the advice given by the veterinary surgeon and the two must work in partnership. The owner must be prepared to instigate ruthless culling of diseased, old or poorly performing birds and adhere to any prophylactic regimes that are suggested for the flock.

Parasite and disease control

Plans for parasite control need to be drawn up and carried out on a routine basis. This should encompass roundworm control as well as surveillance and prophylaxis against protozoan parasites, such as *Trichomonas* and coccidians, and ectoparasites. Good prophylaxis should greatly reduce the likelihood of disease outbreaks. Good parasite control schemes will be part of the overall health strategy of the flock owner and this will also include the quarantine and treatment of newly acquired birds, not taking in stray birds, vaccination and the prompt isolation of sick pigeons. Veterinary input should also extend to advice on breeding and monitoring reproductive performance. Infertile and 'dead in shell' eggs should be submitted for post-mortem examination. It should be emphasized that parasitic treatments on a regular basis without proper diagnosis are not recommended, as they weaken the birds and resistances may develop; in any event, they are unnecessary.

Isolation of sick pigeons

Any bird that appears off colour or shows signs of disease should be isolated immediately and veterinary advice sought. The veterinary surgeon must endeavour to establish a specific diagnosis and then decide what treatment to prescribe. This may involve sending samples for laboratory testing before a decision can be made on the most appropriate therapy.

Specific therapy based on diagnosis

It is essential that therapy is based on a specific diagnosis. Many pigeon diseases will entail whole-flock treatments and the medicines given should be appropriate and if possible specific for the disease that has been diagnosed. Only with a specific diagnosis can a prognosis and risk assessment be given. It is also imperative that treatment is carried out for a suitable length of time and at the correct dose rate. Veterinary input on medicament use should decrease the possibility of iatrogenic and owner-induced toxicity problems and lessen the likelihood of resistant organisms developing.

The veterinary surgeon must not only advise on the above control measures but should also endeavour to visit the premises on a routine basis. If disease control and measurement procedures are in place and adhered to, the overall performance of the flock should improve.

References and further reading

Altman RB, Clubb SL, Dorrestein GM and Quesenberry K (eds) (1997) *Avian Medicine and Surgery.* WB Saunders, Philadelphia

Carpenter JW (2001) *Exotic Animal Formulary.* WB Saunders, Philadelphia

Coles BH (1997) *Avian Medicine and Surgery, 2nd edn.* Blackwell Scientific, Oxford

Hooimeijer J (2006) Management of racing pigeons. In: *Clinical Avian Medicine,* ed. G Harrison and T Lightfoot, pp. 849–860. Spix, Palm Beach, FL

Howard LL *et al.* (2002) Fenbendazole and albendazole toxicity in pigeons and doves. *Journal of Avian Medicine and Surgery* **16,** 203–210

Lumeij DT (2003) Pathophysiology and clinical features of avian cardiac disease, with an emphasis on electrocardiology. In: *Proceedings of 7th European Association of Avian Veterinarians Conference Tenerife 2003,* pp. 407–415

Olsen GH and Orosz SE (2000) *Manual of Avian Medicine.* Mosby, St Louis

Palmer D (1999) *Race Fit.* Petron Lofts, Dewsbury

Pennycott T (2000) *Some Diseases of Racing Pigeons.* SAC Veterinary Science Division, Avian Health Unit, Auchengruive, Ayrshire

Petrak ML (1969) *Diseases of Cage and Aviary Birds.* Lea and Febiger, Philadelphia

Powers L (2005) Veterinary care of Columbiformes. In: *Proceedings of the Association of Avian Veterinarians, Monterey 2005,* pp. 171–182

Redrobe S (2002) Pigeons. In: *BSAVA Manual of Exotic Pets, 4th edn,* ed. A Meredith and S Redrobe, pp.168–178. BSAVA, Gloucester

Ritchie BW, Harrison GJ and Harrison LR (eds) (1994) *Avian Medicine: Principles and Application.* Wingers, Lake Worth, FL

Rosskopf WJ and Wierpel R (1996) *Diseases of Cage and Aviary Birds, 3rd edn.* Lea and Febiger, Philadelphia

Rupley AE (1997) *Manual of Avian Practice.* WB Saunders, Philadelphia

Samour J (2000) *Avian Medicine.* Mosby (Harcourt Publishers), London

Tudor DC (1991) *Pigeon Health and Disease.* Iowa State University Press, Ames

Vogel C (1994) Columbiformes. In: *Avian Medicine and Surgery,* ed. BW Ritchie *et al.,* pp. 1207–1208. Wingers Publishing, Lake Worth, FL

29

Pigeons: infectious diseases

Tom Pennycott

Viral disease

Paramyxovirus infection

Avian paramyxoviruses can be divided into nine different serotypes, the most important of which is paramyxovirus serotype 1 (PMV-1), the causal agent of classic Newcastle disease in poultry. When this was causing heavy losses in the UK poultry industry in the 1970s the virus occasionally spread to pigeons, causing depression, incoordination, leg and wing weakness, twisted necks and death. Disease in pigeons was, however, unusual and represented a spill-over of classic Newcastle disease from poultry.

In 1977 a 'new' disease struck pigeons in Iraq, spreading to Egypt in 1978, Italy in 1981 and Sudan in 1982. This disease caused depression, muscle tremors, loss of appetite, abnormal head carriage, circling, paralysis of the wings or legs, diarrhoea and high mortality. A viral cause was suspected and initially suspicion fell on pigeon herpesvirus. Eventually it was shown that the causal virus was PMV-1, but a variant strain that was slightly different from the classic Newcastle disease virus. This variant strain is now referred to as pigeon PMV-1, or PPMV-1, and can be differentiated from classical PMV-1 using a panel of monoclonal antibodies. Disease in pigeons spread through Europe in 1982 and reached Great Britain in 1983.

PPMV-1 has also periodically spread from pigeons to poultry flocks and game birds, and so the disease in pigeons has been made notifiable (see below). In addition, because of the risk that pigeons may become a reservoir of infection for poultry flocks, all pigeons being raced or shown must be vaccinated against PPMV-1.

Epidemiology

PPMV-1 has been found in wild birds such as feral pigeons, woodpigeons and collared doves. Racing pigeons and show pigeons may be exposed to PPMV-1 through direct or indirect contact with infected wild birds or by contact with infected racing pigeons during training, racing or showing. Vaccinated birds may pick up the virus on their feathers and feet and transport it back to the loft, infecting unvaccinated birds such as young birds or breeding birds. Birds bred late in the season may be particularly vulnerable because such birds are often left unvaccinated for a longer period. Immunosuppressive conditions of young birds such as pigeon circovirus infection (see

later) may predispose to PMV infection or reduce the response to the PMV vaccine. Even healthy birds vaccinated against PPMV-1 may succumb to disease if the viral challenge is sufficiently high. Unlike certain other diseases, infected birds do not become lifelong carriers but stop excreting virus within 6–8 weeks of the initial infection.

Clinical signs

Clinical signs can be seen as early as 5 days after picking up the virus, or as long as 6 weeks after acquiring infection. PPMV-1 causes an interstitial nephritis, resulting in polyuria in a high proportion of susceptible birds. The birds drink more than normal and produce watery green faeces consisting of a pool of clear urine surrounding a core of green material. Fanciers often comment that the floor of the loft becomes very wet and describe the faeces as 'green diarrhoea', but the wet green faeces result from a combination of polyuria, polydipsia and increased excretion of bile.

When the disease was first seen in the 1980s nervous signs were frequently observed, such as loss of balance, inability to pick up feed, torticollis (Figure 29.1), unilateral or bilateral paralysis of legs or wings, loss of righting reflexes, circling, somersaulting, attempting to fly backwards, or tremors of the head and neck. Mortality in adults was usually low, but could be high in young birds as a result of secondary malnutrition or kidney failure. In recent years the pattern of clinical signs appears to have changed, with higher mortality in some outbreaks and smaller numbers of birds showing nervous signs. In general, most birds continue to eat and weight loss is not severe. Recovery from the diarrhoea and mild nervous signs can take 3–8 weeks. The outcome in birds with severe nervous signs cannot be predicted but some birds eventually recover.

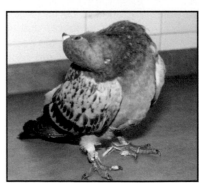

29.1 Torticollis in a pigeon with PPMV-1 infection.

Diagnosis

PPMV-1 infection can be diagnosed by demonstrating significant (the laboratory should be contacted for points of reference) serum antibody levels in live birds relative to the vaccination history, or by isolating PPMV-1 from the tissues of birds that have died or been culled. Virology and serology may give inconclusive results and material from several pigeons should ideally be examined. Findings at post-mortem examination tend to be non-specific, though histopathology may provide supporting evidence of a non-suppurative encephalitis and interstitial nephritis.

Treatment

Different countries have different strategies for the control of this disease, but in the UK Animal Health, formerly the State Veterinary Service must be informed of the suspected presence of PPMV-1 and birds must be prevented from flying out. If disease is confirmed, movement of pigeons into or out of the loft will be prohibited for at least 60 days. Electrolytes in the drinking water are beneficial, and birds with neurological signs should be placed in small groups and assisted to feed and drink. Severely affected birds should be culled if they do not show any signs of improvement within 2 weeks. Hygiene and the efficient use in the loft of approved disinfectants are essential to limit the spread of PPMV-1 and to control secondary conditions.

Control

In addition to the other statutory control measures, vaccination of pigeons taking part in shows or races is now a legal requirement in the UK. There are two licensed vaccines, both of which are inactivated, and also a combined PMV-1/pigeon pox vaccine. Live vaccines do not produce adequate protective antibodies in pigeons and are not licensed for use in pigeons in the UK.

Manufacturers' directions should be followed, but in general terms young birds should be vaccinated against PPMV-1 from 3–4 weeks of age onwards, and adults 3–6 weeks before the onset of breeding, racing or showing. Annual re-vaccination is required. If using the combined PMV–pox vaccine, vaccination of young birds should be delayed to 6 weeks of age.

Vaccine is administered by subcutaneous injection in the lower part of the neck. A very small proportion of birds may develop small lumps or large subcutaneous abscesses. These reactions will be minimized by using good hygienic practices when vaccinating birds. Very rarely a bird may collapse and die shortly after vaccination; at post-mortem examination the blood vessels under the skin of the neck are found to be engorged with blood. This adverse reaction is probably due to the unusually rich blood supply to this part of the neck, with many tiny veins and sinuses, especially in cock birds. Such adverse reactions can be minimized by vaccinating at the base of the neck rather than behind the head, with the neck stretched out and the needle pointing towards the tail of the bird.

Summary

Despite the legal requirement to vaccinate racing and show pigeons against PPMV-1, outbreaks of disease still occur on a regular basis. The 20–40 outbreaks confirmed annually in the UK are probably the 'tip of the iceberg', with many other incidents going unreported or unconfirmed. The possible involvement of PPMV-1 should be considered if birds are presented with very watery 'diarrhoea' or high mortality, even in the absence of neurological signs. A full vaccination history should be taken, but in some circumstances disease may be seen in pigeons that have been vaccinated against PPMV-1.

Pigeon circovirus infection

'Young bird sickness' is a common syndrome of young racing pigeons, usually seen between the ages of 4 weeks and 4 months. Affected birds are lethargic, with loss of appetite, the production of green watery faeces, and sometimes retention of food in the crop. Many birds return to health within 5–7 days but some deteriorate, resulting in the death or culling of the bird. The cause or causes of this syndrome probably vary with time, but currently a primary circovirus infection with other secondary infections is thought to be one of the major causes. Circoviruses are small non-enveloped viruses with a single strand of circular DNA. Measuring around 14–24 nm, they are the smallest viruses known to affect animals. Important members of the family include psittacine beak and feather disease virus (PBFDV), chicken anaemia virus (CAV) and porcine circoviruses I and II (PCV I and II). Circovirus-like viruses have also been described in other avian species such as canaries, finches, ostriches, Senegal Doves, ducks, geese and pheasants.

Pigeons infected with circovirus were first reported in North America in 1993, but retrospective studies demonstrated cases in Canada in 1986 and in Australia in 1989. Cases were seen in Northern Ireland in 1994 and subsequent investigations revealed evidence of circovirus infection in 42 of 64 (66%) sick young pigeons examined between 1995 and 2000. Similarly, in Scotland, circovirus inclusions were seen in 27 of 36 (75%) sick pigeons in 2000, and in 24 of 37 (65%) sick pigeons in 2002. However, such inclusions can also be found in healthy pigeons, and the precise significance of the circovirus remains unproven.

Epidemiology

Most circoviruses target the immune system of the host and this appears to be true for pigeon circovirus, which attacks the bursa of Fabricius, making birds more susceptible to infectious disease and reducing their ability to respond to vaccines. The bursa is only active in young birds and regresses as the birds mature.

Secondary infections seen in 24 young pigeons with circovirus examined by SAC Veterinary Services in 2002 included: viruses, such as paramyxovirus, herpesvirus and adenovirus; bacteria, such as *Escherichia coli*, *Salmonella typhimurium* and *Chlamydophila psittaci*; fungi, such as *Candida albicans* and *Aspergillus fumigatus*; and the protozoans that cause spironucleosis (hexamitosis), trichomoniasis and coccidiosis.

Several papers published in 2005 and 2006 (see 'Further reading') have increased the understanding of this disease. These studies, using PCR tests, have shown that pigeon circovirus DNA can be detected in the internal organs of a high proportion of apparently healthy adult birds, but in cloacal swabs of only a few of the adults. Viral DNA has also been detected in unhatched eggs and in newly hatched squabs, suggesting that some of these carrier birds can pass infection vertically. No evidence was found that crop milk was a major route of transmission. These studies also detected viral DNA in blood and cloacal swabs from a high proportion of young birds, including healthy birds, and sequential studies suggested that most young pigeons became infected between 2 and 10 weeks of age and then continued to excrete the virus. These findings suggest that carrier adults are present in lofts and that some young birds become infected from their parents, with subsequent direct and indirect spread to other young birds.

Clinical signs ('young bird sickness')
Circovirus infection has been demonstrated in birds showing signs such as ill thrift, loss of appetite, weight loss, 'diarrhoea' or poor racing performance. Less commonly, signs of vomiting, respiratory disease or central nervous signs are seen. The role of circovirus in 'young bird sickness' remains to be proven, and it is difficult to separate out the primary effects of the virus (if any) and the results of immunosuppression and secondary diseases. The nature and severity of the clinical signs will vary depending on the secondary infections, and mortality approaching 100% has been reported in a few severely affected lofts.

Diagnosis
Circovirus DNA can be demonstrated by PCR in tissues, cloacal swabs and blood samples from infected birds. Viral DNA can also be detected in apparently healthy birds, therefore additional evidence is required to establish the significance of positive results and tests for other pathogens should be carried out. Gross post-mortem examinations of birds that have died or been culled usually only show evidence of a range of secondary infectious diseases, but histopathological examination typically reveals damage to the immune system. Lymphoid depletion commonly occurs in the bursa and also in spleen, caecal tonsil and gut-associated lymphoid tissue. Some of the bursal follicles may be almost devoid of lymphoid cells and may be cystic. Numerous characteristic botryoid intracytoplasmic inclusions are seen within the macrophages of the bursa, especially in the medulla but also in the cortex.

Treatment
There is no specific treatment for circovirus infection, and it must instead be supportive and aimed at controlling any secondary infections identified at post-mortem examination. Feeding a light diet and the addition of electrolytes to the drinking water may be beneficial. It has been suggested that cider vinegar in the drinking water for 5 days may help to control secondary yeast infections in the crop, and a probiotic or live yoghurt may help to restore the normal intestinal bacterial flora.

Control
The mechanics of pigeon racing make it likely that young birds will at some time be exposed to this virus. If the birds are only exposed to small numbers of viruses, and if they are not subjected to other stresses or pathogens, clinical signs may be minimal or absent. Control must therefore focus on keeping virus numbers in the loft and pigeon transporters to the minimum and on reducing stress factors. Controlling other conditions, such as paramyxovirus and trichomoniasis, will reduce the likelihood of secondary involvement of such pathogens.

Summary
The involvement of circovirus should be suspected if young pigeons are presented with 'young bird sickness', if multiple infectious diseases are causing problems in young birds in the loft, or if infectious diseases occur despite vaccination (e.g. PPMV-1) or despite standard preventive treatments (e.g. trichomoniasis). Major problems can occur if young birds from several different sources are brought together, for example in 'one-loft' races, exposing young susceptible birds to circovirus and to a wide range of potential secondary pathogens.

Pigeon adenovirus infection
Inclusion body hepatitis associated with an adenovirus infection became a significant cause of disease in young racing pigeons in continental Europe in the 1980s and 1990s. In the summer of 1993 there was a marked increase in the number of cases of adenovirus infection in young pigeons in the UK, referred to as 'young bird sickness', the 'vomiting syndrome' or 'adenovirus type I'. This form of 'young bird sickness' has become less common again in the UK and has been replaced by a 'young bird sickness' associated with pigeon circovirus (see above). In addition, a severe necrotizing hepatitis associated with an adenovirus and affecting pigeons of all ages has been described in continental Europe (adenovirus type II).

Epidemiology
Several different strains of adenovirus have been isolated from diseased (and healthy) pigeons, including pigeon adenovirus and several strains of fowl adenovirus. The significance of the different strains is currently unclear. The 'classical' form of adenovirus inclusion body hepatitis characteristically affects young birds under a year old. Disease may be seen before the onset of young-bird racing, but outbreaks commonly occur a few days after the birds return from racing. It seems likely that the stress of being transported to the race site and possible delays before liberation increase excretion of the virus and subsequent spread to other birds in the basket, with further spread to other young birds in the loft when the infected birds return home. Damage to the intestine and crop, intestinal stasis and alterations to the normal flora of the alimentary tract may result in secondary overproliferation of bacteria and yeasts, most often *E. coli* and *Candida albicans*. Infection is acquired through the oral–faecal route. Vertical spread is important in some adenovirus infections of poultry but the significance of this route in pigeons is unclear.

Clinical signs

The adenoviruses damage the cells of the intestine and then the liver, resulting in the production of green faeces, excessive drinking, vomiting, and failure of the birds' crops to empty properly. Most birds recover within 4–6 days but in those with secondary yeast infections of the crop there may be substantial loss of weight, and death within 24 hours can occur due to secondary *E. coli* septicaemia. Recovered birds are often reluctant to exercise, and if such birds are sent training or racing they may not be fit enough to return home.

Diagnosis

A history of sudden onset of crop stasis, regurgitation and diarrhoea in birds a few days after their return from racing is suggestive of adenovirus inclusion body hepatitis. Post-mortem examination is often unspectacular, but there may be a catarrhal enteritis and moderate to marked hepatomegaly with haemorrhages and occasionally pinpoint liver necrosis. Evidence of concurrent infections such as crop candidiasis, trichomoniasis and colisepticaemia may be found. Confirmation of the role of adenovirus is based on the histopathological appearance of the liver, in which significant numbers of large intranuclear inclusions can be found in the hepatocytes, hence the name 'inclusion body hepatitis'. The majority of the inclusions are basophilic, filling most of the nucleus. Eosinophilic inclusions are seen less frequently, surrounded by a halo and marginated nuclear chromatin, and may be confused with the eosinophilic inclusions caused by herpesvirus infections. Unlike infections with pigeon herpesvirus and adenovirus type II, extensive liver necrosis is not usually seen. Attempts to isolate pigeon adenovirus are frequently unsuccessful, therefore laboratories experienced with this virus should be chosen. A PCR that detects this virus has been developed and is available in some countries.

Treatment and control

See comments on the treatment and control of pigeon circovirus infection.

Necrotizing hepatitis (adenovirus type II)

A necrotizing hepatitis of racing pigeons associated with an adenovirus infection has been described in pigeons in Belgium and neighbouring countries, affecting birds of all ages. Affected birds are severely depressed and die within 24–48 hours. Vomiting and yellow diarrhoea may be seen prior to death and overall mortality in the loft can be high – often 30% and sometimes even higher. An enlarged pale yellow liver with a red sheen has been described at post-mortem examination, and basophilic or eosinophilic intranuclear inclusion bodies can be found on histopathology. Unlike the classical inclusion body hepatitis, the inclusions tend to be relatively small and few in number, but are accompanied by extensive hepatic necrosis.

Summary

'Young bird sickness' may be the result of a circovirus infection (see earlier), an adenovirus infection, or even a combination of both viruses. Post-mortem examinations, including histopathology of the bursa of Fabricius

and liver, are required to establish the involvement of these viruses, but treatment and control measures are similar for both viruses. Acute necrotizing hepatitis is a less common manifestation of adenovirus infection, but liver histopathology (and possibly virology) should ideally be carried out when investigating problems of increased mortality in pigeon lofts.

Pigeon herpesvirus infection

Pigeon herpesvirus, related to but distinct from other avian herpesviruses, was first described in the UK in 1964 and still causes problems in pigeons of all ages. The virus appears to be widespread in Europe, with one survey showing that over 60% of clinically normal pigeons had encountered the virus.

Epidemiology

Some clinically healthy adult birds carry this virus, intermittently excreting it and infecting their progeny and other in-contact birds. Transmission of virus into the egg probably does not occur, but infected adults shed virus in their faeces and from the oropharynx, passing virus to their offspring during feeding. The stress of rearing multiple rounds of young birds may increase viral shedding as the breeding season progresses, resulting in further spread of virus to other young birds in the loft. Once infected, birds may become carriers for life, intermittently excreting the virus during periods of stress. Clinical disease typically occurs when the birds are aged 1–6 months, possibly after maternal immunity has waned. Clinical disease may follow the introduction of purchased carrier birds to the loft, and disease has also been seen in feral pigeons, providing another possible source of virus. Concurrent bacterial, viral, yeast and trichomonad infections may be seen in birds with pigeon herpesvirus infection.

Clinical signs

Pigeon herpesvirus damages the upper digestive tract, the respiratory tract and the liver. Discharges from the eyes and nostrils may be seen, and the tongue and oral cavity can become coated with yellow or white necrotic debris similar to that seen in cases of severe trichomoniasis, candidiasis or 'diphtheritic' pox (Figure 29.2). Necrotic material can accumulate

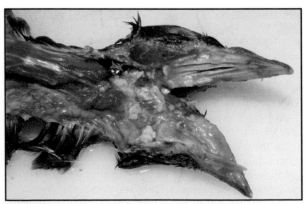

29.2 Pigeon herpesvirus: necrotic debris in the oropharynx. Trichomoniasis, candidiasis and the diphtheritic form of pigeon pox must be considered in the differential diagnosis.

in the oropharynx, causing difficulties in breathing and swallowing. Birds may vomit, stop feeding or only eat small seeds, and produce green watery faeces. Death can occur within 24–48 hours. A high percentage of the birds may appear unwell, breeding performance is reduced, and mortality can reach 15%.

Diagnosis
Confirmation of the diagnosis is usually made at post-mortem examination. Plaques of necrotic debris may extend from the oral cavity to the crop and larynx. The liver is often enlarged and mottled, sometimes with foci of necrosis and haemorrhage. Pericarditis and airsacculitis may be present, and the intestine may be distended with green fluid. Histopathological examination of the liver typically demonstrates foci of hepatocyte degeneration and necrosis associated with eosinophilic intranuclear inclusion bodies.

Treatment
Treatment is based on the provision of electrolytes in the drinking water to combat the effects of any vomiting and diarrhoea, and the control of secondary infectious diseases, especially trichomoniasis. Severely affected birds seldom respond to treatment, and birds with advanced oropharyngeal lesions should be culled.

Control
The virus is most likely to be introduced to the loft by a carrier bird. New stock should be obtained from reputable sources and ideally should undergo a period of quarantine before being admitted to the main loft. Loft management should aim to minimize stress in the birds, thus reducing virus shedding, and good loft hygiene is essential to limit herpesvirus numbers and to control other infectious agents.

Summary
Deaths in birds with green diarrhoea and lesions suggestive of advanced trichomoniasis or candidiasis should make one suspicious of pigeon herpesvirus infection. This is one of the few diseases of pigeons in which severe depression followed by death within 24 hours can be seen in several birds.

Pigeon pox
Several different members of the genus Avipoxvirus, including fowl poxvirus, turkey poxvirus, canary poxvirus and pigeon poxvirus, can cause disease in birds. Pigeon poxvirus produces only a mild infection in chickens and turkeys, and canaries are resistant to the virus. Pigeon poxvirus infection in pigeons is also often a fairly benign disease but its appearance in a pigeon loft during the racing season can create major difficulties because affected birds will not be permitted to race.

Epidemiology
Poxviruses are shed from the lesions and saliva of infected pigeons and can persist in the environment (including loft and baskets) for many months. Other birds usually become infected through minor wounds and abrasions to the skin and mucous membranes, especially around the eyes and wattles, in the oropharynx, and on the feet. Such damage can occur when birds are basketed for training or racing, or during confrontations in the loft, when feeding and drinking. A secondary viraemia may follow, leading to the development of lesions in other parts of the body. In some regions of the world arthropod vectors such as pigeon flies and mosquitoes transmit poxvirus, but the significance of arthropods such as red mite in the UK is unclear. The initial source of poxvirus is usually naturally infected birds but may be birds that have been vaccinated with certain live vaccines: poxvirus can be shed from the site of vaccination for around 3 weeks.

Clinical signs
Birds of all ages can be affected. Yellow wart-like swellings develop at the site of infection, becoming pustules that form scabs and eventually fall off after 3–6 weeks, leaving healthy skin underneath. Typically pox lesions are seen on the eyelids, on the ceres (Figure 29.3), around the eyes, on the wattles around the nostrils, and at the corners of the beak. Similar lesions are seen less commonly on the unfeathered areas of the legs and feet, around the vent, and at the navel of young birds. The lesions may be single or multiple, and range in size from a few millimetres to over a centimetre. If yellow proliferative lesions develop on the hard palate and other parts of the oropharynx the condition is referred to as 'diphtheritic pox', and concurrent trichomoniasis is common in such cases.

Another form of the disease, sometimes called 'atypical pox', or 'pox melanoma', is characterized by the formation of one or more large (several centimetres) black growths on the skin of the neck, chest (Figure 29.4), back or wings. These growths fall off after 3–4 weeks but frequently become ulcerated and infected by secondary bacteria.

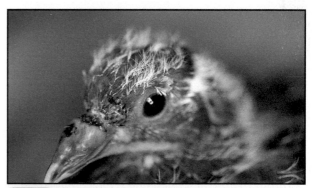

29.3 Cutaneous form of pigeon pox in a nestling. (© Michael Lierz)

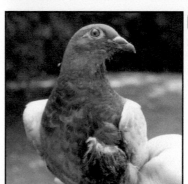

29.4 Atypical pigeon pox: large black mass on the breast.

Pigeons with pox often remain bright, though a transient viraemia may temporarily cause lethargy and lesions in the oropharynx can impair breathing or swallowing. Nodules and pustules can result in local discomfort and extensive lesions at the ceres and wattles can interfere with vision and respiration. Occasionally deformities of the eyelids, tongue or beak may be seen in recovered birds. Secondary excoriation or ulceration of lesions of atypical pox can sometimes cause substantial haemorrhage.

Diagnosis

Most fanciers recognize the gross lesions of pigeon pox without consulting their veterinary advisers. Oropharyngeal lesions could be confused with those of trichomoniasis, candidiasis and pigeon herpesvirus infection. Confirmation of disease can be achieved by lesion biopsy and histopathology, when typical eosinophilic intracytoplasmic inclusion bodies can be seen (Figure 29.5). Pox-like virus particles may also be detected if nodules or pustules are examined by electron microscopy. In some countries a PCR test is available to detect poxvirus. The virus can also be isolated in cell cultures and in chicken embryos.

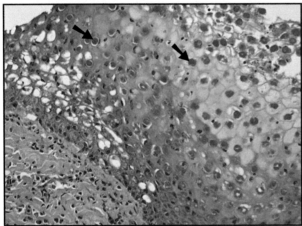

29.5 Intracytoplasmic inclusions (Bollinger bodies) in a section of palpebral conjunctiva. (Courtesy of Alistair Lawrie)

Treatment

Mild lesions will resolve without treatment within 3–4 weeks, and even the large lesions of atypical pox will dry up and fall off within this period. Topical applications of a mild antiseptic or weak tincture of iodine, or the administration of antibiotics in the drinking water, may be helpful in controlling secondary infections. If there is an outbreak of pox during the racing season it may be necessary to separate birds with lesions from apparently healthy birds, and vaccination of the latter birds should be considered. Birds should not be entered for races for at least 3 weeks after the development of clinical disease.

Control

Control of pigeon pox may be desirable because of the implications of an outbreak of pox during the racing season, and until recently two live vaccines have been available in the UK. One vaccine is a combined pigeon paramyxovirus/pigeon pox vaccine and is administered by injection under the skin of the neck. The other vaccine was applied by a stiff brush to the feather follicles of the lower leg or breast after removal of a few feathers, but this vaccine is no longer authorized for use in the UK although used elsewhere. It seems that this very useful vaccine may no longer be produced in future.

A small transient swelling may occur at the site of subcutaneous injection and swelling, discoloration and scabbing are likely to be seen at the site of follicular application. The directions of the vaccine manufacturers must be followed, but adult birds should be vaccinated at least 3 weeks before the onset of breeding, racing or showing. Vaccination at this stage should confer protection during the period of greatest risk – showing or racing – but immunity will not persist for a full 12 months and annual revaccination will be required. All healthy birds in the loft should be vaccinated at the same time. Young birds can be vaccinated from 5–6 weeks of age, but vaccinated birds should not mix with unvaccinated birds for at least 3 weeks and emergency vaccination during the racing season could seriously disrupt the training and racing programme.

Summary

Pigeon pox is a disease that interferes with training and racing but is seldom life threatening, and fanciers usually recognize the condition without the need for veterinary consultation. Although a vaccine against pigeon pox is available, many fanciers do not routinely vaccinate their birds. However, outbreaks of pox affecting several lofts in the same club may occur, prompting the need for emergency vaccination and sometimes the cessation of racing.

Bacterial disease

Salmonellosis

Salmonellosis, often referred to as 'paratyphoid' by pigeon fanciers, can result in a wide range of presenting signs. Although there are over 2000 different serovars of *Salmonella*, the great majority of isolates from racing, show and feral pigeons are *Salmonella enterica* serotype Typhimurium definitive phage types 2 and 99 (*S. typhimurium* DT 2 and DT 99). For example, of 70 isolates from pigeon lofts in Scotland between 1992 and 2006, 58 were DT 2 and 10 were DT 99, with DT 2 strongly predominating in recent years. These phage types appear to be host-adapted to pigeons, but because of the low risk that infection could spread to humans, it is a legal requirement in the UK that all isolations of *Salmonella* from racing or show pigeons must be reported to Animal Health.

Epidemiology

Apparently healthy pigeons can carry this organism, intermittently excreting it in their faeces. Purchased birds, stray racing pigeons or feral pigeons could therefore bring *Salmonella* into the loft, or the organism could be introduced after contact with infected birds during training, racing or showing. The fancier, visitors, vaccinating teams, etc. could also be the source of infection, carrying the bacteria on contaminated clothing, footwear or equipment, and rodents such as rats and mice could mechanically spread the organism from other infected pigeon lofts. Clinical disease may not be immediately apparent and some infected birds remain as carriers. Increased excretion may occur subsequently when birds are paired up for breeding, carrier birds passing the organism into their eggs and 'crop milk' in addition to the faeces, causing disease in the next generation of birds.

Clinical signs

After ingestion of the bacteria and colonization of the intestine there is often a bacteraemia or septicaemia, with subsequent localization of *Salmonella* organisms in tissues such as liver, lung, spleen, pancreas, kidney, gonad and joints. Loss of appetite, green diarrhoea and increased mortality or culling are typically seen, affecting all age groups. Weight loss can be rapid and severe. The fancier may report more 'clear' eggs than normal and increased dead-in-shells and mortality in the first week of life. A small proportion of the birds may develop abnormalities of the central nervous system such as loss of balance, circling and lateral recumbency. Some birds cannot hold their head in the normal position and have difficulty in picking up their food. In some birds the joints of the wings and legs may be hot, swollen (Figure 29.6) and painful, causing the bird to be lame or to droop a wing.

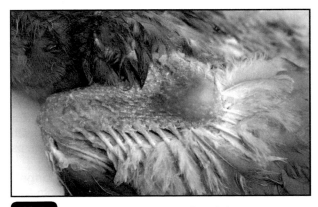

29.6 Salmonellosis: swollen elbow joint.

Diagnosis

Faeces, either from individual birds or pooled from the loft, can be cultured for the presence of *Salmonella*. Selective or enrichment media (see Chapter 21) may be required, especially when screening faecal samples. However, because of the intermittent excretion of the organism, a negative faecal sample does not rule out salmonellosis, and post-mortem examination of birds that have died or been culled should be carried out. Enlargement of the liver and spleen may be seen, sometimes with a purulent pericarditis and perihepatitis. Pale foci of necrosis or granulomas up to 10 mm in diameter in the liver, lung (Figure 29.7) or intestine are frequently seen, and less often in other organs such as spleen, pancreas and kidney. A purulent arthritis affecting one or more joints (especially the elbow joints) may also be seen, and in some chronic cases there can be substantial

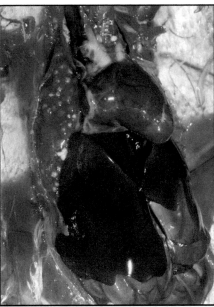

29.7 Salmonellosis: enlarged liver, nodules in lungs.

periarticular fibrosis. Bacteriology, including selective cultures for *Salmonella*, should be made from a wide range of post-mortem tissues. Similar to the situation with faecal examination, the causal organism may not be readily demonstrated in all infected birds, and a combination of pooled faeces and several dead birds may need to be examined before the diagnosis can be confirmed.

Treatment

All the birds in the loft should be treated with an appropriate antibacterial such as amoxicillin or enrofloxacin, selected on the basis of an antimicrobial sensitivity test. Treatment should be given in the drinking water for at least 10 days, and preferably for about 3 weeks, combined with thorough cleansing and disinfection of the loft, feeders and drinkers. This could be followed by a course of probiotics in the drinking water. It is advisable to cull birds with swollen joints or showing advanced central nervous system signs and those with severe weight loss. Following treatment and loft disinfection, pooled faecal samples should be screened for *Salmonella* on several occasions, including before the onset of breeding, with a repeat of the treatment programme if required.

Control

Good hygiene, avoiding overcrowding, obtaining new stock from reputable sources and excluding stray and feral pigeons from the loft will help to reduce the risk of salmonellosis. These measures should be coupled with routine screening of pooled faeces, especially before the onset of breeding. Vaccines (live and inactivated) against salmonellosis are used in some countries, for example in adults before the onset of breeding in lofts that have previously experienced problems with salmonellosis, but the vaccines are not marketed in the UK. It is very important to follow the vaccination instructions of the manufacturers. For example, use of the live vaccine in breeding birds should at the latest be 6 weeks prior to pairing, as a shorter interval might lead to poor breeding performance.

30

Pigeons: respiratory disease

Bob Doneley

Introduction

Respiratory disease is a 'blanket' phrase used to describe a multitude of diseases and syndromes that cause similar clinical signs in pigeons: sneezing, swollen sinuses, oculonasal discharge, dyspnoea, etc. It is a common and often serious problem in pigeons and pigeon lofts. Its impact on the individual bird and on the performance of a racing team cannot be underestimated. Unfortunately there is a tendency for some pigeon fanciers – and some veterinary surgeons – to consider antibiotics and other drugs to be the sole or best solution, and a great deal of money, time and effort is devoted to treating, rather than preventing, this problem.

Predisposing factors

Figure 30.1 gives a checklist of factors that predispose pigeons to respiratory disease.

Loft design	Stocking density; ventilation; climate control; drainage; ease of cleaning
General management	Stock selection; 'life stage' management; hygiene; biosecurity; medication programmes; vaccination programmes; insect and pest control; veterinary involvement
Nutrition	Diet for age and purpose; supplements; food and water dishes (type, number, location)
Physiological stress	Climate extremes; breeding; rearing young; weaning; training
Racing and shows	Exposure to pathogens; stress
Concurrent disease	Parasites; bacterial infections; viral infections; fungal infections

30.1 Checklist for factors predisposing to respiratory disease.

Loft design

Loft design can have a major impact on the spread and severity of respiratory disease in pigeons. Racing pigeons are housed in lofts, ideally with a stocking density of 20 birds per 2–2.5 m³. The design of the loft must take into consideration four basic design criteria: the loft must be dry; it must be well ventilated; it must minimize extreme variations in temperature and humidity; and it must be easy to clean (Figure 30.2).

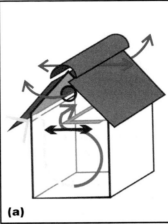

30.2

(a) The optimal fresh air flow direction to prevent respiratory disease. (b) Ventilation is essential to reduce incidence of respiratory disease. (c) Removable roofs can be used for setting up an air flow within the pigeon loft. (d) Solid floor. (a,c, courtesy of E and R Schmölz; b, courtesy of Colin Walker)

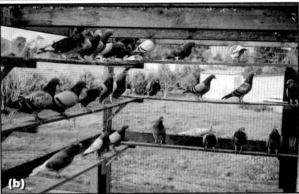

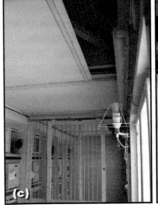

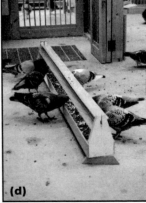

There are almost as many designs and management systems as there are fanciers, but these basic criteria must be assessed by the veterinary surgeon when inspecting premises. Most fanciers have different lofts for different life stages, i.e. young bird lofts, stock lofts and racing lofts (see Chapter 3). Each of these presents different problems in husbandry and disease control and must be assessed separately.

When lofts are overcrowded or poorly ventilated, and dust and droppings are allowed to accumulate, a bird's respiratory system is regularly exposed to a variety of noxious agents, including dust, aerosols and ammonia and other chemicals. This can cause low-grade chronic irritation of the respiratory mucosa, lessening its ability to deal with infectious agents. If the loft's biosecurity is then breached by respiratory pathogens, the penalties for 'foul air' can be magnified many times.

General management

How a loft is managed will have a major impact on the incidence of respiratory infections. As described above, it is inevitable that birds will be exposed to infectious agents. How they are managed will often determine the likelihood of infectious disease occurring and whether (and how) it will spread throughout a loft.

Stocking density, selection of stock, the use of quarantine flights, the level of hygiene maintained within a loft, the use (and misuse) of medications, vaccination programmes (pigeon pox, PMV-1 and *Salmonella*, as appropriate), parasite control, insect and other pest control and the degree of veterinary involvement in loft management are just some of the key management factors that will have an effect on the incidence of respiratory disease within a loft.

Nutrition

Pigeons are traditionally fed a mix of grains and legumes. Some greens are offered and are usually relished. Various vitamin–mineral tonics and blocks are provided, as is grit. Formulated foods are available and are being slowly accepted. Fanciers will vary the proportions of different foodstuffs to meet perceived differing needs for racing, breeding and rearing young. As with any other species, avian or otherwise, malnutrition can lead to a compromised immune system and increased susceptibility to infection (see Chapter 27).

Physiological stress

The normal stresses that a bird is subjected to in its lifetime, such as temperature extremes, weaning, breeding, rearing young, flying and racing, will impose a certain degree of immunosuppression on an individual bird or flock. In normal conditions this stress is to be expected and the birds should cope without any difficulty. However, when combined with other stressors such as overcrowding or poor hygiene, they can become major contributing factors to a flock's susceptibility to disease.

Racing and shows

The very nature of pigeon racing and showing predisposes birds to infection, in that birds under stress are exposed to other birds from many and varied sources – all of them a potential reservoir of infectious agents. The close contact between birds in trucks en route to a release point, or on a show bench, makes the transmission of disease between birds virtually inevitable (Figure 30.3).

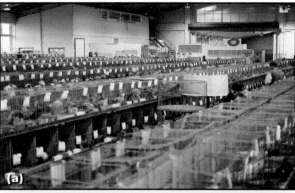
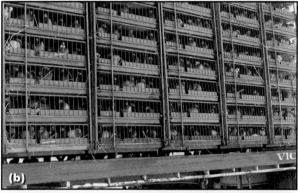
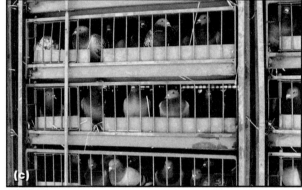

30.3 Times of risk of disease transmission: **(a)** at a pigeon show; **(b)** travelling in pigeon crates; **(c)** travelling in racing baskets. (Courtesy of Colin Walker)

Concurrent disease

Another factor predisposing pigeons to respiratory disease is the immunosuppression caused by the presence of concurrent diseases. Bacterial, fungal, viral and parasitic infections, unrelated to respiratory infections, are often diagnosed in birds presented for respiratory disease. A responsible veterinary surgeon will look past the presenting complaint and examine the bird and flock for the presence of other diseases that may be having an indirect effect on the disease status of the birds.

Clinical signs and diagnosis

As mentioned earlier, the term 'respiratory disease' covers a multitude of disease problems and, as such, does not constitute a diagnosis. The detection of the presence of respiratory disease is merely the first step in determining the diagnosis and, from there, applying a specific and appropriate therapy.

History

A complete history obtained from the fancier is a vital first step in establishing a diagnosis (Figure 30.4). A thorough understanding of the loft layout and design, the daily management, feeding regimes, recent purchases, training cycles and racing performance should be obtained. A visit to the loft is a recommended part of gathering a good history, as many seemingly minor errors in design and management can become apparent to a 'fresh' eye. The use of medications and vaccinations in the flock, whether under veterinary direction or not, must also be investigated; the illicit supply and misuse of drugs is rife within the pigeon fancy and it is the rare fancier who seeks veterinary advice before trying various medications supplied by friends and neighbours.

Physical examination

Armed with a thorough understanding of the loft and flock, a physical examination is the next step. On many occasions a fancier (perhaps seeking to reduce costs) will present a single bird, requesting a diagnosis of a flock problem. This approach should be discouraged as there is always a strong possibility that a single bird may not be representative of the flock as a whole. Instead fanciers should be asked to present three to six birds from each group in the loft: the racing team, the stock birds and the juveniles. These birds should include a mix of both clinically affected and apparently healthy birds.

At a flock level the presence of respiratory disease may be suspected with a 'loss of form' when tossing or racing. Standing quietly in the loft listening to the birds' respiratory noises it may be possible to detect an increased number of birds sneezing. Walker (2000) considered that more than three sneezes in five minutes from 100 birds warrants closer examination.

Clinical signs

This closer examination of individual birds will result in the detection of individual birds with some or all of the clinical signs described in Figure 30.5.

What is the function/purpose of this flock?
- Racing
- Show
- Hobby

Map of facility, showing:
- Loft layout
  - Entire facility
  - Boundary fences
  - Lofts
  - Food storage and preparation areas
- Age groups
  - Squabs
  - Juveniles
  - Adults
- Lofts for different purposes
  - Breeding
  - Training
  - Stock
  - Racing
- Traffic flow
  - Daily movements by owner
  - Pigeons

Loft construction
- Flooring
- Walls
- Roofing
- Ventilation

Management practices
- Diet
- Stocking density
- Quarantine
- Cleaning
  - What with?
  - How often?
- Parasite control
- Medication
- Vaccinations
- Pest control

Stock
- Selection criteria
- Source
- Quarantine protocol, including treatments and vaccinations
- Recent acquisitions

Previous medical problems
- What?
- How diagnosed?
- By whom?
- Treatment?
- Results

This problem
- Description of clinical signs
- When did it start?
- Where did it start?
- How fast is it spreading?
- Any treatments trialled by the owner or other veterinary surgeons?
- Response?

30.4 Checklist for assessing a flock respiratory problem: collecting a thorough history.

Clinical signs	Differential diagnosis
Upper respiratory tract	
<ul><li>Sneezing and yawning</li><li>Ocular discharges</li><li>Periocular alopecia or matting of feathers around the eyes</li><li>Face wiping on perches and wings, or scratching at the face and head with feet</li><li>Conjunctival hyperaemia and chemosis</li><li>Eyelid thickening</li><li>Nasal discharge</li><li>Sinus swellings</li></ul>	<ul><li>Chlamydophilosis</li><li>Mycoplasmasmosis</li><li>Pigeon pox</li><li>Pigeon herpesvirus</li><li>Parasitic rhinitis/sinusitis</li><li>Ammonia toxicosis</li><li>Trichomoniasis</li></ul>
<ul><li>Diphtheritic membranes in the oropharynx</li></ul>	<ul><li>Pigeon pox</li><li>Trichomoniasis</li></ul>
Lower respiratory tract	
<ul><li>Open-mouth breathing</li><li>Loss of body condition</li><li>Coughing</li></ul>	<ul><li>Aspergillosis</li><li>Pulmonary granulomas (bacterial, fungal, chlamydial, etc.)</li><li>'Extra-respiratory' disease – any coelomic condition compressing the abdominal and thoracic air sacs</li></ul>

30.5 Checklist for assessing a flock respiratory problem: localizing clinical signs.

The clinical signs of respiratory disease in the individual bird are as varied as the number of aetiological agents. Early signs may be as subtle as a loss of performance during racing or training. As the condition, regardless of the cause, progresses, the clinical signs become more obvious.

Diagnosis

While a good history and physical examination may detect or confirm the presence of respiratory disease within a flock or in individual birds, they rarely reveal a specific diagnosis; laboratory testing is required to do this.

A thorough evaluation should begin with relatively inexpensive and non-invasive tests, progressing to more expensive and invasive tests as diagnostic possibilities are narrowed (Figure 30.6). Initial testing should include faecal examination (wet smear preparations and faecal flotation) and crop washes or swabs to detect parasites such as *Trichomonas*, other protozoa such as coccidia, or nematodes (*Capillaria*, ascarids). Even if not directly involved in the disease problem confronting the birds, these parasites may have an immunosuppressive effect and it is important to know whether or not they are present. Bacterial and fungal cultures from sinus aspirates or the choana are the next step; once again, they should be collected from several affected birds to determine whether a pattern of infection exists. If the problem appears to be located deeper in the respiratory tract, tracheal swabs or lung washes can be performed.

After these relatively inexpensive and non-invasive tests it is usually necessary to decide in which direction laboratory investigations should continue. The extent and type of testing is often restricted by the fancier's budget and this must be taken into consideration when deciding whether to pursue relatively expensive 'individual' diagnostics. In many cases it may be more appropriate to consider the loft and flock as the patient, and the individual bird as a 'laboratory test'.

In flock problems, or with less valuable birds, it is often faster, more accurate and less expensive to euthanase several birds and perform thorough autopsies, submitting cultures and tissue samples to a veterinary laboratory. Again, it is important to 'test' several birds to confirm a disease pattern. As well as formalinized tissues submitted to the laboratory, frozen tissues should be retained in case PCR is indicated by the laboratory results. For the same reason it may be advisable in certain cases to retain frozen plasma for serological testing.

In the case of valuable show birds, breeders or racers, where the cost of testing is perhaps less important than the survival of the individual (a decision that must be left to the fancier), diagnostic tests such as radiology, endoscopy, serology, biopsy and PCR testing can be employed as they would with any other avian patient to achieve a diagnosis.

	Step	Comment
1.	Collect a thorough history (see Figure 30.4)	These two steps should allow the veterinary surgeon to gain an insight into factors predisposing to the problem (see Figure 30.1)
2.	If possible, visit the facility	
3.	Conduct a basic physical examination and diagnostic tests to: • Detect background problems • Assess whether the problem is an upper respiratory problem, lower respiratory problem or both • Detect possible aetiological agents	1. Physical examination 2. Crop smears 3. Faecal smears 4. Cultures – sinus, tracheal
4.	If a tentative diagnosis has been made at this stage, a treatment trial can be utilized	Failure to make a tentative diagnosis, or failure to respond to a treatment trial, indicates the need for further diagnostic testing. Are the affected birds individually valuable to the client, or is this a general flock problem?
5.	Valuable individual birds	Physical examination and diagnostic tests as recommended for a pet bird, i.e. • Radiology • Endoscopy • Biopsy • Cultures
6.	Flock problem	1. Serology of several birds or culture for *Mycoplasma*. If finances are an issue, frozen plasma can be stored until other diagnostic options have been exhausted 2. Necropsy of at least three affected birds, with the following tests requested from the laboratory: • Histopathology of multiple tissues, especially the cloacal bursa of young birds • Bacterial and fungal culture of liver and lung • PCR of liver for *Chlamydophila psittaci*
7.	Once a diagnosis has been confirmed, appropriate treatment and preventive measures can be instituted	
8.	Once the presenting problem has been identified and controlled/eliminated, it is important to discuss with the client future preventive measures that need to be implemented	Preventive measures include: • Selection and quarantine of new stock • Husbandry changes in design, ventilation and cleaning of lofts • Strategic use of medications • Continued monitoring of the flock to isolate and diagnose new cases promptly

30.6 Suggested protocol for diagnosing respiratory disease.

A thorough and exhaustive investigation should allow the clinician not only to arrive at an accurate diagnosis, but also to determine what factors predisposed the flock or individual birds to the resultant infection. Some of the more significant agents causing respiratory disease in pigeons are described in the next section.

Diseases

Chlamydophilosis

This disease, due to *Chlamydophila psittaci*, is very common in pigeon lofts (see also Chapter 29). A 1983 survey in England and Wales (Parsons, 1996) showed that 83% of the surveyed lofts had serological evidence of exposure. Fortunately, the virulence of this disease appears to be lower in pigeons than it is in psittacine birds; lower grade chronic infections are more common than explosive outbreaks with high mortality. Transmission is by inhalation or ingestion of infected faeces or respiratory secretions. Clinical signs include swollen eyelids, ocular discharge, discoloration of the cere, conjunctivitis (Figure 30.7), keratoconjunctivitis and dyspnoea. More acute cases may present with wasting and green diarrhoea. Concurrent infections (e.g. paramyxovirus-1 (PMV-1), inclusion body hepatitis and salmonellosis) are common. Often the primary presenting complaint is decreased racing performance. A variety of serological tests and PCR are available for diagnosis. Treatment with doxycycline is usually efficacious, but attention must be given to loft hygiene and ventilation. The zoonotic aspects of this disease must be stressed to the fancier.

One-eyed cold

This is the lay term given to a (usually) unilateral conjunctivitis and infraorbital sinusitis in pigeons. Despite a tendency for doxycycline to be prescribed on the assumption that this is caused by either *Chlamydophila* or *Mycoplasma* spp., other pathogens may be involved. Herpesvirus, *Trichomonas* spp. or bacterial infections have all been implicated. The recommended treatment is doxycycline and chlortetracycline eye ointment. Enrofloxacin is also used by some veterinary surgeons as a broad-spectrum treatment. Affected birds should be screened for trichomoniasis. If there is no response to 'standard' treatments, more exhaustive testing should be used to determine the aetiology.

Mycoplasmosis

Mycoplasma is often regarded by fanciers as a major cause of respiratory disease. In contrast, researchers have yet to determine the role played by *Mycoplasma* spp. in respiratory infections. Three species have been isolated from both sick and healthy pigeons: *Mycoplasma columborale*, *M. columbinum* and *M. columbinasale*. *Mycoplasma* is shed in respiratory secretions and transmission is by inhalation or ingestion. Treatment with doxycycline or enrofloxacin is recommended.

Aspergillosis

Aspergillosis (Figure 30.8) is common in poorly ventilated lofts. Affected birds usually present for poor performance, weight loss and dyspnoea. Occasionally a caseous sinusitis is present. Diagnosis is based on autopsy findings, histopathology and culture of affected tissues. While individual treatment is feasible, it is not usually carried out by fanciers as complete recovery and return to racing, breeding or show form is unlikely. Underlying factors, such as immunosuppressive diseases and poor ventilation, should be identified and eliminated.

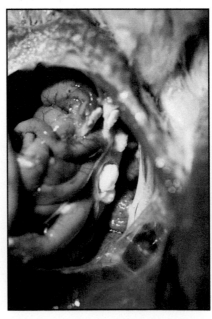

30.8
Aspergillosis in the air sacs. (Courtesy of Colin Walker)

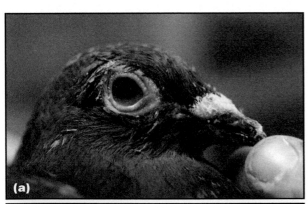

(a)

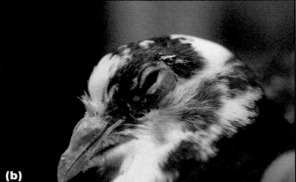

(b)

30.7 **(a)** Conjunctivitis. **(b)** Ocular discharge. (Courtesy of Colin Walker)

Pigeon pox

Pigeon pox presents as two syndromes in pigeons (see also Chapter 29). The dry form is seen as discrete scabby lesions on unfeathered parts of the body, especially the beak and eyelids. The wet form, with fibronecrotic diphtheritic lesions in the oropharynx, is less commonly seen. The presenting syndrome is determined by the strain of the virus, the mode of transmission and the age, species and health of infected bird (Ritchie, 1995). In the absence of secondary infections, most lesions will heal within 3–4 weeks, but diphtheritic lesions may persist for several months. Although the disease is usually self-limiting, the lesions may become infected and painful and may interfere with eating, respiration and vision. If lesions are secondarily infected, antibiotics and gentle cleansing are indicated. Forceful removal of scabs may result in scarring and deformity.

Paramyxovirus 1

PMV-1 in pigeons is not the classic Newcastle disease as seen in poultry, although the pigeon virus can cause disease in poultry. In pigeons it has an incubation period of a few days to a few weeks. In an infected loft new cases can appear for 5–8 weeks after first diagnosed.It usually presents as a neurological disease, although rapid breathing and facial oedema can occur. Affected birds display polydipsia, then watery to haemorrhagic diarrhoea and then neurological signs (head tremor, torticollis, paralysis of wings or legs, and blindness). Respiratory signs are minimal. The mortality rate in adults is low, with birds recovering in about 6 months (although they can have persistent diarrhoea for several months). In young birds malnutrition and renal damage can lead to higher mortality rates.

Pigeon herpesvirus

The pigeon is the primary host and reservoir for the columbrid herpesvirus 1 and 2, with squabs aged 4–16 weeks the most susceptible age group (older birds show milder signs that may go unnoticed and resolve within 1–2 weeks). The virus is spread by faecal and pharyngeal discharges; latently infected carriers are common and transmission occurs during periods of stress. The mild form is seen as a respiratory disease (mild rhinitis, tracheitis and conjunctivitis) with small ulcerations on the mucous membranes of the larynx, pharynx, cere and commissure of the beak. The more severe form of the disease is seen as dyspnoea, anorexia, biliverdinuria, diarrhoea, vomiting, protrusion of the third eyelid and neurological signs. Pathology reveals tracheitis, multiple focal degenerative lesions of the liver (diffuse hepatic necrosis with intranuclear inclusions) and diphtheroid foci on the mucosa of upper airways, pharynx and occasionally crop and intestines. Diagnosis is usually based on finding intranuclear inclusion bodies in the liver and other organs. There are no reliable means of ante-mortem diagnosis. A vaccine is not commercially available; trials indicate that experimental vaccines (at this stage) do not provide protection, but may reduce the degree and duration of viral shedding. The virus is unstable outside the host and is susceptible to most disinfectants.

Parasites

Parasites occasionally occur in the respiratory system. Trichomonads can be found in the sinuses of some birds. Nasal mites (*Neonyssus columbae*, *N. melloi* and *Sternostoma striatus*) and air sac mites (*Cyodites nudus*) have also been found, though the nasal mites are generally regarded as non-pathogenic. Heavy infestations with any mites could lead to decreased performance. *Syngamus trachea* (gapeworm) infection has been recorded, but is regarded as rare (Parsons, 1996). Typical Y-shaped paired worms are found in the trachea of affected birds, which present for gaping and sneezing. Treatment with appropriate anti-parasiticides is recommended.

Ammonia toxicosis

Ammonia toxicosis occurs in poorly ventilated unhygienic lofts. The build-up of ammonia from the nitrogen wastes in accumulated droppings (at concentrations above 100 ppm) initially causes irritation of the conjunctiva and respiratory epithelium, leading to ocular discharge, head shaking and sneezing. If the concentration reaches levels >500 ppm and is not identified and remedied, affected birds become lethargic and perform poorly. Growth rates are reduced and bacterial clearance from the lungs is decreased. Concentrations >1000 ppm cause progressive airway and alveolar disease (Osweiler, 2003). Diagnosis can sometimes be made on examination of the loft; if the veterinary surgeon's eyes begin to water and the smell of ammonia is strong, a presumptive diagnosis of ammonia toxicosis can be made. Commercial gas analysers, as used in the pig and poultry industries, can detect lower concentrations and measure precise concentrations. Ammonia toxicosis can be a predisposing factor for other respiratory infections.

Treatment

One of the biggest problems confronting veterinary surgeons dealing with pigeons is the indiscriminate and often inappropriate use of antibiotics by fanciers. With drugs often available over the internet, through pigeon clubs and friends, and even from other veterinary surgeons (usually supplied without a diagnosis and with minimal instructions and understanding of their use), it is hardly surprising that suboptimal results are the norm. This is the background against which many veterinary surgeons find themselves operating, i.e. fanciers wanting the 'perfect' drug without the expense of veterinary involvement. This attitude must be overcome if a successful treatment plan is to be implemented.

When developing a treatment plan for either individual birds or a loft affected by respiratory disease, there is more to consider than which medication to use. While it is obviously important to use the correct medication, the veterinary surgeon must also:

- Identify and, where possible, eliminate predisposing factors
- Understand the effect of the medication itself on the birds

- Determine the most appropriate route to deliver that medication to the patient.

The selection of the correct medication must be based on the correct diagnosis; the pharmacokinetics of the drug (what the body does to the drug); and the pharmacodynamics of the drug (what the drug does to the body). The route of administration needs to be considered when selecting a therapeutic regime (Figure 30.9). This in turn is determined by:

- The value of the individual bird
- The nature and severity of the illness
- The pharmacokinetics, pharmacodynamics and chemical nature of the selected drug
- The ability of the fancier to medicate the birds.

Prevention and control

It must be emphasized to pigeon fanciers that by the time clinical signs of respiratory disease are present within a flock, the window of opportunity to prevent disease has passed. Additionally, the very nature of pigeon racing and showing makes it unlikely that infectious diseases will be excluded from a loft. While a 'closed' loft would be an ideal situation, the requirements for racing and showing make such an ideal unattainable.

Pigeons are predominantly kept as racing birds or show birds. Either activity stresses the birds while at the same time increasing the individual bird's exposure to a variety of pathogens – and therefore increasing the likelihood of disease introduction into the loft. However, there are many precautions that can be taken to minimize the likelihood of a pathogen being introduced or gaining a foothold within a flock.

Biosecurity

An important role for veterinary surgeons servicing the pigeon fancy is educating their clients about biosecurity. Without a sound loft design and a solid understanding of biosecurity, it is unrealistic to expect a preventive health programme to work: the introduction of disease and flock performance become random events, outside the control of the client or the veterinary surgeon.

Biosecurity in a loft revolves around adherence to two basic principles: that there are *designated areas* within a loft; and that there is a controlled *flow of traffic* (of people, birds, and equipment) between these areas. Strict adherence to these principles (virtually impossible in an active pigeon loft where birds are either racing or showing) should minimize the introduction of disease and, in the event it does get into a loft, minimize the spread of that disease within the loft. But even if strict adherence is not possible, these two principles need to be employed as much as is practical.

- In a pigeon loft the *designated areas* include a racing loft, a breeding loft and a juvenile loft, each ideally geographically distinct from the others. A separate quarantine area should be available to handle new birds and racing/show birds to be returned to the breeding lofts. It is obviously vital to prevent strange birds entering the loft during a race.
- *Traffic flow* must be designed to minimize the spread of disease and to avoid time wasting. 'Back tracking' between areas should be avoided. It is important to avoid the mechanical transmission of disease on clothing and equipment by keeping to clearly defined 'traffic' routes and routines.

Route of administration	Advantages	Disadvantages	Indications
In-water	Easy to administer. Allows simultaneous medication of large numbers of birds	Not all drugs are stable in water. Subject to contamination, de-activation by sunlight, settling out, etc. Therapeutic tissue levels not always achieved. If the medication is unpalatable it may not be consumed. Dehydration may become an issue in some circumstances (e.g. hot weather)	Flock situations where individual treatment is impractical. Examples: doxycycline for chlamydophilosis; parasite treatments (e.g. ronidazole for trichomoniasis)
In-feed	Less risk of contamination, de-activation, etc. More reliable tissue levels usually achieved	Because most pigeons are on grain-based diets, precise dosage is difficult to achieve	Best used in situations where birds are accustomed to eating formulated diets and will readily accept a medicated diet
Aerosol	Delivers medication directly into the respiratory tract. Humidifies respiratory tract	Difficult to treat large numbers of birds precisely	Individual treatment of valuable birds. Flock treatment with aerosol medications if a confined area can be used
Parenteral	Very precise dosage and administration	Labour intensive	Individual treatment of valuable birds
Direct oral administration	Precise dosage and administration	Labour intensive	Individual treatment of valuable birds

30.9 Routes of drug administration for respiratory disease. See Appendix 1 for doses.

Veterinary involvement in the design and implementation of biosecurity measures and husbandry changes in shows and races, particularly in areas such as transport vehicles, is an important aspect of prevention and one that many fancier organizations neglect.

Antibiotics and air ionizers

Antibiotics are not a substitute for sound husbandry and good management. As mentioned earlier, the indiscriminate and inappropriate use of such medications is common within the fancy, but it must be discouraged. This does not mean that the strategic use of medications, under veterinary guidance, cannot be employed as part of the disease prevention measures within a flock.

Air ionizers to 'de-dust' the air in pigeon lofts are widely advertised in some countries. They enrich the air with negative ions, resulting in purified air. A bacterial growth inhibitor is also advertised. Even though not scientifically demonstrated in aviaries, these aids are often used and no negative effect has been reported. Prices depend on the size (air volume) and breeders need to decide whether the positive effect that might occur is worth the price. Air ionizers definitely do *not* replace good hygiene measures.

The bigger picture

The flow chart in Figure 30.10 summarizes the investigation of respiratory problems in a pigeon loft.

Respiratory disease is a common and significant problem in pigeons. The very nature of pigeon keeping, racing and showing produces a number of factors that predispose pigeons to disease, and then offers the opportunity for exposure to a variety of infectious agents. Veterinary surgeons need to look past the obvious 'diagnosis *x* = treatment *y*' scenario that many pigeon fanciers desire and instead look at the bigger picture: 'Why do these birds have this infection?' Drugs alone are not the answer to respiratory disease. When predisposing factors are modified or eliminated and good biosecurity and management are employed, the incidence and effect of respiratory disease can be markedly reduced.

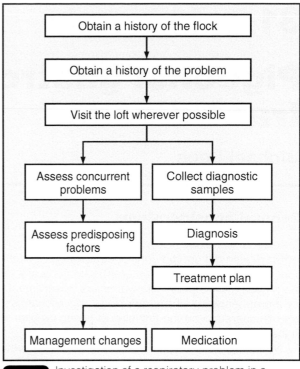

30.10 Investigation of a respiratory problem in a pigeon loft.

References and further reading

Hooijmeijer J (2006) Management of racing pigeons. In: *Clinical Avian Medicine, Vol. II*, ed. G Harrison and T Lightfoot. Spix, Palm Beach, FL

Osweiler GD (2003) Toxic gases and vapors. In: *Proceedings of the Western Veterinary Conference, 2003*

Parsons DG (1996) Respiratory diseases. In: *BSAVA Manual of Raptors, Pigeons and Waterfowl*, ed. PH Beynon *et al.*, pp. 259–266. BSAVA, Gloucester

Ritchie BW (1995) Poxviridae. In: *Avian Viruses: Function and Control*, ed. BW Ritchie, pp. 285–312. Wingers, Lake Worth, FL

Rupiper DJ (1998a) Diseases that affect race performance of homing pigeons. Part 1: husbandry, diagnostic strategies and viral diseases. *Journal of Avian Medicine and Surgery* **12**, 70–77

Rupiper DJ (1998b) Diseases that affect race performance of homing pigeons. Part 2: bacterial, fungal and parasitic diseases. *Journal of Avian Medicine and Surgery* **12**, 138–148

Walker C (2000) *The Flying Vet's Pigeon Health and Management.* Knox Veterinary Clinic, Wantima South, Victoria, Australia

31

Pigeons: gastrointestinal tract disease

Michael Pees

General considerations

Disease of the digestive system is a common problem in pigeons. It can be connected to weight loss or poor performance (see Chapter 28) and generally to many systemic diseases. Many fanciers closely monitor the appearance of the droppings, since changes are considered to be the first sign of health problems in the flock.

Normal pigeon droppings consist of a semisolid part from the intestines and the urate part from the kidneys. The intestinal part (faeces) is of pasty consistency with a greenish or brownish colour. The urate part is attached as a white cap. The droppings of healthy pigeons contain little fluid (see Chapter 7). Abnormally loose faeces can be caused by intestinal problems, but may also be due to polyuria. It is not easy to differentiate between the two conditions, therefore any kind of fluid faeces is normally considered to be 'diarrhoea' by the fancier.

Alterations of the droppings can be caused by many infectious diseases, but may also be due to stress, sexual activity (egg laying in female pigeons) and drug applications. Individual pigeons can suffer from transport stress, trauma, foreign bodies, hormonal imbalances, neoplasia and organ insufficiencies. However, diagnostics and treatment normally focus on diseases that affect several pigeons, with the potential to become a problem for the whole loft.

Clinical signs in pigeons are often caused by more than one agent. Pigeons are known to be infected with various types of parasite without showing clinical signs, but in combination with management problems, stress, and viral or bacterial infections, these parasites can cause clinical problems as secondary infections. On the other hand, the presence of endoparasites in a faecal sample should not lead to a definite diagnosis of primary disease. Further tests might be necessary to diagnose the underlying diseases.

It is therefore advisable to check pigeon flocks regularly for endoparasites. Treatment against trichomoniasis and worm infestation is recommended in apparently healthy animals with endoparasites to prevent future flock problems. This is also vital for the maintenance of optimal flight performance in racing pigeons, but regular treatment regimens can lead to drug resistance, especially in *Trichomonas* spp.

Treatment of intestinal diseases should always be combined with flock hygiene management checks and vitamin supplementation to increase the general resistance and health status of the birds.

Clinical signs often seen alongside faecal abnormalities include emaciation, swollen abdomen, swollen joints (salmonellosis) and incoordination (salmonellosis, paramyxovirus 1).

This chapter focuses on clinical signs that are associated with primary disorders of the gastrointestinal system. For systemic diseases that can also affect the GI tract, see Chapter 29.

Diagnostics

History

A complete history should be taken (see Chapter 7). Vaccinations, hygiene management, recent health checks and preventive drugs are of special interest. Observed alterations in droppings should be described, including the time of disease and the number of pigeons affected.

Important points to be evaluated and discussed include:

- Flock size and structure
- Type and size of aviary
- Feeding management
- Hygiene management
- Vaccination programme
- Prophylactic treatments
- General health/performance problems
- Number of birds affected or dead
- Treatments.

Clinical examination

The clinical examination can give information about the nature and the extent of the disease process. Emaciation is often an indication of a chronic problem.

Examination of the head and palpation of the crop will give hints about diseases of the upper alimentary tract. This includes discharges of the eyes and nostrils and alterations in the pharynx. Yellowish-white plaques in the pharynx can be caused by a herpesvirus (Figure 31.1), poxvirus, candidiasis or trichomoniasis. In the latter case, the odour from the mouth is often sweetish. Both infections can also cause thickening of the crop wall. The crop should be examined for traumatic alterations (e.g. crop perforation due to bite wounds).

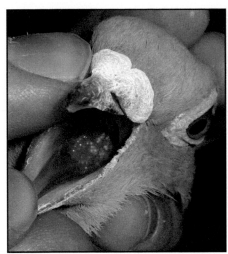

31.1

White plaques (sialoliths) in the pharynx of a pigeon. These plaques are often caused by herpesvirus infections (differential diagnoses trichomoniasis, candidiasis, poxvirus).

Examination of the abdomen gives hints about space-occupying lesions (e.g. due to hepatitis, neoplasia or egg laying). The cloaca should be clean and closed. Dirty feathers indicate diarrhoea.

The clinical examination should also include palpation of the joints, especially of the wings. Swollen joints as well as diarrhoea can be caused by salmonellosis.

Abnormalities of the central nervous system (incoordination, torticollis) can be caused by salmonellosis, paramyxovirus 1 or intoxication, but can also be the result of general debilitation.

Diagnosis

A diagnostic guide to some common infectious diseases of the gastrointestinal tract in pigeons is given in Figure 31.2.

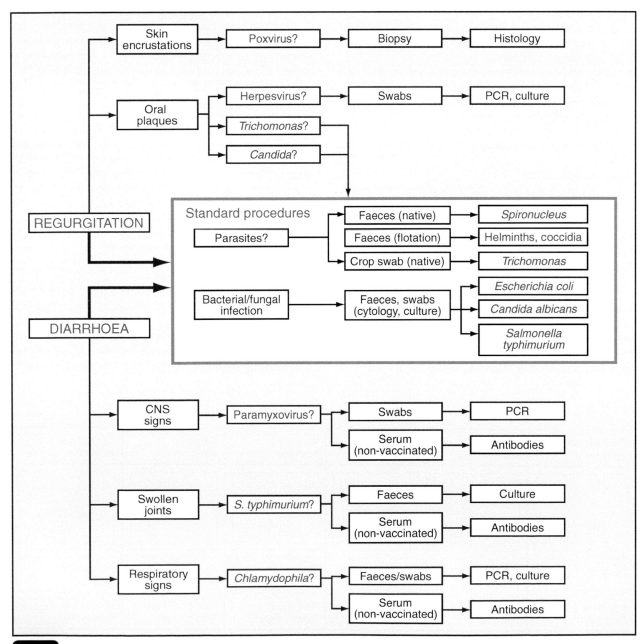

31.2 A diagnostic guide to some common infectious diseases of the gastrointestinal tract in pigeons.

Further diagnostic tools include:

- Faecal examination:
  - Fresh and flotation for parasites (*Spironucleus*, coccidia, nematodes, cestodes, trematodes)
  - Culture for bacterial and fungal infections (including enrichment for *Salmonella* and culture/PCR for *Chlamydophila psittaci*)
  - Culture, PCR and electron microscopy for viral infections (circovirus, PMV-1, adenovirus, reovirus)
- Crop swab:
  - Fresh for parasites
  - Culture/PCR for herpesvirus (pharynx and/or crop)
- Blood examination:
  - Antibodies
    - *Chlamydophila psittaci* (paired serum samples)
    - *Salmonella typhimurium* var. Copenhagen (only in non-vaccinated pigeons or paired serum samples)
    - PMV-1 (only in non-vaccinated pigeons or paired serum samples)
  - Blood chemistry, haematology
- Imaging techniques (radiography, ultrasonography, endoscopy)
- Post-mortem examination.

Faecal examination

Faecal examination is a basic procedure in pigeons and should be carried out regularly in every flock. To check for *Spironucleus columbae* the faecal sample has to be fresh and wet. It can be diluted with some drops of water and should be examined immediately for parasite movement. To check for other endoparasites (e.g. coccidia) and worm eggs, the faecal sample should be mixed with a saturated saline solution in order to float the oocysts and eggs. It is recommended to use samples from different times of the day, since some parasites (e.g. coccidia) are shed irregularly during the day. Commonly found parasite eggs and oocysts are shown in Figure 31.3.

Trematodes are not common causes of gastrointestinal problems in pigeons. A more reliable way to diagnose trematode eggs in faecal samples is the sedimentation method.

Faecal samples can be examined microbiologically. However, in cases of suspected bacterial or fungal infection a swab should be taken rather than a faecal sample, in order to minimize the risk of contamination and overgrowth. It has to be taken into account that the normal flora of pigeons consists of a variety of Gram-negative bacteria (including *Escherichia coli*) and also that the presence of yeasts is considered normal.

Examination for *Salmonella typhimurium* can be done using faecal samples. An enrichment of this bacterium in special solutions is necessary before culture (see Chapter 21). Examination for *Chlamydophila psittaci* can be done with swabs or faecal samples, either in a culture or using a PCR, which is faster and more reliable.

Further faecal examinations include checking for viral infections. The sample that is necessary for the respective examination depends on the laboratory, and its requirements should be checked in advance.

Crop swabs

Examination of a crop swab is mainly to check for the presence of *Trichomonas* (Figure 31.3). A wet swab is inserted via the mouth to the crop and palpated directly under the skin. It is turned several times to scrape some material from the crop wall. The swab is then squeezed between two microscope slides to press the parasites with the fluid on to one of the slides, which is then covered with a cover slip and examined immediately. The parasites are easy to identify by their size and movements.

Post-mortem examination

Necropsy (see Chapter 9) should be performed whenever there are casualties of unknown origin. Regular post-mortem examinations are also important tools for flock health surveys. Where several pigeons are affected, consideration should be given to sacrificing one or more pigeons for post-mortem examination.

Trichomonas gallinae	*Spironucleus columbae*	*Eimeria columbae*	*Ascaridia columbae*	*Capiliaria obsignata*	*Hymenolepis spp.* (cestode)
Crop swab	Fresh faeces	Faeces: fresh/flotation	Faeces: fresh/flotation	Faeces: fresh/flotation	Faeces: fresh/flotation
Size: 6 x 14 μm Tenacity: low	Size: 3 x 8 μm Tenacity: low	Size: 18 x 20 μm Tenacity: high	Size: 90 x 50 μm Tenacity: high	Size: 50 x 30 μm Tenacity: high	Size: 90 x 70 μm Tenacity: high

31.3   Overview of common parasitological findings in pigeons.

Common diseases

Diseases discussed in this chapter primarily affect the digestive tract. Many systemic diseases can also affect the gastrointestinal tract and result in clinical signs of this organ system, such as diarrhoea (Figure 31.4). See Chapter 29 for further details of infectious diseases. Drug doses are given in Appendix 1.

Disease	Clinical signs
Paramyxovirus	Watery green faeces ± CNS signs
Salmonellosis	Diarrhoea ± arthritis and CNS signs
Ornithosis (chlamydophilosis)	Diarrhoea + respiratory signs, conjunctivitis ± CNS signs
Herpesvirus	Oropharyngeal plaques ± secondary GI infection (immunosuppression)
Circovirus	Secondary GI infection (immunosuppression)

31.4 Clinical signs of some systemic infections.

Trichomoniasis ('canker')

Trichomoniasis is caused by the flagellated protozoan *Trichomonas gallinae*. It is a very common disease worldwide. The parasite can be found in approximately 80% of all pigeons examined. The infection is normally subclinical in adult birds (carriers), but young or immunosuppressed pigeons are susceptible to clinical signs. Some strains can cause a high mortality in pigeon populations.

T. gallinae has a direct life cycle and because it has no cyst form it is very sensitive to a dry environment. Infection is normally via the oral route (drinking water, feed). Transmission occurs from parent to offspring (via crop milk) or within transport cabins when pigeons from different flocks use the same water.

Clinical signs and diagnosis

Trichomonas infections normally affect the upper digestive tract (mouth, pharynx, oesophagus, crop). Clinical signs include lethargy, anorexia, ruffled feathers, regurgitation, dyspnoea and sometimes diarrhoea. During clinical examination, white to yellow plaques or caseous material can be found in the mouth and the crop wall often is thickened. A sweetish odour from the mouth is typical. In young birds, the umbilicus and the liver can also be affected. These alterations are normally diagnosed during necropsy.

Diagnosis is by taking a wet swab sample from the crop content. Although staining is possible, the swab should be examined fresh to diagnose the parasites by their motility. The organisms have four flagella and an undulating membrane (see Figure 31.3).

Treatment

Treatment should include the whole flock since infestation can be caused by poor hygiene and poor health control management. Several drugs are available, such as metronidazole, ronidazole and carnidazole. Treatment should include vitamin supplementation to increase general resistance and, if necessary, treatment of accompanying or secondary infections. Disinfectants are not absolutely necessary, since drying out of water containers for approximately 48 hours is sufficient, but hygiene management should be improved. A strict water hygiene routine is advisable, including a daily change of water containers (they can be reused after 1 day of drying) and provision of a sufficient number of containers.

Affected flocks should be rechecked after 2 weeks. Resistances to drugs have been described. To reduce the risk of drug resistance, pigeons should be checked regularly for parasites and treated only on positive findings. Unnecessary treatments may also weaken the bird and may reduce racing performance.

Spironucleus columbae (hexamitiasis)

The causative agent of hexamitiasis is *Spironucleus columbae* (formerly *Hexamita columbae*, see Figure 31.3). It can cause severe diarrhoea in young pigeons. Adult birds play a role as asymptomatic carriers. Infestation with clinical signs is normally the result of a combination of poor hygiene and accompanying bacterial, viral or parasitic infections. The parasite lives in the duodenum and small intestine and is spread by the faeces. *Spironucleus* lacks a cyst form and is therefore very sensitive to a dry environment.

Clinical signs and diagnosis

Clinical signs are diarrhoea of varying extent, with greenish loose to watery faeces, general depression, dehydration and weight loss. Sometimes undigested seeds are seen in the faeces. Vomiting is also possible. Mortality in young pigeons is up to 80%, depending on immune status and secondary infections.

Spironucleus columbae can be demonstrated in fresh warm wet faecal samples. The organisms are identified by their motility (rapid darting motion, in contrast to the jerky motions of trichomonads).

Treatment

Therapy includes vitamin supplementation and hygiene control. Metronidazole and ronidazole can be used.

Coccidiosis

To a small extent coccidians can be found in most pigeons and are not considered to be harmful. There is ongoing debate on whether or not coccidia should be treated if found only in low numbers without clinical signs. Undoubtedly small numbers of the protozoan will induce immunity, but the racing season is stressful for the bird and a few coccidians might become a large problem within a few days, resulting in a loss of racing performance. Therefore, treatment is advisable in racing pigeons during the season, though in young pigeons or breeders there is induction of immunity and no treatment should be considered.

In contrast, high concentrations of the organism can negatively affect performance and also cause severe clinical signs. Under crowded conditions and poor hygiene, coccidiosis can become a problem for the whole loft.

Two species are common in pigeons: *Eimeria columbae* (see Figure 31.3) and *E. labbeana*. They have a direct life cycle with a faecal–oral infection route. They live and reproduce within the mucosa in the intestinal tract. They replicate in the host cells and can cause severe damage to the mucosa. Young pigeons are more susceptible to clinical signs. Development of clinical signs might depend on variations of the pathogenicity.

The oocysts that are shed with the faeces are very resistant in the environment and can survive for more than a year.

Clinical signs and diagnosis

Clinical signs develop rapidly (4–7 days) after ingestion of a relatively large number of sporulated oocysts. Moderate to severe diarrhoea can occur, with watery, dark or even bloody faeces. Depression, anorexia, lethargy and emaciation can also be seen.

Diagnosis is based on the examination of the faeces in combination with the results of the anamnesis and clinical signs. Large numbers of oocysts normally can be found (flotation method), but the number of oocysts seen has little relationship to the extent of the clinical signs. The absence of oocysts does not exclude coccidiosis, since clinical signs can develop faster than the shedding of the parasite (prepatence). Droppings should be collected in the morning, since it has been reported that at this time of the day oocyst concentrations are higher. It is also advisable to collect several samples.

Treatment

Treatment should include all pigeons in the loft. Vitamins (especially vitamins A and B) should be supplemented. Strict hygiene and the use of disinfectants are essential. Toltrazuril, sulphonamides or clazuril can be used to treat the flock.

After infection, a local immunity develops and normally prevents further clinical signs, though reinfection is common. There is no cross-immunity between different coccidian species, but the clinical picture is normally mild after reinfection.

Helminth infestations

Nematodes are the most commonly diagnosed intestinal worms, while cestodes play a minor role in the development of gastrointestinal disease in pigeons. Clinical signs in birds with worm infestation are poor performance, weight loss, anorexia and diarrhoea. *Capillaria* spp. can also cause vomiting and sudden death (from haemorrhage).

The two most important nematodes in pigeons are *Ascaridia columbae* and *Capillaria obsignata*. Both have a direct life cycle. Ascarid eggs are thick-shelled and ovoid; *Capillaria* eggs are smaller and have bipolar plugs (see Figure 31.3). Both eggs are very resistant, even to disinfectants. Adult ascarids are up to 3 cm in length and can be found occasionally in the faeces. *Capillaria* adults are only 1 cm long, with a very small diameter, making diagnosis difficult, even during necropsy. Ascarids live in the small intestine, whereas *Capillaria* can be found from the crop to the caecum. Since they burrow into the mucosal lining and suck blood, *Capillaria* species are considered to be more harmful for the host.

Although diagnosis of worm infestation is normally by faecal egg counts, this method can be misleading: shedding of the parasite eggs depends on several factors and the correlation between eggs found in the faeces and clinical signs is rather low.

Faecal samples are examined using the flotation method.

Cestode eggs are found occasionally in faeces. Because cestodes have an indirect life cycle, they are not considered to be a flock problem, but they can cause clinical signs in individual birds. Proglottids can sometimes be seen in the faeces. Eggs (see Figure 31.3) can be found using the flotation or sedimentation method.

Treatment

Treatment of nematodes is possible using fenbendazole, levamisole or ivermectin. Cestodes can be treated using praziquantel. Strict hygiene control and disinfection are necessary. Nematode eggs are very resistant to disinfectants. New birds should be kept in quarantine before joining the loft.

Bacterial infection

The normal intestinal flora in pigeons consists of a variety of Gram-positive and Gram-negative bacteria. Therefore it is difficult to interpret microbiological results from faecal examinations. However, some bacteria are considered to cause clinical diseases. *Salmonella typhimurium* and *Chlamydophila psittaci* can cause severe diarrhoea and are discussed in Chapter 29. *Escherichia coli* can be found in normal faeces but, depending on the strain and accompanying immunosuppression (adenovirus, circovirus), it can also be the cause of severe disease, especially if obtained in pure culture. However, treatment of *E. coli* in pigeons is only indicated in birds showing clinical signs (severe diarrhoea, flock mortality). General treatment of *E. coli* infection does not make sense and will induce drug resistance. Another bacterium reported to cause gastrointestinal disease is *Streptococcus gallolyticus*.

Treatment should be done following sensitivity testing (excluding *Chlamydophila* infection); for dosages see Appendix 1. The extent of necessary disinfection depends on the bacterium. Hygiene management should be checked and improved, and vitamin supplementation should be given.

Candidiasis

Candidiasis is a mycotic disease that is normally caused by *Candida albicans* and might affect young pigeons. Since yeasts can be found regularly in pigeon faeces, treatment is only necessary in birds with clinical signs (e.g. voluminous faeces, yeasty odour from the mouth or the faeces, thickened crop wall). *Candida* infections should always be considered to be a secondary problem, and underlying diseases should be diagnosed.

Treatment is possible using nystatin (orally to individuals, 100,000 IU/kg over 10 days). For treatment of the flock, chlorhexidine added to the drinking water (2.5 ppm) can help to resolve clinical signs, but is not a specific treatment.

Crop perforation and trauma

Trauma is normally caused during free flight and can be due to raptors or accidents. Trauma of the digestive system mainly concerns the crop.

Crop perforation is a common finding in pigeons; food passes through the opening, causing soiled feathers in this area. In many cases the general condition of the pigeon is not affected, but emaciation and debility are the result of the inability to digest food.

Diagnosis is easy, due to the typical clinical picture. Therapy includes surgical closure of the wound and anti-infective therapy. For general considerations about soft tissue surgery see Chapter 14. The feathers in the wound area are carefully plucked (beware: the skin in pigeons is very thin). The area is cleaned and then the crop wall is separated from the skin. This can be difficult if the wound is not fresh, since both organs might be connected closely to each other, forming a crop fistula. It is important to suture the crop wall with inverting patterns separately before closing the skin. The bird should be fasted for the next 24 hours, then given some fluids. After 48 hours, small amounts of solid food can be offered.

References and further reading

Gelis S (2006) Evaluating and treating the gastrointestinal system. In: *Clinical Avian Medicine, Vol. I*, ed. GJ Harrison and T Lightfoot, pp. 411–440. Spix, Palm Beach, FL

Hooijmeijer J and Dorrestein GM (1997) Pigeons and doves. In: *Avian Medicine and Surgery*, ed. RB Altman *et al.*, pp. 886–909. WB Saunders, Philadelphia

Vogel C, Gerlach H and Löffler M (1994) Columbiformes. In: *Avian Medicine: Principles and Application*, ed. BW Ritchie *et al.*, pp. 1200–1217. Wingers, Lake Worth, FL

32

Pigeons: systemic and non-infectious diseases

Alistair Lawrie

Hepatic disease

Pigeons do not have a gall bladder. Bile drains directly through the right hepatic duct into the duodenum. If this duct gets blocked and then becomes dilated, it may resemble a gall bladder on ultrasound or at post-mortem examination.

Physical findings with liver disease are often non-specific unless there is major hepatomegaly or the presence of ascites. The presence of either or both of these signs is likely to cause a degree of dyspnoea, due to pressure on the lungs and air sacs. Other features associated with liver disease are polydipsia and polyuria and the passing of green urates in the droppings.

Investigations

Clinical biochemistry

The results of clinical biochemistry can be quite difficult to interpret in birds. The plasma bile acid level is the single most useful test for determining liver dysfunction in racing pigeons and, as in other animals, dynamic testing may be of more value. Elevation of other 'liver enzymes' (e.g. AST, GGT) can indicate recent damage to liver cells but gives no indication of the functional ability of the liver. AST will be elevated in cases with muscle damage. Cholinesterase is also an important enzyme for liver disease diagnosis.

Although glutamate dehydrogenase (GLDH), a mitochondrial enzyme, is the most liver-specific enzyme in the racing pigeon and elevations can indicate severe liver damage where cellular necrosis has taken place, it is not a particularly sensitive test. It must be remembered that plasma enzymes may be within normal limits in cases of chronic liver fibrosis. In these instances, however, bile acid levels are likely to be raised and total plasma protein and albumin levels will usually be low. Dehydration or inflammatory disease may artificially raise plasma protein levels.

Imaging and biopsy

Radiology and ultrasonography may provide valuable information, especially in cases with hepatomegaly and internal liver masses. Ultrasonography may be easier to perform in the ascitic bird. Liver echogenicity has been shown to change (more focal and less homogeneous) in birds with gastrointestinal disease (see Chapter 12).

Definitive diagnosis can only be made by either endoscopic, surgical or ultrasound-guided liver biopsy (see Chapters 12, 13 and 14). It is relatively easy to obtain a wedge biopsy sample by ventral midline laparotomy. Post-biopsy haemorrhage may be a significant complication in the bird with a congested liver or which has compromised clotting factor production.

Hepatitis and neoplasia

Hepatitis is a very common feature of many systemic diseases affecting the pigeon and may be viral, chlamydial or bacterial in origin. The hepatic pathology and therefore potential therapy depends upon the causative agent (Chapter 29). Non-infectious liver disease has not been well documented in the racing pigeon. Hepatic changes may be seen in circulatory disorders (portal hypertension and hepatomegaly) and also after hepatic 'insults' from plant or fungal toxins. Pigeons are relatively selective grain and pea eaters and with a few exceptions are unlikely to eat poisonous plants (see Toxicology section, below).

Neoplasia is encountered and may be part of a systemic syndrome (e.g. disseminated lymphoma) or may be a primary liver tumour (e.g. bile duct carcinoma).

Haemochromatosis

Haemochromatosis is not a common condition in pigeons but occurs where there is excessive accumulation of iron causing pathological changes in the liver and other major organs. The condition arises from an altered intestinal absorption of iron, possibly from an inherited defect, and also from high dietary iron content (sometimes by excessive iron supplementation by the fancier).

Clinical signs

Clinical signs relate to the physical changes in the liver, namely hepatic enlargement, ascites and swollen abdomen. Fluid accumulation by pressure on air sacs can lead to weakness and respiratory signs (e.g. coughing). Sudden death without previous signs occurs.

Diagnosis

Definitive diagnosis is by liver biopsy and use of Perle's iron stain. Plasma biochemistry may show an increase in AST levels and a decreased level of plasma proteins. Radiography may reveal hepatomegaly, ascites and sometimes cardiomegaly. Ascitic fluid is a yellowish transudate. Blood iron levels are not diagnostic.

Treatment

Ascitic fluid should be removed if the bird is dyspnoeic, but not too much fluid should be removed at one time since the procedure may induce shock. Phlebotomy is useful and 1–2% of the bird's blood volume can be removed daily until either there is a clinical improvement or the haematocrit reaches the lower end of the range for the species (PCV not lower than 30%). Thereafter, weekly phlebotomy may need to be carried out at volumes of about 1% of body weight. Serum albumin should also be monitored.

Deferoxamine has been used to reduce the level of iron in body tissues. The bird needs to be on a low-iron diet and should not be given supplemental iron by the fancier.

Other parenchymal hepatic conditions can be diagnosed by liver biopsy.

General therapy for hepatic disorders

Treatment of liver disorders is mainly symptomatic and supportive unless a specific infectious agent has been identified that will respond to antibiotics or antiviral treatment. Fluids and easily digested/assimilated foods (e.g. Critical Care Formula, Vetark) should be given by crop tube. A good diet should be offered and vitamin B support of the remaining liver function is essential. In other avian species, lactulose has been found to be useful (to decrease enteric ammonia production) and milk thistle extract is thought to help hepatic cell function and regeneration and to decrease the degree of hepatic fibrosis. Colchicine combined with dandelion extract may also be useful for this purpose.

Renal disease

Renal disease is probably under-diagnosed in the pigeon since signs are mild or non-specific until the advanced stage of the disease. An owner's description of 'diarrhoea' is often polyuria. Some signs of renal disease may appear to relate to other systems, including lameness in cases of renal swelling (pressure on the ischiadic nerve), dyspnoea where there are large renal tumours, ascites compressing the air sacs or even constipation. The presence of articular gout is due to hyperuricaemia from renal disease. A survey of pathological findings in a colony of pigeons (Klumpp and Wagner, 1986) found that salmonellosis and nephritis were the commonest causes of death in 1–3-year-old pigeons. In addition, the monthly mortality from end-stage renal disease and atherosclerosis with secondary complications was greater (2–4%) in birds fed a diet containing cholesterol than in those on non-cholesterol-containing pellets (0.9%).

Anatomy and physiology

The avian kidney differs significantly from the mammalian kidney in both anatomy and physiology (see Chapter 5).

The main nitrogenous waste product of the bird is uric acid, generally regarded as being a non-toxic insoluble substance (compared with urea and ammonia in mammals), most of which has been synthesized by the liver. Some is filtered through the glomeruli, but in a normal healthy bird over 90% is secreted by the cells of the proximal convoluted tubule. Once in the urine, it combines with proteinaceous mucus to become the familiar white colloidal condensate.

Uric acid secretion is barely affected by the glomerular filtration rate until very low levels of urine flow result in the precipitated materials being unable to flow through the tubules.

Since blood uric acid levels do not tend to rise in birds until dehydration is severe, elevated uric acid concentrations indicate either severe dehydration or extensive proximal tubular damage (renal function is below 30% of normal function).

Uric acid concentrations above 600 µmol/l may result in tophi (uric acid crystals) being deposited in and around joints (articular gout) or internal organs (visceral gout).

Some birds with extensive renal damage can have normal uric acid concentrations because: (i) some uric acid is eliminated by filtration even though there is secretory tubular damage; (ii) renal failure cases will often be polydipsic/polyuric and thus will have an increased filtration rate; and (iii) uric acid production may be decreased by compromised liver function or anorexia. In general terms, tubular lesions may lead to hyperuricaemia or polydipsia, whereas glomerular lesions will lead to protein loss and hypoalbuminaemia.

Regulation of sodium and water excretion is by the aldosterone–vasotocin–renin–angiotensin system.

In the face of water deprivation, birds (unlike mammals) are also able to increase their plasma osmolarity gradually. In dehydrated birds up to 15% of urine may be reabsorbed from the colon, but this reabsorption is markedly decreased in stressed birds or those with polyuria.

In cases of renal failure, plasma potassium and phosphorus levels do not tend to rise significantly, nor plasma calcium levels decrease. Potassium levels must be measured patient-side or a spun sample should be sent to the laboratory.

Urine

Most healthy pigeons produce a small amount of urine containing white urates. The urates may become coloured for a number of reasons (Figure 32.1).

Colour	Possible causes
White	Normal
Green	Biliverdinuria – severe hepatic disease (Figure 32.2) (e.g. *Chlamydophila*, hepatitis)
Brownish yellow, golden yellow	Hepatic disease, vitamin administration, hepatitis
Red/brown/chocolate	Nephritis, haemolysis, warfarin-type poisons

32.1 Pigeon urates.

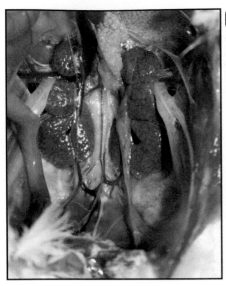

32.2

Green urates in the kidneys of a dove with hepatic necrosis.

- The pH ranges from 5.5 to 6.9 and a trace of protein may be present (0.11–1.99 g/l).
- Urobilinogen is not present in urine.
- Occasionally a trace of glucose may be detected (0–3.2 mmol/l). This may be stress associated, or evidence of proximal tubular damage.

Polyuria is not necessarily a sign of renal disease and may have many causes, including stress (Figure 32.3).

Clinical signs of renal disease

In most cases, there will only be mild clinical signs and renal disease may not even be suspected. In pigeons, most urinary tract diseases are part of systemic diseases affecting many organs.

Abnormal urinary output can be polyuria, anuria or oliguria. Polydipsia will often accompany polyuria and there may be depression, dehydration and/or convulsions. Polydipsia can be the *cause* of polyuria (behavioural) or the *result* of polyuria (renal, endocrine). It is a non-specific sign and needs investigation.

Some renal cases have no change in urinary output. 'Normal' urinary output varies with age, species and physiological state and these factors must also be taken into account in the suspected 'renal patient'.

Diagnosis

In most cases, renal involvement and observed polyuria will be part of a generalized systemic pigeon disease where other more obvious signs (e.g. neurological signs) may point to the diagnosis. Renal biopsy or necropsy may be the only way to achieve a positive diagnosis (Figure 32.4).

Because of the close association with urates and faeces, analysis of urine alone can be difficult. Examination of the urinary sediment is worthwhile if renal disease is suspected. The normal sample may reveal the presence of casts (very few), some cells (e.g. from the cloacal epithelium), small numbers of Gram-positive bacteria (from the faeces/cloaca) and some erythrocytes and leucocytes (normally not more than three per high-power field). The presence of many casts indicates renal pathology. Pigeon urine may be collected directly by cloacal cannulation (Halsema, 1998).

- Pigeon urine has a lower specific gravity (1.005–1.020 g/ml) than that of mammals.

Type	Possible causes
Dietary	Excess salt or minerals, nephritis from feeding high-protein turkey pellets, changing young squabs on to seeds
Psychogenic	Stress, fear, excitement (especially cock birds) and after transport
Hypocalcaemia	Egg-laying females (possibly also in males if they are feeding squabs), lack of feed additives
Systemic infections	Bacterial (e.g. salmonellosis), viral (e.g. PMV-3)
Hepatitis	Liver disease (e.g. adenovirus infection) or generalized infections, toxins
Renal disease	Nephritis, neoplasia, gout
Toxins	Ingested toxins (e.g. mycotoxins, excess salt), pesticides, herbicides
Iatrogenic	Antibiotics (aminoglycosides), steroids, diuretics. Oliguria has been recorded with gentamicin toxicity
Physiological	Egg-laying hens, gastrointetstinal disease

32.3 Causes of polyuria in pigeons.

Method	Comments
Urinalysis	Collect uncontaminated sample on cellophane or by cloacal cannulation
Haematology and biochemistry	Routine blood analysis to differentiate diseases of other organs and to establish renal parameters
Radiography and ultrasonography	Can visualize kidney size and density. Can vary with dehydration (smaller and dense) or nephritis and gout (swollen)
Colour and form (endoscopy)	Visualized on endoscopy. Cysts, neoplasia, renal gout
Biopsy (generally endoscopic)	Easier to get more representative sample than in mammal, due to arrangement of nephrons
Uric acid, albumin, total protein, PCV	Assess degree of dehydration. Filtration must decrease by 70–80% before uric acid levels are elevated; can therefore have serious renal disease before levels are increased. Hyperphosphataemia is not a feature of avian renal disease

32.4 Investigation of renal disease.

Visceral gout

Visceral gout occurs when uric acid crystals (as white flecks) are deposited on the serosal surface of the liver and other organs (e.g. kidneys and pericardium), death following soon after. It is often a post-mortem diagnosis.

It may follow an episode of severe dehydration or nephritis and is an acute and serious disease with a poor prognosis. Tubular secretion of uric acid stops, anuria or oliguria is seen and plasma uric acid levels rise rapidly. Signs of gout are non-specific and may include weight loss, anorexia and emaciation. Sudden death is common and may relate to cardiac embarrassment from the pericardial and epicardial urates or hyperkalaemia (Lumeij, 1994).

Diagnosis

Plasma uric acid levels are usually elevated (though if the uric acid crystals are deposited on the serosa, the plasma level can decrease and might be within normal range) but these are not diagnostic since other conditions can also cause raised uric acid levels. Laparoscopy is the single most useful investigative procedure, but many cases will only be diagnosed at post-mortem examination.

Treatment

In the acutely ill bird intensive supportive therapy (especially fluids) and allopurinol administration may, in some cases, reduce the plasma levels of uric acid but will have no effect upon the previously deposited urates. (Allopurinol reduces the production of uric acid from purines and is unlikely to be of great benefit in cases with nephron or ureteral obstruction.)

Articular gout

In articular gout, uric acid crystals are laid down in and around joints and in tendon sheaths. Once uric acid deposits have occurred they can 'grow', forming larger accumulations of uric acid called tophi. Deposition occurs when the plasma uric acid level is slightly above the solubility of sodium urate in the plasma. It is an extremely painful condition for the bird, resulting in lameness (Figure 32.5) or drooping of the wings.

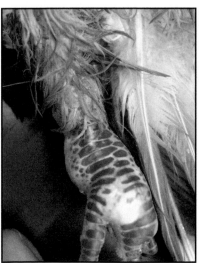

32.5 Articular gout in a Woodpigeon. (Courtesy of Kevin Eatwell)

Diagnostic techniques include aspiration of tophi: needle-shaped uric acid crystals are seen under the microscope. A murexide test involves adding one drop of nitric acid to the material on a slide and heating until dry, then adding one drop of ammonia. A mauve colour indicates the presence of urates.

Treatment of renal disease

Supportive therapy with fluids, heat and nutritional support should be given until a specific diagnosis is reached. Parenteral fluids may be indicated in the most severe cases (see Chapter 8).

In anuric or oliguric pigeons, the fluid should initially be restricted to the daily insensible fluid loss of 20 ml/kg and diuretics (furosemide) given. Monitoring body weight accurately will give an indication of over- or under-hydration. The hydration status of polyuric pigeons must be monitored and fluid given as needed.

Antibiotics should be administered since there is a higher susceptibility to renal invasion from portal vein-carried enteric organisms. Antibiotics that are potentially nephrotoxic should not be used but multivitamin support should be given. Allopurinol or colchicine can be considered in the most severe cases but long-term use may cause renal damage.

A more detailed description of renal diseases, diagnoses and treatment can be found in Lierz (2003).

Endocrine disease

Few endocrine diseases have been documented in pigeons.

Thyroid gland hyperplasia (goitre) has been reported. Birds tend to have very low resting T4 levels and anorexia can lower T3 and T4 levels significantly. Thyroid-stimulating hormone is not widely available and so confirmation of hypothyroidism is difficult. Response to supplementation does not confirm the diagnosis since stress and drugs can also make birds functionally euthyroid. If treatment is attempted, oral supplementation in other birds has been given at 0.01–0.02 mg/kg q12h (Rosenthal, 2005).

In adrenal disease, corticosterone (not cortisone) is the major glucocorticoid in the bird, therefore ACTH stimulation testing must be for corticosterone levels. There are no recorded cases but experimental work has been carried out in pigeons (Westerhof *et al.*, 1994).

Cardiovascular disease

Clinical cases of cardiovascular disease are not often seen in free-flying pigeons. A combination of exercise, fitness and genetic selection for athletic ability has produced birds with healthy cardiovascular systems. Nevertheless, cardiac disease may be observed in systemic infections where myocarditis and pericardial effusion can both occur (e.g. *Chlamydophila* and *Mycoplasma* infections) (see Chapters 29 and 30).

Pigeons on high-cholesterol diets have been shown to develop atherosclerosis and chronic nephritis (Klumpp and Wagner, 1986). Lymphocytic inflammation in the myocardium secondary to viral infection has also been seen leading to poor performance (John Chitty, personal communication).

Clinical signs of heart disease

Signs of heart disease become more obvious with increased severity of the cardiac disease. Hepatic congestion, dyspnoea, ascites and poor performance can be seen (though dyspnoea and ascites have many other causes in birds), but coughing is not usually a feature. Sudden death without premonitory signs can occur.

Diagnosis of heart disease

Cardiovascular examination can be challenging, since the rapid heart rate makes detection of murmurs and arrhythmias difficult and there is often difficulty in peripheral pulse detection. Examination under anaesthetic with the use of ECG and echocardiography is probably the most useful way of obtaining a diagnosis.

Diagnosis is based upon:

- History
- Physical examination (which may have to be brief)
- Auscultation (murmurs can be difficult to classify as systolic or diastolic and there may be cardiac muffling due to liver enlargement or pericardial effusion)
- Complete haematology and plasma biochemistry (including estimation of high- and low-density lipids)
- Radiography, ECG, ultrasonography (see Chapters 11 and 12)
- Blood pressure measurement (using a Doppler unit and appropriately sized cuff on the femur or humerus).

Electrocardiography

Electrocardiography must be able to use a paper speed of 100 mm/s and 1 cm = 1mV. Recordings are made by placing the patient in dorsal recumbency under anaesthetic and attaching the four limb leads to the wings and legs by the use of 25-gauge needles placed through the skin (propatagium and medial thigh). Lead II is normally used for monitoring and interpretation.

The amplitude of the waves tends to be low in avian patients and there is little information correlating cardiac pathology and changes in the ECG. It is assumed that the significance of major abnormalities will be similar to that in mammals, e.g. atrial fibrillation, ventricular premature complexes, AV block. Figure 32.6 lists ECG abnormalities and suggests possible causes.

It should be noted that hypothermia can easily induce arrhythmias, accompanied by a drop in blood pressure, in otherwise healthy birds and this can be fatal if birds become hypothermic when undergoing anaesthesia.

Blood pressure

The arterial pressure is assumed to be much higher than that of mammals, often quoted as being 300–400 mmHg. In reality, blood pressure measurements on anaesthetized birds are nearer to those of mammals and systolic pressures of 90–140 mmHg (Lichtenburger, 2005) are considered to be relatively normal. Maintenance of this blood pressure is helped by the relatively firm structure of the arteries. Peripheral blood flow is thus improved but at increased susceptibility to atherosclerosis and blood vessel rupture when stressed.

Pathological cardiac conditions

Myocarditis, pericarditis and pericardial effusion have been recorded together with ascites in cases of congestive cardiac failure. Infectious agents (e.g. *Chlamydophila*, *Mycoplasma* and *Pasteurella*) can also cause pericardial effusion. Valvular bacterial endocarditis and valvular insufficiencies may be seen.

Treatment of cardiac disease

Figure 32.7 outlines possibly therapies for cardiac disease.

Abnormality	Possible causes
Atrial premature contractions, fibrillation or flutter	Serious atrial dilatation due to valvular insufficiency
Ventricular premature contractions	Hypokalaemia, thiamine deficiency, vitamin A deficiency, paramyxovirus, avian influenza, myocardial infarction, lead toxicity, digoxin toxicity
Ventricular tachycardia, fibrillation and premature contractions	Hypoxic conditions. Changes in T wave indicate hypoxia and more serious abnormalities may follow
Atrioventricular (A-V) block	After drug administration (e.g. xylazine). Also seen in congestive heart failure and atherosclerosis
Small T waves and increasing R waves	Deepening anaesthesia
Arrhythmias	Hypothermia can predispose birds to arrhythmias
Sinus bradycardia	Anaesthetics and hypothermia

32.6 ECG abnormalities.

Therapy/action	Reason	Comments
Digoxin	Treat tachycardia and poor contractility	Once every 24 hours. Use with care and monitor response with ECG, since digoxin can cause serious side effects such as AV block, bradycardia and atrial fibrillation. Discontinue or reduce therapy if any arrhythmias develop or once bird is stabilized
Furosemide	Reduce ascites	0.1–0.2 mg/kg/day
Enalapril	ACE inhibition	5 mg/kg/day reducing to 1 mg/kg/day after improvement in cardiac function has been obtained
Monitor weight	Prevent hypovolaemia	
Monitor potassium levels	Prevent hypokalaemia	
Pericardiocentesis	Decrease cardiac embarrassment and aid venous return	Pericardial fluid can be removed using ultrasound-guided drainage and a median sternal approach (10 ml/kg/day maximum)
Supportive care	Reduce stress	Be aware of positioning risks when investigating birds with congestive failure. Give fluids to prevent circulatory collapse and dehydration. Keep patient in warm and relatively humid (> 60%) environment

32.7 Therapy for cardiac disease.

Eye disease

Conditions around the eyes include traumatic injuries from fighting, insect bites or pigeon baskets, sometimes allowing infections to supervene (e.g. poxvirus, streptococci and staphylococci) (see Chapter 29).

Conjunctivitis is an exceedingly common sign in many infectious systemic diseases affecting the pigeon (see Chapter 29). Other ocular problems include traumatic and inflammatory conditions and abscessation around the lids arising from conjunctival inflammation and infection. Acquired ectropion has been recorded in pigeons that have experienced severe ocular infections.

Neurological disease

Neurological signs present in a number of diseases and conditions, and a detailed history with a full clinical examination is imperative. These signs may vary from dullness, ataxia, paresis and drooping of a wing to torticollis and seizures.

Causes may be infectious or toxic, from hypoglycaemia or related to head trauma. Relevant aspects of the bird's history will include determining whether it is a flock or individual problem, and whether the bird has access to free flight, is young or older, what its sex is, stage of breeding, recent drug administration, the vaccination history, the disease situation in surrounding lofts and evidence of trauma.

Where possible, a specific diagnosis must be made (see later). Some diseases may be notifiable or reportable and others will be expected to respond to appropriate therapy. On diagnosis, a decision can be made on whether to treat the whole flock or just an individual bird (e.g. hypocalcaemic hen).

The major infectious diseases causing nervous signs and their diagnosis and treatment are dealt with in detail in Chapter 29.

Clinical signs of neurological diseases are described in Figure 32.8 along with possible causes, aids to diagnosis and suggested therapy and control/prevention measures. Some of the conditions that present with clinical signs for neurological disease are discussed below.

Toxins

The pigeon owner may have administered medications that can induce nervous signs. These drugs include ivermectin, dimetridazole, levamisole, fenbendazole, quinolones (e.g. enrofloxacin) and aminoglycoside antibiotics.

Free-flying birds might have had access to agricultural pesticides and herbicides, including alphachloralose, metaldehyde and organophosphates. They may also have had the opportunity to ingest poisonous seeds such as those of laburnum or broom shrubs.

Treatment for toxicoses is often supportive and symptomatic, involving fluid therapy, warmth, darkness and administration of diazepam to control seizures (see below).

Deficiencies

Hypocalcaemia and thiamine deficiency are discussed in Chapter 27.

Tick bite syndrome

Tick bites have been recorded as causing a fatal neurological syndrome in a Collared Dove. Because of their management and lifestyle, racing pigeons are not likely to encounter many ticks, but it should be borne in mind when dealing with wild members of the Columbiformes.

Disease/infection	Aids to diagnosis	Therapy, control and prevention
Seizures, torticollis and ataxia		
Paramyxovirus PMV-1	Many birds with polyuria, also tremors, limb paralysis, etc.	Vaccination, culling or symptomatic treatment
Salmonella typhimurium	Swollen joints, diarrhoea, loss of balance, holding head at an angle	Appropriate antibiotics. Culling, vaccination
Influenza	Upper respiratory signs, sinus swellings, deaths	Culling
Ivermectin	History of drug administration	Fluids and nursing
Dimetridazole	History	Fluids and nursing
Organophosphates or carbamates	Free-flying birds or access to (or recent contact or treatment with) poisons	Atropine q4h, diazepam, activated charcoal and fluid therapy
Metaldehyde	Free-flying birds with access to slug bait	Crop flushing and anticonvulsants
Laburnum or broom seed ingestion	Time of year and finding seeds in crop	Empty crop. Fluids and symptomatic therapy
Thiamine deficiency	Intercurrent illness or malnutrition	Administer vitamin B1 and correct underlying causes
Tremors and ataxia		
Paramxyovirus PMV-1	See above	Vaccination, culling
Salmonella infection	See above	Antibiotics
Dimetridazole	History of administration	Fluids and nursing
Levamisole	History	Nursing and anti-emetics
Quinolones	History	Fluids and nursing
Aminoglycosides	Undergoing treatment with	Fluids and nursing
Organophosphates	Access to poison	Atropine, diazepam, activated charcoal
Heat stroke	Warm weather and overcrowding in baskets with poor ventilation	Cool bird in cold water and give fluids
Alpha-chloralose	Birds may become rapidly comatose and die	Warmth and fluids
Drooping wings and lameness		
PMV-1	See above	Vaccination and culling
Salmonella infection	See above	Appropriate antibiotic treatment Vaccination and culling
Streptococcus gallolyticus	Access to contaminated water or food	Antibiotics
Hypocalcaemia	Laying hens or feeding young	Administer calcium and correct the husbandry Vitamin D/sunlight
Thiamine deficiency	See above	Administer vitamin B1
Renal enlargement	Lameness, paresis may be seen where nerves of lumbosacral plexus or ischiadic nerve are compressed by renal swelling/tumours	Establish specific diagnosis. Treatment may not be possible
Articular gout	Lameness or drooping wings may be present. Swollen joints, uric acid tophi present, raised plasma uric acid levels	

32.8 Neurological disease by clinical signs.

Reproductive and paediatric disease

All Columbiformes species are monogamous and the male bird is involved in both the incubation of eggs and the feeding of the chicks (squabs). In the wild the majority will make nests of twigs and may nest in colonies. Some genera are ground or cavity nesters.

Racing pigeons kept in lofts are immensely territorial birds and can be quite aggressive, sometimes with fatal results. Each pair needs its own breeding area or space. Normal breeding behaviour is discussed in Chapter 3.

Although pigeon eggs can be easily incubated artificially, hand-rearing is difficult since crop milk (see Chapter 27) is essential for rearing healthy squabs; their birth weight can be doubled within 34 hours on the rich milk. The quality and quantity of crop milk can be adversely affected by disease (e.g. trichomoniasis or systemic infections); thus prophylactic treatments before breeding are advisable.

Infertility

Infertility can be a major problem for the pigeon fancier and diagnosis of the exact cause can be difficult. It is often a problem of the older pigeon or of the late-born young pigeon (which should not be bred from the following winter).

Collecting semen samples is possible, but endoscopic testicular biopsy will provide the most useful diagnostic information. Endoscopy is also useful for investigation of female infertility, which can include ovarian dysfunction, oviductal infection, inflammation and blockage. Figure 32.9 summarizes possible causes of infertility.

Failure to breed pigeons successfully can be due to poor management and also the presence of subclinical disease in the flock (e.g. PMV-1 or bacterial, *Chlamydophila* or protozoal infections). Heavy endo- or ectoparasite burdens will also have an adverse effect. Prophylactic treatments may be desirable but drug therapy should be avoided during breeding (though trichomoniasis treatments should be given when the birds are actually sitting on the eggs).

Birds that are in poor feather condition should not be bred from. They should be 'race fit' at breeding time and free-flying birds will generally be more fertile than those kept in flights. Lack of sunshine and winters with high humidity and temperatures have been associated with greater breeding problems.

Birds with faeces-caked vents, overgrowth of feathers around the vent or with arthritis or gout may not be able to mate successfully. Pairs also need to be compatible and to have some 'privacy' for mating, i.e. no interference from other cock birds.

Toe nails or broken leg feathers may puncture eggs, especially if they have thin shells due to low calcium content. Territorial aggression may have the same result. Soft-shelled eggs can be the result of nutritional or disease problems. Deformed misshapen eggs may be due to an inherited predisposition.

Treatment of infertility

Treatment is directed at the cause, whether management or from disease. Hormone treatments have been tried on an empirical basis, including follicle-stimulating hormone (FSH), luteinizing hormone (LH) and gonadotrophin-releasing hormone (GNRH) (with anecdotally reported success in older males).

Artificial insemination is possible by obtaining semen from reproductively active males that have been with hens for at least 8 days and inseminating females that have been stimulated by (sterilized) males.

Possible cause	Comments
Lack of condition	Poor husbandry or diet, not in breeding condition, under-exercised, poor weather conditions, vitamin deficiency
Age	Older birds or very young birds
Subclinical disease	PMV, bacterial (especially *Salmonella*), chlamydial, protozoal
Endo/ectoparasites	
Drugs	Anthelmintics and antibiotics, especially fenbendazole and sulphonamides
Physical factors	Too fat, tumours, oviductal abnormalities, hormonal imbalances. Pairing two males or females
Lack of fertilization (clear eggs)	Cloacal obstruction with faeces or feathers. Infertile cock bird. Incompatibility, arthritis, hormonal problems, pairing of two females
Damaged eggs	Trauma from nails. Thin-shelled eggs
Thin-shelled eggs	Calcium and vitamin D deficiencies (lack of sunlight); intercurrent disease
Deformed eggs	Inherited predisposition, salpingitis
Double yolks	Twin embryos can live almost until the point of hatching
No yolk present	Ovarian dysfunction or blockage of proximal oviduct
Dead-in-shell	Bacterial infection of egg (e.g. *Salmonella* or *E. coli*); absorption of chemicals through shell; lack of oxygenation (e.g. egg pores blocked – use straw instead of sawdust); genetic abnormalities. Eggs cracked – clumsy birds or disturbances when sitting (e.g. irritation from red mite infestation), chilled eggs, nutritional deficiencies, loft humidity too low, temperature too high (lethal if overheated)
Inability to hatch	Humidity too high during incubation or too low at hatching; wrong positioning within egg. Weak chicks – nutritional problems

32.9 Causes of infertility.

Hypocalcaemia

Affected birds will appear to 'swim' on the floor using their wings as paddles and will eventually become weaker, comatose and may die. Diagnosis can be confirmed by measurement of blood calcium levels, the ionized calcium level being of particular importance. Administration of calcium and warmth will usually correct the situation. Both cocks and hens can be affected by hypocalcaemia when they are feeding the young.

Egg retention and dystocia

Failure to pass an egg results in the hen becoming egg bound. Causes may be low calcium, intercurrent disease, malnutrition or hormonal problems, or simply that the hen is older and weak.

Obstruction of the oviduct may also be a factor (e.g. inspissated egg or tumour). The oviduct can be too dry due to dehydration or the egg itself is of abnormal shape, size or texture. Diagnosis is by radiography (Figure 32.10), ultrasonography and haematology. A rough estimation of dehydration can be arrived at by 'tenting' of skin, refill time and lack of volume of the basilic vein and measurement of packed cell volume and blood albumin levels. The pectoral muscles of dehydrated pigeons appear 'firm' when palpated. The sternum may also be slightly prominent. Treatment is as for raptors (see Chapters 14 and 21).

32.10 Egg binding in a pigeon. The medullary bone (arrowed) indicates adequate calcium. The deformed egg is clearly visible.

Cloacal prolapse

This can happen after egg laying (and may also be as a result of other causes, such as cloacitis, enteritis and tumours) and requires emergency treatment. After replacement of the cloacal prolapse a cloacopexy or cloacal sutures are needed (see Chapter 14). In chronically prolapsing cases an alternative treatment of cloacal reduction or salpingohysterectomy can be performed.

Salpingitis and oviductal problems

Diagnosis is on the basis of reproductive history, radiography, ultrasonography and endoscopy. A soft tissue enlargement with displacement of other abdominal organs may be seen in the lower abdominal area.

Ovarian cysts and tumours

Diagnosis is usually after investigation of abdominal distension (loss of performance or respiratory compromise) and laparotomy. Oviductal tumours may be cured by surgery. Ovaries and ovarian tumours, which are difficult to excise, may be suspected because of abdominal distension in the hen. They may have ascites and cytology of ascitic fluid obtained by paracentesis can reveal the presence of tumour cells.

Paediatric problems

There are numerous problems that can affect juveniles (Figure 32.11). These may be congenital malformations or caused by disease. Chilling, hygiene and infections must be all considered in the first few days after hatching.

Category	Comments
Death (young squeakers)	Chilling, predation, severe mite infestation, starvation (if both parents aren't feeding the young) or cannibalism due to crowding and stress. Infection (e.g. *Salmonella*; or navel trichomoniasis, which spreads to internal organs), especially after first 4 days of life. Bacterial yolk sac infection may occur (often *E. coli*). Viral infections
Congenital and genetic abnormalities	Partial kidney agenesis. Albino eyes, microopthalmia, absence of eyes, defective vision (clumsy pigeon syndrome), retinal degeneration, cataracts. Polydactyly, webbed toes. Crossed beaks. Lethal achondroplasia. Hermaphroditism. Hereditary ataxia. Featherlessness. Tumbler and roller syndrome. Atherosclerosis
Feather abnormalities	Young squabs (approximately 10 days of age) that have been overdosed with fenbendazole at an early stage of life. Their feathers break along the shafts when they are 'growing in' about 7–10 days later
Skeletal problems	Splay leg fairly common; may be result of inadequate nesting material, metabolic bone disease, or single chick having no lateral support in nest. Slipped tendons and stifle hyperextension may result; has also been associated with nutritional deficiencies (manganese, choline, biotin, pantothenic acid, niacin, folic acid, calcium) as well as genetic components
Vitamin deficiencies	Some abnormalities may be associated with specific nutritional deficiencies (see Chapter 27)
Polydipsia/ polyuria	May be associated with paramyxovirus, adenovirus or *Spironucleus* infection. Also seen when squabs switched from soft foods to seeds

32.11 Paediatric problems.

Oncology

Neoplasms can be classified according to their tissue origins (muscle, fibrous, connective tissue etc.), their activity and cellular composition or by the site at which they occur. The cause of most tumours is unknown. Some tumours have been associated with leucosis, epithelial papillomas and herpes papillomas in other species. Rous sarcoma virus has been recorded in pigeons. Some tumours will present as obvious masses (e.g. cutaneous tumours), while others may be within major organs and difficult to detect at an early stage. Eventually their presence may become obvious through the development of abdominal distension (e.g. gonadal or hepatic tumours). Tumour incidence in the racing pigeon may well be higher than it seems, because of early euthanasia and disposal of underperforming or affected birds by their owners. Reported tumours in pigeons are listed in Figure 32.12 and examples shown in Figure 32.13.

Definitive diagnosis is by biopsy and histopathology. Fine-needle aspiration and abdominal paracentesis are useful aids for diagnosis in the live bird. Ultrasonography, radiography, endoscopy, clinical chemistry and biopsy are needed when there is a suspicion of internal neoplasia.

Therapy is usually limited to the excision of discrete masses, both superficial and abdominal. Except in research programmes, other treatment modalities (e.g. chemotherapy and radiotherapy) have not been recorded in racing pigeons.

Poisoning

In general terms, the treatment of toxicoses in members of the Columbiformes is similar to the treatment in other birds or mammals: remove the bird from the source of the toxin, eliminate the toxin from the bird's body, administer a specific antidote if possible and give supportive treatment (see Chapter 7).

The avian respiratory anatomy makes it a much more efficient gas exchange system than that of the mammal and thus they are much more sensitive to inhaled toxicoses, including inhalation of mycotoxins in poorly maintained lofts. Fortunately, because most pigeons and doves are kept in extensive systems, they are less likely to be affected by domestic inhaled toxins (e.g. from overheated non-stick utensils) and will not be exposed to household plants and food items; also, being granivorous, they are unlikely to ingest significant amounts of lead unless metal particles or shot have been dropped or scattered in grit that the birds may be picking up. Because of their plumage, pigeons are less prone to cutaneous absorption of toxins than mammals, but they may ingest toxins from their feathers during preening or may even inhale particulate toxins from the plumage when sleeping. The lifestyle of the free-flying pigeon puts it at greater risk of being exposed to agricultural pesticides, herbicides and rodenticides.

The majority of pigeons are reasonably selective feeders and will reject any grain that appears 'spoiled'. However, pigeons feeding in fields and picking at

Group	Examples reported
External and musculoskeletal tumours	Rhabdomyosarcoma on the ventral surface of a wing and invading into the pectoral muscles. Leiomyoma. Fibrosarcoma. Lipoma. Xanthoma (Figure 32.14). Capillary haemangioepithelioma (vigorously growing tumour on neck and wing that can regress, seen after pox outbreaks; resolves naturally). Basal cell carcinoma of skin
Internal and disseminated tumours	Synovial sarcoma and epithelial hyperplasia in air sac. Malignant lymphoma under eye with gross nodular lesions throughout major organs. Multicentric lymphosarcoma (birds lack encapsulated lymph nodes so this is multi-organ rather than being a lymphadenopathy). Granulocytic leukaemia. Bile duct carcinoma. Adenocarcinoma of bronchus
Urogenital system tumours	Seminoma in Collared and Turtle Dove. Ovarian papillary adenocarcinoma. Oviductal adenocarcinoma
Congenital conditions	Embryonal nephroma. Thymic epithelial cysts in pigeon chicks. Retention cysts in kidney and pancreas. Polycystic kidneys. Wolffian cysts (developmental cysts from right oviduct)
Other cysts	Tendon and bursal fluid-filled cysts. Air-filled 'cysts' from ruptured cervical air sacs. Feather cysts

32.12 Tumours reported in pigeons.

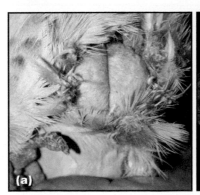
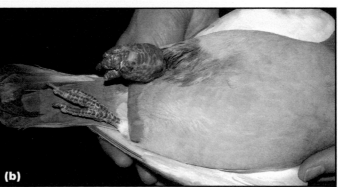

32.13
(a) Abdominal xanthoma.
(b) Foot tumour.

moss and debris in gutters are at the greatest risk. Spoiled food items are more likely to be found in aviaries containing the more exotic varieties of doves and pigeons that also live on fruit.

The risk from owner-administered drug treatments is quite high. Because fanciers will dose their birds with everything that is on the market, toxicoses are often a flock rather than an individual event.

Depending upon the toxin, signs of poisoning include incoordination, seizures, respiratory distress, weakness, diarrhoea, polyuria or sudden death. They must be differentiated from infectious disease with similar signs.

Whatever the cause of the toxicosis, there are some first aid measures that are universal (Figure 32.14).

Mycotoxins

Mycotoxins are produced as chemical metabolites by some fungi. The conditions for the production of mycotoxins may be very specific for a particular fungus. Unfortunately, they are undetectable by sight, smell or taste. Mycotoxins may be present with no visible signs of mould (fungus) growth. The amount of toxin produced may vary and is also variable within different parts of a batch of food.

Type	Signs	Diagnosis	Treatment
Iatrogenic toxicoses			
Ivermectin	Seizures, blindness, death	History of administration	Fluids, warmth, supportive therapy
Dimetridazole	Tremors, ataxia, weakness, seizures	History. Excessive consumption of medicated water fed to nestlings	Fluids
Levamisole	Vomiting, ataxia, catatonia, dyspnoea and death	Vomiting is immediate clinical sign	Nursing
Fenbendazole	Feather abnormalities. Vomiting, neurological signs and death		
Quinolones	Dyspnoea, muscle tremors	History of injectable doses > 70 mg/g	Nursing and fluids
Aminoglycosides	Nephrotoxicity or neuromuscular blockade	High doses given to dehydrated birds	Fluids and supportive treatment
Herbicides, rodenticides and agricultural poisons			
Organophosphates and carbamates (chlorpyrifos, diazinon, carbaryl, malathion, dichlorvos)	Weakness, muscle tremors, ataxia, seizures, paralysis, death in young birds	Contaminated water sources, insecticides and fertilizers. Cholinesterase in plasma and brain	Atropine every 4 hours; pralidoxime chloride; wash affected feathers; activated charcoal, fluids, diazepam and nursing
Alpha-chloralose (avicide)	Coma or death	2.5% causes anaesthesia and hypothermia; > 2.5% is lethal	Warmth and anticonvulsants
Coumarins: warfarin-type	Depression, anorexia, petechiation, epistaxis		Vitamin K
Coumarins: second generation	Similar signs		More toxic, more difficult to treat
Metaldehyde	Fits, ataxia, coma	Slug bait	Flush crop; anticonvulsants; keep in darkness
Fungal toxins			
Various (e.g. ochratoxin, tricothenes, vomitoxin, ergot)	Depression, anorexia, vomiting, polyuria, haemorrhage, paralysis, etc.	Eaten mouldy grain or food. Diagnosis can be very difficult – find toxin in food or GI tract contents	Symptomatic nursing
Plant poisoning			
Laburnum (*Laburnum anagyroides*) and Broom (*Cytisus* spp.)	Fitting, vomiting, ataxia, dyspnoea, death	Time of year and exposure to seed pods	Empty crop of seeds; fluids and symptomatic therapy
Other potential toxicoses			
Sodium chloride	Polydipsia/polyuria	History of exposure to excessive intake of salt	Usually returns to normal in 12 hours. IV fluids if hypovolaemic
Heat	Vomiting, incoordination, ataxia and death (unlike dogs)	Inadequate ventilation in pigeon basket; shut in vehicle in hot weather	Cold bathing: immerse bird in cold water

32.14 Toxicoses: clinical signs, diagnosis and treatment.

There are many mycotoxins. The clinically significant ones for the pigeon are ochratoxin, deoxynivalenol (vomitoxin) and the tricothenes. Contact dermatitis is a possibility with the tricothenes.

Clinical signs

These relate to hepatoxicity, prolonged clotting times, kidney dysfunction and depressed immune system function. Depression, haemorrhages, anorexia, polyuria, erosive lesions of the oral mucosa, constriction of digits, immunosuppression and neurological disorders can all be seen.

Diagnosis

Diagnosis of mycotoxicosis in the live bird is difficult since clinical signs are non-specific and vague or because they mimic other diseases. Diagnosis is based on the finding of mycotoxins in the food or the gastrointestinal tract. Unfortunately, the food may not be available for testing, since it may all have been ingested, consumed some time previously or eaten whilst away from the pigeon loft. Culturing the fungi and identifying mycotoxins can be a lengthy process.

- Tricothenes (*Fusarium* spp.): necrotic lesions from ulceration of the orophharynx and gastrointestinal tract.
- Ochratoxin (*Pencillium* and *Aspergillus* spp.): non-specific and often secondary infections present due to immune system depression and secondary infections (e.g. air sacculitis). It is both hepatotoxic and nephrotoxic. There is no specific treatment and the history of a change in food may be a diagnostic indicator. It is essential that a new food source is given to the birds if mycotoxicosis is suspected.

Post-mortem examination: Some fungal toxins cause hepatic cell degeneration and bile duct necrosis. An enlarged pale liver and enlargement of the spleen and pancreas is thus seen on post-mortem examination. Gastrointestinal haemorrhage from altered clotting ability is common.

Insecticides

The risk from residual pesticides applied to foodstuffs is unknown. Pyrethrins (often combined with piperonyl butoxide) have the lowest toxicity for birds when applied topically. They can be toxic if applied at high concentrations or following inhalation.

Clinical signs

Clinical signs include weakness, anorexia, central nervous system signs, dyspnoea and death.

Organophosphates: Signs of OP poisoning are related to inhibition of acetylcholinesterase and may vary with the age of the bird and the degree of exposure, with chronic exposure possibly resulting in poor hatchability. Delayed toxicosis can occur 7–10 days after exposure to OPs. These signs are due to an organophosphorus ester-induced neuropathy rather than inhibition of acetylcholine activity.

Diagnosis

History of possible exposure to insecticides and clinical signs form the basis for diagnosis. Assay of cholinesterase levels in plasma (to measure depression of cholinesterase) and also in tissue at post-mortem examination (especially brain) may confirm organophosphate and carbamate toxicity. However, 'normal' values for pigeons may be difficult to find. Post-mortem diagnosis from gastrointestinal contents or tissues is possible.

Treatment

For acute OP toxicosis, atropine and pralidoxime chloride (2-PAM) are administered, or atropine alone for carbamate poisoning.

Feather disease

Feather quality can be affected by intercurrent disease, administration of drugs or poor nutrition at the time of moulting or growing new feathers. Once they have grown in, feathers are essentially 'dead' and are then only affected by external physical, infection or parasitic factors.

Initial quality is dependent upon a good diet, health, day length, any drugs administered, genetic factors, physical damage to feather follicles and temperature. Drugs of any sort are best avoided during periods of feather growth. Benzimidazoles, sulphonamides and corticosteroids have commonly been implicated in poor or damaged feathering. Any stress or alteration to the health status or reduction in the amount or quality of the pigeon's diet can result in stress or 'fret marks' across the feathers. These are not going to change and are historical evidence of past events.

Damaged or missing feathers will affect the pigeon's ability to fly or retain heat. Damaged or broken flight feathers can be 'imped' (see Chapter 8) and bent feathers may be gently steamed in order to straighten them (Figure 32.15). Other feathers may be plucked and allowed to regrow if the above measures are not possible. Causes of feather and skin problems and treatment for them are outlined in Figure 32.16.

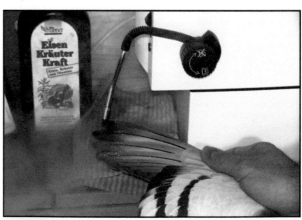

32.15 Preparing for a race. A water mist can be used to straighten the flight feathers. (Courtesy of E and R Schmölz)

Group	Organism/cause	Comments
Ectoparasites	Fleas	Hygiene and environmental control
	Lice	Eggs laid in groove between feather shafts and the barbs. Pinprick damage to feathers. Treatment: cypermethrin and permethrin
	Depluming mite	In skin at base of quill, causes baldness. Treatment: cypermethrin, permethrin, ivermectin
	Quill mite	Within feather shaft, causing baldness. Very inaccessible to treatment
	Red mite	Sucks blood and causes skin irritation and anaemia. Nocturnal; environment must also be treated
	Northern fowl mite	Most of life cycle on bird
	Scaly leg mite	Crusting on legs
Viral	Pigeon pox, PMV-1	Typical pox lesions mainly around eyes and beak. Damaged feather follicles and abnormal or even no feather growth. Pigmentation disturbances (e.g. white vanes) – normal at next moult. Quill may grow almost without any vane; result is 'flag' feather with normal tip and vaneless quill
Bacterial	*Staphylococcus* or *Erysipelothrix* infection, mycobacteria	As infections secondary to skin trauma or irritation. Hard yellow nodules, especially undersides of wings
Fungal	*Trichophyton megnini*	Bare areas of skin. Scaly white crusty patches
Drugs	Benzimidazoles, corticosteroids, sulphonamides	If used during moulting or when feeding feather-growing squabs
Nutritional	Ill health or poor diet	Ensure good diet and vitamin supplements when moulting
Toxic	Drugs or mycotoxins	
Traumatic	From fighting or collisions	Appropriate wound treatment
	Feather damage from drinkers and feeders	Baldness below crop on ventral neck
Neoplastic and other	Capillary haemangioendothelioma	Highly vascular rapidly growing masses. Will resolve in 3–4 weeks. Pox outbreak related? May need cautery and ligation
	Lipomas	
	Xanthomas	
	Feather cysts	May need excision if producing abnormal feathers or lumps

32.16 Causes of feather and skin problems.

References and further reading

Fudge AM (2000) Avian liver and gastrointestinal testing. In: *Laboratory Medicine: Avian and Exotic Pets*, ed. AM Fudge, p. 53. WB Saunders, Philadelphia

Garner M (2003) Air sac adenocarcinomas in birds: 7 cases. In: *Proceedings of 24th annual conference of the Association of Avian Veterinarians*, pp. 55–57

Gfeller RW and Messonnier SP (2004) *Small Animal Toxicology and Poisonings, 2nd edn.* Mosby, St Louis

Gill FB (1995) *Ornithology, 2nd edn.* WH Freeman, New York.

Halsema WB (1998) Collection and analysis of urine in racing pigeons. *Avian Pathology* **17**, 221–225

Hawk CT and Leary SL (1999) *Formulary for Laboratory Animals, 2nd edn.* Iowa State University Press, Ames

Kemba LM, Linden EC, Jones MP and Daniel GP (2003) Quantitative renal scintigraphy in domestic pigeons (*Columba livia domestica*) exposed to toxic doses of gentamicin. *American Journal of Veterinary Research* **64**(4), 453–462

Klumpp, SA and Wagner WD (1986) Survey of the pathological findings in a large production colony of pigeons, with special reference to pseudomembranous stomatitis and nephritis. *Avian Disease* **30**(4), 740–750

Kollias GK (1984) Liver biopsy techniques in avian clinical practice. *Veterinary Clinics of North America* **14**(2)

Lichtenburger, M (2005) Emergency medicine for the avian patient. In: *Association of Avian Veterinarians Proceedings, Monterey 2005*, p. 121

Lierz M (2003) Avian renal disease: pathogenesis, diagnosis and therapy. *Veterinary Clinics of North America: Exotic Animal Practice* **6**, 29–55

Lumeij JT (1994) Nephrology. In: *Avian Medicine Principles and Application*, ed. BW Ritchie *et al.*, p. 540. Wingers, Lake Worth, FL

Lumeij JT (2003) Pathophysiology and clinical features of avian cardiac disease, with an emphasis on electrocardiology. In: *Proceedings of 7th European AAV Conference Tenerife* pp. 407–415

Pees M, Keifer I, Krautwald-Junghanns E *et al.* (2006) Comparative ultrasonographic investigations of the gastrointestinal tract and the liver in healthy and diseased pigeons. *Veterinary Radiology and Ultrasound* **47**, 370

Pennycott TW (1996) Nervous conditions of pigeons. In: *BSAVA Manual of Raptors, Pigeons and Waterfowl*, ed. PH Beynon *et al.*, pp. 267–271. BSAVA, Cheltenham

Petrak ML (1969) *Diseases of Cage and Aviary Birds.* Lea and Febiger, Philadelphia

Phalen DN (2000) Avian renal disease. In: *Laboratory Medicine: Avian and Exotic Pets*, ed. AM Fudge, pp. 61–67. WB Saunders, Philadelphia

Powers L (2005) Veterinary care of Columbiformes. In: *Proceedings of the Association of Avian Veterinarians, Monterey* pp 171–182

Proctor NS and Lynch PJ (1993) *Manual of Ornithology.* Yale University Press, New Haven

Rae M (2000) Avian endocrine disorders. In: *Laboratory Medicine: Avian and Exotic Pets*, ed. AM Fudge, pp.76–88. WB Saunders, Philadelphia

Redrobe S (2002) Pigeons. In: *BSAVA Manual of Exotic Pets, 4th edn*, ed. A Meredith and S Redrobe, pp. 168–178. BSAVA Publications, Gloucester

Rosenthal K (2005) Clinical implications of endocrine disease in avian patients. In: *Proceedings of Association of Avian Veterinarians Conference Monterey* pp. 3–9

Schmidt RE (2003) *Pathology of Pet and Aviary Birds.* Iowa State Press, Ames

Smith FM, West NH and Jones DR (2000) The cardiovascular system. In: *Sturkie's Avian Physiology*, pp. 148–151. Academic Press, San Diego

Tudor DC (1991) *Pigeon Health and Disease.* Iowa State Press, Ames

Westerhof I, van den Brom WE, Mol JA, Lumeig JT and Rijnberk A (1994) Sensitivity of the hypothalamic-pituitary-adrenal system of pigeons (*Columba livia domestica*) to suppression by dexamethasone, cortisol, and prednisolone. *Avian Disease* **38**(3), 435–445

33

Passerine birds: nutrition and nutritional diseases

Brian Stockdale

Introduction

Few of the passerine species commonly kept in aviculture could be described as totally specialist feeders but, for reasons of convenience, species are generally categorized according to their principal dietary component (Figure 33.1) (see also Chapters 1 and 4). Many species switch their food types with either food availability or physiological needs. For example, many primarily insectivorous temperate birds become frugivores in the autumn. Similarly, a large number of granivorous finches feed almost exclusively live food to their chicks.

Basic nutrition group (capitals indicate principal diet)	Examples
CARNIVORES/OMNIVORES	Crows, ravens, magpies, birds of paradise, orioles
FRUGIVORES/Insectivores	Waxwings
FRUGIVORES/Nectivores/ Insectivores	Tanagers
GRANIVORES/Insectivores	Sparrows, weavers, estrelid finches, buntings
GRANIVORES/Insectivores/ Frugivores	Old and New World seed-eaters, cardinals
INSECTIVORES	Wagtails, pipits, accentors
INSECTIVORES/FRUGIVORES	True thrushes, chats, robins, bulbuls, white-eyes, warblers, babblers, parrotbills
INSECTIVORES/FRUGIVORES (Omnivores)	Starlings, mynahs, mockingbirds
NECTIVORES/Insectivores	Sugarbirds, sunbirds, spiderhunters

33.1 Overview of feeding behaviour in the order Passeriformes. Many species are insectivorous when young.

General principles of a captive diet

The wide range of foods that birds consume reflects the varied nutrients available within those foods and the fact that a single class of food is generally insufficient to provide all the necessary nutrients, especially at times of nutritional stress. Chemical analysis of individual foods commonly provided to captive passerine birds confirms that many of the essential nutrients are either absent, or only minimally provided, or provided in excess. A bird's nutritional status is a balancing act between its nutrient needs, the nutrients that are available and the metabolic, physiological and behavioural adaptations that the bird can bring into play to avert or minimize discrepancies. Nutrient levels in any diet given to captive birds should be adjusted to meet the demands of different stages in the bird's lifecycle and to provide the minimum required levels of all necessary nutrients.

Assessment of nutrient values

Many essential dietary nutrients are known, but there is a lack of accurately assessed nutrient values in relation to species-specific levels of digestive efficiency and absorption capabilities. For example, whilst the energy or mineral levels of individual foodstuffs can be determined, these levels may not be applicable to pet birds in general, or to a particular species of bird. Nor are the levels and quality of nutrients within a particular food fixed. For example:

- Mineral levels in seeds may be affected by mineral levels in the growing medium
- Nutrient levels in a crop may be affected by poor harvesting techniques, condition of the crop at harvest (e.g. under-ripe or too wet seed heads) and post-harvest over-drying
- Vitamin levels (especially vitamin E tocopherols and pro-vitamin A carotenes) degrade during prolonged storage
- Poor storage conditions may allow forage mite and beetle contamination (possibly requiring chemical control)
- Seeds may have been stored in plastic bags or containers, encouraging 'sweating' and increasing the potential for mycotoxin production (paper bags are preferable for storage)
- Genetic modification of crops may or may not have an effect on nutrients.

Nutrient requirements

Using the small amount of data that is available, a basic minimum maintenance provision for both macro- and micronutrients for 'generic passerines' can be achieved and makes a valid starting point (Figure 33.2).

Nutrient	Minimum	Maximum
Gross energy (kcal/kg)	3500	4500
Total protein (%)	14	
Amino acids (%)		
Arginine	0.75	
Lysine	0.75	
Methionine	0.35	
Methionine + cysteine	0.58	
Threonine	0.46	
Vitamins		
Vitamin A activity (IU/kg)	8000	
Vitamin D3 (ICU/kg)	1000	2500
Vitamin E (ppm)	50	
Vitamin K (ppm)	1	
Biotin (ppm)	0.25	
Chloine (ppm)	1500	
Folic acid (ppm)	1.5	
Niacin (ppm)	50	
Pantothenic acid (ppm)	20	
Pyridoxine (ppm)	6	
Riboflavin (ppm)	6	
Thiamine (ppm)	4	
Vitamin B12 (ppm)	0.01	
Minerals		
Calcium (%)	0.50	1.20
Phosphorus (%)	0.50	
Calcium:total phosphorus ratio	1:1	2:1
Chlorine (%)	0.12	
Magnesium (ppm)	600	
Potassium (%)	0.40	
Sodium (%)	0.12	
Trace minerals (ppm)		
Copper	8	
Iodine	0.40	
Iron	80	See ISD section
Manganese	65	
Selenium	0.10	
Zinc	50	

33.2 Nutrient profile recommendations for passerine birds.

The precise levels of each of the nutrients required for optimal health for each of the species being considered, at all periods of its life, have not yet been defined. The basis for captive-bird diets at present is on the principle of 'minimal levels', relying on information available from analysis of diets consumed by free-ranging birds, extrapolation of data from the poultry industry, the small amount of direct experimental evidence, general nutritional principles and trial and error.

In practice, aviculturalists provide their birds with foods that are readily available, cheap, willingly consumed and have historically been shown to be 'suitable' for that type of bird.

It is not within the scope of this chapter to discuss all the complex nutritional inter-relationships between macro- and micronutrients, nor the physiological actions of these nutrients on the avian body. The aim is to highlight areas of an avian life cycle where additional nutrition is required above 'sustainability' and to discuss the consequences of malnutrition in its widest form.

Unlike their wild conspecifics, where gross deficiency of food may be an issue, it is the *quality* of the food in terms of available nutrients rather than *quantity* that dictates the nutritional status of captive passerines (Figure 33.3).

Wild birds	Captive birds
Diversity of diet allows for nutrient complementation by chance or design	Diet fixed by provision
Feeding level driven by endogenous energy demand Increased energy expenditure results in higher feeding rate and increased likelihood of micronutrient acquisition	Lower energy expenditure results in less food eaten Generally, birds do not over-consume large amounts of energy to obtain adequate amounts of specific nutrients
Commonly foods that are low in protein are also low in ME, resulting in protein-to-calorie ratios that enhance the overall nutrient 'quality' of the food	High-calorie (cultivated) seeds result in low protein-to-calorie ratios; these are the type commonly fed to captive granivores and are of 'poor quality'
Nutritional plasticity at times of altered nutritional demand A change to protein rich foods (invertebrates) during breeding	Diet fixed by provision
Limited food resources can compromise life history patterns	Food quantity should never be an issue

33.3 Comparison of factors involved in nutrient provision in wild and captive passerine birds.

Seed as a food source

Nutritional shortfalls

The range of seeds available is reasonably extensive (Figure 33.4) but in captivity most species confine themselves to a narrow selection of 'favourite' seed types. Seed selection is based primarily on the bird's ability to handle the shape of the seed and this is a function of the bird's bill structure.

As seed-eating birds remove the outer husk of the seed prior to consumption, the more appropriate the seed shape is to bill structure, the faster the handling time and the greater the foraging returns. Little consideration is given to the macro- or micronutritive quality of the seeds provided, though a single study (Murphy and King, 1989) showed the ability of a

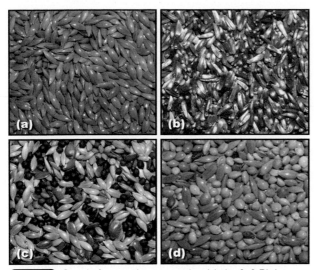

33.4 Seeds for captive passerine birds. **(a)** Plain canary seed. **(b)** Niger seed. **(c)** Mixture including canary seed, red and black rape seed (small round seeds), linseed (brown, flat and tear-shaped) and hemp (buff, round and the largest). **(d)** Mixed foreign finch (canary seed with mixed millets – red, white and panicum).

seed-eating passerine bird to select preferentially feeds with a higher level of sulphur-containing amino acids during the moult. Where nutritive value is assessed in seeds of similar size, selection may depend upon macronutrient composition, preference being given to seeds with high starch or oil content (Diaz, 1996; Schaefer *et al.*, 2003; van der Meij, 2005). Feeding is usually driven by energy needs (the optimal diet theory).

Seeds are generally energy rich but poor in other nutrients. The seeds commonly provided fall into two classes according to their main energy supply: either carbohydrate (canary seed, millets) or oils (sunflower, rape, hemp, linseed). Both classes are generally low in protein, especially essential amino acids, and grossly deficient in minerals (with the exception of phosphate, which further adds to the Ca:P imbalance) and the majority of the vitamins (Figure 33.5).

Vitamins	Vitamin A, vitamin D3, vitamin E, vitamin K, choline, niacin, pantothenic acid, riboflavin (B2), folic acid, cyanocobalamine (B12), biotin (H)
Minerals	Calcium, phosphorous (70% tied up as non-digestible phytates in plant products), sodium
Trace minerals	Selenium, iron, copper, zinc, manganese, tin, iodine, boron, chromium, vanadium, bismuth
Pigments	Chlorophyll, canthaxanthin
Essential amino acids	Lysine, methionine
Fibre	Mucopolysaccharides (soluble and insoluble)
Vitamin precursors	Beta-carotenes converted to vitamin A in the liver
Fatty acids	Deficiency and imbalance of omega-3 and -6

33.5 Essential nutritional ingredients from eight groups are missing from seeds (adapted from McDonald, 2006).

Maintaining granivores on an exclusively seed-based diet may lead to nutritional deficiencies, signs of which may be clinical, behavioural or more subtle (Figure 33.6).

Clinical signs
Loss of feather colour and quality. Protracted moults. Hyperkeratosis, especially feet and legs. Soft-shelled eggs and egg binding. Obesity
Behavioural signs
Poor parenting. Failure to sing or court. Nutritional pica (grit ingestion)
Other signs
Suppression of the immune system leading to greater susceptibility to disease and parasitism. Intestinal malabsorption and dysfunction (pH change predisposing to avian gastric yeast *Ornithogaster macrorhabdus* formerly 'megabacteriosis'). Reduced reproductive performance (smaller clutches, dead-in-shell, poor sperm quality). General malaise or premature death from pansystemic organ dysfunction

33.6 Signs of nutritional deficiency.

Correction of seed-based diets

Trace minerals and vitamins
Powder and liquid preparations containing varying levels and ranges of minerals and vitamins are commercially available to correct the shortfall in micronutrients in seed-only diets.

Powders are often sprinkled over seeds in the hope that sufficient adheres to the seed husk and is ingested by the bird as it shells the seed. The majority falls to the bottom of the dish and is discarded. A more satisfactory method is to include vitamin powders in a proprietary eggfood, which will already contain a certain level of added micronutrients. Most breeders do not feed eggfoods year-round.

Soluble mineral and vitamin preparations added to the drinking water, once or twice weekly, provide a convenient method of administration, though some vitamins (e.g. vitamin A) are not stable in solution and rapidly degrade. The high mineral and vitamin content of the water is also conducive to promoting bacterial and algal growth.

Control over the levels of ingestion of micronutrient supplements remains problematic.

Soluble calcium
This is usually provided in the form of cuttlefish bone or soluble grit (powdered oyster shell) or as a water-soluble supplement. The actual solubility and availability to the bird of calcium given in these forms is questionable. Calcium availability and absorption are multifactorial, depending not only on the actual levels of calcium in the diet but also on the amount of lipids ingested, vitamin D3 (usually provided in the vitamin supplement) and the conversion of endogenous vitamin D2 under the influence of ultraviolet (UV) light. The majority of finches are kept in indoor accommodation and do not have access to natural sunlight. Provision of UV-emitting bulbs within the bird room may help to remedy this, but for UV to be effective the birds should not be more than around 60 cm away from the source.

Problems arising from inadequate calcium absorption in passerine birds fall into two areas:

- Osteodystrophic conditions, mainly seen in nestlings, which develop with bent long bones and kinky spines and sternums. Calcium deficiency has also been indicated in the condition of splay or straddle leg
- Reproductive disorders, such as thin-shelled eggs, egg binding, smaller clutches, poor recycling ability and as one of the possible causes of dead-in-shell.

As well as the recognized need in bone and egg-shell mineralization, calcium is essential during the moult, when a cyclical osteoporosis and renovation of the skeleton takes place.

Calcium for softbills: Calcium is also an additional dietary requisite for softbills. Many softbills actively consume snail shells and small bones prior to egg laying (Graveland and Drent, 1997). Provision of calcium to softbills can be achieved by mixing a balanced calcium supplement with a Ca:P ratio of 1.5–2:1 (or ground-up cuttlefish bone) with their soft food.

Grit
Passerine birds hull their food prior to swallowing and so there is less need for active grinding to take place in the gizzard. The insoluble grit, flint and quartz chips often seen in pet-bird cages are now generally considered not to be essential for seed-eating passerine birds (Taylor, 1996). If available, grit will often be consumed as a soluble calcium substitute, resulting in digestive disorders.

Green food
Various green foods, fed in limited quantities, will provide additional dietary fibre, carotenoids, essential fatty acids, vitamins, trace minerals and antioxidants and should be included in the diet of seed eaters. Plants with dark green leaves tend to provide higher levels of minerals, vitamins and carotenoids.

Formulated diets
Formulated extruded or pelleted diets are an integral part of dietary management for many captive birds, particularly members of the orders Galliformes and Psittaciformes, and are gaining popularity in the feeding of passerine birds. Formulated diets provide all the necessary macro- and micronutrients in a balanced and readily absorbable form. The majority of seed eaters and softbills seem to be willing to eat these diets.

Nutritional excesses

Oil seeds
Seed mixtures, often augmented with mineral and vitamin supplements, are usually fed to seed-eating passerine birds. This practice allows birds to choose the seed varieties they prefer and in many cases these are the 'fat' or oil-based seeds such as oilseed rape, sunflower, linseed and hemp. Excessive consumption can result in obesity, fatty liver and kidney disease.

In obese birds large pads of fat can be visualized and palpated overlying the pectoral muscles and in the region of the cloaca. Enlarged liver lobes may also be seen extending below the level of the sternum (though this is not specific to fatty liver disease). To avoid these problems, canary and European finch breeders usually reduce the levels of 'oil' seeds in the diet once the moult is complete, preferring to keep their birds 'fit' over the winter months. Obesity can be a problem for individual caged pet birds, canaries on 'mixed canary' seed and small finches such as Zebra Finches on a constant supply of millet sprays.

Excessive hemp seed is said to result in the loss of the red pigmentation on the breast feathers of male Bullfinches, with patchy areas of black (the base melanin pigmentation) being visible. The red coloration returns at the next moult if hemp is withheld. Hemp can also be responsible for producing a respiratory wheeze (asthma-like) in individual canaries. Respiration returns to normal once access to hemp seed is removed. However, when presented with such a case it is important that other differential diagnoses are investigated (see Chapter 34).

Mealworms
The excessive feeding of mealworms in particular to softbills and buntings (Emberizidae) can also lead to fatty liver disease.

Vitamin supplements
The use of mineral and vitamin supplementation is common amongst finch keepers. Levels of both vitamin A and vitamin D in many of these supplements are very high compared with the required daily intake. Excessive administration or intake of supplements can result in overdosing. At 4–10 times the recommended levels of vitamin D, effects can include increased calcium and bone absorption, hypercalcaemia, decreased parathormone (PTH), mineralization of soft tissues, nephrocalcinosis and polyuria (see sections on vitamin A and recessive white canaries; and on iron storage disease in softbills).

Areas of additional nutritional demand

The cyclical nature of a bird's life – reproduction, egg laying, feeding chicks and moulting – is mirrored by the need for additional dietary provision.

Breeding and rearing
The production of eggs is a nutritionally demanding process, particularly for small passerines, some of which lay a clutch of eggs weighing more than the female's own body weight. Egg quality is directly determined by the quality of the nutrients deposited in them by the female bird. This in turn is a direct reflection of dietary provision.

Demand for protein
The increased demand for protein (up to 235% of maintenance) (Robbins, 1981) required for the development of the female reproductive tract, accretion of yolk lipoproteins during the week

preceding oviposition and secretion of albumen during oviposition is met from both exogenous dietary sources and endogenous body reserves. For wild birds of northern temperate regions, this demand may be met by a change from a principally seed-based diet to a diet with a greater level of protein-rich invertebrates and the higher protein-containing seeds of leguminous plants.

For birds from neotropical regions, food availability is a much stronger breeding cue than photoperiodic change. Breeding is timed to coincide with the production of ripening seeds, usually following periods of rain. Ripening seeds have a milky consistency when crushed and a much higher essential amino acid level than dried seeds (Figure 33.7).

Seed		Lysine (g/100 g protein dry matter)
Canary[a] (*Phalaris canariensis*)	Dry	1.9
	Ripe	5.5
Millet[a] (*Panicum milioceum*)	Dry	2.6
	Ripe	4.1
Whole egg (chicken)[a]		7.6
Muscle (White-crowned Sparrow)[b]		7.18

33.7 Comparison of relative levels of the essential amino acid lysine in green and dry seeds. [a] Allan and Green (1997), [b] Murphy 1994

Unless provided with additional dietary protein sources, captive birds are unable to reach the levels of essential amino acids required to adequately fund optimal reproductive activities. Endogenous protein reserves, mainly the larger pectoral muscle mass, are utilized to provide an additional amino acid supply. Excessive 'body plundering' debilitates the bird and limits further reproductive effort.

Additional protein can be provided in the form of eggfood and 'livefood'.

Eggfood

Traditionally, aviculturalists provided their breeding birds with a range of home-made recipes based around hard-boiled eggs. Several brands of mineral- and vitamin-enriched powdered egg and cereal-based 'eggfoods' are now commercially available. Commercial eggfoods, usually with a crude protein content of 16–20%, generally come as a dry granular powder which is moistened with water, soaked seed or grated carrot to give a moist crumbly consistency.

Eggfood is fed in small quantities – about 5 g per bird. Feeding is usually started in the pre-breeding period to accustom the bird to the food, when it may be fed once or twice weekly. The frequency is increased to daily during pairing up and egg laying. Care has to be taken that the food does not become stale, especially during hot weather. Once incubation starts, many canary fanciers stop feeding eggfood, especially if the cock bird is maintained with the hen. It is thought that the continued high plane of nutrition will encourage the cock to bully the hen into deserting her current nest so that he can re-mate and start another nest (the author believes that quality nutrition should continue to be fed during this period, making it easier for the hen to replenish lost nutrients and body tissues catabolized during egg production). Eggfood is then reintroduced once the chicks have started to hatch and may be provided two or three times a day, though the parent birds tend not to feed the newly hatched chicks for the first 12 hours or so, allowing the remnants of the yolk sac to provide the initial nutrition. They do provide the chicks with fluids.

Livefood

Many foreign finches do not readily accept eggfood and are encouraged to come into breeding condition by supplying fresh seeding grasses if available, or by feeding livefood. For the small finches, fruit flies (*Drosophila* spp.) and 'mini' mealworms (small soft-skinned larvae of the flower beetle *Tenebrio molitor*) are often supplied. Livefood is also essential for the successful rearing of many of the nominally granivorous finches, e.g. the majority of waxbills, sparrows and buntings. For larger birds, crickets can also be fed.

Whilst invertebrates are relatively high in fats and protein, and the feeding of invertebrates would seem essential for the successful breeding and rearing of many of the small passerines and softbills, their overall balanced nutritional value is questionable (Figure 33.8).

Gut-loading: Invertebrates are generally low in vitamins and calcium (with a very poor Ca:P ratio) and a lot of their nutritional value can be attributable, particularly in the case of earthworms, to the nutritional value of their gut contents. 'Gut-loading' of the live invertebrates by providing them with a high quality

Species	Crude fat	Protein[a]	Vitamin A (IU/kg)	Ca	P	Ca:P ratio (approx.)
Mealworm (*Tenebrio molitor*)	31	45–50	810 ± 325	0.12	1.42	1:12
Crickets, adult (*Acheta domesticus*)	23	57–60	810 ± 850	0.21	0.78	1:4
Waxworm (*Galleria mellonella*)	51.5	37–40	150 ± 160	0.06	1.20	1:20
Fruit fly (*Drosophila*)	18	48–50	Not detected	0.14	1.10	1:8
Earthworms[b]	12.6	45–55	2400 ± 300	1.0	0.8	1.25:1

33.8 Approximate composition of invertebrates commonly fed to passerine birds. [a] Protein % derived from (total nitrogen – non-protein nitrogen) × 6.25, [b] Earthworm values variable, depending on quality and quantity of gut contents.

food prior to feeding them to the birds assists this. Dusting crickets with a calcium-based mineral supplement prior to feeding is an appropriate method of mineral administration. Livefood can also be used as a vehicle for administering drugs (especially wormers and anti-protozoal drugs) to softbills.

Problems encountered with livefood: One of the most commonly used livefoods is mealworms. Although newly moulted larvae are softer skinned, and seed eaters tend to kill and additionally soften them prior to feeding them to their young, digestion by chicks can still be a problem. Deaths occur due to crop and gizzard impaction with the chitinous skins or the solid heads. Many birds will only breed if livefood is available and will feed it almost exclusively to their chicks. This exclusive feeding will often directly lead to deficiencies of both calcium and vitamins, thiamine deficiency in particular being commonly reported. Chicks develop with limb disorders and are often abandoned by the parents or die.

Maggots are also fed. These, whilst having similar nutritive values to mealworms and having the same problems with their chitinous exoskeleton, have the added disadvantage of potentially poisoning the birds by carrying *Clostridium botulinum* toxins.

Worms (usually the tiger worm *Eisenia foetida* and *Dendrobaena* sp.) are also supplied as live food to some groups of birds. Where these are bred in home wormeries the potential for introducing *Syngamus trachea* may be increased.

Fatty liver disease may also be a consequence of excessive consumption of invertebrates, mealworms in particular (Macwhirter, 1994).

Soaked seed

Soaking and germinating seeds and small legumes is a traditional method of providing additional nutrients to breeding birds. The seeds selected for soaking are usually those with a rapid germination time (2–3 days) and mainly consist of wild weed and grass seed mixtures with oilseed rape often added.

The process of soaking seeds to the point of chitting does not increase the *level* of nutrients within the seed, but it does initiate enzymatic processes altering the nature of the stored nutrients, inactivating digestive inhibitors (a range of proteases) and making the nutrients more easily absorbed and digested, especially by nestlings. The softening of the husk also makes seeds more easily hulled and eaten by newly weaned chicks, which still have relatively soft beaks.

As well as stimulating germination the process of soaking the seeds stimulates bacterial and fungal growth. Strict hygiene, frequent washing of the seed during soaking and prevention of souring during feeding are required to avoid contamination. Some fanciers wash the seeds with a weak solution of bleach or disinfectant to 'sterilize' the outside of the seeds prior to soaking, but this seems to have little effect on the level of yeasts and fungi on the seeds once they are re-exposed to the air. The risk of problems increases with the time that the seeds remain uneaten. Organisms can then build up to unmanageable levels and disease, usually in the form of enteritis, occurs. Problems arise mainly from toxins produced on the seed whilst in the food bowl. These may directly cause illness or produce gut stasis, allowing colonization by potentially pathogenic enteric bacteria such as *Escherichia coli* to cause enteritis, diarrhoea and death due to a combination of toxaemia, bacteraemia and dehydration. For this reason some fanciers avoid using it.

Soaked seed is fed to breeding birds in a similar fashion to eggfood and is continued through the post-weaning period.

Nutritional dead-in-shell

Because all the nutrients required for embryonic development and survival must be placed within the egg prior to shell formation, there is a heavy onus on the nutritional status of the female bird. The causes of death at the point of pipping (dead-in-shell) are multi-factorial. Nutritional underfunding of the egg, especially with antioxidants (vitamins E, A and C and carotenoids), greatly increases the oxidative stress within the egg, leading to embryonic death. In poultry, it has been shown that increased dietary levels of these antioxidants greatly increase hatchability. Trace minerals and other vitamins also have a profound effect on avian embryogenesis; deficiencies result in a variety of fatal physical and metabolic abnormalities (Wilson, 1997).

Moult

For a large number of canary and finch breeders, feather quality is paramount to producing show winners and a 'good moult' is fundamental in achieving feather quality. Feathers constitute in excess of 10% of the body mass of a small passerine bird and renewing this amount of tissue in a relatively short period of time (a canary moult lasts about 10 weeks) places a high metabolic and nutritional demand on a bird.

Protein

Protein, mainly in the form of keratins, makes up approximately 90% of the dry matter content of feathers (which can represent 25% of the total protein content of the body). Structurally, keratins contain a higher level of the sulphur-containing amino acids, methionine and cysteine, than normal body or egg protein. To supply a sufficiently high level of these essential amino acids (although birds are capable of forming endogenous stores of cysteine as the tripeptide glutathione, which can act as a short-term nutritional buffer) requires a much higher protein intake than that which would account solely for the additional protein mass of the feathers. For the majority of captive seed eaters, additional sources of protein should be provided to ensure a successful moult. Eggfood, wild seeding grasses where available and livefood are often supplied.

Moulting in the majority of northern temperate birds such as canaries and European finches is photo-induced (via an endocrine cascade). There is no indication that (mal)nutrition has any proximate control over the onset of the moult. Moult will proceed irrespective of the nutritional status of the bird. However, inadequate nutrition before or during the moult will result in the bird adjusting its moult by:

- Delaying or interrupting the moult
- Reducing the rate of feather production (to meet nutritive intake or reduce daily needs)
- Sustaining the production at the cost of other body functions
- Some combination of the above.

The result of these effects may be any of the following:

- A protracted moult
- Poor quality feathers (pigmentation changes, structural defects to the barbs, 'thin' feathers, stress bars)
- Increased nutritional stress and increased susceptibility to disease (the moult is often the time when small captive passerine birds die).

Carotenoids and antioxidants

The increased metabolism involved in new feather production and the catabolism of body tissues during this time produces increased levels of oxidative stress within the body. It is essential that the diet provides adequate levels of antioxidants in the form of vitamin E, vitamin C, vitamin A and carotenoids.

For the majority of the small passerines, carotenoids provide the exogenous supply of pigments that create the colours of many birds. An inadequate supply of the appropriate dietary carotenoids may leave the feathers (and in many cases the bare skin of the legs, face patches and beak) of low colour intensity, giving a washed-out appearance. The bird also uses many of these carotenoids pigments as metabolic antioxidants. The moult places an additional burden on the division of these carotenoid between the new feathers and the immune system. This conflict between body and feather for dietary carotenoid resources often leads to poor coloration and a potentially compromised immune system.

Feather colour

Birds are unable to produce carotenoids endogenously and must absorb them from their food. Lutein, zeaxanthin and the β-carotenes are the carotenoids most commonly found in foodstuffs (leaves, flowers, fruit, seeds and insects). Many avian species absorb these carotenoids and deposit them in their plumage directly without modifying their structure. Others modify the structure and with it the colour. One of the modified yellow groups is 'canary xanthophyll' which imparts the yellow colour to the domesticated Canary and many other finches.

Coloured canaries, having received a 'red factor' from their Red Siskin ancestry (see Chapter 4), are able to metabolize other carotenoids, which are deposited as a red colouring. These are the same pigments (4-oxo-carotenoids) that impart the red colouring to the Bullfinch.

Colour feeding

Maintaining good coloration can be difficult in some captive birds. Most grains and seeds provide the basic yellow pigments, lutein and zeaxanthin, but the red-producing pigments, contained in a number of hedgerow berries and fruits, are less easy to supply. Many breeders provide a commercially available substitute, canthaxanthin, to provide the dietary pigments necessary to produce good feather colour. These are fed to enhance the feather appearance of coloured canaries, mules and hybrids, and European finches. The colouring agent is supplied either through the drinking water or in soft-food during the moult. Overdosing can result in a 'burnt' colour, which is marked down on the show bench. Following colour feeding, the loss of a feather, especially a tail or primary feather, will result in the re-growth of a pale feather, again counting against the bird on the show bench.

Provision of vitamins

Adequate levels of all the essential vitamins are required by birds for healthy maintenance, feather growth and reproduction as outlined above and appropriate diets should reflect these levels.

Vitamin C

Vitamin C (L-ascorbic acid) has very diverse physiological functions within the avian body and is an essential requirement for some birds. It forms part of the redox system and is active at a cellular level in maintaining cell wall integrity. It is also secreted into eggs and functions as part of the anti-oxidative processes involved in yolk metabolism. Vitamin C is synthesized by the action of L-gulonolactone oxidase (GLO) on glucose and takes place principally in the liver and kidneys. The enzyme GLO has been lost by several avian (and mammalian) lineages and for some birds exogenous supplies of vitamin C are required. GLO is present in all *non*-passerine birds studied to date but absent in several passerine species. Evolutionary loss has been suggested to have occurred in species where ample levels of ascorbic acid are available in their food. In passerine birds, however, the pattern of GLO loss is not obviously associated with dietary shifts, being present in some frugivores and absent in omnivores within the same family. It is estimated that up to half of the birds of the order Passeriformes may be unable to synthesize vitamin C.

The levels of dietary vitamin C required for normal growth and health and reproduction in captive birds must be determined on a species-by-species basis. Sources of vitamin C are widespread among food items, especially those of plant origin (though seeds and grain are generally low). Recommended levels for vitamin C in bird diets are 50–150 mg/kg (dry matter basis). For the majority of softbills that have fruit included in their diet, dietary vitamin C levels should not be a problem. For granivorous birds, salad leaves, dandelion leaves, chickweed or similar green foods should be provided.

Vitamin A and recessive white canaries

Recessive white canaries have been developed from strains of coloured canaries. The effect of this mutation, a single autosomal recessive, is the total inhibition of carotenoid colouring in the plumage and adipose tissue (compared with dominant white canaries, which show evidence of lipochrome colouring on their flight feathers). Unlike normal canaries, which convert β-carotenes to vitamin A, recessive white canaries are totally unable to utilize β-carotene (Wolf *et al.*, 2000). They are also much less efficient at utilizing retinol, requiring three times the level of normal canaries. Vitamin A provision to these canaries should be based on this knowledge. Care should be taken not to induce hypervitaminosis A in normal coloured canaries if housed together. The recommended daily levels of vitamin A for recessive canaries is 18,000 IU/kg of food, compared with a level of 6000–8000 IU/kg for normal canaries. This level would seem appropriate for most types of the finch.

Nutrition of softbills

Softbills, by definition, eat a diet that consists of relatively soft food items (compared with the hard-coated seeds consumed by granivorous birds). Adaptations to this type of diet include a finer, usually less robust bill structure, a wider gape, reduced crop size, a smaller less muscular gizzard for those that eat fruit, reduced intestinal length and a more rapid intestinal transit time.

Softbills can be further divided into those species that predominately eat invertebrates or meat, those that are omnivorous, those that eat predominately fleshy fruits and berries and a small number of species that are predominantly nectar feeders.

Fruit

Few birds are exclusively frugivorous. Fruit pulp typically contains simple hexose sugars, such as glucose and fructose, or lipids (fatty acids and waxes). Fruits contain low levels of protein (generally 3–7%) and with few exceptions this limits fruit as a complete dietary source. Although fruit-eating birds seem to exist on a diet lower in protein than most birds, those maintained exclusively on an all-fruit diet lose weight and the majority of fruit-eaters need to supplement their diet with protein, usually by eating invertebrates.

Fruit sugars

The levels of sugars (simple and complex) and lipids vary between the many hundreds of fruits that birds eat. Sugars are water soluble and readily absorbed by both passive and active mechanisms. Lipids are hydrophobic and must be emulsified and hydrolysed prior to passive absorption. The process of lipid digestion requires a longer intestinal transit time and increased bile production for adequate digestion. Birds that are used to eating a high proportion of (fat-rich) insects have the digestive mechanisms in place to deal efficiently with lipid-rich berries. Individual birds are able to modulate their digestive function according to the nutritional composition of their diet. The lipid portion of the fruits and berries is important not only as a source of nutrition but also as a carrier for the lipid-soluble vitamins and carotenoid pigments contained within both the pulp and cuticle of the fruit. As the level of proteins, lipids or carbohydrates alters within the range of foods that the birds are eating, so do the respective levels of appropriate digestive enzymes. This is a rapid response allowing a high level of nutritional flexibility.

Sucrose intolerance in softbills: Many of the wild fruits eaten and dispersed by birds are rich in monosaccharide sugars (hexoses). Cultivated fruits often contain high levels of complex sugars, sucrose for example, which gives them a sweeter taste. For birds of the sturnid–muscicapid lineage, which lack expression of the intestinal enzyme sucrase, sucrose is not only a useless energy source but can cause osmotic diarrhoea (Malcarney *et al.*, 1994). This should be borne in mind when hospitalizing any of these birds.

Protein: invertebrates

Diets for captive softbills should, regardless of the level of fruit eaten, include an additional source of protein. The natural protein source for wild softbills is invertebrates. Many of these may be found within the plants or leaf litter of the aviary and additional natural supplies can be encouraged by having a pile of rotting fruit or compost on the aviary floor. Additional supplies are usually required and should be supplied especially if breeding is to be considered. The livefoods commonly supplied are locusts, house crickets, earthworms, maggots, fruit flies and mealworms, waxmoth larvae (see Figure 33.8) and, where appropriate, baby mice and dead day-old chicks (see Figure 33.8).

'Meating off': alternatives to livefood

As has been discussed, livefood in captivity does not provide a balanced diet and the provision of excessive amounts (which are usually eaten in preference to other foods) will lead to malnutrition.

Good health and longevity can be achieved without large quantities of livefood and so artificial prepared diets have been developed to replace a large percentage of the livefood eaten. Commercially available 'insectivorous' foods are available and, depending on the species of bird, these are usually augmented with a range of minced meats, fish-based products (roe or brine shrimp), cheese (hard and soft), tinned and pre-soaked cat, dog and ferret complete diets, and koi or trout pellets (though care must be taken with the iron content of many of these prepared diets).

Encouraging birds to convert to an artificial diet can often be achieved by coating livefoods with a honey or sugar glaze or a light coating of corn oil and mixing them with the prepared foods. Birds eating the livefood are 'encouraged' to taste the new food sticking to the insect's body. Softbills tend to be very active birds and where livefood is given it acts to increase environmental enrichment.

Iron storage disease

Iron storage disease (ISD) is a life-threatening condition affecting several avian species. Storage of iron, in the form of haemosiderin, in the cells of the liver, spleen and other organs is part of normal metabolism. However, when accumulation becomes excessive, liver disease, heart failure and ultimately death will ensue. ISD is principally a disease of captivity, being rarely reported in free-living birds. Within the order Passeriformes it is most commonly reported in mynahs, tanagers, birds-of-paradise and starlings.

The aetiology of ISD is complex and not fully understood, with several factors being implicated (Mete *et al.*, 2001, 2003).

Species differences

In most taxa, iron load never reaches levels that cause health problems. In birds, iron overloads are most commonly found in species that, in the wild, feed primarily on fruits and insects. Both insects and fruit are, in general, poor sources of dietary minerals. With natural diets low in iron, some bird species may have developed physiological mechanisms to extract and absorb dietary iron very efficiently. Mechanisms to compensate for scarcity of dietary iron might produce iron overloads when challenged with iron levels found in 'normal' captive diets. However, there are also many frugivorous species in which ISD has never been recorded, suggesting some evolutionary predisposition in those species that are susceptible.

Diet and stress

Commercial diets are generally higher in available iron than those diets consumed in the wild. Maintaining a low level of dietary iron is very difficult with the composition of any natural food varying according to soil, weather and other variables, including contaminants or additional supplements. Ascorbic acid (vitamin C), which occurs in many of the fruits and vegetables fed to frugivores, enhances the absorption of iron from non-haem sources (iron from haem sources is already highly available) (Olsen *et al.*, 2006).

Supplementation with high levels of vitamin A also increases dietary iron uptake. Vitamin A is low in the natural diet of fruit eaters and is absorbed without a natural feedback mechanism. Conversion of dietary carotenoids to vitamin A has, however, a regulatory mechanism in place. ISD may simply be the result of protracted exposure to excess dietary iron.

Stress has been indicated as a catalyst in the precipitation of ISD as a clinical disease.

Prevention

As the treatment of ISD is generally not very rewarding, involving regular phlebotomy and the administration of chelating agents such as deferoxamine (see Chapter 34), control of the condition is aimed at prevention.

- Be aware which species are susceptible and maintain such birds on a low-iron diet. A diet containing less than 50 ppm iron is recommended; commercial diets formulated to achieve this level are available. Avoid the addition of foods high in available iron (e.g. meat-based products, raisins).
- The addition to the diet of plant-based iron chelators such as phytates and tannins has been suggested. These compounds bind up the dietary iron within the gut, preventing absorption. The addition of brewed tea to the drinking water has been used. Many of the wild fruits (e.g. wild figs) that are consumed by birds susceptible to ISD are high in iron but are also high in tannins, limiting the amount of available iron. It should be noted that these chelating agents are non-specific and chelate other (essential) heavy metals. Their use should be undertaken with caution and excessive use avoided.
- Feed fruits containing vitamin C at a different time to foods containing significant iron, as vitamin C has a role in converting the oxidation state of iron from the +3 to +2 form (i.e. from Fe^{III} to Fe^{II}), thus increasing solubility and absorption.
- Avoid supplements high in vitamin A (a level of 1000–1500 IU vitamin A/kg diet is recommended for susceptible species). Replace these with high levels of carotenoids.

References and further reading

Allan LR and Green ID (1997) The importance of green seed in the nutrition of the Zebra Finch. *Australian Journal of Ecology* **22**, 44, 412–418

Bairlein F (1996) Fruit-eating in birds and its nutritional consequences. *Comparative Biochemistry and Physiology A* **113**, 215–224

Brue R (1994) Nutrition. In: *Avian Medicine: Principles and Application*, ed. BW Ritchie *et al.*, pp. 63–78. Wingers, Lake Worth, FL

De Nagy H, Hrabar K and Perrins M (2002) The effect of bill structure on seed selection by granivorous birds. *African Zoology* **37**(1), 67–80

Diaz M (1990) Interspecific patterns of seed selection among granivorous passerines: effects of seed size. Seed nutritive value and bird morphology. *Ibis* **132**, 467–476

Diaz M (1996) Food choice by seed-eating birds in relation to seed chemistry. *Comparative Biochemistry and Physiology, Part A: Physiology* **113**(3), 239–246

Graveland J and Drent RH (1997) Calcium availability limits breeding success of passerines on poor soils. *Journal of Animal Ecology* **66**(2), 279–288

Harper EJ and Turner CL (2000) Nutrition and energetics of the canary (*Serinus canaries*). *Comparative Biochemistry and Physiology Part B* **126**, 271–281

Houston DC, Donnan D, Jones P *et al.* (1995) Changes in the muscle condition of female Zebra finches during egglaying and the role of protein storage in bird skeletal muscle. *Ibis* **137**, 322–328

Klasing KC (1998) *Comparative Avian Nutrition.* CAB International, Wallingford, Oxford

McDonald D (2006) Nutrition and dietary supplementation. In: *Clinical Avian Medicine*, ed. G Harrison and T Lightfoot, pp. 86–102. Spix, Palm Beach, FL

Macwhirter P (1994) Passeriformes. In: *Avian Medicine: Principles and Application*, ed. BW Ritchie *et al.*, pp. 1172–1199. Wingers, Lake Worth, FL

Malcarney HL, Martinez Del Rio C and Apanius V (1994) Sucrose intolerance in birds: simple nonlethal diagnostic methods and consequences for assimilation of complex carbohydrates. *The Auk* **111**, 170–177

Martinez Del Rio C (1997) Can passerines synthesise Vitamin C? *The Auk* **July**

Mete A, Hendriks HG, Klaren PH *et al.* (2003) Iron metabolism in mynah birds (*Gracula religiosa*) resembles human hereditary haemochromatosis. *Avian Pathology* **32**, 625–632

Mete A, Dorrestein GM, Marx JJ *et al.* (2001) A comparative study of iron retention in mynahs, doves and rats. *Avian Pathology* **30**, 479–486

Murphy ME (1994) Amino acid composition of avian eggs and tissues – nutritional implications. *Journal of Avian Biology* **25**, 27–38

Murphy ME and King JR (1989) Sparrows discriminate between diets differing in valine and lysine concentration. *Physiology and Behaviour* **45**, 423–430

Olsen GP, Russell KE, Dierenfeld E, Falcon MD and Phalen DN (2006) Impact of supplements on iron absorption from diets containing high and low iron concentrations in the European Starling (*Sturnus vulgaris*). *Journal of Avian Medicine and Surgery* **20**, 67–73

Robbins CT (1981) Estimation of the relative protein cost of reproduction in birds. The Condor **83**(2), 177–179

Schaefer HM, Schmidt V and Bairlein F (2003) Discrimination abilities for nutrients: which difference matters for choosy birds and why? *Animal Behaviour* **65**, 531–541

Stockdale BC (2005) The nutritional implications of producing the 'optimal egg' in captive birds. In: *Proceedings 9th Meeting of the European Association of Avian Veterinarians, Arles*, pp. 340–347

Taylor EJ (1996) An evaluation of the importance of insoluble versus soluble grit in the diet of canaries. *Journal of Avian Medicine and Surgery* **10**, 248–251

van der Meij MAA (2005) A tough nut to crack. Adaptations to seed cracking in finches. Doctoral thesis, Leiden University, Faculty of Mathematics & Natural Sciences, Institute of Biology

Vezia F and Williams TD (2003) Plasticity in body composition in breeding birds: what drives the metabolic cost of egg production? *Physiological and Biochemical Zoology* **76**, 716–730

Wilson HR (1997) Effects of maternal nutrition on hatchability. *Poultry Science* **76**(1), 134–143

Wolf P, Bartels T, Sallmann HP *et al.* (2000) Vitamin A metabolism in recessive white canaries. *Animal Welfare* **9**, 153–165

34

Passerine birds: approach to the sick individual

J.R. Best

Introduction

For a veterinary surgeon the treatment of the single pet passerine bird raises many fascinating challenges, especially with diagnosis and therapy. Although the treatment of these birds is unlikely to have a serious impact on a practice's time or economics, it is important to appreciate the emotional value of these birds to their owners who, more often than not, are elderly people living on their own.

This chapter is devoted to the problems a veterinary surgeon might face when presented with an individual passerine bird kept as a companion. The patient is most likely to be a member of the finch family, more particularly a domesticated Canary or one of the commoner species of captive-bred finches, such as the Zebra Finch and Gouldian Finch, and is likely to be kept in an indoor cage, either on its own or with a small number of companions. Mynah birds, especially Indian Hill Mynahs, are often kept as companion birds and have specific management and disease problems.

As patients, individual passerine birds place some constraints on the veterinary surgeon.

- Their small size reduces the scope of a clinical examination and limits the investigations that are practicable.
- Costs of treatment and investigations are frequently an important factor in the approach to a case.

The approach to the examination of such companion birds and their mode of presentation will differ from that of an aviary bird.

- As the bird is a pet, the owner often has a very close emotional attachment with it and will keep it under close scrutiny, so any change in its behaviour, however slight, might be noticed by the owner sooner than with a bird in a aviary.
- As the bird is likely to be kept in a fairly closed environment, any disease it has is unlikely to be caused by a newly acquired infectious agent (unless the bird has been obtained recently, and especially if it a young bird) and is more likely to be due to husbandry factors or an age-related degenerative condition, the life expectancy of most captive passerine birds being 8–12 years.

Clinical history and examination

Details on the collection of a clinical history, handling and a clinical examination are given in Chapter 7; however, history taking and examination of an individual pet passerine bird does present a few features that might require special attention.

- Being caged birds it is important that they are presented in their normal cages, together with any companions, as this will reduce the stress on the bird and allow it to be examined from a distance. If the bird has to be admitted for investigation and treatment, it will be under less stress if in its own cage and with its companions.
- Ideally the cage should have any loose substrate and absorbent paper removed from the floor and not have been cleaned for at least 12 hours. This will allow an assessment to be made of the standard of husbandry and an examination made of the droppings and any regurgitated ingesta (see Figure 34.8).
- The precise location of the cage within the house is often important to assess the risk of toxic fumes and the adverse effects of cold air and draughts when close to a window, or of dry air from a domestic heating system.
- The amount of exercise, if any, that the bird is allowed outside the cage should be ascertained.
- Capture of a small bird within a cage is easier and safer if the perches have been removed and, if possible, the lighting in the room reduced.
- The weight of the bird, together with its body condition, gives an important indication of the progress of a case. Small birds can be restrained in washable cloth bags or small plastic top-loading hamster boxes and weighed on digital pan scales, ideally registering at intervals of 2 g. Spring balances, as used in the field by bird ringers, are accurate and ideal for small birds.

There are a few physical features that might appear to be abnormalities and cause concern to the owner or an inexperienced clinician.

- In many small passerine birds the crop, when full of seed, will appear on the side of the neck or even on the dorsal aspect of the neck. This is normal and the swelling can be seen to be a full crop as the seed is clearly identified through the thin skin and crop wall.

- Females in breeding condition develop a brood patch, which is a large area of featherless skin on the ventral abdomen.

Stabilization of a sick passerine bird

The stabilization of any anorexic bird is a vital part of the treatment regime (see Chapter 7) and this becomes even more critical in a small bird. The smaller the bird, the higher the metabolic rate and, if not eating or drinking, the faster its energy reserves will be depleted and the sooner it will become dehydrated. Maintaining the patient at a temperature within its thermoneutral range will help to conserve energy reserves; and the administration of fluids, together with a suitable energy source, will counteract dehydration and hypoglycaemia. The thermoneutral range of small birds is between 25° and 35°C and the smaller the bird the higher the range (Figure 34.1) (Dawson and Whitow, 2000). Such temperatures can be maintained in a suitable hospital cage or by placing a heat lamp (preferably with a dull heat-emitting bulb) on or close to the bird's own cage,

so creating a heat gradient that will allow the bird to choose its optimum temperature.

The daily maintenance requirement for fluid in birds weighing more than 100 g is 5–10% of their body weight, rising to 50% of the body weight for small birds weighing 10–20 g (Goldstein and Skadhauge, 2000). Similarly energy requirements for small birds are much higher than for larger species and small passerine birds may not survive more than 48–72 hours without food (Perrins, 1979).

It is safe to assume that an inappetent bird will have lost at least 5–10% of its body fluids and depleted its energy reserves. These deficits should be replaced within the first 24–48 hours of treatment, using a proprietary rehydration preparation or a glucose solution (containing at least 4% glucose). For very small birds the most accessible and least stressful route of administration of fluids for stabilization is orally, using a suitable crop tube. Small birds weighing less than 30 g can be given no more than 0.5 ml of fluid at a time by gavage. Subcutaneous injections of sterile isotonic fluids (4% glucose/0.18% saline solution) can be repeatedly administered in the loose skin of the groin (see Chapter 8).

Critical care of a sick individual can only be given effectively with the bird hospitalized, as few owners of companion birds will have the necessary skills or equipment.

Diagnostic procedures

Figure 34.2 gives a guide to differential diagnosis for sick passerine birds; Figure 34.3 lists common syndromes in such patients, with suggestions of probable causes and action to be taken.

Clinical pathology
Although the size of the bird and financial constraints may often limit the extent of investigations, routine microscopy of crop washes, faeces and blood films should be well within the scope of most veterinary practices and are frequently very helpful in establishing a diagnosis (Figure 34.4).

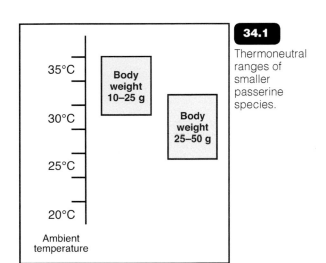

34.1 Thermoneutral ranges of smaller passerine species.

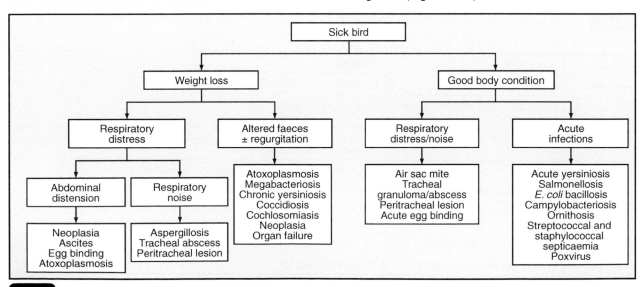

34.2 Guide to differential diagnosis of an individual sick passerine bird.

Syndrome	Causes	Investigation	Action/Treatment
Sudden death	Inhaled toxins (CO, kitchen fumes); spontaneous internal haemorrhage; acute infections; apparent 'sudden death' due to poor observation by owner	Autopsy	Check gas appliances, check location of kitchen in relation to bird
Plumage problems	Abnormal moult; feather pecking by mate; feather cysts; external parasites	Review husbandry practices. Examination and microscopy of affected feathers and skin	Separation. Surgical excision, removal. Identify and local treatment with ivermectins or pyrethroids
Skin disease	*Cnemidocoptes* on face/beak and legs; *Ornithonyssus* on the body; papillomavirus infection on feet; dry necrosis of digits	Examination and microscopy of skin scrapings	Local treatment with ivermectins. Local treatment with ivermectins. Amputation
Stops singing	Male bird in moult; debilitating disease	Clinical examination, and if weight loss, investigate	
Weight loss	Atoxoplasmosis; megabacteriosis; chronic yersiniosis; coccidiosis; cochlosomiasis; trichomoniasis; neoplasia; organ failure; starvation	Microscopy of crop washes and faeces	Toltrazuril (prophylaxis in breeding unit). Amphotericin, citric acid. Broad-spectrum antibiotic of use only in early stages. Toltrazuril. Metronidazole. Metronidazole. Poor husbandry or inability to pick up and dehusk seed
Ocular discharges	Conjunctivitis, local infection may be associated with lower respiratory tract infection; pox lesions; chlamydiosis		Local, and systemic antibiotics if indicated
Respiratory noises	Air sac mites; tracheal/bronchial infection	Trial therapy with ivermectin	Ivermectin, 1% in propylene glycol, 2–3 treatments at 10-day intervals. Broad-spectrum antibiotic – enrofloxacin
Respiratory distress	Acute respiratory infections; space-occupying abdominal lesions, including egg binding	Examination of abdomen	Suitable systemic antibiotic (fluoroquinolone) and ivermectin
Regurgitation	Trichomoniasis; candidiasis; bacterial crop infection; crop impaction	Microscopy of crop wash	Metronidazole. Nystatin. Broad-spectrum antibiotic
Undigested seed in faeces	Malabsorption	Investigate chronic alimentary tract infections	
Soft faeces/ diarrhoea	Atoxoplasmosis; cochlosomiasis; coccidiosis; candidiasis; megabacteriosis; bacterial enteritis; female during egg laying	Microscopy of crop washes and faeces. Examination of abdomen	Toltrazuril (prophylaxis in breeding unit). Metronidazole. Toltrazuril. Nystatin. Amphotericin, citric acid. Neomycin, broad-spectrum antibiotic
Neurological signs	Head tilt/ataxia; fits	Detailed history and examination. Trial calcium and vitamin therapy	Aetiology uncertain: inner ear disease; CNS damage (e.g. intracerebral haemorrhage, abscess). Possibly hypocalcaemia. CNS infections, poisoning (heavy metal, pesticide)
Lameness	Fractures; temporary nerve damage; ill fitting leg ring; articular gout; arthritis		

34.3 Common syndromes of individual sick passerine birds: probable causes and action to be taken.

Sample	Preparation	Diagnosis
Crop wash	Wet preparation	Flagellates – trichomonads. *Candida* – budding yeasts and pseudomycelia. Bacterial flora
	Gram stain or rapid Romanowsky-type stains	Bacterial flora and yeasts
Faeces	Wet preparation	Protozoan cysts – coccidia. Flagellates – *Cochlosoma*. Megabacteria (*Macrorhabdus ornithogaster*). Bacterial flora
	Gram stain	Megabacteria (*Macrorhabdus ornithogaster*). Bacterial flora
Blood	Centrifuged heparinized capillary tube	Anaemia and level of hydration. Extent of buffy coat
	Rapid Romanowsky-type stain	Indication of type of anaemia. Rough indication of total white cell count and differential. Presence of haematozoa
Skin scraping	Wet preparation in liquid paraffin or KOH	Ectoparasites – *Cnemidocoptes*
Feathers	Attached to a slide by adhesive tape	Ectoparasites – e.g. lice

34.4 Microscopy and laboratory tests as aids to diagnosis in an individual sick passerine bird.

Staining of heat-fixed crop washes and faecal smears with Gram stain is useful in determining the extent and nature of the microbial flora.

Small amounts of blood can be collected directly into heparinized capillary tubes by pricking the caudal tibial vein. The right jugular vein can be used for venepuncture in passerine species weighing in excess of 50 g; it is located running under a featherless tract of skin and care must be exercised to minimize the stress of handling the patient and the risk of haemorrhage from a damaged vein. The morphology of blood cells, estimations of leucocyte abundance and relative differentiation, and presence of haematozoa can be obtained from air-dried thin blood films stained with a rapid Romanowsky-type stain (ideally smears for staining should be made from fresh whole blood, as heparin affects staining, but for practical reasons a heparinized tube is suggested in this situation). If sufficient blood is available (1% of the bird's body weight is regarded as the amount that can be collected safely), centrifugation will give an indication of the haematocrit and the depth of the buffy coat and, using a refractometer, total plasma proteins can also be estimated. Sufficient blood might be collected from larger passerine birds to be submitted to laboratories for total leucocyte counts and biochemistry.

Crop washes and faeces may be examined as wet preparations with a small amount of material suspended in an isotonic solution under a cover slip. It will show motile flagellates, often in large numbers, especially in the faeces of nestlings in cases of cochlosomiasis; they may be visible under low power but are clearly identified under a high-power dry lens. Fresh material must be examined, as flagellate numbers and their activity will rapidly decline after collection. The characteristic budding yeast cells of candidiasis are clearly seen under the high-power dry lens but the hyphae of a pseudomycelium, which can occur in acute cases, could be overlooked. So-called megabacteria (*Macrorhabdus ornithogaster*) (see Figure 35.2) might be found in crop washes from affected birds, but they are more usually found in faeces, often in vast numbers, and are easily recognized in wet preparations; however, the absence of megabacteria in the faeces does not always preclude their presence and examination of smears of proventicular mucus collected during an autopsy is more accurate. Staining of air-dried and heat-fixed smears of material from the alimentary tract with Gram stain or one of the rapid Romanowsky stains will demonstrate some significant microorganisms, including *M. ornithogaster* and other yeasts, and also show details of the bacterial flora. Most healthy passerine birds will have few or no bacteria in their faeces; hence large numbers of bacteria, especially if mostly of one type (e.g. all Gram-negative rods or Gram-positive cocci) might well be highly significant. For faecal examination, it is important to ensure that a droppings sample contains mainly faecal material, as large amounts of urate crystals complicate examination. Examination of a wet preparation is greatly improved by lowering the substage condenser of the microscope and in doing so simulating a 'phase contrast' image. Parasitic ova and protozoan cysts may be demonstrated using standard flotation methods.

Radiology (see Chapter 11) is also a very valuable tool in passerine birds.

Autopsies are always of value, especially in the case of an unexplained death. An autopsy, backed up with laboratory techniques that could be available in most practices, will often give an indication of the cause of death, which may put an owner's mind at rest and will certainly increase the clinician's experience

Therapeutics

The size of small birds presents some considerations regarding the administration of medication.

- The maintenance of therapeutic blood levels of medicines in small birds will require higher dose rates and more frequent administration than in larger birds with lower metabolic rates. Wherever a range of dose rates for birds is quoted, the highest dose rate should be considered for small birds. Unfortunately few therapeutic agents have product licences that include dosage details for birds. For therapeutic dose calculations the use of allometric scaling is recommended (see Appendix 1).
- The method of administration of a medicine is critical in ensuring that a patient receives an effective therapeutic dose. Indirect administration by the addition of medicine to the drinking water is only effective if (i) the medicine is capable of adequate intestinal absorption, and (ii) the bird is able to drink sufficient water containing a concentration high enough to ensure an effective and lasting therapeutic blood level (polydipsic birds run the risk of over-dosage). Direct administration (either orally with a gavage tube or parentally) is more effective in ensuring the certain delivery of a measured dose, though potentially more stressful for the patient. Parenteral administration by injection into the caudal half of the pectoral muscle mass is tolerated but repeated injections are best avoided due to the resultant tissue damage, with further medication being continued by the oral route.

Anaesthesia

Inhalation anaesthesia, using isoflurane or sevoflurane, is the method of choice for small birds (see Chapter 10). Anaesthesia for short periods is induced and maintained with the patient restrained and its head held within a small mask made from a 1.0 or 2.0 ml plastic syringe case.

Common surgical procedures

During any surgical procedure, haemostasis is critical as only a small loss of circulating volume (4–6 drops for a 20 g finch) could induce hypovolaemic shock. For soft tissue surgery see Chapter 14 and for orthopaedics Chapter 15.

Egg binding

Female pet birds will come into breeding condition, ovulate and lay eggs without the presence of a male. Dystocia is common but often the problem is not recognized by the owner. The egg is usually easily identified by palpation of the caudal abdomen as a smooth firm mass. If the egg is soft-shelled, as is often the case, crepitus may be felt when pressure is applied to the thin shell; if the egg is shell-less, only a soft fluctuating discrete mass is palpated.

In acute egg binding, where the presence of an egg is causing obstruction to the rectum and ureters and possibly compressing the pelvic blood vessels and nerves, the bird might suddenly show all the signs of a sick bird and be unable to perch. This is life-threatening and requires urgent attention first to stabilize the patient with fluids and heat (see above) and then physical removal of the egg if it has not been passed within a few hours of the bird being held within its thermoneutral range. Under general anaesthesia, attempts can be made to express the egg from the oviduct using gentle external digital pressure. Egg binding is often associated with a roughened and thin-shelled egg, and such manipulation frequently leads to collapse of the egg, with its contents and the remnants of the shell being passed within a few hours. Aftercare depends on the condition of the patient, but must involve supportive treatment until the bird regains its appetite, heated accommodation and antibiotic therapy (to control salpingitis and peritonitis).

A chronic form of egg binding can occur when the retained egg does not interfere with the functioning of other organs. In such cases the bird gradually loses weight and presents with a swollen abdomen, due to the retained egg and, possibly, inspissated pus within the oviduct and an accompanying peritonitis. Diagnosis can be assisted by radiography to demonstrate the calcified egg shell and 'ground glass' appearance of a peritonitis, together with paracentesis and cytological examination of any resultant peritoneal fluid to demonstrate the presence of inflammatory cells. In such cases the prognosis is poor: surgery is impracticable and the condition is beyond the help of medical treatment.

Diseases of the integument

Feather cysts

Abnormal feather development is frequently found with canaries and takes the form of either thickened 'tufts' of dysplastic feathers or smooth spherical cutaneous masses that often ulcerate to reveal an accumulation of inspissated feather material (Figure 34.5). This lesion has been classified as a benign neoplasm, trichofolliculoma. The lesions, which are often recurrent, are usually found on the feather tracts of the back and wings. The cause is considered to be genetic and occurs most frequently in certain types of crossbred birds. Small lesions rarely cause problems but larger ulcerated lesions appear to cause discomfort and could become infected. If excised early in development, before ulceration has occurred, there is a risk of haemorrhage from the base of the cyst

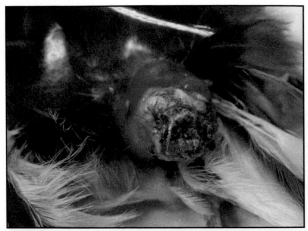

34.5 Canary with feather cyst on tail. (Courtesy of Neil Forbes)

contents and in many cases it might be preferable to leave lesions until they have ulcerated before manual expression of the inspissated material. Lesions frequently recur and cauterization of the base of the lesion with silver nitrate sticks can be effective. In cases with frequent recurrence, especially involving body feather tracts, resection of the skin carrying the lesions can be successful.

Abnormal moults

Most adult passerine birds have a complete annual moult that follows the period of sexual activity. Juveniles have a complete moult of the juvenile plumage that starts about 4 weeks after fledging. Some species might moult more often or only partly. These moults should only last for about 6–9 weeks. The control of moulting is complex and is under hormonal control (thyroid and sex hormones) affected by external factors such as the photoperiod, ambient temperature and nutrition.

Abnormal feather loss is usually associated with abnormal moulting patterns and commonly involves the contour feathers of the head. Some birds may appear to have an interrupted moult (so called stuck-in-moult) and others appear to be in a continual moult (soft moult). In an individual caged indoor pet bird abnormal moults frequently correct themselves but indicate that attention could be paid to the general level of husbandry (nutrition, photoperiod and ambient temperature). Increasing the length of the photoperiod and the ambient temperature, although not easy to produce in a normal household, might tend to induce feather growth in a bird with an interrupted moult and decreasing these parameters might stop a moult in a bird showing a continual moult. Ideally changes to the photoperiod should be made by 30-minute increments or reductions every 2–3 days and should vary within the range of 12–18 hours of illumination daily.

Ectoparasitic infections

Infections with ectoparasites in individual pet birds are likely to be existing infections present before the bird was obtained, or could be acquired from wild birds if the cage is placed out of doors during the summer.

Cnemidocoptes spp.

Cnemidocoptes spp. commonly infect the scaly skin of the tibiotarsus and digits, and occasionally the beak and the adjacent skin of the face (Figure 34.6). The diagnosis is confirmed with microscopy of skin scrapings. *Cnemidocoptes* spp. will not survive off the host for any significant length of time. The infection is treated with 1% ivermectin diluted 1:50 in propylene glycol and applied to the lesions with a cotton bud or percutaneously at the rate of one drop for a small bird, or similarly using proprietary preparations (Alpharma, 1:10 ivermectin), the medication being applied every 7–10 days for three applications.

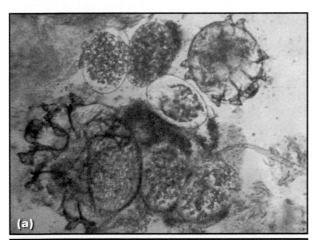

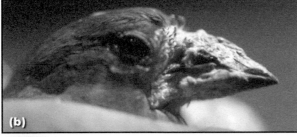

34.6 **(a)** *Cnemidocoptes* mites. **(b)** Severe scaly face in a finch.

Epidermoptid and northern mites

Epidermoptid mites and *Ornithonyssus* spp. (Northern mite) (Figure 34.7) can cause disturbance to the bird due to irritation and the infestation can be extremely heavy, especially in birds that are in poor condition. The life cycle occurs entirely on the host's body, hence treatment with ivermectin or fipronil should be applied every 7–10 days for three applications.

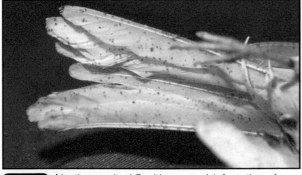

34.7 Northern mite (*Ornithonyssus*) infestation of a canary.

Dermanyssus gallinae

Dermanyssus gallinae (red mite) is less likely to infest an individual pet bird, as the mites are only present on birds at night, spending the day away from the host in crevices in the bird's surroundings. However, birds acquired during the summer from a heavily infested aviary may carry some mites, as would any fomite acquired with the birds. Heavy infestation can cause severe irritation to the bird and a regenerative anaemia through blood loss, as the mites feed on blood. Control requires destruction of the cages or their treatment with a suitable insecticide.

Diseases of the respiratory tract

Dyspnoea and tachypnoea in birds may be caused by primary respiratory disease but are also commonly associated with space-occupying lesions within the abdominal cavity; lesions such as hepatomegaly, ascites and neoplasia compress the air sacs and thus compromise respiration.

Small birds showing respiratory distress must be handled with great care and kept in ventral recumbency whenever possible. The small size of most companion passerine birds prevents the use of many valuable diagnostic procedures that can be employed in larger birds.

In birds showing tachypnoea with an abdominal swelling, abdominal radiography (especially following oral administration of barium sulphate contrast medium) is helpful in determining the position and size of abdominal viscera. Choanal and conjunctival swabs submitted for bacteriological examination might identify potential pathogens and indicate suitable treatment regimes. Submission of choanal, conjunctival and faecal swabs for PCR testing for *Chlamydophila psittaci* would be indicated if there is a history of acquisition from a possible source of infection or of human illness. If sufficient blood could be collected safely, limited haematological and biochemical parameters could be obtained.

Infectious conjunctivitis

Canaries commonly show signs of conjunctivitis, which is often unilateral (so-called one-eyed cold). The birds show a catarrhal discharge (often bubbly), mild blepharospasm and self-trauma, with the bird rubbing the affected eye with its wing, leading to staining and disruption of the covert feathers of the wing. This condition is most likely to be infectious and associated with mycoplasmosis, chlamydophilosis or primary or secondary bacterial infections and is commonly associated with an infection of the lower respiratory tract. Treatment is usually successful with a broad-spectrum antibiotic either systemically (orally in drinking water, or preferably by gavage) or as an ophthalmic preparation (without corticosteroid).

Infectious conjunctivitis must be differentiated from other causes of ocular discharges, blepharospasm and ocular discomfort, such as traumatic lesions, foreign bodies, corneal damage or intraocular disease.

Air sac mites (*Sternostoma tracheacolum*)

Respiratory ('knocking') noises, especially in Gouldian Finches but also in canaries, are commonly associated with air sac mites. The mites, whose life cycle is entirely within the host, live in the air sacs and will enter the bronchi and trachea, where they can then cause respiratory noise, mouth breathing, head shaking and dyspnoea. The mites are likely to pass to young birds being fed by infected adults.

Diagnosis can be made by transillumination of the trachea, when the mites can be seen as black dots. Diagnosis is usually made, however, by response to treatment with ivermectin given either orally or by percutaneous administration, the treatment being repeated at least twice at 10-day intervals. Treatment of heavy infections can lead to a temporary increase in respiratory distress whilst the mites are being expelled; severe cases can result in death following treatment, due to occlusion of the airways with dead and dying mites.

Lack of response to treatment of the respiratory signs might indicate an alternative cause, such as lower respiratory tract infections, tracheal and bronchial granulomas or abscesses and peri-tracheal masses.

Diseases of the alimentary tract

Regurgitation

Owners might not be aware that their bird is regurgitating seed and a careful examination of the cage might reveal clusters of regurgitated seed adhering to surfaces within the cage. Investigations of alimentary tract disease (crop swab, parasitology) are described above (see clinical pathology).

Non-infectious causes of regurgitation may be associated with crop impaction as the result of inappropriate feeding (for example, eggfood fed as a very stiff mixture whilst the bird does not have adequate access to water).

Abnormal droppings

True diarrhoea is not a common finding in individual pet birds but polyuria, with an excessive amount of the urinary component of the dropping, is commonly mistaken for diarrhoea. Polyuria can be associated with many conditions; it may be the result of a primary polydipsia, a diet with a high moisture or salt content or impaired tubular reabsorption in renal disease. It is also commonly seen when a bird is stressed; for example, a bird placed in unfamiliar surroundings, or transported, will often pass very wet droppings. Investigation requires a critical review of the bird's husbandry, including diet, and a clinical examination and abdominal radiography.

Due to the size of most companion passerine birds the scope of investigations into the causes of polyuria is limited. If sufficient blood (minimum 0.2 ml) can be collected, uric acid can be an indication of renal disease. Urinalysis is rarely helpful in the investigation of polyuria in a small bird and it is difficult to collect an uncontaminated sample, though microscopic examination of sediment might reveal casts.

It is common to be presented with a bird that is polydipsic and polyuric, yet appears to remain healthy in other respects, though regular clinical examinations and monitoring of body weight would indicate the need for further investigation. For a more detailed view of avian renal disease and diagnosis see Lierz (2003).

Some of the more frequently seen causes of diarrhoea are shown in Figure 34.8. True diarrhoea would appear as droppings that are loose and usually without white urates or clear urine. Microscopic examination of wet preparations and Gram-stained smears will indicate the presence of flagellates, parasitic cysts, yeasts or megabacteria (*Macrorhabdus ornithogaster*) and the extent and nature of the bacterial flora (e.g. sparse or large numbers, comprising predominately Gram-positive cocci and rods, or Gram-negative rods). Faeces from most apparently normal passerine birds contain low numbers of enteric bacteria. Selective bacteriological culture techniques can demonstrate potential pathogens, especially *Campylobacter*, *Clostridium*, *Salmonella*, *Escherichia coli* or *Yersinia*. Diarrhoea can also occur as a sign of organ failure, especially in hepatopathy.

Appearance of droppings	Probable causes
Firm, dark faecal component, with an equal or smaller amount of pure white urates and a minimal amount of moisture	Normal
Green staining droppings with minimal faecal component	Anorexia/starvation
Undigested seed in faeces	Malabsorption associated with alimentary tract infections; megabacteriosis
Soft faeces/diarrhoea	Atoxoplasmosis; cochlosomiasis; coccidiosis; candidiasis; megabacteriosis; bacterial enteritis; female during egg laying
Wet droppings with normal formed faecal component	Stress; renal disease; polydipsia
Excess urates in droppings	Renal disease
Frank blood	Cloacolith; cloacal infection; egg-laying injury

34.8 Appearance of droppings from pet passerine birds and their possible causes.

Neurological problems

A sudden-onset ataxia and head tilt is a frequent finding, especially in young finches. The aetiology is unclear. Most birds remain alert and are able to feed. A pragmatic approach to such cases might include parenteral treatment with calcium and multivitamins to correct any deficiencies, antibiotic for any localized infection within the brain and corticosteroids to reduce any intracerebral swelling. Some birds recover but in many the signs persist.

Neoplasia

Although neoplastic lesions are not seen as commonly in captive passerine birds as in psittacine birds (especially the Budgerigar), they do occur and should always be borne in mind as a potential diagnosis, especially in cases of emaciation together with abdominal distension in the older bird.

Lymphosarcoma of the liver and spleen and adenocarcinoma of the kidney or gonad may lead to abdominal distension and emaciation, often associated with respiratory distress caused by compression of the air sacs by the growing tumour. Renal neoplasia might be associated with lameness due to pressure on the nerves of the lumbosacral plexus. Lymphosarcoma of the liver and spleen could superficially resemble the hepatomegaly and splenomegaly of infectious disease, especially atoxoplasmosis (though atoxoplasmosis is primarily a disease of the young bird). In canaries, superficial masses on the wing, especially in the region of the carpus, are most commonly caused by feather cysts but they do need to be differentiated from tumours (e.g. fibromas), as the inspissated material of a feather cyst may simply be 'shelled out', whereas surgical removal of a neoplastic mass would be more complicated, often resulting in severe problems with postoperative haemostasis.

Nutritional diseases

Nutritional diseases in passerine birds are discussed in detail in Chapter 33.

Iron storage disease (haemochromatosis) in mynahs

Iron storage disease is a common and serious problem in a wide range of softbill species whilst kept in captivity, especially mynahs, and should be considered whenever such birds are presented.

In a pet bird, due to most owners' close observation, the first signs of illness are often noticed sooner than would happen in an aviary bird and early recognition is important in successful control of the disease. Severe cases present with progressive lethargy, loss of pectoral muscle mass, abdominal swelling due to ascites and an associated dyspnoea (due to compression of the air sacs). Severely affected and emaciated birds must be handled with care, especially those with advanced ascites, as respiration is easily compromised during lateral and dorsal recumbency.

A tentative diagnosis can often be made on the presenting signs but confirmation requires radiography to demonstrate hepatomegaly (Figure 34.9) (after drainage of the ascitic fluid, preferably in a conscious patient gently restrained in a vertical position), biochemistry to demonstrate elevated liver enzymes and blood iron levels and, if indicated, histopathological examination of a liver biopsy. Normal levels of blood iron are quoted as approximately 35 µmol/l, with levels in excess of 161 µmol/l indicating disease.

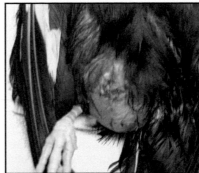
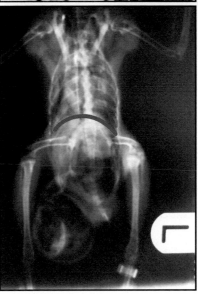

34.9

Abdominal hernia in a Greater Hill Mynah. The liver is enlarged (red line) due to haemochromatosis and the resulting increased abdominal pressure has 'induced' the hernia. (© John Chitty)

Treatment
Treatment requires control of the ascites, if present, and reduction of the iron load in the body tissues.

Abdominal paracentesis: Ascites, and the associated dyspnoea due to compression of the air sacs, is controlled by abdominal paracentesis. With the patient gently restrained in an upright position an intravenous catheter (19 or 21 gauge) is introduced into the swollen abdomen in the midline, well below the caudal edge of the sternum, to avoid penetrating the liver. The needle is withdrawn from the catheter once the abdominal wall has been penetrated, to avoid damaging the viscera, and the ascitic fluid is then slowly drained. This procedure is repeated as required.

Phlebotomy: Although it is reported that chelating agents, such as deferoxamine (100 mg/kg q24h s.c.), have been used with variable effects, the most commonly advocated therapy is phlebotomy. The regular removal of blood will stimulate erythropoiesis and this will gradually deplete the stores of iron. Various protocols are described for the withdrawal of blood (such as 1% body weight weekly), but the progress should be monitored and the amount and frequency of phlebotomy indicated by regular haematocrit determinations and, ideally, blood iron levels. A diet with low levels of iron, although never an effective form of control in itself, will be an adjunct to treatment.

Prevention
This is discussed in Chapter 33.

Obesity

Obesity is the commonest nutritional problem for a caged companion bird. Affected birds have a body weight that is considerably higher than the mean weight for captive birds of its species and large subcutaneous fat depots, especially over the pectoral muscles, which can be palpated and also visualized through the skin. Obesity is associated with poor exercise tolerance and frequently with an abdominal distension associated with both intra-abdominal fat and hepatomegaly (caused by hepatic lipidosis). Once a bird has become obese, the condition can only be controlled effectively with the full compliance of the owner and all persons involved with its care. This requires time spent by the veterinary surgeon in explaining the rationale of obtaining weight loss, i.e. feeding less than the maintenance ration, offering a balanced diet and introducing an exercise regime. Goals need to be set, the ideal parameter to monitor being the bird's body weight measured on a weekly basis. The accuracy of weight measurement is ensured by weighing at the same time of day in relation to feeding times and using a weighing balance that, for a small bird, registers at intervals of 1 g. The amount of food presented to the bird should be reduced gradually over a period, with the aim of determining the bird's daily consumption, and then this amount can be further reduced, the reduction being guided by the rate of loss of body weight. At the same time the bird should be encouraged to exercise outside the cage, but in many grossly obese pet birds the ability to fly may have been lost permanently.

References and further reading

Dawson WR and Whittow GC (2000) Regulation of body temperature. In: *Sturkie's Avian Physiology, 5th edn*, ed. GC Whittow, pp. 343–390. Academic Press, San Diego

Goldstein DL and Skadhauge E (2000) Body fluid composition. In: *Sturkie's Avian Physiology, 5th edn*, ed. GC Whittow, pp. 343–390. Academic Press, San Diego

Kirkwood JK (1983a) Dosing exotic species. *Veterinary Record* **112**, 486

Kirkwood JK (1983b) Influence of body size on health and disease. *Veterinary Record* **113**, 287

Lierz M (2003) Avian renal disease: pathogenesis, diagnosis and therapy. *The Veterinary Clinics of North America: Exotic Animal Practice* **6**, 29–55

Perrins C (1979) *British Tits*. Collins, London

Pokras MA, Karas AM, Kirkwood JK and Sedgewick CJ (1993) An introduction to allometric scaling and its uses in raptor medicine. In: *Raptor Biomedicine*, ed. PT Redig, JE Cooper, D Remple and BD Hunter. Chiron Publications, Keighley, Yorkshire

35

Passerine birds: going light

Ron Rees Davies

Introduction

'Going light' is a term used by breeders of passerine birds for those that are losing body condition with few (or often no) other outward signs. A bird is often discovered to be going light when it is caught and handled for routine husbandry reasons (transferring to a show cage, outdoor flight aviary, breeding pen) or may be discovered to have 'gone light' when it finally starts displaying other, end-stage signs of cachexia such as being 'fluffed' (lethargic and with feathers held away from the body – a form of behavioural heat retention) or having cloacal 'clagging' (faecal accumulation on the feathers around the vent due to either diarrhoea or failure to groom properly).

Although fanciers often perceive going light to be a specific condition, because of the non-specific presentation and often unknown timescale it is possible for any bird with a chronic disease process to present in this way. In particular, birds with protein-losing conditions (enteritis, nephropathy, peritonitis), abnormal hepatic function (hepatic lipidosis, iron storage disease) and subacute to chronic infective processes (mycobacteriosis, yersiniosis, salmonellosis, parasites) are likely to present with loss of weight or, more importantly, of body condition and muscle mass (ascites would be an important adjunctive clinical finding in several of these conditions).

The general work-up of a sick passerine bird is described fully in Chapter 34 and should be considered in every case. Figure 35.1 lists differentials and features of some common diseases that can present with weight loss as the only or predominant presenting sign.

Disease	Cause	Species affected	Predisposing factors	Notes
Aspergillosis	*Aspergillus* spp. (occasionally other fungi cause similar disease)	Any, but particularly mynahs, ramphastids, corvids, recently captured wild birds	Stress Humid or dusty environments	
Mycobacteriosis	*Mycobacterium avium*; other mycobacteria	Any, but Red-hooded Siskins may be particularly susceptible	Stress Exposure to organism	Often no gross tubercles at post-mortem examination; microscopic granulomas in intestinal wall or lungs
Candidiasis	*Candida albicans*	Any	Usually secondary to other stressors or disease	Thickening and inflammation of upper GI tract; usually associated with regurgitation
Trichomoniasis	*Trichomonas* spp. of flagellate protozoa	Any	Housing with or near infected pigeons or budgerigars; open-topped aviaries	Regurgitation usually obvious
Iron storage disease	Excessive uptake of dietary iron	Mynahs, toucans, touracos	Stress factors High iron dietary components	Ascites usually obvious
Acanthocephalans, cestode infections	Various tapeworm or acanthocephalan species	Any		Require invertebrate intermediate hosts so generally only seen in wild-caught birds; often asymptomatic
Nematode infections	*Ascaridia* spp; *Porrocaecum* spp; *Capillaria* spp.	Earthworm-eating species (*Porrocaecum*) Any (*Ascaridia / Capillaria*)	*Ascaridia* and *Capillaria* have direct life cycles (though earthworms may act as paratenic hosts) *Porrocaecum* needs earthworms as intermediate hosts Earthworms may be present in earth-floored aviaries or may be fed as live food	Earthworm control as well as direct medication of infested birds will be needed
Salmonellosis and pseudotuberculosis	Various species of *Salmonella* and *Yersinia*	Any	Rodent or wild bird contamination of feed	More usually present as acute or subacute illness, often death with no weight loss.

35.1 Diseases of passerine birds that can present with weight loss as the sole or predominant sign.

Although some individual birds presented by fanciers as going light will have some of the above conditions, there are two groups that are particularly a concern for fanciers and breeders as they potentially affect several birds in a collection: *Macrorhabdus ornithogaster* yeast infection (previously known as megabacteriosis); and the coccidiosis/atoxoplasmosis group. Unfortunately, as well as the presenting sign of wasting, the two conditions are linked by both confusion over nomenclature and difficulties over effective therapy, making 'going light' a frustrating syndrome to diagnose and treat.

Macrorhabdus ornithogaster

So-called megabacteriosis has now been identified not as a bacterial condition but as a proventricular/ventricular disease (PVD) condition associated with infection with the yeast *Macrorhabdus ornithogaster*. PVD associated with *Macrorhabdus* has been reported in a variety of species, including canaries, Gouldian Finch, Zebra Finch and European Goldfinch (Herck *et al.*, 1984; Filippich, 1994).

The exact relationship between the organism and PVD is not well established. The organism is present in many asymptomatic birds, including wild European fringillid finches, and may be a normal commensal inhabitant of the gastrointestinal tract (one study of Goldfinches captured in the wild in Australia showed 60% to be positive for the organism) (Herck *et al.*, 1984; Pennycott *et al.*, 1998). The possibility remains that the yeast is simply an opportunist invader of an already compromised proventricular environment, and this is supported by the finding that some *Macrorhabdus*-negative birds remain negative even when housed in the long term with positive conspecifics (Filippich, 1992). Birds with PVD often have an elevated proventricular pH, with associated softening of the koilin layer of the ventriculus. *Macrorhabdus* organisms are often found in the proventricular glands of such cases, but the question of whether they cause the pH alteration or take advantage of it has not been adequately answered (although *Macrorhabdus* can also be found in birds with normal proventricular pH). Clinically, PVD-affected birds sometimes, but not invariably, show a lymphoplasmacytic enteritis, though this is not specifically associated with the locality of yeast organisms, which are found only in the lumen and do not invade the mucosal epithelium (Greenacre *et al.*, 2000; Filippich, 1994). However, the facts that the majority of birds with PVD can be confirmed to be infected with large numbers of *Macrorhabdus* and that some birds clinically improve after treatment with amphotericin B suggest that the organism is indeed playing a pathological role.

Clinical signs and diagnosis

In passerine cases, weight loss is the predominant clinical sign. Birds have both a decreased appetite (they will often exhibit 'sham eating' behaviour, sitting by the food bowl picking up seeds but not swallowing them) and also a decreased ability to digest food (droppings may become voluminous and contain pieces of undigested seeds).

Diagnosis of *Macrorhabdus*-associated PVD is by microscopic demonstration of the organisms on a faecal (live) or proventricular (post-mortem) smear (Figure 35.2). If present in high numbers, the organisms can be seen simply on a wet mount specimen, but they are far more readily demonstrated using cytology stains. They stain positive with both Gram's and periodic acid–Schiff staining techniques. Even severely affected birds may shed the organism only intermittently in the faeces and so 'false negative' results are possible with this technique.

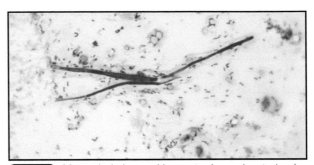

35.2 *Macrorhabdus ornithogaster* (megabacterium) in a proventricular smear. Gram stain.

The yeasts form large 'rod' organisms of variable length but noticeably larger (20–200 μm in length) than surrounding bacteria (common bacteria being 2–6 μm in length) and often form parallel bundles.

Treatment

Treatment of individual passerine birds with *Macrorhabdus*-associated PVD is usually unrewarding, though there are reports of successful use of nystatin in Goldfinches. Although amphotericin B is widely regarded as more effective against *Macrorhabdus* than nystatin, published data on its use in passerine birds is lacking and in any case oral amphotericin B suspension (Fungilin®, Squibb) has recently become unavailable in the UK (though may still be available as a human medication elsewhere). In severely affected flocks the disease may to some extent be suppressed by intermittent use of in-water amphotericin B, but there can be regulatory problems (in the UK) with this approach as the most useful formulation (Megabac-S, Vetafarm, Australia) has to be imported under authorization from the Veterinary Medicines Directorate on an individual case basis.

Coccidial diseases

A variety of coccidial parasite species affect passerine birds, including species of *Dorisella*, *Eimeria* and *Wenyonella*, but most importantly a range of morphologically similar *Isospora* species. The exact classification is a matter of debate. Canaries are hosts to the intestinal coccidian parasite *Isospora canaria*. Other species of passerine bird host intestinal *Isospora* organisms referred to as *Isospora lacazei*, but current morphological evidence suggests that this is a group of many (over 50 have been described) probably host-specific *Isospora* species, and that some passerine species host more than one *Isospora*: sparrows in

Normandy, for example, have at least 12 (Grulet *et al.*, 1982). Finally there is much debate over the status of 'atoxoplasma'. Once grouped along with a parasite of amphibians as *Lankesterella*, the organism was then classified as *Isospora* and later reclassified as avian *Toxoplasma* and *Atoxoplasma*; current molecular and morphological work replaces it as *Isospora serini*, despite a marked difference in life cycle from the intestinal species (Barta *et al.*, 2005). A further complication is that although earlier work suggested possible cross-infection of sparrow and canary 'atoxoplasma' infections, current work suggests that the systemic *Isospora* species are again host specific.

To summarize: there are therefore two important, clinically distinct coccidial syndromes in passerine birds, intestinal coccidiosis and systemic coccidiosis ('atoxoplasmosis'), with similar characteristics in different hosts although probably caused by host-specific *Isospora* species.

Intestinal coccidiosis

Life cycle

Isospora canaria has a conventional coccidian life cycle (presumably the other intestinal *Isospora* species in other hosts are similar). All of the endogenous stages take place within the epithelium of the small intestine: there are three asexual generations (shizogony) and a sexual generation (gametogony) described in the duodenal epithelium. Oocysts are shed in the faeces and sporulate outside the host after a period of several days, the actual time varying depending on environmental temperature and humidity (Box, 1975). The prepatent period is 4–5 days for *I. canaria* and patency lasts for 10–13 days. The life cycle is direct, with transmission via the faeco-oral route (Figure 35.3).

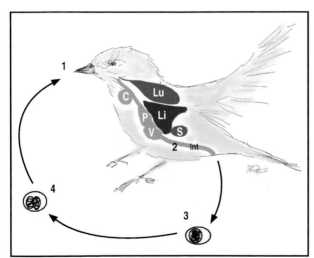

35.3 The life cycle of a passerine intestinal coccidian species, such as *Isospora canaria*. (1) Infective oocysts are ingested. (2) Three asexual generations and one sexual reproductive generation occur in the duodenal epithelium. (3) Unsporulated oocysts appear in the faeces 4–5 days after infection and continue to be shed for 13 days. (4) After several days outside the host the oocysts sporulate and are then infective. (C = crop; P = proventriculus; V = ventriculus; Lu = lung; Li = liver; S = spleen; Int = intestine).

Pathology

Clinical effects are worst in youngsters soon after weaning. Clinical infection is probably related largely to captive husbandry and hygiene factors, as wild fringillid finches have been found to be infected, presumably incidentally (Pennycott *et al.*, 1998). In canaries, fledglings of 8 weeks of age onwards are affected. Inflammatory response to the parasites causes oedema and haemorrhage in the duodenal wall and the associated malabsorption leads to diarrhoea (sometimes haemorrhagic), emaciation and death.

Diagnosis

Large numbers of unsporulated oocysts can be seen in fresh faecal smears (Figure 35.4) but accurate identification of species involved may require both sporulation of the oocysts and careful morphological examination and measurement. The length to width ratio of *I. canaria* oocysts is 1.13, compared with 1.05 for *I. serini* (Box, 1975). At post-mortem examination, oocysts may be present in intestinal content and cytology of scrapings of duodenal mucosa will reveal parasitic trophozoites. Those of *I. canaria* sit within the cell between the nucleus and the basement membrane, whereas those of *I. serini* are found on the luminal side of the nucleus (Box, 1977).

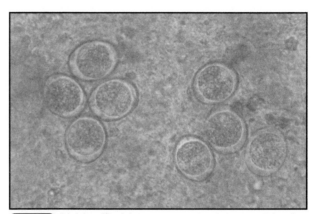

35.4 Unidentified *Isospora* oocysts in an unstained faecal smear.

Treatment

A variety of standard treatments for coccidiosis in poultry or pigeons can be used to treat or prevent intestinal coccidiosis in passerine bird colonies. Protocols of particular use include in-water medication with amprolium at 50–100 mg/l for 5 days or longer, toltrazuril at 75 mg/l on 2 days a week for 4 weeks, or sulfachlorpyridazine at 150–300 mg/l on 5 days a week for 2–3 weeks. Intestinal coccidiosis is less likely to be seen in individual pet birds, but where the above medications are not available, or where the bird's illness makes water intake unpredictable, oral dosing using trimethoprim/sulphonamide combinations may have some suppressant effect on the infestation.

Systemic coccidiosis (atoxoplasmosis)

Passerine host species commonly affected by systemic coccidiosis include canaries and other finches, notably Siskins, Goldfinches, Greenfinches and Bullfinches, along with Grosbeaks, Starlings and Mynahs (Anwar, 1966; Ball *et al.*, 1988; Cooper *et al.*, 1989; McNamee *et al.*, 1995; Giacomo *et al.*, 1997).

Life cycle

Despite early work suggesting that atoxoplasmosis is spread via blood-sucking parasites, current evidence suggests a faeco-oral infection route (Figure 35.5). Once sporulated oocysts are ingested, the sporocysts enter the bloodstream via the small intestinal wall where they are ingested by mononuclear phagocytes. During the course of five asexual reproduction cycles (schizogony) the infected phagocytes become distributed throughout the body, particularly the liver and spleen, which both become severely swollen. The organism then returns to intestinal epithelial sites (possibly after being coughed up from the lungs and swallowed) for a further two shizogony cycles before completing a sexual (gametogony) phase and passing in the faeces as oocysts before finally undergoing sporogony outside the host. The prepatent period is 9–10 days and patency can persist for several months (Box, 1977). Because of the widespread dissemination of the systemic stages of the organism and the longevity of avian macrophages, infection and shedding can be prolonged.

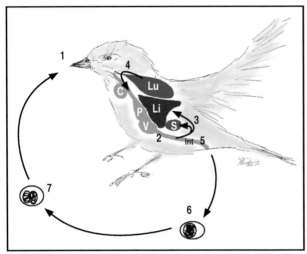

35.5 The life cycle of a passerine systemic coccidian species such as *Isospora serini* ('atoxoplasma'). (1) Infective oocysts are ingested. (2) Sporocysts cross the small intestine wall and enter circulating phagocytes. (3) Infected phagocytes spread through the body, particularly to the liver and spleen. Five asexual reproduction cycles take place. (4) The organism returns to the intestinal epithelium, probably through being coughed up and swallowed. (5) Two further asexual and one sexual generations occur in the intestinal epithelium. (6) Unsporulated oocysts begin to be shed in faeces 9–10 days after initial infection. (7) After several days sporulation occurs and the oocysts are now infective. (C = crop; P = proventriculus; V = ventriculus; Lu = lung; Li = liver; S = spleen; Int = intestine).

Pathology

'Atoxoplasmosis' affects young canaries, usually between 2 and 9 months of age. Clinically birds present generally 'fluffed' with severe debilitation, emaciation, sometimes diarrhoea or neurological

signs, and eventually death. Within an infected colony up to 80% of chicks may become affected and die, sometimes without showing marked pre-mortem abnormalities. As with *I. canaria*, *I. serini* causes oedema and inflammation of the duodenum but also severe swelling of the liver (which is sometimes mottled due to necrosis) and spleen (which is usually dark red). The hepatic enlargement is such that the liver can be clearly seen through the skin, projecting well beyond the sternum as a blue or black structure, giving rise to common names of 'black spot disease' and 'thick liver disease'. Myocardium and skeletal muscle may also be damaged. Cytology and histopathology reveal granulomatous and lympho-histiocytic inflammation of the myocardium, intestine, spleen and liver.

Diagnosis

Microscopically parasites can be found as inclusions in the cytoplasm of monocytes and macrophages either in smears of liver, spleen or lungs or sometimes in buffy coat smears of a blood sample from a live bird. The nucleus of the host leucocyte is indented to a crescent shape by the parasite, which stains pink with Romanowsky-type stains such as Giemsa or Diff-Quik. Shedding levels in intestinal content or faeces are low (100–200 per 24 hours) and so faecal microscopy is not a reliable way of confirming a diagnosis; in any case faecal oocysts cannot readily be differentiated from intestinal *Isospora* species, except for a few hosts such as Bali Mynahs where intestinal coccidians are rare (Norton *et al.*, 2003). PCR testing methods are now available in some countries to increase test sensitivity, particularly when testing asymptomatic birds.

Treatment

Intracellular stages are not generally responsive to treatment (though primaquine may have some suppressant effect (Greiner and Ritchie, 1994)) and so clinical recovery of severely affected birds is poor. Intestinal stages, and therefore oocyst shedding, can be suppressed by the use of sulpha drugs, particularly sulfachlorpyridazine at 150–300 mg/l drinking water on 5 days a week for several months (usually until the bird is completely moulted). Other anticoccidials may also suppress faecal shedding and have been suggested as routine pre-breeding and post-weaning treatments to reduce shedding from asymptomatic parent stock and transfer between infected youngsters. Other treatment measures include general nutritional support (the use of soft foods to improve digestion and absorption within the inflamed upper gastro-intestinal tract) and general hygiene measures (cleanliness, particularly of cage floors and bathing/drinking water).

General recommendations

Figures 35.6 and 35.7 recommend logical approaches to the investigation of individual or flock cases of 'going light'.

Step	Notes
History taking and full clinical examination	To rule out other illnesses, particularly noting ascites, abnormal masses, urate output
Faecal wet preparation microscopy (faecal portion of a dropping mixed with 1 drop saline)	Particularly looking for coccidial oocysts as well as helminth ova or *Giardia*
Faecal cytology (remove cover slip from sample above, allow to dry and stain with Gram's or other cytology stain)	Particularly looking for *Macrorhabdus ornithogaster*, but also assess relative proportions of bacteria and yeasts in the faeces
Blood sample	Depending on patient size, test availability and finances tests carried out could vary from simple smear examination from one drop of blood for intra-phagocyte coccidial parasites as well as approximation of absolute and differential white blood cell counts, through to full haematology, biochemistry and PCR testing for *Isospora serini*

Where no specific diagnosis has been reached during the above evaluation protocol, it may be necessary to start a broad-spectrum treatment approach using trimethoprim/sulpha combinations (in case of systemic bacterial disease but also providing some suppression of coccidial activity) along with amphotericin B (or if not available, nystatin) in an attempt to suppress *Macrorhabdus*. General supportive therapy should also be instituted, possibly including fluid therapy and nutritional support

35.6 Recommended diagnostic steps for individual birds 'going light'.

Step	Notes
History taking and husbandry evaluation	For large colonies a site visit is recommended
Examination where possible of both live affected birds and recently dead birds	
Faecal flotation on a large pooled faeces sample	Looking for helminth ova and particularly coccidial oocysts
Multiple Gram-stained faecal smears from affected and contact birds	Looking for *Macrorhabdus ornithogaster*
Post-mortem examination of recently dead or sacrificed birds	Particularly looking at cytological features of proventricular and intestinal contents and mucosa, where necessary followed by histopathological evaluation of proventriculus, intestine, spleen, liver, lungs and other organs
Where no definite diagnosis has been reached consider PCR testing	Blood samples from affected and in-contact birds and spleen, liver or lung samples taken during post-mortem examination

35.7 Recommended diagnostic steps for a flock outbreak of several birds 'going light'.

References and further reading

Anwar M (1966) *Isospora lacazei* (Labbe, 1893) and *I. chloridis* sp. n. (Protozoa: Eimeriidae) from the English sparrow (*Passer domesticus*), greenfinch (*Chloris chloris*) and chaffinch (*Fringilla coelebs*). *Journal of Protozoology* **13**(1), 84–90

Ball SJ, Brown MA, Daszak P *et al.* (1988) Atoxoplasma (Apicomplexa: Eimeriorina: Atoxoplasmatidae) in the greenfinch (*Carduelis chloris*). *Journal of Parasitology* **84**(4), 813–817

Barta JR, Schrenzel MD, Carreno R *et al.* (2005) The genus *Atoxoplasma* (Garnham 1950) as a junior objective synonym of the genus *Isospora* (Schneider 1881) species infecting birds and resurrection of *Cystoisospora* (Frenkel 1977) as the correct genus for *Isospora* species infecting mammals. *Journal of Parasitology* **91**(3), 726–727

Box ED (1975) Exogenous stages of *Isospora serini* (Aragao) and *Isospora canaria* sp. n. in the canary (*Serinus canarius* Linnaeus). *Journal of Protozoology* **22**(2), 165–169

Box ED (1977) Life cycles of two isospora species in the canary, *Serinus canarius* Linnaeus. *Journal of Protozoology* **24**(1), 57–67

Cooper JE, Gschmeissner S and Greenwood AG (1989) Atoxoplasma in greenfinches (*Carduelis chloris*) as a possible cause of 'going light'. *Veterinary Record* **124**(13), 343–344

Filippich LJ (1992) Megabacteria and proventricular disease in birds. In: *Proceedings of the Australian Association of Avian Veterinarians*, pp. 1–12

Filippich LJ (1994) Megabacteria and proventricular/ventricular disease in psittacines and passerines. In: *Proceedings of the Annual Conference of the Association of Avian Veterinarians*, pp. 287–293

Giacomo R, Stefania P, Ennio T *et al.* (1997) Mortality in black siskins (*Carduelis atrata*) with systemic coccidiosis. *Journal of Wildlife Diseases* **33**(1), 152–157

Greenacre CB, Wilson GH and Graham JE (2000) The many faces of megabacterium. In: *Proceedings of the Association of Avian Veterinarians*, pp. 193–196

Griener EC and Ritchie BW (1994) Parasites. In: *Avian Medicine, Principles and Application*, ed. BW Ritchie, GJ Harrison and LR Harrison, pp. 1007–1029. Wingers, Lake Worth, Florida

Grulet O, Landau I and Baccam D (1982) Les *Isospora* du moineau domestique; multiplicité des espèces. *Annales de Parasitologie Humaine et Comparée* **57**(3), 209–235

Herck H, van Duyser T, Zwart P *et al.* (1984) A bacterial proventriculitis in canaries (*Serinus canaria*). *Avian Pathology* **13**(3), 561–572

McNamee P, Pennycott T and McConnell S (1995) Clinical and pathological changes associated with atoxoplasma in a captive bullfinch (*Pyrrhula pyrrhula*). *Veterinary Record* **136**(9), 221–222

Norton TM, Neiffer DL, Seibels R *et al.* (2003) Atoxoplasma medical protocols recommended by the passerine atoxoplasma working group. *Atoxoplasma workshop; Eastern Regional American Zoological Association*. Available online: http://www.riverbanks.org/subsite/aig/Atoxo-recommendations.htm (accessed 28 May 2007)

Pennycott TW, Ross HM, McLaren IM *et al.* (1998) Causes of death of wild birds of the family Fringillidae in Britain. *Veterinary Record* **143**(6), 155–158

36

Passerine birds: investigation of flock mortality/morbidity

Kevin Eatwell

Clinical approach to flock mortality/morbidity

Clinical history

Given the wide range of passerine species, having suitable reference texts available to allow an assessment of appropriate husbandry techniques is essential. Figure 36.1 provides a checklist of appropriate questions when taking a history and notes the potential significance of the answers given.

Examination of the environment

Site visit

If possible, a site visit to make a direct assessment of the birds' environment and husbandry should be arranged. If this is not possible, some photographs or videos of the set-up at home will help to get a feel for how the birds are kept. It is important to stress to the owner that the environment should be in a typical state, as many individuals make everything spotless before a veterinary visit.

Points worth checking are the size of the enclosure, hygiene levels, substrate, perch design, breeding facilities, and food and water provision (see Chapter 4). The source of the water may also be an important factor, as it will affect the bacterial load and likelihood of contamination (e.g. heavy metals). Any evidence of vermin should be noted. Natural plants should be identified in case any of them are toxic (plants that have been reported as potentially toxic include azalea, avocado, buttercup, cherry, clematis,

Clinical history questions	Significance
• Numbers and species of birds owned? • Numbers and species of birds ill?	May suggest that only certain susceptible species are affected and gives indication of percentage of birds falling ill
• Clinical signs?	Will help to create shortlist of potential conditions
• Age spread of ill birds?	Some agents (e.g. polyomavirus) may lead to high mortality in juveniles
• Death rate and timing (overnight *versus* over a few days)?	Sudden mass mortality would suggest a husbandry or toxic event. A more chronic history would suggest an endemic disease
• Normal diet offered? • Supplementation types and amounts? • Any additional food sources? • Any novel food given or change in diet?	Passerines have a high metabolic rate and presenting correct diet appropriately is important: one day of dietary change could lead to mortality due to starvation
• Water provision, including drinker type and position?	Water needs to be accessible all the time
• Supplemental lighting and heating offered?	Passerines need to feed for longer hours than the natural photoperiod and to be kept warmer during winter months in cooler climates
• Any possibility of vermin?	Can transmit pseudotuberculosis
• Any nesting sites provided and breeding attempts noticed?	Competition for nesting sites can lead to trauma. Viruses such as polyomavirus are more prevalent in a breeding population
• Any new additions (numbers and species)? • When was the last bird added to the collection? • Any contact with other birds (birds on holiday or on loan)? • Any exhibitions attended? • Any contact with wild birds?	May identify if there is any correlation between mortality and introduction of carrier birds, or transmission of disease due to mixing of birds between collections
• Any medications already given, and dose? • Any vaccines administered?	Many fanciers will have already treated their birds; this may lead to false-negative results when performing faecal analysis, cultures or PCR testing. Drug toxicity also a possibility (e.g. dimetridazole)
• Aviary layout and routine?	May suggest route of transmission of diseasse

36.1 Checklist of clinical history questions and potential significance.

iris, ivy, lily-of-the-valley, lobelia, mistletoe, laurel, oleander, parsley, privet, rhododendron, rhubarb, virginia creeper, wisteria and yew).

A site visit also gives the opportunity for calm observation of the general activity of all birds in the collection and subtle signs of ill health may be detected during this time. Sick birds should be isolated and examined further.

Practice visits

Financial limitations may prevent a site visit. Faecal material from the birds' boxes or cages can be obtained and examined. The nature of the container may indicate the level of care at home. Samples of food and water may be required and can be assessed for their suitability.

If there is poor reproductive performance, eggs and chicks may be presented for examination. Dead birds should be subjected to a full post-mortem examination (see Chapter 9).

Clinical examination

In the group situation close individual observation by the owner may not be possible and many birds, given their high metabolic rate, will simply be found dead after a short period of being 'fluffed'. Some birds may be presented alive but in a critical condition.

A decision has to be made regarding the economics of trying to save the individual bird (and the likelihood of success) or instead considering whether to euthanase the bird and perform a full post-mortem examination immediately. In most situations of group or flock mortality the latter is to be preferred and is the approach taken in this chapter. The approach to an individual sick bird (which may well be suffering from an infectious disease or group illness) is given in Chapter 34 and clinical examination is covered in detail in Chapter 7.

Common conditions encountered are shown in Figure 36.2 and discussed in Figure 36.3. Differentials to consider based on clinical signs are listed in Figure 36.4.

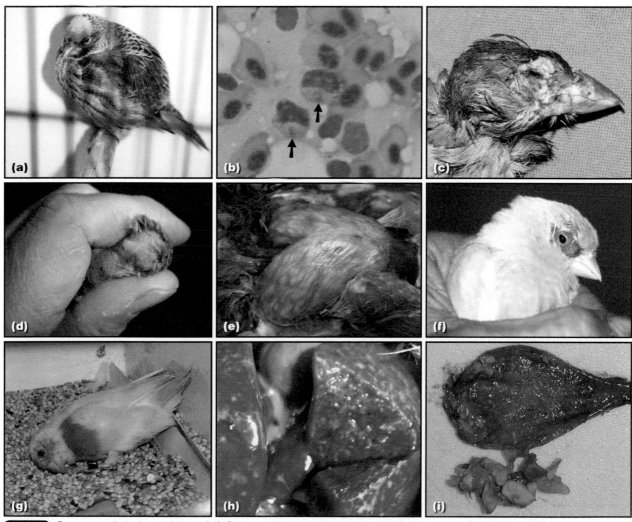

36.2 Common clinical conditions. **(a)** Canary with atoxoplasmosis, showing non-specific 'fluffing'. **(b)** 'Atoxoplasma' inclusions (arrowed) within the leucocytes on a blood smear. **(c)** House sparrow affected with avian poxvirus (dry pox).**(d)** Zebra Finch with feather loss over the crown. This bird was housed with larger, more aggressive, Java Sparrows. **(e)** Leucocytozoonosis in an Orange-headed Thrush (note striping of muscle). **(f)** Sinusitis in a canary. This presentation could be due to a variety of pathogens, including *Mycoplasma* spp. **(g)** Mutation Gouldian Finch with PMV-III infection. **(h)** Pseudotuberculosis (*Yersinia pseudotuberculosis*) in post-mortem image of liver. **(i)** Gross pathology of a crop from a Greenfinch showing caseated lesions of trichomoniasis. (a,b,g, courtesy of Alistair Lawrie; c, © Michael Lierz; e, © John Chitty; i, courtesy of B. Lawson/Zoological Society of London)

Condition	Clinical signs	Suggested diagnostics	Notes
Atoxoplasmosis ** (*Isospora serini*) 'thick liver disease'	Sudden deaths, diarrhoea, neurological signs, red vent, swollen liver, emaciation	Haematology of buffy coat for inclusions (see Figure 36.2b). Post-mortem examination: hepatosplenomegaly, oedematous duodenum. Histopathology and cytology of liver, spleen and lungs: parasites found in leucocyte cytoplasm	Young birds in first year of life mortality up to 80%, particularly canaries, European finches and Bali Mynahs. Transmission by faeco–oral route (see Chapter 35)
Avian pox *** (starling pox, sparrow pox, juncopox, mynahpox, canary pox)	Cutaneous form (dry pox): crusting lesions on eyes, beak (see Figure 36.2c), wing webs, legs and toes; erosions and ulcerations, depigmentation when area heals. Diphtheroid form (wet pox): lesions on tongue and pharynx, dysphagia and dyspnoea. Septicaemic form: severe dyspnoea, cyanosis and depression, most common form presented in passerines	Post-mortem examination: diphtheritic lesions and exudates within respiratory tract (wet pox). Histopathology to confirm Bollinger bodies within epithelial cells. PCR test of residue	Endemic problem in canaries and fringillid finches; also found in mynahs. Can lead to 100% mortality in canaries due to development of septicaemic form. Usually after introduction of new latently infected bird to naive population. Transmission by ectoparasites or due to skin trauma. Incubation period up to 4 weeks. Vaccination possible with attenuated live vaccine, every 6 months starting when the young fledge. Vaccinate in wing web (not licensed within UK). Usually immune to infection within 14 days.
Campylobacteriosis *** (*Campylobacter* spp.)	Yellow droppings, high nestling mortality, ill birds	Post-mortem examination: intestinal tract filled with yellow contents. Cytology and culture of organism	Bengalese Finches can be carriers. Improve hygiene to reduce incidence rates
Chlamydophila **	Dyspnoea, nasal discharge, conjunctivitis, diarrhoea, ill birds	Post-mortem examination. Impression smears of liver and spleen, Macchiavello or Giemsa stain. PCR of tissues	Usually transmitted from infected psittacines, waterfowl or wild birds
Coccidiosis *** (*Isospora* spp.)	Diarrhoea, distended abdomen and emaciation, sudden death	Faecal examination for parasites	Common in canaries
Cochlosomosis ** (*Cochlosoma* spp.)	Mild diarrhoea in adult finches, ill nestlings, poor feathering, yellow droppings, passing whole seeds	Post-mortem examination: yellowing and shrivelled appearance. Histopathology of intestinal wall. Examination of wet preparation of fresh faeces for flagellates	Usually death of fostered Australian finch chicks being raised by Bengalese Finches. Also occurs in mixed aviaries
Endoparasitic infections *** (e.g. *Capillaria* spp.)	Diarrhoea, ill birds, emaciation	Post-mortem examination: creamy plaques throughout upper digestive tract, thickened bowel loops. Cytology. Faecal examination for ova	
Feather lice **	Irritation, restlessness, feather plucking if severe	Lice visible on feathers with human eye. Cytology can be used for confirmation	Common in canaries, more typically on debilitated birds
Feather plucking (behavioural) ***	Feather loss over back of head (see Figure 36.2d) and rump most typical. Usually inflicted by another bird	Rule out other causes and based on clinical history	Common in certain species of imported passerines (e.g. Lavender Finches) and also in breeding groups
Gapeworm *** (*Syngamus trachea*)	Gasping, wheezing, coughing, sneezing, head shaking	Transillumination or endoscopic examination of trachea if species large enough to examine safely. Faecal examination for typical eggs. Post-mortem examination: red adult worms within trachea and bronchi	Commonly found in both wild and captive birds, in particular, European Starling, mynahs and corvids. An essential aspect is invertebrate intermediate hosts required for parasite transmission
Leucocytozoonosis * (*Leucocytozoon* spp.)	High nesting mortality, anorexia, anaemia	Blood smear: parasites within leucocytes. Post-mortem examination (see Figure 36.2e): hepatosplenomegaly. Impression smears of viscera	Requires high density of insect vectors
Macrorhabdus ornithogaster *** (megabacteriosis, avian gastric yeast)	Passing whole seeds, ill birds, regurgitation, emaciation	Post-mortem examination: enlarged proventriculus with thick mucous layer, ulceration and haemorrhages possible. Cytology of proventriculus (see Chapter 35). May also be identified on faecal examination. Large, variable staining rods	Common in canaries, estrildid finches and reported in wild finches (Gentz, 2003). Amphotericin B usual recommended treatment but nystatin has been effective in Goldfinches (Gerlach, 2001)

36.3 Common clinical conditions of passerine birds. (*** = commonly found; ** = occasionally seen; * = rarely presented) (continues) ▶

Condition	Clinical signs	Suggested diagnostics	Notes
Mycobacteriosis (*Mycobacterium avium, avium-intracellulare* or *genavense*) *	Ill birds, diarrhoea, weight loss, sudden death	Post-mortem examination unrewarding, classical tubercles often not present in passerines. Cytology of impression smears of liver and intestine	Requires acid-fast staining. Starlings and sparrows more susceptible
Mycoplasmosis *** (*Mycoplasma* spp.)	Conjunctivitis, sinusitis (see Figure 36.2f), sneezing, nasal discharge, starvation due to blindness	Post-mortem examination. Histopathology and cytology of lesions. Response to appropriate therapy, e.g. tylosin	Outbreaks in wild finches reported with *Mycoplasma gallisepticum*
Papillomavirus *	Skin nodules on feet and legs	Histopathology of lesions	Found in wild Chaffinches and Bramblings. Highly host-specific and unlikely to be encountered in other species but has been reported in canaries
Paramyxovirus **	PMV-1: diarrhoea, dyspnoea. PMV-2: Upper respiratory tract disease PMV-3: torticollis (see Figure 36.2g), dyspnoea, conjunctivitis, yellowish diarrhoea	Post-mortem examination usually unremarkable. Histopathology: pancreatitis, encephalitis, myocarditis with inclusion bodies. Virus isolation and serology	PMV-3 is most common serotype to infect passerines. Common in Estrildidae. Incubation period up to 6 weeks
Polyomavirus *	High nestling mortality, skin lesions, poor feather development, abdominal haemorrhages, beak deformities	Post-mortem examination: hepatosplenomegaly, internal haemorrhages. Histopathology: intranuclear inclusion bodies, liver and spleen necrosis	Can also affect older birds. Vaccination possible in America. Stopping breeding along with environmental hygiene can stem flow of outbreaks
Pseudo-tuberculosis *** (*Yersinia pseudotuberculosis*)	Sudden deaths, debility, emaciation, diarrhoea, respiratory signs	Clinical history: most infections over winter. Post-mortem examination (see Figure 36.2h): hepatosplenomegaly with abscessation throughout organs. Histopathology, cytology. Culture of the organism: ideally use selective *Yersinia* CIN medium and cold enrichment; will also grow on blood agar	Can lead to high mortality. Transmitted by rodents: eliminate these from environment; prevent contamination of food and water; vigorous attention to hygiene. Feral birds can infect captive populations
Red mite ** (*Dermanyssus gallinae*)	Pruritis, pale mucous membranes, respiratory distress, depression	Environmental assessment: mites are motile and live off host; photophobic and can be found in crevices between perches and cage or in nest boxes. Can live in environment for months. Cytology and visual inspection	Common – most significant parasite found. Usually only a problem in birds housed intensively. Attention to environmental control is as important as treating the birds
Scaly face mites ** (*Cnemidocoptes pilae*) 'Tassle foot'	Scaly crusts over feet, eyes and beak, pruritus, depigmentation	Cytology of lesions in 10% KOH for characteristic mites	Treatment of birds alone is sufficient
Septicaemia due to salmonellosis, colibacillosis, pasteurellosis and other Gram-negative infections ***	Matted feathering around face and head, regurgitation, dysphagia, dyspnoea, diarrhoea, nestling mortality, rhinitis, conjunctivitis	Post-mortem examination: yellow nodules throughout gastrointestinal tract, liver and spleen. Crop wash cytology (stain for Gram-negative rods and inflammatory response), culture and histopathology	Contact birds likely to be infected. Common finding in wild UK finches – must be differentiated from trichomoniasis. Vigorous hygiene to reduce reinfection rates. Can be secondary to other immunosuppresive infections, such as polyomavirus
Starvation **		History: birds found dead in morning following cold night in winter. May well be adequate food and water sources available. Post-mortem examination confirming empty gastrointestinal tract	Prolonged adverse weather possible in wild birds. In captive birds, due to low temperatures and prolonged periods of darkness
Toxicoses *	Respiratory signs	Clinical history of exposure. Carbon monoxide: minimal post-mortem signs. PTFE: red or haemorrhagic lungs	Other examples: carpet freshener, glues, paints, smoke
	Neurological signs	Nitroimidazole toxicity (e.g. metronidazole): irreversible neurological signs. CNS histopathology	Other examples: heavy metals, ethanol (rotting fruit)
	Anorexia, diarrhoea, ataxia, tremors, seizures	Organophosphorus toxicity: cholinesterase activity reduced on blood sample	Commonly used routinely for environmental parasite control
	Gastrointestinal signs	Avocado toxicity, toxic plants	

36.3 (continued) Common clinical conditions of passerine birds. (*** = commonly found; ** = occasionally seen; * = rarely presented) (continues) ▶

Condition	Clinical signs	Suggested diagnostics	Notes
Toxoplasmosis *	Dyspnoea, blindness, ataxia, torticollis	Post-mortem examination: severe hepatosplenomegaly and pneumonia. Histopathology and cytology of tissues	Transmitted by cat faeces. Common in canaries. Usually asymptomatic
Tracheal mites *** (*Sternostoma tracheacolum*)	Dyspnoea, nasal discharge, change in voice, head shaking, wheezing, gasping, excessive beak wiping, loss of condition	Endoscopy to visualize parasites in species large enough to examine safely. Transillumination of trachea. Eggs in faeces (must be differentiated from *Dermanysuss* spp.). Post-mortem examination: identify black mites. Microscopic examination (see Figure 36.5)	Common finding in passerines, particularly Gouldian Finches and canaries. Transmission from parents when feeding young. Treat parental stock prior to breeding or use resistant species to foster chicks
Trichomoniasis *** (*Trichomonas gallinae*)	Regurgitation, respiratory signs, nasal discharge, emaciation, salivation, dysphagia	Post-mortem examination: thickened crop wall (see Figure 36.2i) and oesophagus, yellow nodules throughout upper gastrointestinal tract. Crop wash cytology for motile organisms	In-contact birds likely to be infected. Epidemic proportions in wild UK finches at the time of writing (Cunningham *et al.*, 2005; Pennycott *et al.*, 2005; Holmes and Duff, 2005)

36.3   (continued) Common clinical conditions of passerine birds. (*** = commonly found; ** = occasionally seen; * = rarely presented)

Main clinical sign	Differentials	Other clinical signs
Dyspnoea	Tracheal mites	Change in voice, head shaking, beak wiping, emaciation
	Gapeworm	Coughing, sneezing, head shaking
	Avian pox (wet pox)	Lesions on tongue and pharynx, cyanosis, depression
	Trichomoniasis	Nasal discharge, emaciation, salivation, dysphagia
	Chlamydophilosis	Nasal discharge, conjunctivitis, diarrhoea, ill birds
	Red mites	Pruritis, pale mucous membranes, depression
	Paramyxovirus infection	PMV-1 diarrhoea PMV-3 torticollis, conjunctivitis, yellowish diarrhoea
	Toxoplasmosis	Blindness, ataxia, torticollis
	Gram-negative septicaemia	Diarrhoea, nestling mortality
	Toxicosis	CO, PTFE, carpet freshener, glues, paints, smoke
Diarrhoea (unusual presenting clinical sign, may well represent polyuria instead)	Campylobacteriosis	High nestling mortality, ill birds
	Endoparasitic infections	Ill birds, emaciation
	Coccidiosis	Distended abdomen and emaciation, sudden death
	Macrorhabdus ornithogaster	Passing whole seeds, ill birds, regurgitation, emaciation
	Cochlosomosis	Mild in adults, ill nestlings, poor feathering
	Chlamydophilosis	Nasal discharge, conjunctivitis, dyspnoea, ill birds
	Toxicosis	Avocado toxicity, toxic plants
	Pseudotuberculosis	Debility, emaciation, respiratory signs
	Paramyxovirus infection	PMV-1 dyspnoea PMV-3 torticollis, dyspnoea, conjunctivitis
	Avian pox (dry and wet pox)	Crusting lesions on skin and mucous membranes
	Mycobacteriosis	Ill birds, weight loss, sudden death
	Septicaemia	Nestling mortality, rhinitis, conjunctivitis
	Atoxoplasmosis	Neurological signs, red vent, swollen liver, emaciation
Facial swellings or discharges	Mycoplasmosis	Sneezing, nasal discharge, starvation due to blindness
	Chlamydophilosis	Nasal discharge, dyspnoea, diarrhoea, ill birds
	Paramyxovirus infection	PMV-2 upper respiratory tract diseases

36.4   Differential diagnosis of group morbidity/mortality based on presenting clinical signs. (continues) ▶

Main clinical sign	Differentials	Other clinical signs
Feather loss or mutilation	Behavioural	Feather loss over back of head and rump most typical
	Scaly face mites	Scaly crusts over feet, eyes and beak, pruritis
	Red mites	Pale mucous membranes, respiratory distress, depression
	Feather lice	Irritation, restlessness, feather plucking if severe
	Viral papilloma	Skin nodules on feet and legs
	Polyomavirus infection	High nestling mortality, abdominal haemorrhages
Neurological signs	Paramyxovirus infection	PMV-3 dyspnoea, conjunctivitis, yellowish diarrhoea
	Toxoplasmosis	None
	Atoxoplasmosis	Diarrhoea, red vent, swollen liver, emaciation
	Toxicosis	Nitroimidazole, heavy metal, ethanol, OP toxicity
Regurgitation	Gram-negative septicaemia	Matted feathering, dysphagia, dyspnoea
	Trichomoniasis	Respiratory signs, emaciation, salivation, dysphagia
Sudden deaths, ill birds (fluffed up)	Pseudotuberculosis	Debility, emaciation, diarrhoea, respiratory signs
	Septicaemia	Diarrhoea, nestling mortality, rhinitis, conjunctivitis
	Atoxoplasmosis	Diarrhoea, neurological signs, red vent, emaciation
	Starvation	Fluffed up birds
	Mycobacteriosis	Ill birds, diarrhoea, weight loss
	Polyomavirus infection	Skin lesions, abdominal haemorrhages, beak deformities
	Leucocytozoonosis	Anorexia, anaemia
	Toxicoses	Varies depending on agent

36.4 (continued) Differential diagnosis of group morbidity/mortality based on presenting clinical signs.

Euthanasia

Euthanasia is best performed by an overdose of a gaseous anaesthetic delivered by mask or by placing the bird in a sealed container with some gaseous anaesthetic on a cotton wool ball (the open drop method). Should there be a need for intravenous pentobarbital injection, the right jugular vein can be accessed most easily under anaesthesia for euthanasia.

Zoonotic diseases

Transmission of diseases to humans is unusual from passerine birds. Chlamydophilosis and salmonellosis are potential zoonoses. Red mites can also bite humans.

Disease control

Good hygiene practices can lead to a significant reduction in disease. General recommendations include the following.

Aviary design

- Cover the aviary roof and trim any overhanging branches to reduce exposure to wild birds and minimize the risk of transmission of infectious agents and parasites (Figure 36.5).
- Concrete the aviary floor and provide plastic skirting around the base of the aviary to limit

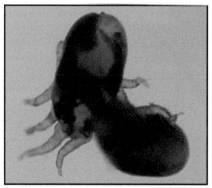

36.5 Tracheal mites from a Gouldian Finch. (Courtesy of Alistair Lawrie)

entry of vermin (mice and rats) and to limit exposure to pseudotuberculosis. Rodenticides or traps may need to be used in severe infestations, in which case caution should be advised and birds must be kept away. Concreting the base of the aviary will also reduce pathogen build-up, prevent any growth of toxic plants and allow more thorough disinfection.
- Double-wire the enclosure to prevent any trauma from wild birds (such as Sparrowhawks) and to reduce the likelihood of ingesting external toxic plants.
- Remove top layer of the aviary substrate to remove any potential pathogens such as ascarid ova, pseudotuberculosis or *Macrorhabdus* organisms.

Feeding areas

- Place food in small amounts at multiple sites to minimize faecal contamination around the food source and to prevent build-up of potential pathogens in one area of the aviary. This also reduces competition for food and water.
- Rotate the positions of feeding areas around the aviary to reduce faecal contamination in the same sites.
- Position feeding areas away from any potential perching sites, to reduce faecal contamination of the food.
- Use suspended feeders with no flat surfaces or ledges.
- Clean all feeding areas regularly and remove all uneaten food.
- Disinfect water bowls and feeding areas regularly, followed by thorough rinsing of the area.
- Prepare all food in a separate hygienic area before entering any enclosures.
- Wear gloves when feeding or cleaning. Change gloves between feeding each group of birds and disinfect footwear to minimize cross-contamination between enclosures.

Therapeutics

Ideally a definitive diagnosis should be achieved prior to medications being administered, though it is of course possible that treatment for the likely cause of illness will be required prior to a definitive diagnosis being reached.

Many agents are not licensed for use in exotic animal species and this should be mentioned and written consent obtained from the owners prior to treatment. Individual medication may be difficult, due the stress of repeated capture (both on the birds and owner) and trauma from repeated oral dosing or injections. Thus treatment of the flock will be via a limited number of routes:

- Medicated drinking water
- Medicated feed
- Nebulization.

In-water medication

Typically in-water medication is used while limiting access to other water sources (bathing bowls, rain, high moisture content food items) where this is possible. Problems associated with this route include reduced intake, irregular intake and no intake overnight, all leading to sub-therapeutic levels. Toxicity is possible in hot weather due to increased levels of water consumption and this has been reported with nitroimidazoles. Dehydration is also possible when only set amounts of medicated water are offered. Many diseased individuals may still succumb to the disease process despite medication, because time may be required for therapeutic levels to be achieved and many sick birds may be too ill to consume sufficient medicated water.

In-food medication

Seed should not be top-dressed because medicines can be lost when the seed is dehusked by the birds. The addition of drugs to other food items, such as softfood, fruit or insectivorous mixes, can be performed but is haphazard as selective feeding, conspecific aggression and interspecific aggression can lead to a marked variation in intake.

Nebulization

Nebulization is another possible route for treatment, usually reserved for respiratory disease alongside systemic therapy. Ideally the birds should be kept in a smaller enclosure (e.g. a cage). Fogging the aviary with disinfectants, along with vigorous hygiene, can help to limit pathogen build-up.

Drug dosages

Passerines have a higher metabolic rate compared with other birds and their water and feed consumption are elevated as a result. This means that drugs delivered in water or food may be more effective in passerine birds than in most birds seen in general practice. Despite this, the elevated metabolic rate of passerines may lead to sub-therapeutic levels if doses are extrapolated from other avian families. This is because they may excrete drugs more quickly and require larger doses to obtain therapeutic levels. Dosages may need to be higher and more frequent as a result. See Appendix 1 for dosages.

Acknowledgements

The author is grateful to Miss Suzetta Billington, who kindly read and commented on early drafts of this chapter.

References and further reading

Cunningham AA, Lawson B, Bennett M *et al.* (2005) Garden bird health. *Veterinary Record* **156**, 656

Dorrenstein PM (2000) Passerine and exotic softbills. In: *Avian Medicine*, ed. TN Tully *et al.*, pp. 144–179. Butterworth-Heinemann, Oxford

Gentz EJ (2003) Passeriformes (songbirds, perching birds). In: *Zoo and Wild Animal Medicine, 5th edn*, ed. ME Fowler and RE Miller, pp. 267–275. WB Saunders, Philadelphia

Gerlach H (2001) Megabacteriosis. *Seminars in Avian and Exotic Pet Medicine* **10**(1), 12–19

Holmes P and Duff P (2005) Ingluvitis and oesophagitis in wild finches. *Veterinary Record* **157**, 455

Pennycott TW, Cinderly A, Park A *et al.* (2002) *Salmonella enterica* subspecies *enterica* serotype Typhimurium and *Escherichia coli* 086 in wild birds at two gardens in south west Scotland. *Veterinary Record* **151**, 563–567

Pennycott TW, Lawson B, Cunningham AA *et al.* (2005) Necrotic ingluvitis in wild finches. *Veterinary Record* **157**, 360

Ritchie BW (1995) *Avian Viruses*. Wingers, Lake Worth, FL

Sandmeier P and Coutteel P (2006) Management of canaries, finches and mynahs. In: *Clinical Avian Medicine Volume II*, ed. GJ Harrison and TL Lightfoot, pp. 879–913. Zoological Education Network, Palm Beach, FL

Further information on trichomoniasis in wild UK finches can be obtained at http://www.ufaw.org.uk/gbhi.php

37

Legal, zoonotic and ethical considerations

Peter Scott

Introduction

This chapter covers UK legislation concerning raptors, pigeons and passerine birds. It looks at trading in CITES 'A' species, the import and export of birds within and outside the European Union (EU), methods and legal aspects of bird identification, the control of zoonoses and, finally, ethical issues such as tethering of raptors and the breeding of mutation passerine birds. Some of the important points of the more significant pieces of legislation are outlined in Figures 37.1 to 37.4. Some of the implications for those who keep, handle, treat or advise on the species in this Manual are considered further below.

Animals Act 1971	To make provision with respect to civil liability for damage done by animals. It places liability on the keeper, who at the time may not be the owner
Pet Animals Act 1951 **Pet Animals Act 1951 (Amendment) Act 1982**	BVA and local authority consultative groups have Guidelines for Inspections under the Pet Animals Act which specify cage dimensions and standards for shops. Considerations during an inspection should include: • The basic five freedoms (see Zoo Licensing Act in welfare section) or five principles as outlined • Suitable food • The cage size requirements from the WCA • Isolation/separate accommodation available if necessary • Signs of behavioural problems (e.g. feather plucking/picking)
Wildlife and Countryside Act 1981	There are several areas where this impinges on bird owners. The term 'wild bird' should be taken to mean any bird of a species that is ordinarily resident in or is a visitor to the European territory of any EU Member State in a wild state (Section 27(1), as amended by SI 1487/2004 The Wildlife & Countryside Act (England & Wales) (Amendment) Regulations 2004)). The protection provided makes it an offence to: • Take, injure, kill or sell a protected species • Disturb a protected species in its nest or place of shelter • Possess a protected species • Release a Barn Owl without Defra authorization • Release or allow to escape into the wild any non-indigenous species or a species listed in Schedule 9 • Various methods of trapping, netting or hunting are prohibited or restricted Species of European bird are listed as protected: • Schedule 1, Part 1, lists those that are protected by special penalties at all times, i.e. they may not be killed or taken from the wild at any time • Schedule 1, Part 2, lists those that may be sold alive at any time if bred in captivity and close ringed • Schedule 1, Part 4, lists birds that may be kept in captivity

37.1   Important points of the more significant pieces of legislation regarding keeping birds.

| Directive 92/65 EEC (the 'Balai' Directive) (continues) | Certification of birds for import/export is complex and requires consultation every time with Defra. Export papers often require certification that an area is clear of Newcastle disease; this cannot be certified without the prior confirmation and permission of Defra. This Directive requires an official export health certificate.
From 1 July 2007, new rules came into effect indefinitely; these will ban imports of wild-caught birds but allow captive-bred birds from approved breeding establishments in some countries outside the EU.
There are three categories of birds: poultry, captive birds and pet birds. Import and quarantine requirements are laid down in EU legislation.
Poultry and captive birds imported into the EU from third countries must enter at designated Border Inspection Posts, where they are subject to veterinary inspections. All consignments are subject to documentary and identity checks to ensure that the conditions of import, set out by EU legislation, are met.
All birds imported from third countries must undergo a period of quarantine. From the time of import, live poultry (or eggs once hatched) must be held for six weeks in an approved quarantine establishment to ensure they are not carrying any disease. |

37.2   Important points of the more significant pieces of legislation regarding import and export of birds. (continues) ▶

Directive 92/65 EEC (the 'Balai' Directive) (continued)	Captive birds may be imported from other EU Member States provided that they do not come from any area under official restrictions because of an avian influenza outbreak. Quarantine for imports of captive birds from other EU Member States is not required. Import of captive birds from third countries has been suspended by the EU until further notice because of the avian influenza situation. Pet birds may be imported from either EU or third countries subject to a specific licence under which they will be required to spend 35 days in domestic quarantine.
CITES ('Washington' Convention on International Trade in Endangered Species of Wild Fauna and Flora)	CITES aims to protect certain plants and animals by regulating and monitoring their international trade to prevent it reaching unsustainable levels. The Convention came into force in 1975 and the UK became a Party to it in 1976. There are now over 150 Parties. The CITES Secretariat is administered by the United Nations Environment Programme.
Council Regulation (EC) No. 338/97 (deals with the protection of species of wild fauna and flora by regulating the trade in these species) **Commission Regulation (EC) No. 1808/2001** (replaced **Commission Regulation (EC) No. 939/37**)	CITES has been implemented in the European Union since 1984 through a number of regulations. These set out the rules for the import, export and re-export of the species to which they apply. The regulation of trade is based on a system of permits and certificates that may only be issued when certain conditions are met. In the European Union the CITES Appendices I–III are replaced by Annexes A–C to EC Regulation 338/97. Current species lists are held at by the UNEP World Conservation Monitoring Centre and can be viewed by visiting their website http://www.unep-wcmc.org/species/trade/eu/tradereg.html • **Annex A** includes all species listed in **Appendix I** of CITES, plus certain other species included because they look the same, need a similar level of protection, or to secure the effective protection of rare taxa within the same genus. • **Annex B** includes all the remaining species listed in **Appendix II** of CITES, plus certain other species included on a 'lookalike' basis, or because the level of trade may not be compatible with the survival of the species or local populations, or because they pose an ecological threat to indigenous species. • **Annex C** includes all the remaining species listed in **Appendix III** of CITES. • **Annex D** includes those non-CITES species not listed in **Annexes A** and **C** which are imported into the EC in such numbers as to warrant monitoring.
COTES (Control of Trade in Endangered Species (Enforcement) Regulations 1997	COTES enforces CITES in the UK. It was widely felt by conservation groups that the weak powers of this legislation account for the relatively few prosecutions under it. This resulted in harsher penalties being introduced in 2003. There are provisions within COTES for power of entry and provision for offences by corporate bodies. It is advisable to check current lists and requirements via the internet or with Defra, as these change fairly frequently.

37.2 (continued) Important points of the more significant pieces of legislation regarding import and export of birds.

Animal Welfare Act 2006	This replaced various pieces of legislation which were out of date or not fit for purpose. The new Act introduces a 'Duty of care' – a legal term meaning that someone has an obligation to do something. Prior to the Animal Welfare Act 2006, there was only a duty to ensure that an animal didn't suffer unnecessarily. The new Act keeps this duty but also imposes a broader duty of care on anyone responsible for an animal to take reasonable steps to ensure that the animal's needs are met. This means that a person has to look after the animal's welfare as well as ensure that it does not suffer. The Act says that an animal's welfare needs include: • A suitable environment • A suitable diet • The ability to exhibit normal behaviour patterns • Any need it has to be housed with, or apart from, other animals • Protection from pain, suffering, injury and disease. A 'protected animal' under the AWA is one that is: • Normally domesticated in the British Isles • Either permanently or temporarily under a person's control, or • Not living in a wild state. The duty of care (the need to provide for an animal's welfare) applies to animals for which a person is responsible. A person is responsible for an animal if that person is: • The owner of the animal • In charge of the animal, for example an owner of boarding kennels • A parent or guardian of a person under 16 who is responsible for the animal • A person responsible for an animal on a temporary basis, perhaps while owners are on holiday. The range of the AWA is great because it has been drafted such that secondary legislation under it can be prepared quickly and in response to specific issues. Guidelines will be published which will need to be considered.
Performing Animals (Regulation) Act & Performing Animals Rules 1968 (This Act will be replaced by secondary legislation under the Animal Welfare Act 2006)	These require any person who exhibits or trains any performing (vertebrate) animal to be registered with a local authority. The term 'exhibit' is defined as 'exhibit at any entertainment to which the public are admitted, whether on payment of money or otherwise ...' and to 'train' means 'train for the purpose of any such exhibition'. This provision applies to situations that involve animal performances. A person who exhibits or trains a performing animal must be registered (e.g. circuses, falconry displays, cabarets, film making). The definitions in the Act also appear to cover some of the training and performance with animals that takes place in zoos. However, it might be expected that training that was carried out to assist in the routine management of an animal (and not intended as preparation of a performance) would not involve registration.

37.3 Important points of the more significant pieces of legislation regarding welfare. (continues) ▶

Zoo Licensing Act 1981 (Amendment) (England and Wales) Regulations 2002	This Act includes all places where animals not normally domesticated in UK are displayed to the public for seven days or more per year whether a charge is made or not. This could range from a conventional zoo/bird garden to a council-operated park with aviaries. This Act was primarily concerned with public safety, although animal welfare issues were also covered. The recent Amendments comply with the EC Zoos Directive (1999/22/EC) to provide for good standards of animal care, and set the framework for the participation of zoos in conservation, research and education. The Secretary of State's Standards for Modern Zoo Practice are the standards to which zoos and public aquaria must operate. The general standards are based around the 'Five Freedoms' presented as Five Principles: • Provision of food and water – requiring attention to nutritional content, method of presentation and natural behaviour of the animal or bird • Provision of a suitable environment – consistent with species requirements, spatial requirements are included as are appropriate 3D environments • Provision of animal healthcare – to protect the animal from injury and disease • Provision of an opportunity to express most normal behaviour – taking into account enrichment and husbandry guidelines • Provision of protection from fear and distress – including group composition, sex ratios, stocking levels.

37.3 (continued) Important points of the more significant pieces of legislation regarding welfare.

Diseases of Poultry (England) Order 2003	Makes avian influenza and Newcastle disease notifiable in any species of bird.
Abandonment of Animals Act 1960	Makes it an offence of cruelty under the 1911 Act to abandon an animal without reasonable excuse in circumstances likely to cause it suffering. Prosecutions have been sought in regard of pet cockatiels released when an owner moved house.
Zoonoses Order 1989 made under the Animal Health Act 1981	Designates organisms of the genus *Salmonella* and the genus *Brucella* as zoonotic, enabling powers (including powers relating to the slaughter of poultry) under the Animal Health Act 1981 to be used to reduce any risk to human health of these organisms. Under this order the term 'poultry' has been extended to include birds of any species. The order provides for the imposition of control measures which include quarantine, movement restrictions, cleansing and disinfection.
Diseases of Animals (Seizure) Order 1993	Lists psittacosis (ornithosis) amongst the diseases to which this order applies (1) An inspector or veterinary inspector shall have power to seize anything (other than a live animal) whether animate or inanimate, by or by means of which it appears to him that a disease to which section 35(1) of the Animal Health Act 1981 applies might be carried or transmitted. (2) An inspector or veterinary inspector exercising powers under this order shall dispose of the thing seized by destruction, burial, treatment or such other method of disposal as he thinks expedient to prevent the spread of disease. This essentially provides for collection of samples, which then allows for the exclusion of Newcastle disease or avian influenza.
Psittacosis or Ornithosis Order of 1953	This provides for the detention and isolation of birds and for other powers to prevent the spread of disease. This order extends the definition of the expression 'disease' for the purposes of the Diseases of Animals Act 1950 to include 'psittacosis' or 'ornithosis'. The order also provides for the detention and isolation of birds affected, or suspected of being affected, with this disease, and for the cleansing and disinfection of premises and utensils for such birds. The order, together with the Diseases of Animals (extension of Definition of Poultry) Order 1953, also enables powers of compulsory slaughter to be used, at the Government Minister's discretion, in respect of poultry affected with, or in any way exposed to psittacosis/ornithosis. This regulation brings 'parrots' within the definition of poultry. Despite all of this, psittacosis in humans is not currently a notifiable disease in the UK. For a time, to gather information, it was made notifiable in three local authorities (Cambridge City, South Cambridgeshire and East Cambridgeshire).
Medicines (restrictions on the administration of veterinary medicinal products) regulations 1994 (SI 1994/2987), as amended by SI 1997/2884 (Amelia 8)	The Regulations establish in UK law the prescribing cascade, and the requirements for minimum withdrawal periods and for record keeping by veterinary surgeons adopted by the European Community in 1990. In summary, when no authorized veterinary medicinal product exists for a condition in a particular species, and in order to avoid causing unacceptable suffering, veterinary surgeons exercising their clinical judgement may prescribe for one or a small number of animals under their care in accordance with the following sequence: (i) A veterinary medicine authorized for use in another species, or for a different use in the same species ('off-label use') (ii) A medicine authorized in the UK for human use (iii) A medicine to be made up at the time on a one-off basis by a veterinary surgeon or a properly authorized person. There are additional requirements for treating food-producing animals. The small number of animals limitation, and the requirement to follow the three stages of the cascade in strict order, do not apply to non-food-producing animals of minor or exotic species. The Veterinary Medicines Directorate suggests that, as a working rule, 'minor and exotic species' is taken to cover all companion, laboratory and zoo animals (other than any whose produce might enter the food chain) other than cats and dogs.

37.4 Important points of the more significant pieces of legislation regarding zoonosis and other health-related matters.

Falconry

As a pastime with a long history, there are several legal requirements associated with falconry.

• The bird being flown may or may not have to be registered (Wildlife and Countryside Act (WCA) Schedule 4 birds must be registered).
• Depending on the quarry species, a quarry licence may be required (necessary unless the quarry is listed in WCA Schedule 2). If game birds are hunted a Home Office certificate is required and prey can only be sold to a game dealer.
• Permission is required to hunt on the land.
• In other EU countries there may be additional controls. For example, in Germany it is necessary to pass state examinations, initially to obtain a hunting licence and then a falconry licence.

Trading in CITES 'A' birds

All European species of raptor are included in Annex A of EC Regulation 338/97 (see Figure 37.2). Aside from trading restrictions, CITES also requires under Article 10 that anyone breeding or displaying for commercial gain any species (including parts, cadavers or hybrids) listed on Annex A requires a licence, referred to as a 'specimen specific' licence. The Global Wildlife Division of the Department for Environment, Food and Rural Affairs (Defra) is the UK CITES Management Authority: it is responsible for ensuring that the Convention is implemented in the UK and it issues Article 10 Certificates.

Such birds must be close-ringed (see below) and identified (EU 1808/2001). Currently, birds bred in captivity must be fitted with a close ring, or if this is not possible due to the physical or behavioural characteristics of the specimen concerned, an unalterable microchip that meets ISO Standards 11784:1996 and 11785:1998(E) can be used. Close rings are continuous metal bands without any breaks.

Sale of a bird requires an Article 10 certificate. Zoos with many such animals usually apply for Article 60 licences (previously called Article 30s), which are collection specific and act as a blanket licence for all of the animals and plants they hold and are designed to deal with transfers between zoos. Each bird needs to have an EU certificate, which is like a passport (including details of ring number, sex, birth date, breeder). Additional certificates regarding health etc. are necessary but vary between different countries.

Import, export and re-export permits are required to authorize trade in CITES species with non-EU countries. Various health certificates will also be required.

CITES information sources

Defra Global Wildlife Division:
http://www.defra.gov.uk/wildlife-countryside/gwd/cites/index.htm
UK CITES:
http://www.ukcites.gov.uk/
UNEP World Conservation Monitoring Centre:
http://www.unep-wcmc.org/

Do not rely solely on the websites. They are often out of date, or buried amongst old ones. Speak to Defra after investigating the websites.

Also see:
Joint Nature Conservation Committee:
http://www.jncc.gov.uk
Red List of Endangered Species
http://www.redlist.org/

Releasing CITES 'A' birds

Rehabilitators have a problem in that if they release a bird that is not likely to survive they may contravene the Abandonment of Animals Act 1960, yet not releasing it may contravene the Wildlife and Countryside Act (WCA). In such circumstances a licence from Defra is required, based on a veterinary report that the bird is disabled or otherwise unfit for release (e.g. imprinted) and individually identified. Section 14 of the WCA, in addition to making it an offence to release non-native species, includes a list (Schedule 9) of animals that are also prohibited, including Barn Owls.

Importation of captive and pet birds

Importing birds into the EU is quite challenging. Apart from proof of a bird's legality, certain health certificates are required. Also importation from certain countries might be prohibited altogether. In the light of certain diseases, such as avian influenza, this situation might change almost daily and the requirements should be ascertained from the appropriate government office in good time.

Import and export: some practical points

Determine the species. This sounds easier than it may be in practice, but could be crucially important in moving a bird to another country.

Action by the owner

- Check with Defra's Global Wildlife Division regarding any CITES requirements. If appropriate, obtain certificates and submit to destination country for its own CITES team to approve importation (failure to do so could lead to confiscation).
- Submit to Defra for CITES approval; Defra will then issue an import certificate.

Action by the veterinary surgeon

- Advise the owner to clarify the situation with Defra's Global Wildlife Division.
- Check with Defra Animal Health Office

Keeping, buying and selling WCA Schedule 3 and Schedule 4 birds

Section 6(1) of the 1981 Wildlife and Countryside Act restricts the sale of any live wild bird to those species listed in the Act's Schedule 3, Part 1. In this respect 'sale' includes possessing, offering, exposing or transporting for the purposes of sale (6(1)(a)), or publishing or causing to be published an advertisement likely to be understood as conveying that the person buys or sells birds (6(1)(b)). Section 6(5) qualifies Schedule 3, Part 1, requiring birds involved to have also been bred in captivity and close-ringed in accordance with SI 1220/1982.

Nothing within the 1981 Act requires any bird, including those listed on Schedule 3, Part 1, to be close-ringed or in any other way ringed if it is not intended for sale or exhibition under Section 6.

The Bird Registration Team deals with all applications to register these birds. This includes applications for captive-bred, disabled wild, and imported birds. The Act places the burden of proof on the keeper of any Schedule 4 bird to show that it has been legally acquired, and documentary evidence to support this should be kept.

Under the Wildlife and Countryside Act 1981, any bird listed on Schedule 3 must be ringed if it is to be sold; those listed on Schedule 4 must be ringed and registered with Defra if kept in captivity. This impacts on both falconers and those who wish to keep and breed 'British' birds. The species covered by Schedules 3 and 4 are listed in Figures 37.5 and 37.6.

Blackbird (*Turdus merula*)
Brambling (*Fringilla montifringilla*)
Bullfinch (*Pyrrhula pyrrhula*)
Bunting, Reed (*Emberiza schoeniclus*)
Chaffinch (*Fringilla coelebs*)
Dunnock (*Prunella modularis*)
Goldfinch (*Carduellis carduellis*)
Greenfinch (*Carduellis chloris*)
Jackdaw (*Corvus monedula*)
Jay (*Garrulus glandarius*)
Linnet (*Carduellis cannabina*)
Magpie (*Pica pica*)
Owl, Barn (*Tyto alba*)
Redpoll (*Carduellis flammea*)
Siskin (*Carduellis spinus*)
Starling (*Sturnus vulgaris*)
Thrush, Song (*Turdus philomelos*)
Twite (*Carduelis flavirostris*)
Yellowhammer (*Emberiza citrinella*)

37.5

Wildlife and Countryside Act 1981: Schedule 3. Note: This list uses names as listed in the Act.

Many of the birds currently listed on Schedule 4 are also protected by CITES. Defra acts as UK Management Authority for CITES. At present keepers of listed birds often have to complete several pieces of paperwork for Defra: (a) to register the bird under Schedule 4; and (b) to comply with CITES controls. This may change.

Some species are recommended for removal from Schedule 4, as they are widely bred in captivity and there is little evidence that they are being taken from the wild. Others are recommended for removal because their wild populations have reached a level where they do not require the additional protection that the registration system provides.

Birds listed on Schedule 4 and CITES Annex A need an Article 10 licence for sale purposes. Those not on CITES 'A' can be sold once ringed and registered. Those with an incorrect ring (perhaps imported birds) need to be specified in a licence issued by Natural England's Wildlife Licensing department as an 'application for a licence to sell captive bred birds not fitted with the correct closed ring'.

Close-ringing

Rings are fitted to recently hatched chicks (3–10 days of age depending on species); after this period the close ring will no longer pass over the foot joint. There may be problems with adult female birds removing their chicks' rings, or damaging the chicks when trying to remove rings, or possibly even ejecting ringed chicks from the nest.

Bunting, Cirl (*Emberiza cirlus*)
Bunting, Lapland (*Calcarius lapponicus*)
Bunting, Snow (*Plectrophenax nivalis*)
Buzzard, Honey (*Pernis apivorus*)
Eagle, Adalbert's (*Aquila adalberti*)
Eagle, Golden (*Aquila chrysaetos*)
Eagle, Great Philippine (*Pithecophaga jefferyi*)
Eagle, Imperial (*Aquila heliaca*)
Eagle, New Guinea (*Harpyopsis novaeguineae*)
Eagle, White-tailed (*Haliaeetus albicilla*)
Chough (*Pyrrhocorax pyrrhocorax*)
Crossbills (all species) (*Loxia* spp.)
Falcon, Barbary (*Falco pelegrinoides*)
Falcon, Gyr (*Falco rusticolus*)
Falcon, Peregrine (*Falco peregrinus*)
Fieldfare (*Turdus pilaris*)
Firecrest (*Regulus ignicapillus*)
Fish-Eagle, Madagascar (*Haliaeetus vociferoides*)
Forest-Falcon, Plumbeous (*Micrastur plumbeus*)
Goshawk (*Accipiter gentilis*)
Harrier, Hen (*Circus cyaneus*)
Harrier, Marsh (*Circus aeruginosus*)
Harrier, Montagu (*Circus pygargus*)
Hawk, Galapagos (*Buteo galapagoensis*)
Hawk, Grey-backed (*Leucopternis occidentalis*)
Hawk, Hawaiian (*Buteo solitarius*)
Hawk, Ridgway (*Buteo ridgwayi*)
Hawk, White-necked (*Leucopternis lacernulata*)
Hawk-Eagle, Wallace (*Spizaetus nanus*)
Hobby (*Falco subbuteo*)
Honey-Buzzard, Black (*Henicopernis infuscatus*)
Kestrel, Lesser (*Falco naumanni*)
Kestrel, Mauritius (*Falco punctatus*)
Kite, Red (*Milvus milvus*)
Merlin (*Falco columbarius*)
Oriole, Golden (*Oriolus oriolus*)
Osprey (*Pandion haliaetus*)
Redstart, Black (*Phoenicurus ochruros*)
Redwing (*Turdus iliacus*)
Sea-Eagle, Pallas (*Haliaeetus leucoryphus*)
Sea-Eagle, Stellers (*Haliaeetus pelagicus*)
Serin (*Serinus serinus*)
Serpent-Eagle, Andaman (*Spilornis elgini*)
Serpent-Eagle, Madagascar (*Eutriorchis astur*)
Serpent-Eagle, Mountain (*Spilornis kinabaluensis*)
Shorelark (*Eremophila alpestris*)
Shrike, Red-backed (*Lanius collurio*)
Sparrowhawk, New Britain (*Accipiter brachyurus*)
Sparrowhawk, Gundlach's (*Accipiter gundlachi*)
Sparrowhawk, Imitator (*Accipiter imitator*)
Sparrowhawk, Small (*Accipiter nanus*)
Tit, Bearded (*Panurus biarmicus*)
Tit, Crested (*Parus cristatus*)
Warbler, Cetti (*Cettia cetti*)
Warbler, Dartford (*Sylvia undata*)
Warbler, Marsh (*Acrocephalus palustris*)
Warbler, Savi (*Locustella luscinioides*)
Woodlark (*Lullula arborea*)
Wryneck (*Jynx torquilla*)

37.6 Wildlife and Countryside Act 1981: Schedule 4 (current list, but under review). Note: This list uses names as listed in the Act.

In the UK, breeders who do not normally deal in birds may see no necessity to fit close rings to their young birds. In other EU countries, such as Germany, it is required by domestic legislation to identify birds by an agreed method; thus a UK breeder who has not fitted a close ring will be prevented from selling the birds.

Statutory requirements regarding the type of close ring required to legitimize sale or exhibition are contained within SI 1220/1982 – Wildlife and Countryside (Ringing of Certain Birds) Regulations 1982. SI 1220/1982 gives internal ring diameter (in millimetres) for each bird species, on a scale from 2.4 mm to 7.1 mm. For ease of use the ring suppliers designate these with letters, in the range A to S. The difference in internal diameter between each of these is 0.1 mm. Larger rings are available for the larger captive raptors.

Rings are of an approved type and in the UK may be issued by one of two Defra-approved suppliers: the British Bird Council (BBC) and the International Ornithological Society (IOA). In other EU countries different manufacturers are approved by the national authorities and sizes and nomenclature also vary.

Any application for a close ring must be made by the keeper or prospective keeper of the bird, who must also provide details of its parents or prospective parents, and in the case of existing birds specify its age and (where known) its sex.

European Commission Regulation 1808/2001 (Ringing)

This EU regulation is sometimes brought into legal arguments concerned with ringing Schedule 3 birds, but it is actually directed at CITES Annex A birds. Species listed on Schedule 3 and most other bird species covered by the 1981 Wildlife and Countryside Act are not also covered by CITES.

Bird gatherings: pigeon racing and falconry

For biosecurity reasons some restrictions have been placed on where birds are permitted to race from. Races are regarded as gatherings of birds, which are now included in Regulation 6(1) of The Avian Influenza (Preventive Measures) (England) Regulations 2006, which bans bird gatherings unless under licence.

Defra has assessed the risks related to avian influenza as being sufficiently low that bird gatherings can currently take place under general licence, granted by Defra's Animal Health offices. This also applies to meetings of falconers who hunt together. A ' bird gathering' for the purposes of the general licence means the arrangement by a person of the collecting together of poultry or other captive birds from different epidemiological groups at one location. These are generally falconry displays, fairs, markets, shows, exhibitions and pigeon races. An event involving a single bird, or birds that are normally kept together, does not pose an increased risk of disease spread and so is not classed as a gathering.

Zoonoses

The Health and Safety at Work etc. Act 1974 and The Control of Substances Hazardous to Health (COSHH) regulations 1988 both apply here. Civil law relating to negligence also has a bearing with regard to clients or indeed veterinary staff who may become infected or injured (Animals Act 1971). It is now necessary to prepare COSHH sheets related to zoonotic diseases.

Ornithosis

Psittacosis (ornithosis) is perhaps the most significant zoonosis associated with birds and it must be noted that people have died following infection from their birds. At the same time it is a popular diagnosis (or misdiagnosis) in humans who have disclosed that they keep birds. Compulsory slaughter of pet birds has never been carried out on the grounds of psittacosis infection. A number of veterinary surgeons have recommended this as a course of action but it is not required in the UK and indeed is rarely necessary (in this author's view) and may lead to claims for compensation.

Other zoonoses

Other zoonotic infections of note include *Campylobacter*, *Salmonella* and *Escherichia coli*. For raptors, these may be associated with prey items. Other potentially zoonotic organisms include *Mycobacterium avium*, *Pasteurella multocida* and *Yersinia pseudotuberculosis*. Avian influenza must be mentioned although pigeons are not considered high-risk species. Newcastle disease has been known to cause conjunctivitis in humans.

Ethical and practical issues

Falconry

There are ethical issues associated with falconry that seriously tax the mind, and about which for some there is no debate at all. First, there is simply the ethics of hunting – using a bird or birds to drive game and kill it. Falconry is not akin to foxhunting, where an animal is pursued perhaps for long distances; the falcon and his handler kill quickly with little preamble, mimicking the natural behaviour.

Flying weight

Another aspect of falconry is the method of training and hunting: the bird is said to be kept 'keen' to work for a food reward; it kills game and receives payment in the form of food. One school of thought suggests that this means that birds are starved and kept hungry and given just enough to maintain the chosen 'flying weight'. Others say that the flying weight concept is incorrect; they suggest that, like mammalian top predators, the birds' weight naturally fluctuates in days of feast and famine, and that maintaining flying weight is an artificial concept to suit the falconer. The general aim should always be to maintain a positive energy balance but, putting it simplistically, hungry birds hunt; if they are not hungry, they rest, since there is little reason to hunt. Out of the hunting season birds are allowed to gain weight. Of course this is a gross simplification and actually some birds will not fly well unless they are actually quite fat and none will fly well starved and cachexic.

Tethering

Tethering is long-established practice with working raptors but has its critics. It has a place in the training of birds but increasingly falconers are 'free-lofting' birds in aviaries. Tethering involves a higher degree of care from the falconer to protect the bird and cater to its needs since its range is restricted.

Shows

There are concerns currently under zoo licensing legislation regarding falconry shows set up during summer months, which may potentially sit outside the legislation. The suggestion has been made that when birds are taken to the falconer's home in the evening, rather than being left at the site of exhibition, they are not 'being kept' at the licensed site for display. It is not the intention of the Act to permit loopholes like this: the farm park owner who decides to keep a tiger should not be able to escape licensing simply by taking the animal home for the evening. The protections offered by the Zoo Licensing Act to the animals involved must be extended to all animals being displayed to the public.

Escapes

As yet another link to falconry (which hardly seems fair), Section 14(1) of the WCA makes it an offence if a person releases or allows the escape of an animal (including bird) of a kind that is not ordinarily resident in and is not a regular visitor to Great Britain in a wild state; or a species listed in Schedule 9. Schedule 9 now includes Barn Owls, not least because of the overenthusiastic breeding and release programmes that were turning birds out in inadequately surveyed areas where they could not find sufficient food. Licences to release are available. This also affects those people who might wish to free-fly their birds (zoos and private keepers) and if in doubt people wishing to do so should contact Defra's wildlife inspectorate for advice.

Cage sizes

There are also provisions in Section 8 of the 1981 WCA that regulate the size of cage in which any bird (excluding poultry) may be kept. The cage or other receptacle must be sufficient in height, length or breadth to permit a bird to stretch its wings freely unless: (a) the bird is being moved by any means; (b) it is being shown or exhibited and is not so kept for longer than 72 hours; (c) it is undergoing treatment or examination by a vet; or (d) it is being trained for exhibition and is not so kept for any longer than one hour in any period of 24 hours.

Sources of further information

Publications

Cooper ME (1987) *An Introduction to Animal Law*. Academic Press, London

Health & Safety Executive: *The occupational zoonoses*

Health & Safety Executive: *Common zoonoses in agriculture* (Leaflet AIS2) (see also www.hse.gov.uk/pubns/ais2.pdf)

Address

Wildlife Licensing Unit
Natural England, Burghill Road, Westbury-on-Trym, Bristol BS10 6NJ (tel. 0845 601 4523; fax 0845 601 3438; email wildlife@naturalengland.org.uk)

Websites

CITES: http://www.cites.org/

Defra Animal Health and Welfare: http://www.defra.gov.uk/animalh/index.htm

Health Protection Agency: http://www.hpa.org.uk/

Joint Nature Conservation Committee: http://www.jncc.gov.uk

Natural England: http:www.naturalengland.org.uk

Red List of endangered species: http://www.redlist.org

UNEP World Conservation Monitoring Centre: http://www.unep-wcmc.org/

World Conservation Union: http://www.iucn.org/

For most important EU legislation in relation to conservation: http://europa.eu.int/eur-lex/en/lif/reg/en_register_15103020.html

Appendix 1

Formulary

Please note that few of these drugs are authorized for use in these species in the UK. Where authorized, the stated drug dose may be different to that included in the following table (in which drug doses recommended by authors within this volume have been included).

It is recommended that clinicians follow the prescribing legislation in their own country and use authorized products at the authorized dose rate in that country before using alternative drugs or alternative dose rates.

Drug	Raptors	Pigeons	Passerine birds
Antibacterial drugs			
Amoxicillin	150 mg/kg i.m. q24h *Long-acting injection* 150 mg/kg orally q12h	150 mg/kg i.m. q24h *Long-acting injection* 100–200 mg/kg orally q6–8h 1–1.5 g or 500–800 mg powder per litre of drinking water for 5–7 days *(Authorized product)*	1.5 g/l drinking water for 5–7 days
Amoxicillin/clavulanate	150 mg/kg orally or i.v. q12h or i.m. q24h *May cause regurgitation if used orally*	As raptor	As raptor
Azithromycin	50 mg/kg orally q24h for 5 days *Chlamydophilosis*		
Cefalexin	40–100 mg/kg i.m. or orally q8–12h	As raptor	As raptor
Chloramphenicol		25 mg/kg orally q12h	
Chlortetracycline		40–50 mg/kg orally q8h 130–400 mg/l water	
Ciprofloxacin		5–20 mg/kg orally q12h 250 mg/l water	
Clindamycin	100 mg/kg orally q24h *Halve dose if used with marbofloxacin*		
Doxycycline	50–75 mg/kg orally q12h 100 mg/kg i.m. for 5–7 days *('Vibravenos' – Special Treatment Certificate required in the UK)*	10–50 mg/kg orally q12–24h for 3–5 days (45 days for chlamydophilosis) 200–500 mg/l water	40 mg/kg orally q12–24h 200–500 mg/l daily in water
Enrofloxacin	15 mg/kg orally or i.m. q12h *Licensed in companion birds. Irritant injection. Care with use in working birds due to muscle damage. May cause regurgitation*	5–15 mg/kg orally or i.m. q12h 100–300 mg/l water	Individual dosing as raptor In water at 100–150 mg/l
Lincomycin	50–75 mg/kg orally or i.m. q12h		
Lincomycin/spectinomycin		500–750 mg combined activity/l daily in water 50 mg/kg orally q24h	
Marbofloxacin	10mg/kg orally, i.m. or i.v. q24h	As raptor	As raptor

Drug	Raptors	Pigeons	Passerine birds
Antibacterial drugs (continued)			
Oxytetracycline	200 mg/kg i.m. q24h *Long-acting preparation* 25–50 mg/kg orally q8h	50 mg/kg orally q6h 80 mg/kg i.m. q48h 130–400 mg/l water	100 mg/kg orally q24h 4–12 mg/l drinking water for 7 days
Piperacillin	100 mg/kg i.m. or i.v. q12h *Often combined with tazobactam; use as above and base dosage on piperacillin dose. Above preparation should be reconstituted with glucose–saline for improved stability. Prepared solution also suitable as a topical flushing agent*		
Trimethoprim/ sulphonamide	30 mg/kg i.m. q12h 12–60 mg/kg orally q12h	60 mg/kg orally q12h 475–970 mg/l water	
Tylosin		50 mg/kg orally q24h 25 mg/kg i.m. q6–8h 800 mg/l water	1 g/l drinking water daily for 7–10 days
Antifungal drugs			
Amphotericin B	1.5 mg/kg i.v. q12h for 3–5 days *Give with 10–15 ml/kg saline*		100,000 IU/kg orally q12h–q8h 1–5 g/l drinking water for 10 days 100 mg/kg orally q12h *For* Macrorhabdus *infection* *Please note that the cheaper suspension of this drug is now unavailable in the UK Suspension can be imported from within the EU on an STC Intravenous forms are available but expensive. A form for flock treatment (Megabac-S, Vetafarm) is licensed in Australia and can be imported using a Special Treatment Authorization*
Enilconazole	Dilute 10% solution 10:1 and give 0.5 ml/kg/day intratracheally for 7–14 days		
Fluconazole	2–5 mg/kg orally q24h		
Itraconazole	10–20 mg/kg orally q24h (prophylactic) 10–15 mg/kg orally q12h (therapeutic)		
Ketoconazole	25 mg/kg i.m. or orally q12h		
Nystatin	300,000 IU/kg orally q12h *Not absorbed from GI tract*	100,000 IU/kg orally q24h for 10 days	5000–300,000 IU/bird q12h for 10 days *For* Macrorhabdus *infection* *There are some doubts as to its efficacy*
Terbinafine	10–15 mg/kg orally q12h		
Voriconazole	12.5 mg/kg orally q12h for 30–60 days		
Antiprotozoal drugs			
Amprolium		28 ml of the concentrate per 4.5 l drinking water for 7 days. In severe outbreaks continue with half-strength solution for a further 7 days	50–100 mg/l drinking water for 5 days or longer
Carnidazole	25–30 mg/kg orally once May repeat the next day if required	12.5–25 mg/bird orally once	
Chloroquine			2 g/l drinking water daily for 14 days

Drug	Raptors	Pigeons	Passerine birds
Antiprotozoal drugs (continued)			
Chloroquine/primaquine	Take one chloroquine tablet 500 mg, add one primaquine tablet 26 mg. Crush them and add 10 ml water. 0.5 ml of this then gives active ingredients of 15 mg chloroquine plus 0.75 mg primaquine. Initial dose (0 hours) is 25 mg/kg chloroquine + 1.3 mg/kg primaquine; then 15 mg/kg chloroquine at 12 h; then 15 mg/kg chloroquine at 24 h; then a final dose of 15 mg/kg chloroquine at 48 h Prophylaxis: 26.3 mg/kg orally weekly from 1 month before until 1 month after mosquito season *Avian malaria*		
Clazuril	30 mg/kg orally once	5–10 mg/kg orally once	
Dimetridazole		50 mg/kg orally q24h or in water for 6 days	
Mefloquine	50 mg/kg orally q24h for 7 days *Avian malaria*		
Melarsamine	0.25 mg/kg i.m. q24h for 4 days *Leucocytozoonosis*		
Metronidazole	50 mg/kg orally q24h for 5 days *Trichomoniasis*	40–50 mg/kg orally q24h for 5–7 days 100 mg/kg orally q48h × 3 200 mg/kg orally once	50 mg/kg q12h oral dosing to individual birds 200 mg/l drinking water daily for 7 days
Paromomycin	100 mg/kg orally q12h for 7 days Repeat after 1 week		
Pyrimethamine	0.5 mg/kg orally q12h for 28 days *Leucocytozoonosis*		
Ronidazole		10–20 mg/kg orally q24h for 7 days 1 g/l in water daily equivalent to 12.5 mg/kg/day	50–400 mg/l drinking water for 5 days
Sulfachlorpyridazine		300–1000 mg/l water for 3 days Then 2 days off before repeating course	150–300 mg/l 5 days a week for 2–3 weeks (several months for systemic coccidiosis)
Sulfadimidine		40–50 mg/kg orally q24h for 7 days or 2 days off and 3 days on	
Toltrazuril	25 mg/kg orally weekly × 3 *Coccidiosis*	75 mg/l water for 5 days 10–15 mg/kg orally twice a week for several weeks	75 mg/l 2 days a week for 4 weeks
Trimethoprim 40 mg/ml + sulfamethoxazole 200 mg/ml	0.15 ml/kg i.m. q24h for 7 days *Leucocytozoonosis*	60 mg/bird orally q24h for 3 days 480 mg/l daily in water	30 mg/kg orally q12–24h
Antiparasitic drugs			
Fenbendazole	*Nematodes and some cestodes:* 25–100 mg/kg orally once *Capillariasis:* 25 mg/kg orally q24h for 5 days *Blood dyscrasias have been reported at higher doses in vultures and some other raptors*	8 mg/bird *(licensed preparation for pigeons in the UK)* 10–20 mg/kg orally q24h for 3 days. Repeat after 2 weeks *Feather damage reported at higher doses*	20 mg/kg by gavage q24h for 3 days
Fipronil	Apply spray preparation via pad to base of neck, tail base and under each wing. *Do not soak the bird* *Do not exceed 7.5 mg/kg = 3 ml/kg*	As raptor	Apply lightly under each wing on to skin of birds

Drug	Raptors	Pigeons	Passerine birds
Antiparasitic drugs (continued)			
Ivermectin Moxidectin Doramectin	Ivermectin 200 µg/kg orally or i.m. Moxidectin 500–1000 µg/kg once for capillariasis; 200 µg/kg once for ectoparasites Doramectin 1000 µg/kg twice 1–2 weeks apart *Serratospiculum*	Ivermectin 200 µg/kg orally or i.m. 0.5 ml of 0.02% solution (in propylene glycol) applied as spot-on Repeat after 2 weeks	As raptor – may also be applied topically to skin at same dose rate (usually diluted to 0.02% solution in propylene glycol) Repeat q7–10 days x3 for mites, q10days x 2 for air sac mites
Levamisole		15–20 mg/bird orally. Repeat after 10 days 200 mg/l water	150 mg/l daily in drinking water for 3 days
Piperazine		1.9 g/l water	3.7 g/l drinking water for 12 hours. Repeat in 2–3 weeks
Piperonal powder	Shake over entire bird	As raptor	As raptor
Praziquantel	10 mg/kg i.m. Repeat after 1 week *Cestodes and trematodes*	10–20 mg/kg orally 7.5 mg/kg s.c. Repeat after 14 days	
Pyrethrum (powder/spray)		Apply powder as directed for feather lice	0.8% spray from 60 cm away Use 2–3 × 1-second bursts
Anti-inflammatory drugs			
Carprofen	1–5 mg/kg i.m. or orally q12–24h *Care in dehydration, shock and renal dysfunction. Higher dose rate appears effective for 24 hours*	As raptor	As raptor
Ketoprofen	1–5 mg/kg i.m. q8–24h	As raptor	As raptor
Meloxicam	0.1–0.5 mg/kg i.m. or orally q24h *Precautions as carprofen*	As raptor	As raptor
Piroxicam	0.5 mg/kg orally q24h	As raptor	As raptor
Sedative, analgesic and emergency drugs			
Adrenaline (epinephrine)	0.5–1 mg/kg i.v., intraosseous, intratracheal or sublingual	As raptor	As raptor
Atropine	0.04–0.5 mg/kg i.m.	0.4 mg/kg i.m. q4h *Toxicities*	Not indicated
Bupivacaine	< 2 mg/kg Mix with DMSO for topical analgesia		
Buprenorphine	0.01–0.05 mg/kg i.m. or i.v. q8–12h	As raptor	As raptor
Butorphanol	0.1–4 mg/kg i.m. q6–12h	As raptor	As raptor
Dexamethasone sodium phosphate	2–6 mg/kg i.m. or i.v. *Care with use of corticosteroids in birds – immunosuppression and other side effects are common*	As raptor	As raptor
Diazepam	0.2–1 mg/kg i.v. or i.m. q12–24h *Control of fitting: lower dose q24h orally may be useful as an appetite stimulant*	0.2–1 mg/kg i.v. or i.m.	0.5 mg/kg orally
Doxapram	5–20 mg/kg i.v., intraosseous or intratracheal	As raptor	As raptor
Glycopyrrolate	0.01–0.03 mg/kg i.m.	As raptor	Not indicated
Ketamine	5–10 mg/kg i.m. once for seizures		
Lidocaine	< 2.5 mg/kg local perfusion	As raptor	Unlikely to be able to dose safely
Midazolam	0.5–1 mg/kg i.v. or i.m. q8–12h		
Prednisolone sodium succinate	10–30 mg/kg i.v. or i.m. *See dexamethasone re precautions*	As raptor	As raptor

Formulary

Drug	Raptors	Pigeons	Passerine birds
Miscellaneous drugs			
Aciclovir	333 mg/kg orally q12h for 7–14 days *Herpesvirus*		
Allopurinol	10 mg/kg orally q12h *Toxicity reported in Red-tailed Hawks at 50 mg/kg*	830 mg/l water	
Colchicine	0.04 mg/kg orally q12h	As raptor	
Deferoxamine		20 mg/kg orally q4h	100 mg/kg i.m. or s.c. q24h
Digoxin	0.02–0.05 mg/kg orally q12h for 2–3 days, then reduce to 0.01 mg/kg q12–24h	0.02 mg/kg orally q24h	
Dimercaprol/BAL (British Anti-Lewisite)	2.5 mg/kg i.m. q4h for 2 days, then q12h until signs resolve		
Edetate calcium disodium	35–50 mg/kg i.m. q12h for 5 days, then stop for 2 days Repeat courses until lead levels normal	As raptor	As raptor
Enalapril	5 mg/kg orally q24h until signs improve then decrease to 1 mg/kg	As raptor	
Furosemide	0.1–6.0 mg/kg orally, i.m. or i.v. q6–24h *Not in dehydrated or hyperuricaemic birds*	0.1–0.2 mg/kg/day	
Isoxsuprine	Small pinch powder/kg orally q12h (Navicox)		
Kaolin/pectin mixture	15 ml/kg orally	As raptor	As raptor
Lactulose	0.5 ml/kg orally q12h	0.3 ml/kg orally q8h	
Metoclopramide	0.3–2.0 mg/kg orally, i.m. or i.v. q8–24h		
Milk thistle extract		33–50 mg/kg orally q8h	
Oxprenolol	2 mg/kg orally q24h		
D-Penicillamine	55 mg/kg orally q12h for 10 days		
2-Pralidoxamine (2-PAM)	10 mg/kg i.m.	10–100 mg/kg i.m.	
Propentofylline	5 mg/kg orally q12h		
Succimer	25–35 mg/kg orally q12h 5 days/week for 3–5 weeks		
L-Thyroxine		0.02 mg/kg orally q12–24h	
Vitamin A		20,000 IU/kg i.m.	
Vitamin B complex	10–30 mg/kg i.m. q24h	1–3 mg/kg i.m.	
Vitamin B1 (thiamine)	10–30 mg/kg i.m. q24h		
Vitamin E/selenium	0.5 mg Se + 1.34 IU vitamin E/kg s.c. Repeat after 72 hours		
Vitamin K1	0.2–2.5 mg/kg orally/i.m. q4–24h	As raptor	As raptor
Topical treatments			
Aloe vera	Apply q24h to skin lesions *For skin infections and polyfolliculosis. May add heparin at 1000 IU heparin/150 mg aloe vera*		
Bacitracin–neomycin–polymyxin 'Vetropolycin' ophthalmic ointment	Ophthalmic use or for topical use at orthopaedic pin–skin interfaces		

Drug	Raptors	Pigeons	Passerine birds
Topical treatments (continued)			
Chlorhexidine	1:50 solution used as spray for skin infections q24h. Can be added to water at 2.5 ppm for candidiasis in pigeons		
Chlorhexidine–miconazole	Use as directed as required for dermatomycosis		
Dimethylsulfoxide (DMSO)	*Anti-inflammatory* *May be combined with other drugs*		
Echinacea cream	Apply q24h to chronic infections *Immunomodulator? Use herbal form*		
F10 ointment	Apply q24h to infected areas *Barrier cream*		
Flurbiprofen	1 drop q12h *NSAID; excellent for uveitis or ocular pain, especially in corneal damage*		
Fusidic acid	Skin: apply q24h Ophthalmic preparations: apply q12–24h *Various formulations.* **Avoid those containing corticosteroids**		
Ofloxacin	1 drop q12h *Fluoroquinolone antibiotic*		
Silver sulfadiazine	Apply to infected areas q24h *Barrier cream*		
Vecuronium	1 drop of 0.8 mg/ml solution in 0.9% saline. Repeat after 2 minutes *Mydriatic: enables examination of posterior segment of the eye.* **Ensure solution does not contain surface-acting penetrating agent**		
Nebulized agents – see Chapter 20			

Allometric scaling

The smaller a warm-blooded animal, the higher is its metabolic rate. Therefore, to obtain effective levels of medication, a higher dose rate and/or more frequent administration is required. *NB The more closely related the species, the more appropriate are the results of these calculations.*

Dose calculation

Improved accuracy in calculating doses can be obtained using formulae based on metabolic energy requirements of an individual rather than its body mass. Energy use is proportional to body mass (M, in kg); the daily energy requirements (minimum energy cost, MEC, in kcal) of a warm-blooded animal can be calculated thus:

$$MEC = K \times M^{0.75}$$

where K is a constant (70 for mammals, 78 for non-passerine birds and 129 for passerine birds).

Using a 'control' species for which the pharmacokinetics of the required therapeutic agent are known, $MEC^{control}$ for a model individual can be calculated. Then, knowing the total dose required for this model individual, the required dose per kcal can be derived:

$$MEC\text{-}dose^{control} = dose \text{ (mg)} / MEC^{control}$$

The total dose for the target individual can be calculated:

$$MEC^{target} = K \times M^{0.75}$$

$$dose^{target} \text{ (mg)} = MEC^{target} \times MEC\text{-}dose^{control}$$

For dose calculation per kg body mass and the determination of the correct frequency for drug application, it is of advantage to use the specific minimum energy cost (SMEC), which is calculated thus:

$$SMEC = K \times M^{-0.25}, \text{ where K is the same constant as above.}$$

Using the control species where the dose/kg is known, the $SMEC^{control}$ is determined to calculate the SMEC-dose ^{control}:

$$SMEC\text{-}dose^{control} = dose \text{ (mg/kg)} / SMEC^{control}$$

Determination of the $SMEC^{target}$ of the target animal allows the calculation of the target dose in mg/kg:

$$dose^{target} \text{ (mg/kg)} = SMEC^{target} \times SMEC\text{-}dose^{control}$$

(continues overleaf) ▶

(continued)

Frequency of administration

Frequency (F) is the number of treatments per 24 hours.

The frequency in relation to the SMEC is calculated for the control animal:

$SMEC\text{-}F^{\text{control}} = F / SMEC^{\text{control}}$

The frequency for the target animal can then be calculated:

$F^{\text{target}} = SMEC^{\text{target}} \times SMEC\text{-}F^{\text{control}}$

Example

The dose of enrofloxacin for a 900 g Peregrine Falcon (control) is 13.5 mg q24h (at 15 mg/kg). What is the dose for a 40 g passerine bird (target)?

Where MEC^{control} and $SMEC^{\text{control}}$ are for the Peregrine Falcon, and MEC^{target} and $SMEC^{\text{target}}$ are for the passerine bird:

For the Peregrine Falcon:

$MEC^{\text{control}} = 78 \times 0.9^{\,0.75} = 72.072$
$SMEC^{\text{control}} = 78 \times 0.9^{\,-0.25} = 80.106$

$MEC\text{-}dose^{\text{control}} = 13.5 / 72.072 = 0.187$
$SMEC\text{-}dose^{\text{control}} = 15 / 80.106 = 0.187$

$SMEC\text{-}F^{\text{control}} = 1 / 80.106 = 0.0125$

For the passerine bird:

$MEC^{\text{target}} = 129 \times 0.04^{\,0.75} = 11.481$
$SMEC^{\text{control}} = 129 * (0.04)^{\,-0.25} = 288.444$

$11.481 \times 0.187 = 2.147$ mg enrofloxacin total dose
$288.444 \times 0.187 = 53.94$ mg enrofloxacin per kg

Frequency: $288.444 \times 0.0125 =$
3.6 applications q24h, i.e. roughly q8h

List of bird names

Family	Common name	Species name
Order Falconiformes (day-hunting raptors)		
Falconidae (falcons)	American Kestrel	*Falco sparverius*
	Brown Falcon	*Falco berigora*
	Common Kestrel	*Falco tinnunculus*
	Crested Caracara	*Caracara cheriway*
	Eleanor's Falcon	*Falco eleonorae*
	Eurasian Hobby (hobby)	*Falco subbuteo*
	Grey Kestrel	*Falco ardosiaceus*
	Gyrfalcon	*Falco rusticolus*
	Lanner Falcon	*Falco biarmicus*
	Mauritius Kestrel	*Falco punctatus*
	Merlin	*Falco columbarius*
	Peregrine Falcon	*Falco peregrinus*
	Prairie Falcon	*Falco mexicanus*
	Saker Falcon	*Falco cherrug*
	Seychelles Kestrel	*Falco araea*
Accipitridae (hawks, including eagles and Old World vultures)	African Fish Eagle	*Haliaeetus vocifer*
	Augur Buzzard	*Buteo augur*
	Ayres's Hawk-Eagle	*Hieraaetus ayresii*
	Bald Eagle	*Haliaeetus leucocephalus*
	Bat Hawk	*Macheiramphus alcinus*
	Bateleur Eagle	*Terathopius ecaudatus*
	Bay-winged Hawk (South American race of Harris' Hawk, *q.v.*)	*Parabuteo unicinctus*
	Bearded Vulture (Lammergeier)	*Gypaetus barbatus*
	Black-chested Buzzard-Eagle	*Geranoaetus melanoleucus*
	Black Kite	*Milvus migrans*
	Black-winged Kite	*Elanus caeruleus*
	Brahminy Kite	*Haliastur indus*
	Cape Griffon Vulture	*Gyps coprotheres*
	Cinereous Vulture (European Black Vulture)	*Aegypius monarchus*
	Cooper's Hawk	*Accipiter cooperii*
	Eurasian Buzzard (Common Buzzard)	*Buteo buteo*
	Eurasian Sparrowhawk (Sparrowhawk)	*Accipiter nisus*

List of bird names

Family	Common name	Species name
Order Falconiformes (day-hunting raptors) (continued)		
Accipitridae (hawks, including eagles and Old World vultures) (continued)	European Honey Buzzard	*Pernis apivorus*
	Ferruginous Hawk	*Buteo regalis*
	Golden Eagle	*Aquila chrysaetos*
	Greater Spotted Eagle	*Aquila clanga*
	Griffon Vulture	*Gyps fulvus*
	Harris' Hawk	*Parabuteo unicinctus harrisi*
	Himalayan Griffon Vulture	*Gyps himalayensis*
	Lappet-faced Vulture	*Torgos tracheliotus*
	Long-crested Eagle	*Lophaetus occipitalis*
	Long-legged Buzzard	*Aquila rufinus*
	Montagu's Harrier	*Circus pygargus*
	Northern Goshawk (Goshawk)	*Accipiter gentilis*
	Oriental White-backed Vulture	*Gyps bengalensis*
	Osprey	*Pandion haliaetus*
	Red-headed Vulture (Indian Black Vulture)	*Sarcogyps calvus*
	Red Kite	*Milvus milvus*
	Red-tailed Hawk	*Buteo jamaicensis*
	Spanish Imperial Eagle	*Aquila adalberti*
	Tawny Eagle	*Aquila rapax*
	White-headed Vulture	*Trigonoceps occipitalis*
	White-tailed Sea Eagle	*Haliaeetus albicilla*
Cathartidae (New World vultures)	Andean Condor	*Vultur gryphus*
	Black Vulture	*Coragyps atratus*
	King Vulture	*Sarcoramphus papa*
	Turkey Vulture	*Cathartes aura*
Sagittariidae	Secretary Bird	*Sagittarius serpentarius*
Order Strigiformes (nocturnal raptors)		
Strigidae (owls)	Burrowing Owl	*Athene cunicularia*
	Eurasian Eagle Owl	*Bubo bubo*
	Ferruginous Pygmy Owl	*Glaucidium brasilianum*
	Great Grey Owl	*Strix nebulosa*
	Great Horned Owl	*Bubo virginianus*
	Little Owl	*Athene noctua*
	Snowy Owl	*Bubo scandiaca*
	Spotted Eagle Owl (African Eagle Owl)	*Bubo africanus*
	Striped Owl	*Pseudoscops clamator*
	Tawny Owl	*Strix aluco*
Tytonidae (barn owls)	Barn Owl	*Tyto alba*
Order Columbiformes (pigeons and doves)		
Columbidae (pigeons and doves)	Bleeding Heart Dove	*Gallicolumba* spp.
	Diamond Dove	*Geopelia cuneata*
	Eurasian Collared Dove	*Streptopelia decaocto*
	Rock Dove (domestic or racing pigeon)	*Columba livia*
	Victoria Crowned Pigeon	*Goura victoria*

Family	Common name	Species name
Order Passeriformes _(passerine birds)_		
Fringillidae (true finches)	Brambling	_Fringilla montifringilla_
	Chaffinch	_Fringilla coelebs_
	Common Redpoll	_Carduelis flammea_
	Eurasian Bullfinch (bullfinch)	_Pyrrhula pyrrhula_
	Eurasian Siskin	_Carduelis spinus_
	European Goldfinch	_Carduelis carduelis_
	European Greenfinch	_Carduelis chloris_
	Island Canary (canary)	_Serinus canaria_
	Red Siskin	_Carduelis cucullata_
	Twite	_Carduelis flavirostris_
Estrildidae (waxbills)	Bengalese Finch (Society Finch) – derived from the White-Rumped Munia (_Lonchura striata_)	Sometimes referred to as _Lonchura domestica_
	Gouldian Finch	_Erythrura gouldiae_
	Java Sparrow	_Lonchura oryzivora_
	Orange-cheeked Waxbill	_Estrilda melpoda_
	Parrotfinch	_Erythrura_ spp.
	Zebra Finch	_Taeniopygia guttata_
Emberizidae (buntings)	Reed Bunting	_Emberiza schoeniclus_
	White-crowned Sparrow	_Zonotrichia leucothrys_
	Yellowhammer	_Emberiza citrinella_
Passeridae/Ploceidae (sparrows)	House Sparrow	_Passer domesticus_
	Red-billed Buffalo Weaver	_Bubalornis niger_
Prunellidae	Dunnock (Hedge Sparrow)	_Prunella modularis_
Turdidae	Eurasian Blackbird	_Turdus merula_
	Orange-headed Thrush	_Zoothera citrana_
	Song Thrush	_Turdus philomelos_
Timaliidae	Red-billed Leiothrix (Pekin Robin)	_Leiothrix lutea_
Sturnidae (starlings)	Bali Myna(h) (Rothschild's Starling)	_Leucospar rothschildi_
	European Starling	_Sturnus vulgaris_
	Hill Myna(h) Greater Hill Myna(h)	_Gracula religiosa_ _G. r. religiosa_
	Purple Starling (Glossy Starling, Purple Glossy Starling)	_Lamprotornis purpureus_
	Superb Starling (Spreo Starling)	_Lamprotornis superbus_
Corvidae (crows)	Eurasian Jackdaw	_Corvus monedula_
	Eurasian Jay	_Garrulus glandularius_
	Raven	_Corvus corax_
Meropidae	European Bee-eater	_Merops apiaster_
Upupidae	Eurasian Hoopoe	_Upupa epops_
Mimidae (thrashers)	(many genera)	
Muscicapidae (flycatchers)	(many genera)	
Nectariniidae (sunbirds)	(many genera)	
Paradisaeidae (birds of Paradise)	(many genera)	
Thraupidae (tanagers)	(many genera)	

Appendix 3

Laboratory reference ranges

Biochemistry

| Parameter | Falcons | | | | | | | |
	Saker Falcon	Gyrfalcon	Peregrine Falcon	Lanner Falcon	Merlin	Kestrel	Gyr–Saker hybrid[a]	Gyr–Peregrine hybrid[a]
Albumin (g/l)	9–12.3 5.2–15.0[b]	6.6–16.8[c]	6.9–14.8[a] 12.7–22.4	9.6–16	8.6–16.1			6.8–14.3
A:G ratio	0.45–0.57			0.44–0.57	0.47–0.58			
Alanine aminotransferase (ALT) (IU/l)	36–55 29–362[b]	32–589[c]	38–303[a] 29–90			35–60	28–393	29–429
Alkaline phosphatase (ALP) (IU/l)	285–450		31–121	180–510	54–310	20–100		
Aspartate aminotransferase (AST) (IU/l)	45–95 40–358[b]	44–471[c]	35–327[a] 34–162	30–118	50–125	100–200	40–544	44–469
Bile acids (µmol/l)	20–90 1.7–13.3		5–69[e]					
Calcium (mmol/l)	2.15–2.61 1.97–2.77[b]	1.98–3.48[c]	1.94–2.54[a]	2.07–2.45	2–2.45	2.1–2.4	1.95–3.12	1.88–2.58
Cholesterol (mmol/l)	4.5–8.6 3.43–7.54[b]	3.42–7.12[c]	3.18–9.97[a]	3–8.8	3–7.8		2.77–10.05	3.06–7.71
Chloride (mmol/l)	114–125							
Creatine kinase (IU/l)	355–651		120–442[d]	350–650	521–807			
Creatinine (µmol/l)	23–75 11–64[b]	14–73[c]	12–64[a]	37–75	16–50		13–75	16–73
Glutamate dehydrogenase (GLDH) (IU/l)			< 8[d]					
Globulin (g/l)	18–28			21.2–21.8	17.2–25			
Glucose	12–14			11–15	9–12			
Gamma-glutamyl transferase (GGT) (IU/l)	0.8–5.9		0–3[d]					
Lactate dehydrogenase (LDH) (IU/l)	551–765 664–3852[b]	870–3871[c]	721–3799[a]	434–897	320–630		662–3720	544–3595
Phosphate, inorganic (mmol/l)	0.72–2.16			0.68–2	0.95–1.79			
Phosphorus (mmol/l)	0.81–2.08[b]	0.45–2.89[c]	0.87–1.88[a] 0.55–1.53				0.78–2.38	0.66–2.21
Potassium (mmol/l)	0.8–2.3 1.6–4.7[b]	1.9–4.9[c]	1.8–5.1[a]	1–2.1	1–1.8		1.8–4.9	1.6–4.7
Sodium (mmol/l)	154–161			152–164	155–170			
Total protein (g/l)	27–366 85–44.6[b]	4.5–46.2[c]	16.0–38.9[a] 24–41	33–42	27.5–39	25–34	5.0–46.7	4.7–40.2
Urea (mmol/l)	0.5–2.6 0–8.3[b]	0–9.5[c]	0.3–9.0[a]	1.3–2.7			0–9.5	0.3–7.8
Uric acid (µmol/l)	320–785 110–1260[b]	80–690[c]	170–1250[a]	318–709	174–800		100–1180	120–1740

▶

Parameter	Hawks							
	Common Buzzard	Northern Goshawk	Sparrowhawk	Harris' Hawk	Black Kite	Marsh Harrier	White-tailed Sea Eagle	Tawny Eagle
Albumin (g/l)	5–14	8.8–12.4		13.9–17	6–23			11.1–13.5
A:G ratio		0.4–0.57		0.46–0.55				0.44–0.55
Alanine aminotransferase (ALT) (IU/l)	0.5–58	0–44	2.5–30.5		35–60 (GPT)	18–58 (GPT)	0–30 (GPT)	
Alkaline phosphatase (ALP) (IU/l)	35–86	15.6–87.5 42–63	103–118	20–96	20–100		7–76	17.1–69.7
Aspartate aminotransferase (AST) (IU/l)	0.5–27 (GOT)	176–409 0–31 (GOT)	140–151 (GOT)	160–348	100–200 (GOT)	140–440 (GOT)	30–160 (GOT)	124–226
Calcium (mmol/l)	2–2.8	2.15–2.69		2.1–2.66	1.8–2.7			2.21–2.66
Cholesterol (mmol/l)		4–11.5		6.6–13.1				7.9–10.7
Chloride (mmol/l)								114–123
Creatine kinase (IU/l)		218–775		224–650				
Creatinine (µmol/l)		41–94		20–59				31–59
Globulin (g/l)		18–29.2		21–29.4				25.3–28.4
Glucose		11.5–15.9		12.2–15.7				10.2–14.5
Gamma-glutamyl transferase (GGT) (IU/l)		3–7.6		2–6.9				1–2.7
Lactate dehydrogenase (LDH) (IU/l)		120–906		160–563				211–369
Phosphate, inorganic (mmol/l)		0.8–1.97		0.8–2.14				1.2–1.78
Potassium (mmol/l)				0.8–2.3				1.5–3.1
Sodium (mmol/l)				155–171				153–157
Total protein (g/l)	33–50	26.3–42		31–45.7	30–41	31–58	28–45	29–41.4
Urea (mmol/l)				0.7–1.9				0.8–2.7
Uric acid (µmol/l)		511–854		533–785				413–576

Parameter	Owls			Pigeons and passerines			
	Northern Eagle Owl	Barn Owl	Tawny Owl	Pigeon	Canary	Finch	Hill Mynah
Albumin (g/l)	11.1–13.5						
A:G ratio				1.5–3.6			
Alanine aminotransferase (ALT) (IU/l)			32.5–40 (GPT)	19–48			
Alkaline phosphatase (ALP) (IU/l)			42.2–215		146–397		
Aspartate aminotransferase (AST) (IU/l)			23.5–103.5	45–123	45–170	150–350	150–350
Bile acids (µmol/l)				22–60			
Calcium (mmol/l)	2.16–2.61	2.2–2.6		1.9–2.6	1.28–3.35		2.25–3.25
Cholesterol (mmol/l)	3.9–7.1						
Creatine kinase (IU/l)				110–480			
Creatinine (µmol/l)	31–49			23–36	8.85–88.5		8.85–53.10
Globulin (g/l)	18.7–22.4						
Glucose (mmol/l)	13.5–21.7			12.9–20.5	16.15–21.7	11.1–24.97	10.54–19.44
Gamma-glutamyl transferase (GGT) (IU/l)				0–2.9			
Lactate dehydrogenase (LDH) (IU/l)				30–205	1300–1816		600–1000
Phosphate, inorganic (mmol/l)	1.15–1.94						
Phosphorus (mmol/l)					0.52–1.80		

Laboratory reference ranges

Parameter	Owls			Pigeons and passerines			
	Northern Eagle Owl	Barn Owl	Tawny Owl	Pigeon	Canary	Finch	Hill Mynah
Potassium (mmol/l)				3.9–4.7	2.7–4.8		0.3–5.1
Sodium (mmol/l)				141–149	125–154		136–152
Total protein (g/l)	30.1–34.5	32		21–35	20–44	30–50	23–45
Urea (mmol/l)	0.9–2.9			0.4–0.7			
Uric acid (μmol/l)	475–832			150–765	4.3–14.8 mg/dl	4–12 mg/dl	4–10 mg/dl

Sources: Appendix 8.1 of *BSAVA Manual of Raptors, Pigeons and Waterfowl* (ed. PH Beynon, NA Forbes and NH Harcourt-Brown, 1996); author; [a] Lierz and Hafez (2006); [b] Lierz (2002); [c] Lierz (2003); [d] Lumeij *et al.* (1998).

Haematology

Parameter	Falcons						
	Saker Falcon	Gyrfalcon	Peregrine Falcon	Lanner Falcon	Lagger Falcon	Merlin	Gyr hybrid[a]
RBC (x10^{12}/l)	2.54–3.96		2.95–3.94	2.63–3.98	2.65–3.63	2.84–4.1	
PCV (l/l)	0.38–0.49		0.37–0.53	0.37–0.53	0.39–0.51	0.39–0.51	
Hb (g/l)	115–165		118–188	122–171	128–163	132–179	
MCV (fl)	124–147		118–146	127–150	123–145	105–130	
MCH (pg)	41.4–45.4		40–48.4	42.3–48.8	38–47.7	36–45.9	
MCHC (g/l)	304–349		319–352	317–353	312–350	340–360	
WBC (x 10^9/l)	3.8–11.5		3.3–11	3.5–11	5–9	4–9.5	
Heterophils (%) Heterophils (x10^9/l)	61.68 ± 11.16[a] 2.6–5.85	60.42 ± 14.68[a] 2.31–8.85	60.95 ± 12.01[a] 1.4–8.55	1.65–8.8	3.5–6.57	3.2–4.03	60.42 ± 14.68
Lymphocytes (%) Lymphocytes (x10^9/l)	31.11 ± 11.46[a] 0.8–4.25	34.37 ± 14.23[a] 0.48–2.36	32.00 ± 11.81[a] 1.1–3.3	1.1–5.13	1.7–4	1.2–1.56	34.37 ± 14.23
Monocytes (%) Monocytes (x10^9/l)	4.72 ± 3.02[a] 0–0.8	4.73 ± 3.67[a] 0.03–0.90	6.23 ± 3.65[a] 0.1–0.86	0–0.9	0–0.85	0–0.5	4.73 ± 3.67
Eosinophils (%) Eosinophils (x10^9/l)	1.12[a] 0–0.2	0.31[a] 0.0–0.68	0.52[a] 0–0.3	0–0.2	0–0.2	0–0.15	0.31
Basophils (%) Basophils (x10^9/l)	0.40[a] 0–0.45	0.04[a] 0.0–0.29	0.26[a] 0–0.6	0–0.45	0.17–0.83	0–0.15	0.04
Thrombocytes (x10^9/l)	12–25		6–46	5–40	12–35		
Fibrinogen (g/l)	< 3.5		< 4.2	< 4	< 4	< 4	
Parameter	Hawks						
	Common Buzzard	Northern Goshawk	Ferruginous Hawk	Red-tailed Hawk	Harris' Hawk	Golden Eagle	Tawny Eagle
RBC (x10^{12}/l)	2.13–2.76	2.6–3.48	2.41–3.59	2.3–3.5	2.63–3.5	1.69–3.21	1.65–2.35
PCV (l/l)	0.32–0.44	0.43–0.53	0.37–0.48	0.35–0.53	0.4–0.55	0.31–0.53	0.37–0.47
Hb (g/l)	101–167	121–177	107–166	123–175	121–171	112–173	108–175
MCV (fl)	151–165	141–156	150–178	157–168	147–163	165–186	163–188
MCH (pg)	48–53	44.5–51.6	46–57.4	43–50.4	45.4–51.1	53.8–67.7	54–62
MCHC (g/l)	307–339	305–343	297–345	312–350	301–330	326–364	206–360
WBC (x 10^9/l)	5–13	4–11	4.5–6.8	3.4–7.5	4.8–10	6.2–17	5–9.5
Heterophils (%) Heterophils (x10^9/l)	3.2–11	3.5–6.97	1.89–3.76	1.9–3.5	2.3–6.71	4.5–15.2	3.58–6.45
Lymphocytes (%) Lymphocytes (x10^9/l)	0.3–3.1	1.38–1.93	0.78–1.74	1.3–1.1	0.6–2.36	0.75–3.37	0.51–2.72
Monocytes (%) Monocytes (x10^9/l)	0.2–0.68	0–0.1	0.24–1.5	0.12–1.2	0.2–1.49	0–0.63	0.2–1.07

▶

| Parameter | Hawks | | | | | | |
	Common Buzzard	Northern Goshawk	Ferruginous Hawk	Red-tailed Hawk	Harris' Hawk	Golden Eagle	Tawny Eagle
Eosinophils (%) Eosinophils (×10⁹/l)	0.1–0.8	0–0.65	0.3–0.7	0.1–0.9	0–0.75	0.1–0.6	0.3–2.1
Basophils (%) Basophils (×10⁹/l)	0–0.9	0–0.35	0.15–0.6	0–0.5	0–1.55	0–0.16	0–0.4
Thrombocytes (×10⁹/l)	8–46	15–35	8–47	4–33	10–59	7–45	19–25
Fibrinogen (g/l)	< 3.6	< 3.5	< 3.5	< 3	< 4.3	< 4.5	< 3.5

| Parameter | Owls | Pigeons and passerines | | | |
	Northern Eagle Owl	Pigeon	Canary	Finch	Hill Mynah
RBC (×10¹²/l)	1.65–2.35	3.1–4.5	2.5–4.5	2.5–4.6	2.4–4.0
PCV (l/l)	0.36–0.52	0.425	0.45–0.60	0.45–0.62	0.44–0.55
Hb (g/l)	107–180	81–99			
MCV (fl)	189–204				
MCH (pg)	64.6–76				
MCHC (g/l)	325–376				
WBC (x 10⁹/l)	3.5–12.1	13–22.3	4–9	3–8	6–11
Heterophils (%) Heterophils (×10⁹/l)	2.2–9.23	4.3–6.2	20–50	20–65	25–65
Lymphocytes (%) Lymphocytes (×10⁹/l)	1.5–5.07	10.9–12.2	40–75	20–65	25–65
Monocytes (%) Monocytes (×10⁹/l)	0–0.48	0.4–1.1	0–1	0–1	0–3
Eosinophils (%) Eosinophils (×10⁹/l)	0–0.48	0.1–0.3	0–1	0–1	0–3
Basophils (%) Basophils (×10⁹/l)	0–0.35	0.1–0.5	0–5	0–5	0–7
Thrombocytes (×10⁹/l)	1–29	7–27			
Fibrinogen (g/l)	< 4.5				

Sources: Appendix 8.1 of *BSAVA Manual of Raptors, Pigeons and Waterfowl* (ed. PH Beynon, NA Forbes and NH Harcourt-Brown, 1996); author; [a] Wernery *et al.* (2004).

References

Lierz M (2002) Blood chemistry values of the Saker Falcon (*Falco cherrug*). *Tierärztliche Praxis*, **30**, 386–388

Lierz M (2003) Plasma chemistry reference values for gyrfalcons (*Falco rusticolus*). *Veterinary Record* **153**, 182–183

Lierz M and Hafez HM (2006) Plasma chemistry reference values in hybrid falcons in relation to their species of origin. *Veterinary Record* **159**, 79–82

Lumeij JT, Remple JD, Remple CJ and Riddle KE (1998) Plasma chemistry in peregrine falcons (*Falco peregrinus*): reference values and physiological variations of importance for interpretation. *Avian Pathology* **27**, 129–132

Wernery U, Kinne J and Wernery R (2004) *Colour Atlas of Falcon Medicine*. Schlutersche, Hanover

Appendix 4

Conversion tables

Biochemistry

	SI unit	Conversion	Non-SI unit
Alanine aminotransferase	IU / l	x 1	IU / l
Albumin	g / l	x 0.1	g / dl
Alkaline phosphatase	IU / l	x 1	IU / l
Aspartate aminotransferase	IU / l	x 1	IU / l
Bilirubin	μmol / l	x 0.0584	mg / dl
Calcium	mmol / l	x 4	mg / dl
Carbon dioxide (total)	mmol / l	x 1	mEq / l
Cholesterol	mmol / l	x 38.61	mg / dl
Chloride	mmol / l	x 1	mEq / l
Cortisol	nmol / l	x 0.362	ng / ml
Creatine kinase	IU / l	x 1	IU / l
Creatinine	μmol / l	x 0.0113	mg / dl
Glucose	mmol / l	x 18.02	mg / dl
Insulin	pmol / l	x 0.1394	μIU / ml
Iron	μmol / l	x 5.587	μg / dl
Magnesium	mmol / l	x 2	mEq / l
Phosphorus	mmol / l	x 3.1	mg / dl
Potassium	mmol / l	x 1	mEq / l
Sodium	mmol / l	x 1	mEq / l
Total protein	g / l	x 0.1	g / dl
Thyroxine (T4) (free)	pmol / l	x 0.0775	ng / dl
Thyroxine (T4) (total)	nmol / l	x 0.0775	μg / dl
Tri-iodothyronine (T3)	nmol / l	x 65.1	ng / dl
Triglycerides	mmol / l	x 88.5	mg / dl
Urea	mmol / l	x 2.8	mg of urea nitrogen / dl

Temperature

	SI unit	Conversion	Conventional unit
	°C	(x 9/5) + 32	°F

Haematology

	SI unit	Conversion	Non-SI unit
Red blood cell count	10^{12} / l	x 1	10^6 / μl
Haemoglobin	g / l	x 0.1	g / dl
MCH	pg / cell	x 1	pg / cell
MCHC	g / l	x 0.1	g / dl
MCV	fl	x 1	μm³
Platelet count	10^9 / l	x 1	10^3 / μl
White blood cell count	10^9 / l	x 1	10^3 / μl

Hypodermic needles

	Metric	Non-metric
External diameter	0.8 mm	21 G
	0.6 mm	23 G
	0.5 mm	25 G
	0.4 mm	27 G
Needle length	12 mm	¹/₂ inch
	16 mm	⁵/₈ inch
	25 mm	1 inch
	30 mm	1¹/₄ inch
	40 mm	1¹/₂ inch

Suture material sizes

Metric	USP
0.1	11/0
0.2	10/0
0.3	9/0
0.4	8/0
0.5	7/0
0.7	6/0
1	5/0
1.5	4/0
2	3/0
3	2/0
3.5	0
4	1
5	2
6	3

Index

Page numbers in *italic* type indicate figures

Index

Index

Index

Index

Index